PHYSICAL THERAPY OF THE CERVICAL AND THORACIC SPINE

THIRD EDITION

PHYSICAL THERAPY OF THE CERVICAL AND THORACIC SPINE

Edited by

Ruth Grant, BPT, MAppSc, Grad Dip Adv Man Ther

Professor of Physiotherapy
Pro Vice Chancellor and Vice President
Division of Health Sciences
University of South Australia
Adelaide, South Australia
Australia

with 123 illustrations

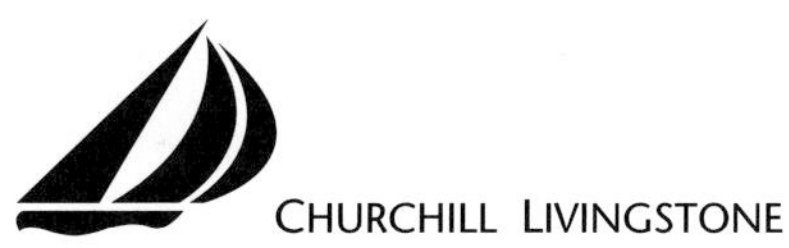

CHURCHILL LIVINGSTONE

An Imprint of Elsevier Science
New York, Edinburgh, London, Philadelphia

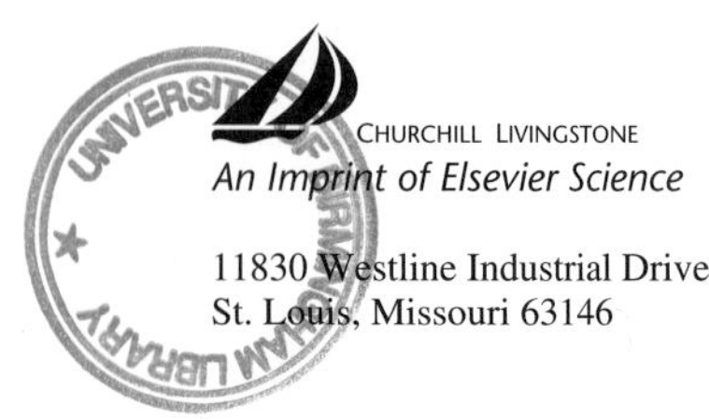

CHURCHILL LIVINGSTONE
An Imprint of Elsevier Science

11830 Westline Industrial Drive
St. Louis, Missouri 63146

PHYSICAL THERAPY OF THE CERVICAL AND THORACIC SPINE 0-443-06564-0

Distributed in the United Kingdom by Churchill Livingstone, Robert Stevenson House, 1-3 Baxter's Place, Leith Walk, Edinburgh EH1 3AF Scotland, and by associated companies, branches, and representatives throughout the world.

NOTICE

Physical therapy is an ever-changing field. Standard safety precautions must be followed, but as new research and clinical experience broaden our knowledge, changes in treatment and drug therapy may become necessary or appropriate. Readers are advised to check the most current product information provided by the manufacturer of each drug to be administered to verify the recommended dose, the method and duration of administration, and contraindications. It is the responsibility of the licensed prescriber, relying on experience and knowledge of the patient, to determine dosages and the best treatment for each individual patient. Neither the Publisher nor the editor assume any liability for any injury and/or damage to persons or property arising from this publication.

Previous editions copyrighted 1994, 1988

Library of Congress Cataloging-in-Publication Data
Physical therapy of the cervical and thoracic spine / edited by Ruth Grant.—3rd ed.
p. cm.
Includes bibliographical references and index.
ISBN 0-443-06564-0
1. Neck pain—Physical therapy. 2. Backache—Physical therapy. 3. Cervical vertebrae—Diseases—Physical therapy. 4. Thoracic vertebrae—Diseases—Physical therapy. I. Grant, Ruth, M. App. Sc.

RD768.P48 2002
617.5′6062—dc21 2002025740

Acquisitions Editor: Andrew Allen
Developmental Editor: Marjory Fraser
Publishing Services Manager: Pat Joiner
Project Manager: Keri O'Brien
Cover Designer: Mark A. Oberkrom
Designer: Rokusek Design

CL/MVY

Printed in the United States of America

Last digit is the print number: 9 8 7 6 5 4 3 2 1

Contributors

Nikolai Bogduk, MD, DSc
Director, Newcastle Bone & Joint Institute, University of Newcastle, Royal Newcastle Hospital, Newcastle, New South Wales, Australia

David S. Butler, BPhty, MAppSc
Adjunct Senior Lecturer, School of Physiotherapy, University of South Australia; Private Practitioner, Goodwood, Adelaide, South Australia, Australia

Judi Carr, AUA, Grad Dip FE
Murray Mallee Community Health Service, Murray Bridge, South Australia, Australia

Nicole Christensen, MAppSc, PT, OCS, FAAOMPT
Orthopaedic Curriculum Coordinator, Department of Physical Therapy, Mount St. Mary's College, Los Angeles, California

Brian C. Edwards, OAM, BSc (Anat), BAppSci (Physio), Grad Dip, Manip Th, FACP, Hon DSc (Curtin)
Specialist, Manipulative Physiotherapist, Mount Medical Centre, Perth, Western Australia, Australia

Ruth Grant, BPT, MAppSc, Grad Dip Adv Man Ther
Professor of Physiotherapy, Pro Vice Chancellor and Vice President, Division of Health Sciences, University of South Australia, Adelaide, South Australia, Australia

Jan Lucas Hoving, PT, PhD
Department of Clinical Epidemiology, Cabrini Hospital, Monash University Department of Epidemiology and Preventive Medicine, Cabrini Medical Centre, Malvern, Victoria, Australia

Vladimir Janda, MD, DSc
Professor Emeritus, Department of Rehabilitation Medicine, Postgraduate Medical Institute, Charles University Hospital, Prague, Czech Republic

Mark A. Jones, BS, MAppSc
Senior Lecturer and Coordinator, Postgraduate Programs in Manipulative Physiotherapy, School of Physiotherapy, Division of Health Sciences, University of South Australia, Adelaide, South Australia, Australia

Gwendolen A. Jull, PhD, MPhty, Grad Dip Manip Ther, FACP
Associate Professor and Head, Department of Physiotherapy, The University of Queensland, Brisbane, Queensland, Australia

Bart W. Koes, PhD
Professor of General Practice, Department of General Practice, Erasmus University, Rotterdam, The Netherlands

Diane Lee, BSR, MCPA, FCAMT
Private Practitioner, Delta Orthopaedic Physiotherapy Clinic, Delta, British Columbia, Canada

Mary E. Magarey, PhD
Senior Lecturer, School of Physiotherapy, Division of Health Sciences, University of South Australia, Adelaide, South Australia, Australia

Stephen May, MA, MCSP, Dip MTD, MSc
Superintendent Physiotherapist, Physiotherapy Department, Walton Hospital, Chesterfield, Derbyshire, United Kingdom

Mary Kate McDonnell, MHS, PT, OCS
Instructor, Program in Physical Therapy, Washington University, School of Medicine, St. Louis, Missouri

Robin A. McKenzie, CNZM, OBE, FCSP (Hon), FNZSP (Hon), Dip MDT
President, McKenzie Institute International, Waikanae, New Zealand

Barbara McPhee, Dip Phty, MPH
Professional Ergonomist and Physiotherapist, The OH&S Services Network, Ryde, New South Wales, Australia

Shirley Sahrmann, PhD, PT, FAPTA
Professor, Physical Therapy, Cell Biology, and Physiology; Associate Professor, Department of Neurology; Director, Program in Movement Science, Washington University, School of Medicine, St. Louis, Missouri

Helen Slater, MAppSc, BAppSc
Lecturer and Coordinator, Sports Clinic 652; Master of Sports Physiotherapy, School of Physiotherapy, Curtin University of Technology, Perth, Western Australia, Australia

James R. Taylor, MD, PhD, FAFRM (Sci)
Adjunct Professor, School of Health Sciences, Curtin University of Technology; Visiting Professor, Australian Neuromuscular Research Institute, Queen Elizabeth II Medical Centre, Perth, Western Australia, Australia

Patricia H. Trott, MSc, Grad Dip Adv Man Ther, FACP
Adjunct Associate Professor, School of Physiotherapy, University of South Australia, Adelaide, South Australia, Australia

Lance Twomey, AM, PhD, BSc (Hon)
President and Vice Chancellor, Curtin University of Technology, Perth, Western Australia, Australia

David R. Worth, PhD, MAppSc, BAppSc (physio)
Senior Consultant, Rankin Occupational Safety and Health, Mile End, South Australia, Australia

Anthony Wright, BSc (Hons) Phty, MPhty St (Manip Ther), PhD
Professor and Head, School of Physiotherapy, Curtin University of Technology, Perth, Western Australia, Australia

Preface

Physical therapists involved in the management of patients with symptoms arising from the cervical and thoracic spine face similar challenges to those in 1994 when the second edition of this book was published, and indeed, to those faced in 1988 when the book was first published. Headache and neck pain affect two thirds of the population and remain as ubiquitous today as they did then.

This third edition of *Physical Therapy of the Cervical and Thoracic Spine*, however, demonstrates the progression in knowledge and understanding that has taken place since the publication of the first edition—increased knowledge and understanding of the structure and function of the cervical spine in particular, of muscle recruitment and the role of muscles in segmental stabilization, of the pain sciences and their underpinning of patient assessment and management, of clinical management approaches and their bases in clinical research, contemporary science, and clinical hypothesis. Our knowledge of the effects and efficacy of manual therapy in the treatment of the cervical spine has increased significantly over these years. In 1988, few randomized controlled trials addressed the efficacy of treatment approaches for neck pain. There are considerably more published today. Two new chapters in this third edition, Chapter 12 by Professor Anthony Wright and Chapter 20 by Dr. Jan Hoving and Professor Bart Koes, illustrate this greater knowledge.

Sackett et al* defined *evidence-based practice* as "the integration of best research evidence with clinical expertise and patient values." Sackett et al emphasize that "when these three elements are integrated, clinicians and patients form a diagnostic and therapeutic alliance which optimises clinical outcomes and quality of life." This is a timely reminder from the "Father of Evidence-Based Medicine" that treatment based on best research evidence *alone*, albeit important, is not evidence-based practice as defined. This third edition provides best research evidence and, concomitant with that, contributions from eminent clinicians based on that research evidence, on contemporary biomedical knowledge and pathophysiological considerations, or on a systematic critically evaluative approach.

The book is presented in three interrelated parts as before. The first part (Chapters 1 to 5) provides up-to-date knowledge of functional and applied anatomy, biomechanics, and innervation and pain patterns of the cervical and thoracic spine, with a new chapter on the biomechanics of the thorax (Chapter 3).

The second part of the book, which is on examination and assessment (Chapters 6 to 11), provides a solid and contemporary base for the practicing clinician and emphasizes inter alia, a clinical reasoning approach to orthopedic manual therapy; a movement impairment approach in the examination of the cervical and thoracic spine, rather than one related to specific structural diagnosis; clear evolution in our under-

*Sackett DL, Straus SE, Richardson WS et al: *Evidence-based medicine*, ed 2, Edinburgh, 2000, Churchill Livingstone.

standing of neurodynamics; and an update and reappraisal of premanipulative testing of the cervical spine.

The third part, on clinical management and evidence-based practice (Chapters 12 to 21), has been expanded and includes six completely new chapters. The chapters are written by eminent clinicians and researchers and will undoubtedly prove valuable to physical therapists in their greater understanding and more effective management of patients who present with upper quarter dysfunction.

The final chapter (Chapter 21) reflects more broadly on the changing nature of professional practice, the knowledge explosion, and the challenges of knowledge management. This chapter considers also the centrality of the patient and of clinical expertise, as well as research evidence, in successful evidence-based practice.

Ruth Grant

Contents

I ANATOMY, BIOMECHANICS, AND INNERVATION

1 Functional and Applied Anatomy of the Cervical Spine, **3**
James R. Taylor and Lance Twomey

2 Biomechanics of the Cervical Spine, **26**
Nikolai Bogduk

3 Biomechanics of the Thorax, **45**
Diane Lee

4 Innervation and Pain Patterns of the Cervical Spine, **61**
Nikolai Bogduk

5 Innervation and Pain Patterns of the Thoracic Spine, **73**
Nikolai Bogduk

II EXAMINATION AND ASSESSMENT

6 Clinical Reasoning in Orthopedic Manual Therapy, **85**
Nicole Christensen, Mark A. Jones, and Judi Carr

7 Examination of the Cervical and Thoracic Spine, **105**
Mary E. Magarey

8 Premanipulative Testing of the Cervical Spine—Reappraisal and Update, **138**
Ruth Grant

9 Combined Movements of the Cervical Spine in Examination and Treatment, **159**
Brian C. Edwards

10 Muscles and Motor Control in Cervicogenic Disorders, **182**
Vladimir Janda

11 Upper Limb Neurodynamic Test: Clinical Use in a "Big Picture" Framework, **200**
David S. Butler

III CLINICAL MANAGEMENT AND EVIDENCE-BASED PRACTICE

12 Pain-Relieving Effects of Cervical Manual Therapy, **217**
Anthony Wright

13 Management of Cervicogenic Headache, **239**
Gwendolen A. Jull

14 Management of Selected Cervical Syndromes, **271**
Patricia H. Trott

15 Sympathetic Nervous System and Pain: A Reappraisal, **295**
Helen Slater

16 Manual Therapy for the Thorax, **320**
Diane Lee

17 Movement-Impairment Syndromes of the Thoracic and Cervical Spine, **335**
Mary Kate McDonnell and Shirley Sahrmann

18 Mechanical Diagnosis and Therapy for the Cervical and Thoracic Spine, **355**
Stephen May and Robin A. McKenzie

19 Neck and Upper Extremity Pain in the Workplace, **374**
Barbara McPhee and David R. Worth

20 Efficacy of Manual Therapy in the Treatment of Neck Pain, **399**
Bart W. Koes and Jan Lucas Hoving

21 Reflections on Clinical Expertise and Evidence-Based Practice, **413**
Ruth Grant

PHYSICAL THERAPY OF THE CERVICAL AND THORACIC SPINE

PART I

Anatomy, Biomechanics, and Innervation

Functional and Applied Anatomy of the Cervical Spine

CHAPTER 1

James R. Taylor and
Lance Twomey

OVERVIEW

The human spine, as a whole, combines the following three important functions:

1. It forms a stable osteoligamentous axis for the neck and torso and for the support of the head, torso, and limbs.
2. It provides a variety and range of movements that are essential for human tasks related to positioning of the upper limbs and hands, varying the direction of vision and contributing to locomotion.
3. It forms a protective conduit for the spinal cord and its nerves, conducting them as closely as possible to the points of distribution of the spinal nerves to the parts they innervate.

The cervical and thoracolumbar regions of the spine show significant contrast in their functions of weightbearing and movement. In the thoracolumbar spine, stability in loadbearing is the primary requirement, whereas the cervical spine is specialized for mobility. The cervical spine not only holds the head up, but it also directs the gaze through a range of 180 degrees in the horizontal plane and a range of about 120 degrees in the vertical plane.[1] The severe handicap posed by neck stiffness (e.g., a person with ankylosing spondylitis driving a car) illustrates the importance of rapid, wide range mobility in the neck.

This functional contrast between the cervical spine and the rest of the spine is reflected by many differences in the shape, size, and structure of its vertebrae and its intervertebral joints. The first two cervical vertebrae are unique, and their synovial joints contribute nearly one third of the flexion-extension and more than half of the axial rotation of the cervical spine. The remainder of the cervical spine, with its six motion segments (from C2-3 to C7-T1), is much more slender and mobile than the six motion segments of the lumbar spine.[2] These cervical joints collectively provide a sagittal range of up to 90 degrees compared to about 60 degrees in the lumbar spine. The lower cervical joints allow a wide range of axial rotation, a movement that is restricted in the lumbar spine.[3,4]

The structural features that determine these contrasts in function between cervical and lumbar regions are the greater slenderness of the cervical spine, marked differences in facet shape and orientation, and the presence of prominent uncinate processes on cervical vertebrae. The uncinate processes project upward from the lateral margins of each cervical vertebral body; there are no uncinate processes in lumbar vertebrae.[5-7] Although the cervical spine is the most slender part of the spine, it has the widest spinal canal, since it carries the thickest part of the spinal cord.

This slender column supports the head, which weighs about 4 kg.[8] The support of a heavy head on a slender, highly mobile stalk makes the neck vulnerable to injury. In our postmortem study of spinal injuries in 385 victims of road trauma, half of all the spinal injuries were to the cervical spine.[9] Control of the motor and sensory functions of the torso and all four limbs is transmitted through the cervical spinal cord, so injury to the cervical cord causes quadriplegia. The blood vessels that supply the brainstem, cerebellum, and occipital lobes of the cerebrum also pass up through the cervical transverse processes and behind the lateral masses of C1. Injury to the vertebral arteries is a rare complication of manipulation of the cervical spine.[10]

These general considerations make it abundantly clear that a sound and practical knowledge of the functional and applied anatomy of the cervical spine is essential for any health professional who would examine it and understand or treat cervical pain or dysfunction. This account begins with a review of spinal development and growth, then provides descriptions of adult anatomy and movements, common features of aging in the cervical spine, and the anatomy of injuries and pain of cervical spinal origin.

RESUME OF DEVELOPMENT

In the third week of embryonic life, the longitudinal axis of the embryo is formed by the growth of the notochord between the ectoderm and the endoderm. The notochord is the precursor of the vertebral column, and the neural tube is formed parallel and dorsal to the notochord. Paraxial mesoderm develops on each side of the notochord and neural tube.[11] The original notochord has an important influence on the ectoderm that is dorsal to it. It induces thickening of the adjacent dorsal ectoderm to form the neural plate, which folds to form the neural tube. At the same time the paraxial mesoderm on each side of the notochord and neural tube is segmenting into regular blocks of mesoderm called *somites*. The notochord and neural tube together induce the mesodermal cells of the somites to form a continuous cylindrical mesodermal condensation around them called the *primitive vertebral column* (Figure 1-1). The medial parts of the somites (sclerotomes) are the raw material from which the original vertebral column is made. The dorsal aorta descends anterior to the original vertebral column, and its regular intersegmental branches supply this mesodermal vertebral column. Vertebral column development is usually described in the following three stages.[12,13]

Mesodermal Stage

The mesodermal column is formed around the notochord by tissue from the ventromedial, sclerotomic portions of the somites. Although formed from the somites, this mesodermal column is continuous and unsegmented. It resegments into alternate light-and-dark bands all the way along its length (Figures 1-1 and 1-2). Neural processes grow around the neural tube from each light band. The aorta sends intersegmental branches around the middle of each light band. The light bands have a better blood supply and grow in height more rapidly than the adjacent dark bands (Figure 1-2).[14]

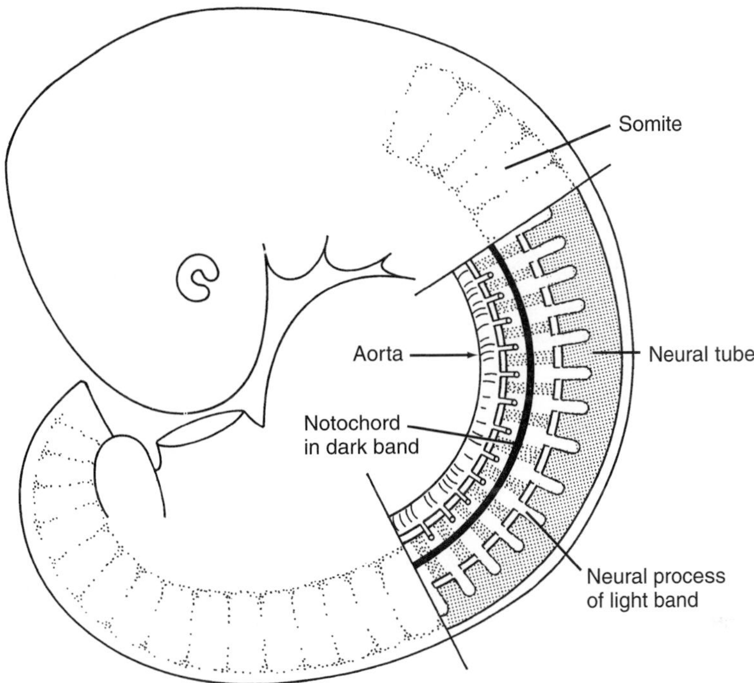

Figure 1-1
Diagram of a 7-mm human embryo with external features removed from the central part to show midline structures, including the notochord enclosed in the primitive vertebral column; the light bands (primitive vertebrae) with their neural processes partly enclosing the neural tube; and the dorsal aorta whose intersegmental branches supply the light bands.
(From Taylor JR, Twomey LT. In Grieve GP, editor: *Modern manual therapy of the vertebral column,* Edinburgh, 1986, Churchill Livingstone.)

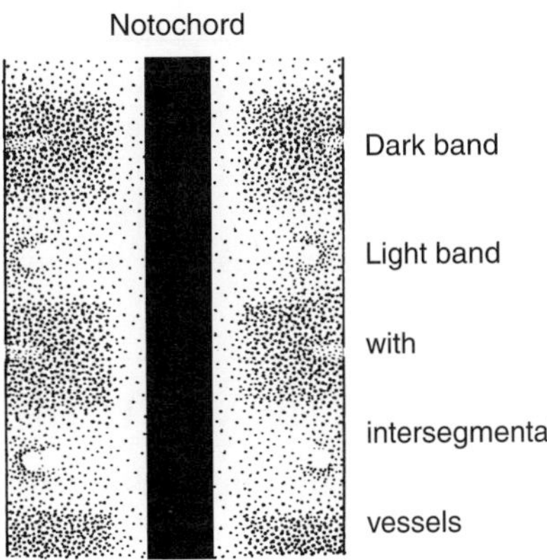

Figure 1-2
Diagram of coronal section of a 7-mm embryo showing the alternating light bands (primitive vertebrae) and dark bands (primitive intervertebral discs). The intersegmental branches of the aorta lie within the periphery of the light bands.
(From Taylor JR, Twomey LT. In Grieve GP, editor: *Modern manual therapy of the vertebral column,* Edinburgh, 1986, Churchill Livingstone.)

Cartilaginous Stage

Each light band, with its neural processes, differentiates into a cartilaginous model of a vertebra at about 2 months' gestation. The differentiation and rapid growth of the light bands into fetal cartilage models of vertebral bodies is accompanied by notochordal segmentation. The cylindrical notochord swells within each dark band or primitive intervertebral disc and constricts and disappears from each cartilaginous vertebra. Each notochordal segment will form a nucleus pulposus at the center of a disc. At the periphery of the primitive intervertebral disc, fibroblasts lay down collagen fibers in outwardly convex lamellae. The cartilaginous stage of vertebral development is a short one, and blood vessels grow into the cartilaginous vertebra, heralding the appearance of the primary centers of ossification.

Osseous Stage

Three primary centers of ossification are formed in each vertebra. Bilateral centers for the vertebral arch appear first, then one center appears for each vertebral body. The earliest vertebral arch centers are in the cervicothoracic region; hence cervical arches ossify relatively early, and sacrococcygeal centers appear last. The single anterior ossification center forms the centrum of each vertebral body. The first centra appear in the thoracolumbar region, and the cervical centra appear relatively late.

Ossification extends from the three primary centers through the cartilage model of each vertebra, replacing cartilage with bone, except for three cartilage growth plates. Bilateral neurocentral growth plates and a single, midline growth plate between the laminae persist in the ring around the spinal canal to ensure continued growth in girth of the canal to accommodate early rapid growth of the spinal cord. When the spinal canal reaches the required girth, the three growth plates around it fuse. The halves of the vertebral arch fuse at about 1 year after birth. The bilateral neurocentral growth plates between the arch and the centrum, on each side, fuse at 3 years of age in cervical vertebrae. The cervical neurocentral growth plates are within the vertebral body, so the lateral quarters of each cervical vertebra are ossified from the vertebral arches and the uncinate processes will later grow upward from these lateral parts.

Growth plates and cartilage plates also cover the upper and lower surfaces of the vertebral body, next to the discs, to ensure growth in vertebral height. Each cartilage plate remains unossified throughout its life, except at its circumference, where a ring apophysis appears. This bony ring apophysis appears between 9 and 12 years of age and fuses with the vertebral body between 16 and 18 years of age, at the completion of vertebral growth, 2 years earlier in females than in males.

GROWTH IN LENGTH OF THE VERTEBRAL COLUMN

Growth is most rapid before birth, and the rate decreases progressively in infancy and childhood, with a final growth spurt at adolescence. The spine contributes 60% of sitting height. A measure of spine length, sitting height increases by 5 cm in the second year of life, by 2.5 cm per annum from 4 to 7 years of age, then by 1.5 cm per annum from 9 to 10 years of age. During the adolescent growth spurt, the spine increases to a growth velocity of 4 cm per annum (peaking at 12 years of age in girls and at 14 years of age in boys). Sitting height reaches 99% of its maximum length by 15 years of age in girls and 17 years of age in boys.[15]

NOTOCHORDAL, NEURAL, VASCULAR, AND MECHANICAL INFLUENCES ON DEVELOPMENT

The notochord and neural tube induce formation of the mesodermal vertebral column around them from the medial parts of the somites. Regular segmentation of the mesodermal column is influenced by the regular arrangement of intersegmental arteries within it. The notochord makes a smaller contribution to the original nucleus pulposus in cervical discs than in lumbar discs, but notochordal tissue atrophies and disappears during childhood in both regions. The smaller notochordal contribution to the cervical nucleus and the greater contribution to the cervical nucleus from surrounding fibroblastic cells means that from an early stage there is more collagen in the cervical nucleus than in other regions.

The persistence of live notochord cells in vertebrae may lead to the formation of chordomas in adults. These rare malignant tumors are usually seen in high retropharyngeal or low sacrococcygeal situations. Congenital fusion of vertebrae, "butterfly vertebra," or hemivertebra, may result from abnormal development of the notochord or the segmental blood vessels. Congenital fusion of vertebrae is quite common in the cervical spine.

Growth of the spinal cord influences growth of the vertebral arches and canal, just as brain growth influences skull-vault growth. An enlarged spinal cord results in an enlarged canal. Spina bifida is a developmental anomaly that varies from a simple cleft in the vertebral arch *(spina bifida occulta)*, which is common and innocuous, to complete splitting of the skin, vertebral arch, and underlying neural tube with associated neurological deficits. In meningomyelocele, abnormal development of the neural tube is the primary event, and the skeletal defects are secondary. It occurs most often in the lumbosacral spine, but it also occurs in the cervical region.

The cervical spine forms a secondary lordotic curve during the first 6 months of postnatal life. When the infant assumes erect posture, a lumbar lordosis appears. These postural changes produce changes in the shape of the intervertebral discs and slow changes in the position of the nucleus pulposus. They also produce changes in the shape of the vertebral end-plates.

Uncinate processes grow upward from the posterolateral margins of each cervical vertebra during childhood, and uncovertebral clefts begin to appear in the lateral parts of each intervertebral disc just before adolescence. These uncovertebral clefts or joints are unique to the cervical spine and are favored by their greater mobility and the narrowing of the lateral parts of the interbody space.

SEGMENTATION AND VERTEBRAL ANOMALIES

NORMAL SEGMENTATION

The mesodermal column is formed from the medial parts of the somites (sclerotomes), which are segmented blocks of mesoderm. However, the column itself is continuous and unsegmented. It resegments into its own sequence of alternate light-and-dark bands so that the vertebrae develop between the *myotomes* (segmental blocks of muscle derived from the middle parts of the somites); thus the muscles will bridge over from vertebra to vertebra. This alternation of muscle and bone is essential to the proper function of the locomotor system.

Regularly spaced intersegmental branches of the dorsal aorta pass around each developing vertebra and provide nutrition for rapid growth (Figures 1-1 and 1-2). Vascular anomalies may result in anomalies of segmentation.[16]

Segmental Anomalies

A hemivertebra develops if one side of the vertebral body fails to grow. Absence of an intersegmental vessel on one side may result in failure to grow on that side; thus only one side grows, and a hemivertebra appears. Absence of a notochordal segment may cause centra to fuse, forming congenital fusion between vertebrae. The relatively high frequency of this occurrence in the cervical spine may relate to the smaller contribution made by the notochord to the nucleus in the cervical region.

Chordoma

Notochordal cells produce substances that loosen and digest the inner margins of the surrounding envelope. This "invasive" characteristic contributes to the growth of the expanding nucleus in fetuses and infants.[11] Notochordal cells do not normally survive beyond early childhood—except perhaps deeply buried in the developing sacrum or at the craniocervical junctional region. If notochordal cells survive, they may be "released" by trauma to the containing tissues and begin to multiply again, causing a malignant chordoma. Fortunately this is a rare tumor.

Butterfly Vertebra

The mucoid streak persists until about 20 weeks' gestation as an acellular notochordal track through the cartilage models of fetal vertebrae. Ossification of the centrum usually obliterates it. If the notochordal track persists through the centrum after birth, it locally inhibits ossification and a butterfly vertebra may be the result.

NORMAL ADULT ANATOMY OF THE CERVICAL SPINE

Upper Cervical Spine

Atlas and Related Structures. The atlas or first cervical vertebra (C1) has a ring structure around a wide vertebral foramen that has to accommodate both the spinal cord and the dens of C2 with its ligaments. Two lateral masses are joined by anterior and posterior arches (Figure 1-3). Anteriorly the anterior arch shows a small, midline tubercle for the upper attachment of the anterior longitudinal ligament; posteriorly it has a small midline facet for the dens. Paired tubercles on the medial aspect of each lateral mass are for attachment of the transverse ligament that holds the dens in place. The atlas has no vertebral body because the embryonic centrum of the atlas fuses with the axis during development to form its dens or odontoid process. The upper and lower articular facets on the lateral masses of C1 form the atlantooccipital joints and the lateral atlantoaxial joints respectively. The lateral articular facets on C1 and C2 do not correspond to those of the zygapophyseal joints below C2 as the lateral masses of C1 and C2 are on a more anterior plane than the zygapophyseal joints.

The atlas has long transverse processes but no spinous process, only a small posterior tubercle on the posterior arch.[17] This posterior tubercle is for the attach-

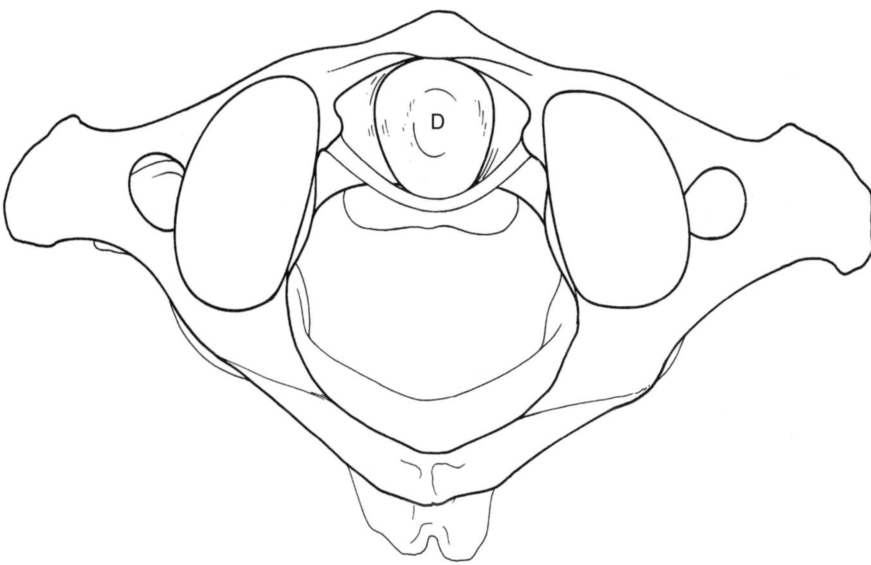

Figure 1-3
Atlas as viewed from above, with the dens of C2 and the transverse ligament. The diagram of C1 shows the concave articular facets for the occipital condyles and the articulation of the anterior arch with the odontoid process *(D)* of C2. The transverse ligament, which holds the dens in place, is attached to two tubercles on the medial aspects of the articular masses. The foramina transversaria and the long transverse processes are seen lateral to the articular masses.

ment of the nuchal ligament and the rectus capitis posterior minor. The tips of the transverse processes may be palpated anteroinferior to the mastoid processes. The vertebral arteries pierce the medial part of each transverse process to wind around behind each lateral mass and groove the upper surface of the posterior arch. The small first cervical nerves pass out over the posterior arch below the arteries, on each side, under cover of the posterior atlantooccipital membrane. This membrane passes from the posterior arch to the posterior margin of the foramen magnum. Deep to this membrane the vertebral arteries course upward and medially to the foramen magnum in the floor of the suboccipital triangle. This triangle, between the rectus capitis posterior major and the superior and inferior oblique muscles, is deeply placed under the overhanging occiput, covered by the semispinalis capitis and the upper fibers of trapezius. The dorsal ramus of C1 supplies the three small suboccipital muscles and the upper fibers of semispinalis. The deeply placed plexus of suboccipital veins behind C1 and C1-2 have extensive connections with vertebral veins, intracranial veins, and deep cervical veins. They are thin walled and may be bruised in severe whiplash injuries.[18]

A thicker anterior atlantooccipital membrane attaches the anterior arch of C1 to the base of the skull just in front of the anterior margin of the foramen magnum. This membrane is covered medially by the longus capitis and laterally by the rectus capitis anterior. The small muscles anterior and posterior to the atlas may be important in cervicocapital postural control. The rectus capitis posterior minor also has a partial attachment to the posterior dura mater that keeps it from buckling in extension movements of the head and neck.[19]

Atlantooccipital Joint. The paired lateral masses of the atlas articulate with the occiput condyles on each side of the foramen magnum. The upper articular surfaces of C1 are concave in the sagittal plane, and they closely fit together with the convex occipital condyles (Figure 1-4). The kidney-shaped C1 facets are elongated from front to back, with their anterior ends closer together than their posterior ends. Their anterior ends also project higher than their posterior ends. This shape provides for more extension than flexion in the atlantooccipital joint.[20] Atlantooccipital dislocation, or fracture dislocation, can occur in severe injuries in motor vehicle accidents. The injury is often fatal because the dislocation may impact on the junction of the brainstem and spinal cord.

The upper facets of C1 are slightly curved in the coronal plane with their lateral margins higher than the medial margins. Functionally the right and left lateral atlantoaxial joints resemble two separated parts of an ellipsoid joint that allows about 10 degrees of lateral bending of the head to each side.[20] Severe axial compression tends

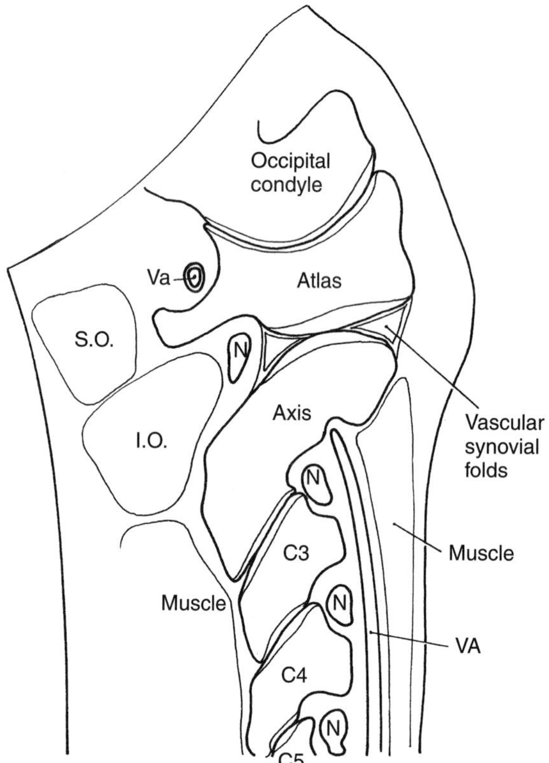

Figure 1-4
This sagittal section from a young adult shows the zygapophyseal joints, whose facets are oriented at 45 degrees to the long axis of the spine. The biconvex atlantoaxial facets are incongruous; triangular, vascular synovial folds occupy the anterior and posterior parts of the joint. The convex occipital condyle fits neatly into the concave facet of the atlas. The vertebral artery *(Va)* is seen in transverse section on the posterior arch of the atlas and in sagittal section, ascending through the foramina transversaria of the cervical vertebrae. The dorsal root ganglion of C2 lies behind the atlantoaxial joint covered by the inferior oblique *(IO)* and the superior oblique *(SO)* muscles. Anterior to the articular masses of C3-5, the dorsal root ganglia of C3, C4, and C5 *(N)* lie behind the vertebral artery.

to force the lateral masses apart, with possible fracture of the slender anterior and posterior arches (Jefferson's fracture).

Each joint is enclosed by a lax fibrous capsule, lined on its inner aspect by synovial membrane. Like the atlantooccipital joint, this joint is often well preserved in elderly people whose cervical zygapophyseal joints have become arthritic and stiff.[21]

Axis Vertebra (C2). The central part of the axis vertebra is formed from the vertebral body of C2 surmounted by the toothlike dens or odontoid process.[22] The lateral masses of C2 project outward from this central part, terminating as small transverse processes that are angled downward and much smaller than those of C1. The vertebral arch of C2 is stronger and thicker than that of C1 with a distinctive, thick, prominent spinous process in the form of an inverted V as viewed from behind. The lateral masses have upper facets for the lateral atlantoaxial joints. On a more posterior plane, the laminae have downward and forward-facing facets for the C2 to C3 zygapophyseal joints.[23]

The short transverse processes of C2 have obliquely directed foramina transversaria for the vertebral arteries, which pass upward and outward at a 45-degree angle through C2 toward the more laterally placed foramina transversaria of C1.

The triangular outline on the anterior surface of the body of C2 reflects the narrowing of the upper end of the anterior longitudinal ligament as it passes up to attach to the anterior tubercle of the atlas.[24] The prominent, upwardly projecting dens is covered behind by the transverse ligament. This is in turn covered by the membrana tectoria, which is the upward continuation of the posterior longitudinal ligament. The membrana tectoria attaches above to the basiocciput inside the foramen magnum.

Atlantoaxial Joint. The vitally important and interesting atlantoaxial joint complex has three parts—two symmetrical lateral parts between the lateral masses of the atlas and axis and a central part formed by the enclosure of the dens between the anterior arch of the atlas and the strong transverse ligament. These joints provide the largest component of cervical axial rotation, which is required for both voluntary and reflex turning of the head to direct the gaze to right or left. The stability of the joint depends on the integrity of the transverse ligament that holds the dens in place.[25] The dens acts as the "axis" around which rotation takes place. Rotation at C1-2 can be tested with the head fully flexed.

The lateral joints are flat in the coronal plane, sloping downward and laterally from the base of the dens, but in the sagittal plane the facets of C1 and C2 are both convex, making them incongruous. The incongruity is further increased by the greater central thickness of the articular cartilages. The gaps between the anterior and posterior parts of the facets are filled by large, vascular, fat-filled synovial folds (Figure 1-4). These triangular meniscoid inclusions are attached at their bases to the inner aspect of the fibrous capsule, and their inner surfaces are lined by synovial membrane. These vascular fat pads are soft and change shape readily, moving in and out of the joints as the head is flexed or extended; however during very rapid movements (e.g., whiplash), they are vulnerable to bruising as they are nipped between the facets. The posterior synovial folds are most often injured in extension injuries.[21]

A well-defined fibrous capsule, about 1 to 2 mm thick, is attached around the articular margins. The roots of the second cervical nerve leave the spinal canal close to the posteromedial capsule. They join as the spinal nerve passes transversely behind the posterior fibrous capsule, in which the large dorsal root ganglion dwarfs the small anterior root. The large dorsal ramus forms the greater occipital nerve, which hooks under the inferior oblique muscle to ascend through the semispinalis capitis into the posterior scalp.[26,27] It can be palpated about 1 cm lateral to the external occipital protuberance.

The inferior oblique muscle passes transversely from transverse process of C1 to the spine of C2, enclosing a space immediately behind the lateral atlantoaxial joint (Figure 1-4). This space behind C1-2 contains the C2 nerve, surrounded by a plexus of large, thin-walled veins. These thin-walled veins may be injured in whiplash, forming a hematoma around the C2 nerve that may track along the nerve. Lateral to the lateral masses of C1 and C2, the slightly tortuous vertebral artery is loosely attached to the joint capsule; its tortuous vertical course allows for stretching during flexion.

The central part of the atlantoaxial joint complex is formed by the articulation of the dens with the anterior arch of the atlas and the enclosure of the dens by the strong transverse ligament, which passes between large tubercles on the medial aspects of the lateral masses of the atlas. Articular cartilage covers the articulations, and there are separate synovial cavities between the dens and the arch and between the transverse ligament and the dens. From near the tip of the dens on each side, strong alar or "check" ligaments pass upward and outward to tubercles on the medial margins of the occipital condyles.[28] A much finer apical ligament passes from the tip of the dens to the anterior margin of the foramen magnum, and an inferior longitudinal bundle passes from the transverse ligament to the back of the body of C2, completing a cruciate ligamentous complex covered behind by the membrana tectoria and the anterior dura mater. The skull and atlas rotate around the axis of the dens, an excessive movement being checked by the alar ligaments, which may be injured in rotational strains.

Upper cervical flexion extension movements are shared almost equally between the congruous atlantooccipital joints and the incongruous lateral atlantoaxial joints as the incongruity between the reciprocally convex lateral masses of C1 and C2 allows rocking with flexion and extension in this joint.[20]

Lower Cervical Spine (C3-T1)

Vertebrae. Cervical vertebrae have the smallest bodies and the largest spinal foramina of the vertebral column (Figure 1-5). The C3 to C6 vertebrae are described as "typical cervical vertebrae," but C6 is atypical in some respects, having a longer spinous process than C3 to C5 and prominent, palpable anterior tubercles called *carotid tubercles* on its transverse processes. A typical cervical vertebra has a small vertebral body whose upper surface is flat centrally but is shaped like a seat with side supports (uncinate processes) and whose lower surface is concave in the sagittal plane (Figure 1-5). From the posterolateral "corners" of this vertebral body, the thin pedicles project posterolaterally. From the pedicles, thin laminae are sharply angled posteromedially to enclose a large triangular spinal foramen. Short bifid spinous processes extend back from C3 to C5. The spinous process of C7 is long and pointed, projecting prominently at the base of the neck so that C7 is called the *vertebra prominens.* The spinous process of C6 is usually not bifid, and it is intermediate in length between those of C5 and C7. Usually all the spinous processes between C2 and C7 are readily palpable, especially with the patient supine and muscles relaxed. With care, each spinous process can be identified.[29]

Lateral to the junction of the pedicles and laminae are the articular masses, with articular facets on their upper and lower surfaces. The upper facets are directed upward and backward, and the lower facets are directed forward and downward (Figures 1-4 and 1-5). These facets are flat and form synovial zygapophyseal joints with the facets of the adjacent vertebrae. The articular masses from C3 to T1 form bilateral articular columns that bear a significant proportion of axial loading.[25] Once again, facet

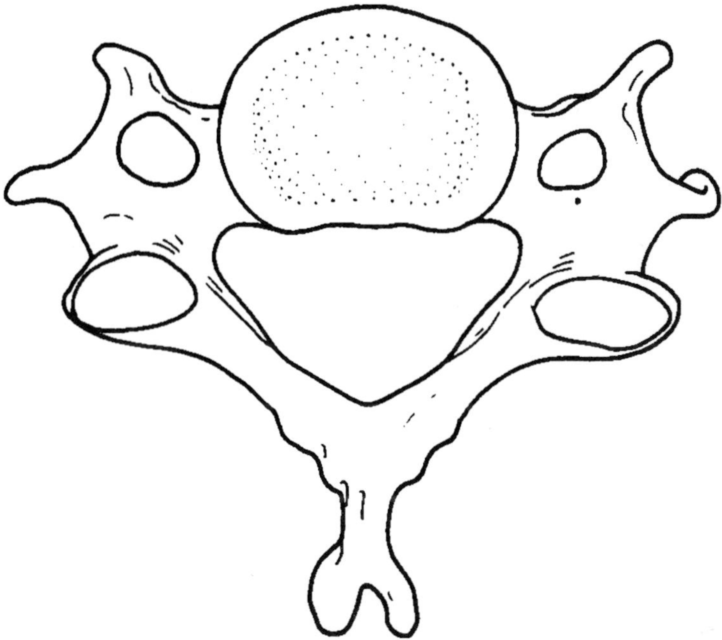

Figure 1-5
Typical cervical vertebra as seen from above. The C3 to C5 vertebrae each show a small vertebral body, bifid transverse and spinous processes, a large triangular spinal canal, and zygapophyseal facets, which lie in an oblique coronal plane, at 45 degrees to the long axis of the spine.

joint levels can be identified by palpation, C2-3 being particularly prominent, and other levels are identifiable with reference to the palpable spinous processes.

Facet Angles. The cervical zygapophyseal facets are described as "lying in an oblique coronal plane."[17] Milne[30] measured the angle between the facets and the superior surface of the corresponding vertebral body in 67 human skeletons. He found the angles to range from an average of 127 degrees at C5 to 116 degrees at C7 and 112 degrees at T1. Considering that the superior surface of each cervical vertebral body slopes downward and forward, these findings would correspond to angles varying from about 45 degrees to the long axis of the spine in the midcervical spine, reducing to just over 30 degrees to the long axis of the spine at T1. In sagittal sections of adult cervical vertebrae, we found these angles to vary considerably, but 45 degrees is close to the average in the midcervical spine, and 30 degrees is close to the average for T1.

The transverse processes project anterolaterally from the front of the articular masses and the sides of the vertebral bodies as two elements enclosing foramina transversaria for the vertebral arteries (Figure 1-5). The anterior costal element of this transverse process projects from the vertebral body. The posterior, or true, transverse element projects from the articular mass. Each transverse process has two small tubercles at its tip in the C3 to C6 vertebrae for attachment of the scalene muscles—scalenus anterior to the anterior tubercles and scalenus medius to the posterior tubercles. The upper surfaces of the transverse processes are concave or gutter shaped for the passage of the cervical spinal nerves. These gutters are wider from C5 down, corresponding to the large size of the dorsal root ganglia and nerves forming the brachial plexus, which passes out behind the vertebral artery into the interscalene plane in the root of the neck.

The atlas, axis, and C7 are atypical cervical vertebrae. The C7 vertebra has a long spinous process and more vertically oriented zygapophyseal facets and lacks an anterior tubercle on its transverse process. The C7 transverse process has a small foramen, but it does not transmit a vertebral artery, only a vertebral vein. There is a gradual transition from the 45-degree angle of typical cervical facets to the 20- to 30-degree angle of thoracic facets.

Vertebral Arteries. The first part of the vertebral artery rises from the subclavian artery and passes upward on longus colli to enter the foramen transversarium of C6. The second part ascends through C6 to C1 inclusive, accompanied by a vertebral venous plexus and a plexus of small sympathetic nerves. The third part curves behind the lateral mass of C1 on to its posterior arch. The fourth part pierces the dura and arachnoid to enter the cranial cavity and the subarachnoid space at the foramen magnum.[31,32] Within the cranial cavity, the two arteries ascend between the base of the skull and the medulla in the subarachnoid space and join to form the basilar artery at the level of the pontomedullary junction. They are usually asymmetrical to some degree. From a study of 150 cadavers, Stopford[33] claimed that 51% showed the left artery to be larger than the right, 41% showed the right artery to be larger than the left, and only 8% of the left and right arteries were equal in size. In an unpublished study based on measurements of the arterial images in magnetic resonance (MR) scans of 267 patients, Kearney[34] found the left artery to be larger in 49% of patients, the right artery to be larger in 29% of patients, and approximately equal in 22% of patients. These findings have relevance in passive movement and manipulative studies. When there is gross asymmetry, there may be a greater risk of depriving the hindbrain of its blood supply from maneuvers that obstruct the larger vertebral artery.[10] Vertebral artery injury is relatively rare in motor vehicle trauma, except in severe fracture-dislocations, but we have observed a small number of instances of intimal damage with dissection and formation of loose inner flaps in traumatized arteries after motion segment subluxation in motor vehicle accidents. In survivors of such accidents, vertebral artery thrombosis is likely.

The vertebral arteries within the cervical spine give off small branches to supply the vertebrae and deep muscles and a few small feeders to the arteries of the spinal cord, the main arteries to the cord (one anterior and two posterior) deriving from the terminal portions of the vertebral arteries within the cranial cavity. Each vertebral artery supplies small branches at the level of C2, which form spiral arteriolar "glomeruli." (These glomeruli enter ampullary veins below the base of the skull in the suboccipital region.[35]) These small arteries, which connect directly to large veins, have a rich autonomic nerve supply that controls blood flow. Injuries that paralyze their nerve supply could cause arteriovenous fistulae.

The vertebral veins have plentiful connections with segmental neck veins and with the internal vertebral venous plexus in the epidural space. The epidural venous sinuses are large and valveless, so blood from their connecting veins can flow in different directions within them (i.e., into the basivertebral veins of the vertebral bodies). Therefore these veins act as routes for the spread of cancer cells—usually to thoracic or lumbar vertebrae.

Motion Segments. Each lower cervical mobile segment consists of "interbody joints" (an intervertebral disc and two uncovertebral joints) and two zygapophyseal (facet) joints. The subaxial cervical mobile segments have an average of about 15 degrees of sagittal range per mobile segment compared to an average of about 10 degrees per mobile segment in the lumbar spine.[3,36] These ranges of movement depend

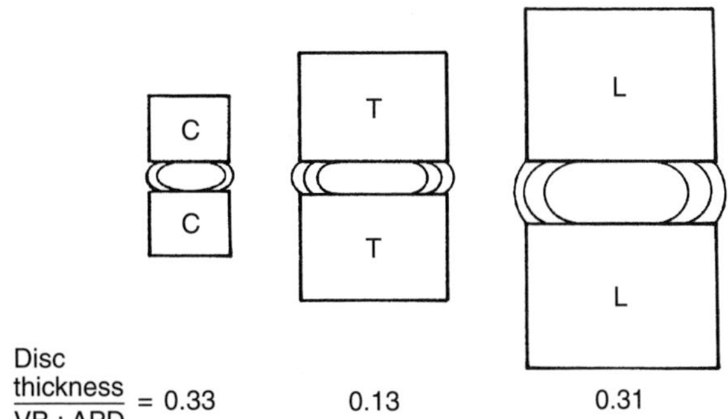

Figure 1-6
Factors controlling movement range. The slenderness of cervical vertebrae and the relative thickness of the discs favor mobility. An index of disc thickness over the anteroposterior diameter *(APD)* of the vertebral body *(VB)* is highest in the cervical spine *(C)*, next highest in the lumbar spine *(L)*, and lowest for the thoracic spine *(T)*.

on the thickness of the intervertebral discs relative to the horizontal dimensions of the vertebral bodies (Figure 1-6). The dimensions and compliance of the intervertebral disc determine the amount of movement possible; the extent and orientation of the zygapophyseal articular surfaces control the types of movement possible and make an essential contribution to stability by restraining excessive movement.

Van Mameren et al[37] showed that in living subjects, the range of active cervical motion in the sagittal plane could vary considerably depending on variation in the instructions given to the subjects. The complex interplay of soft tissue restraints and other factors resulted in the same subjects moving through different ranges in successive attempts to perform essentially the same movement.

Special features of lower cervical mobile segments include the development and natural history of the nucleus pulposus; the growth of uncinate processes, formation of uncovertebral joints, and disc fissuring; the orientation of zygapophyseal facets at 45 degrees to the long axis of the spine; and the age-related formation of uncovertebral osteophytes encroaching on the intervertebral canals together with barlike posterior disc protrusions into the spinal canal.

Development and Natural History of the Nucleus Pulposus. The nucleus pulposus is formed from the interaction of notochordal cells and the surrounding loose connective tissue of the disc. The notochordal segments make a much smaller contribution in cervical discs than in thoracic or lumbar discs. The rapid growth of notochordal segments and their interaction with the surrounding disc tissues forms a large, soft gelatinous mass at the center of each lumbar intervertebral disc. In cervical discs the notochordal segment may remain small and rudimentary at birth; the cervical nucleus of infants and young children owes less to the notochord than to the lumbar disc, and the cervical nucleus contains more collagen than the lumbar nucleus.[11,38]

The more dramatic regional differences between cervical and lumbar discs are due to the growth of cervical uncinate processes (Figure 1-7) and the formation of uncovertebral clefts in the cervical discs of children. This leads to horizontal fissuring of the cervical nucleus and posterior annulus fibrosus (beginning in young adults), so the nucleus pulposus of cervical discs has a relatively brief existence (in childhood and young adults) as a soft "encapsulated nucleus" enclosed by an intact fibrous and cartilaginous envelope. With the advent of fissuring in early adult life, soft nuclear material may "dry out" or be masked by becoming enmeshed in a plentiful collagenous network. Discs also develop regional characteristics in response to different functional demands. Cervical discs bear less axial load than lumbar discs. Proteoglycan and water content relate to load bearing, and proteoglycan concentration is lower in cervical discs than in lumbar discs.[38]

Therefore the cervical disc should not be regarded as a smaller version of a lumbar disc. It is vastly different in many respects. It has less soft nuclear material, in children and what remains is enmeshed in collagen in adults, with universal fissuring of cervical discs in adults. Nuclear prolapse is less likely than in lumbar discs except in severe traumatic incidents, when herniated, cervical disc material is more likely to pass backward into the wide spinal canal than to pass laterally through the uncovertebral joints into the intervertebral canals. Lumbar discs tend to herniate posterolaterally after traumatic rupture of the annulus in relatively young adults, but it is more usual for the already-fissured cervical annulus to show a generalized, barlike posterior ridge as a transverse, annular, and osteophytic protrusion into the spinal canal, seen in middle-aged or elderly cervical spines.

Growth of the Uncinate Processes: the Uncovertebral Joints of Luschka. The lateral parts of a cervical vertebral body are formed by ossification from the neural arch centers of ossification, not from the centrum. The width of the infant intervertebral disc does not extend to the whole transverse extent of the vertebral body. The outer edge of the annulus is said to reach just lateral to the line of fusion of the centrum and vertebral arches. From the upper lateral borders of each vertebral body, processes grow upward toward the vertebral body above, in the loose vascular fibrous tissue at the lateral margins of the annulus.[6] Each process or uncus has grown enough by 8 years of age to form a kind of adventitious "joint" called the *uncovertebral joint*, or *cleft*, on each side of the disc (Figure 1-7). There is some doubt as to whether this joint or pseudarthrosis develops within true disc tissue or whether it appears as a cleft in the looser connective tissue immediately lateral to the annulus.[5,7,36,39] Loose connective tissue in this lateral interbody space

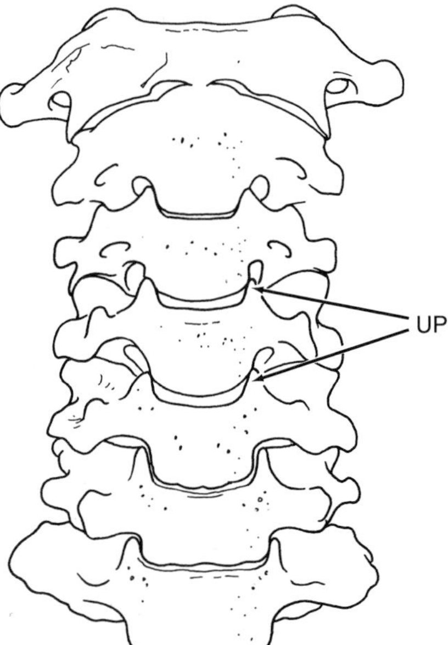

Figure 1-7
Anterior view of cervical spine shows the unique shape of cervical vertebral bodies, which have uncinate processes *(UP)* projecting upward from their lateral edges to form uncovertebral "joints" with the vertebra above.

may be formed into annular lamellae before the uncovertebral clefts appear. The formation of the uncus effectively narrows the lateral interbody spaces in which the translatory movements accompanying flexion, extension, and rotation take place. It "concentrates" the plane of shear to a narrow horizontal band within the lateral annulus. When the clefts appear in adolescence, the tip of the uncus and the groove in the lateral margin of the vertebra above are observed to be lined by a fibrocartilage that is probably derived from the horizontally cleft outer annulus whose lamellae are bent outward and compacted together; a thin fibrous "capsule" limits each cleft laterally.[40]

Cervical Disc Fissuring. The same shearing movements that resulted in uncovertebral cleft formation in adolescents results in medial extension of horizontal fissures into the nucleus and posterior annulus from the uncovertebral clefts in young adults (Figure 1-8). At first, these fine fissures are difficult to observe in postmortem discs from adults in their twenties, except after injection of contrast into the nucleus in living subjects or Indian ink into the center of postmortem discs, when spread through the fissures into the uncovertebral clefts is observed. However, by the time a person is in his or her late thirties, these transverse posterior fissures are more obvious, extending right through the posterior part of the adult intervertebral disc between the two uncovertebral joints, leaving only the anterior annulus and the anterior and posterior longitudinal ligaments intact[6,7,18,40-43] (Figure 1-9).

Such extensive fissuring changes the cervical disc in middle life from a structure that deforms around a central nucleus on movement, to a bipartite disc with a "gliding joint" between its upper and lower parts, which allows translation of several millimeters forward and backward in full flexion and extension (Figures 1-8 and 1-9). This arrangement is related to the wide range of mobility of the cervical spine, which entails much less stability than the thoracolumbar spine. Because the anterior annulus and longitudinal ligaments are the only intact parts of most cervical discs in adults over 35 years of age, the cervical motion segment is heavily dependent on the integrity of the zygapophyseal joints and posterior musculature and ligaments for its stability. The additional loading of the uncovertebral joints that accompanies disc fissuring, loss of

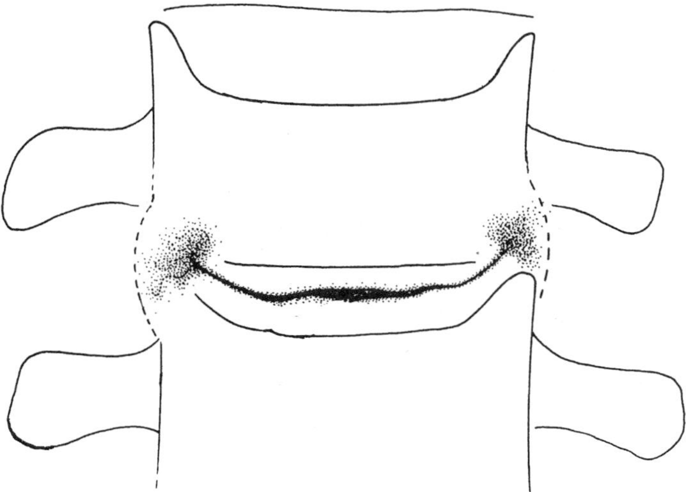

Figure 1-8
This diagram of a normal discogram from a 36-year-old woman shows how contrast, injected centrally, typically spreads transversely through linear fissures in the normal disc into both uncovertebral joints in which expanded cavities allow diffuse spread of the contrast.

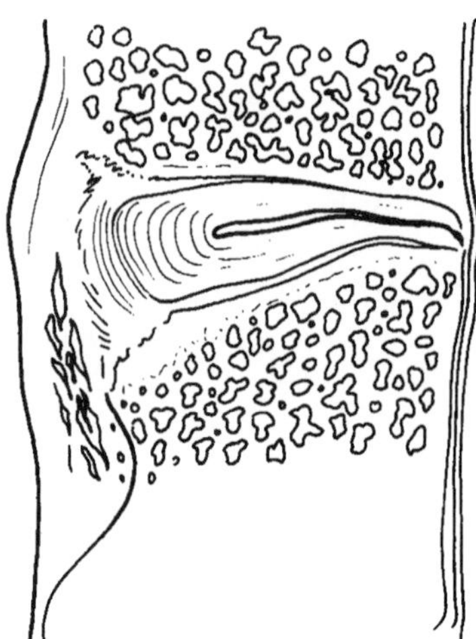

Figure 1-9
This diagram is traced from a sagittal section of a normal elderly cervical disc, near the midline. It illustrates the transverse fissuring, which is a normal feature of most adult cervical discs; the posterior half of the disc is completely fissured; only the anterior annulus and the longitudinal ligaments remain intact.

nuclear material, and "disc collapse," leads to lateral osteophytosis from the uncinate processes into the intervertebral canals (Figure 1-10). In some individuals these osteophytes are very large; they severely limit the space available to the spinal nerves and may compress the anterior part of the spinal cord.[44,45]

Zygapophyseal Joints. By the orientation of their articular facets, zygapophyseal joints determine the directions of intervertebral movements. Their articular surfaces are oriented at about 45 degrees to the long axis of the spine, with a range of 30 to 60 degrees.[36] The cranial facets are directed upward and backward; the caudal facets are directed downward and forward. The facet orientation facilitates sagittal plane movements and requires that axial rotation and lateral bending are always coupled.

The joint capsules are lax, permitting great mobility.[36,46] In our studies of sagittal sections of more than 200 cervical spines of people of all ages, we have found that the lateral joint capsule is lax and fibrous; it is partly formed by the ligamentum flavum anteriorly, but the posterior capsule is very thin, and the large triangular fat pad at the lower posterior joint margin is enclosed by the insertions of the deep multifidus muscles that wrap around the articular column. Where the upper end of the joint adjoins the intervertebral canal anteromedially, the capsule contains very little fibrous tissue and is formed by the synovial fat pad that projects into the joint. Vascular, fat-filled synovial folds project between the articular surfaces from the upper and lower joint recesses as "meniscoid inclusions," which are vulnerable to bruising or rupture in whiplash injuries, forming facet joint hemarthroses (Figure 1-4).[18]

In flexion, a cervical vertebra both tilts and slides forward on the subjacent vertebra, with ventral compression and dorsal distraction of the disc, "spreading the spinous processes like a fan."[46] Forward rotation and translation probably occur together, but Jones[47] maintains that the forward slide is most evident in the later stages of flexion. In full flexion, there may only be about 5 mm of facetal contact remaining.[36] Lateral radiographs of the flexed cervical spine show a "stepped" arrangement of the vertebral bodies because of the forward slide (an appearance that might be associated with instability if observed in the lumbar spine but regarded as normal in the flexed cervical spine). With rotation of 15 degrees or more, there is about 2 mm of translation. Therefore the centers of motion for sagittal plane movements are located in the subjacent vertebra. These centroids are relatively low in the vertebral body for upper subaxial segments and relatively close to the disc in cervicothoracic segments.[36]

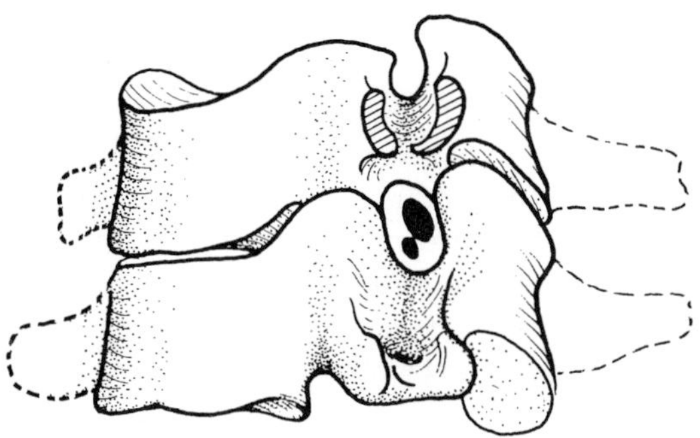

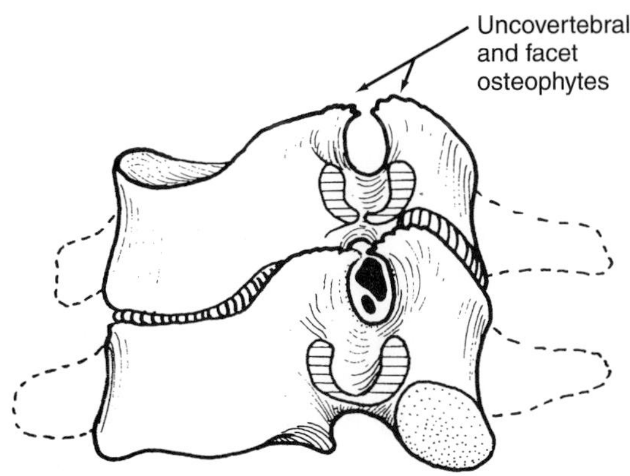

Figure 1-10
Oblique views of normal and arthritic vertebrae. These anterior oblique views look along the intervertebral foramina and show the large dorsal and small ventral roots of the cervical nerves emerging between the zygapophyseal and uncovertebral joints. Note the reduced space for the nerves when uncovertebral and facet osteophytes appear.

The orientation of the cervical facets and the presence of uncovertebral joints both contribute to the process that leads to shearing and posterior fissuring in adult cervical intervertebral discs. These changes would appear to be the price paid in reduced stability for the required range of cervical mobility. The reduced stability in full flexion, which depends on maintenance of a few millimeters of facet contact, obviously requires the strength and integrity of the posterior muscles and ligaments.

Degenerative Pathology. Disc fissuring involves the posterior parts of the disc and extends between the two uncovertebral joints on each side, but the posterior longitudinal ligament usually remains largely intact.[6] Isolated disc thinning is a common degenerative phenomenon, especially in C4-5, C5-6, or C6-7. When the uncus comes to bear more directly and firmly on the lower lateral margin of the vertebra above, the "articular surfaces" of these pseudarthroses become weightbearing and the uncinate processes grow posterolaterally directed osteophytes. Uncovertebral osteophytes frequently project into the intervertebral canals in middle-aged and elderly cervical spines. Anteriorly directed osteophytes from the zygapophyseal superior articular facets are also quite common in elderly subjects.[44]

Disc thinning is accompanied by posterior bulging of the disc as a bar projecting into the anterior epidural space. The uncovertebral osteophytes appear to extend medially along the posterior disc margins so that the disc bulge is accompanied by marginal osteophytes above and below. The structures vulnerable to compression or distortion as a result of this degenerative spondylosis are the cervical nerve roots, the vertebral arteries, and the spinal cord.

Cervical Nerve Roots. The lateral recesses of the spinal canal are wider in the cervical spine than in the lumbar spine but the lower cervical intervertebral foramina are almost filled by the large cervical dorsal root ganglia. The nerve roots and ganglia pass through the foramen at or below the level of the uncovertebral and zygapophyseal joint lines with the large sensory roots above and behind the small motor roots. The lumbar dorsal root ganglia, by contrast, occupy the uppermost parts of large intervertebral canals under the pedicles. Lumbar nerve roots are more at risk of entrapment in the lateral recesses of the lumbar spinal canal, but cervical nerve roots are more at risk of close confinement or entrapment in the intervertebral foramina by a combination of uncovertebral and facet osteophytes (Figure 1-10). They are liable to be squeezed in pincer fashion between the zygapophyseal and uncovertebral osteophytes or squeezed down by the encroaching osteophytes into the lower part of the intervertebral foramen.

Spinal Cord. The posterior bars formed by disc protrusions, flanked by marginal osteophytes, project into the anterior epidural space. The cervical spinal canal is fortunately relatively large in its anteroposterior diameters, ranging from 13 to 22 mm in midsagittal diameter between C3 and C7, with a mean value of about 17 mm.[29] The spinal cord normally occupies about 60% of this anteroposterior space.[36] However, in the extended position, particularly with degenerative changes in the lower cervical region, the combination of disc protrusion and posterior infolding or buckling of the dura and ligamenta flava may imperil the cord. In elderly women with thoracic osteoporotic kyphosis, the upper thoracic kyphosis requires a compensatory cervical lordosis that further narrows the spinal canal.

In postmortem examinations of the cervical spines of elderly subjects, we often find the anterior surface of the spinal cord to be permanently indented by disc and osteophytic bars. These may exist without producing recognized symptoms. However, in cervical injuries, such subjects are more vulnerable to spinal cord damage than young subjects.[48]

Vertebral Arteries. Laterally directed uncovertebral osteophytes also encroach on the course of the vertebral arteries, making the originally straight arteries tortuous. They are often, in addition, observed to be thin walled and dilated in elderly subjects. Such subjects are often osteoporotic. This combination of changes would make cervical manipulation potentially hazardous in elderly subjects.[10]

ANATOMY OF CERVICAL INJURIES

MECHANISMS

In flexion, the posterior elements (facets) are distracted and the anterior elements (discs) are compressed. In extension, the anterior elements are distracted and the posterior elements are compressed. The cervical facet orientation means that translation accompanies these anterior and posterior rotations, with shearing forces in the tissues of the motion segments. Flexion or extension injuries are often accompanied by axial compression, especially in motor vehicle trauma. The cervical spine is quite well protected against flexion injury by the bulk of the strong posterior cervical muscles. In contrast, there are only a few small anterior muscles to protect against extension. The longus colli et cervicis with the prevertebral fascia is small in bulk compared to the posterior muscles and their fasciae. Slender necks are more vulnerable to injury than thick necks. Therefore whiplash symptoms more often lead to chronic pain syndromes in females than in males. Flexion injuries, with single-level fracture dislocation, are more commonly seen than extension injuries in specialist spinal injuries units. In contrast, in clinical practice a clinician sees extension injuries more often. Extension injuries tend to be multisegmental, especially involving C5-6 and C6-7 at the lower end and C1-2 and C2-3 at the upper end.

Nature of Extension Injuries in Severe Whiplash or From Craniofacial Impacts

Extension injury frequently causes transverse tears of the anterior annulus at the disc-vertebral interface as a result of anterior distraction and shear, without rupture of the anterior longitudinal ligament that remains intact. This may occur in several discs because the forces are absorbed partially by each disc. More severe extension injuries may partially avulse the disc from the vertebral margin with tearing of the anterior longitudinal ligament. The small anterior muscles are the last structures to tear because they are more compliant and stretchable than the anterior annulus, with the anterior longitudinal ligament intermediate in its capacity for stretch. At the same time, posterior compression of the articular columns bruises the vascular, intraarticular synovial folds; damages the articular cartilages; or fractures the tip of a facet, which is forced against an adjacent vertebral arch. In the acute injury one may observe facet joint hemarthroses. Such injuries have been commonly observed during autopsy after fatal motor vehicle accidents. They may also be demonstrated if magnetic resonance imaging (MRI) is done at the acute stage, although MRI is not sensitive enough to demonstrate all the lesions. In posttraumatic chronic pain, facet pain is more common than disc pain, and the painful facet may show signs of arthropathy on a bone scan.

We have observed in many fatally injured individuals subjected to violent movements in both flexion and extension, that the main injuries have been sustained in extension. This relates to the inadequate protection given by seatbelts in head-on collisions, in which the majority of drivers and front seat occupants of cars involved in high-speed collisions strike their head on the steering wheel or some other part of the car and sustain a craniofacial trauma with a neck extension injury. More than 90% of these individuals show disc injuries, and about 80% also show soft tissue injuries to the facet joints. Nearly 15% also show intraneural bruises in the dorsal root ganglia.[6,41,42,49,50]

Upper Thoracic Aging and Injuries

The question often arises as to whether interscapular pain is caused by the referral of pain from the neck or by local pain from pathological conditions in thoracic segments.

In postmortem studies of the junctional cervicothoracic region, there is a marked contrast between the spondylosis observed in C5-6 and C6-7, with disc thinning or even spontaneous fusion across degenerate segments and the good preservation of the adjacent upper thoracic segments. This probably relates to the greater stiffness of the upper thoracic segments caused by the short sturdy ribs of the upper rib cage. However, radiographic findings often show widespread thoracic degenerative changes in midthoracic and lower thoracic segments in middle-aged subjects, sometimes related to the so-called Scheuermann's disease.

Upper thoracic segments also show injuries after severe trauma.[43] In flexion compression or axial compression injuries, the anterior elements show end-plate fractures, bone bruising caused by multiple trabecular microfractures, or vertebral wedging or burst fractures in more severe flexion compression injuries. These vertebral injuries are accompanied by bleeding into the adjacent discs, which show less direct injury than in the cervical spine (except for the upper two thoracic discs, which may show injuries similar to the cervical spine).

In the thoracic articular columns, facet injuries are almost as frequent as in the cervical spine.[43] There is an additional risk of facet tip fracture because small ridges of bone jut out from the thoracic laminae below the inferior recesses of the thoracic zygapophyseal joints; in extension trauma, an inferior articular process may impact on this ridge with damage to the facet tip.

INNERVATION OF CERVICAL MOTION SEGMENTS

Intervertebral Disc

The longitudinal ligaments and the annulus of cervical intervertebral discs are innervated from the ventral rami, sinuvertebral nerves, and vertebral nerves (around the vertebral arteries). According to Bogduk et al,[51] only the outer annulus is innervated, but Mendel et al[52] demonstrated nerves through the whole thickness of the annulus. Nerves are not found in the cartilage plates or in the nucleus pulposus of normal discs.

Zygapophyseal Joints

The medial branch of each dorsal ramus contributes to the innervation of two zygapophyseal joints.[27,53] The medial branches of the C4 to C8 dorsal rami curve dorsally around the waists of the articular pillars. There are often two of these branches on each articular pillar. They supply the zygapophyseal joint capsules above and below and innervate the corresponding segments of multifidus and semispinalis. The fibrous capsule and joint recesses are innervated, but the ligamentum flavum does not appear to have any nociceptive nerves.[54-56] The synovial folds projecting into the joints from the polar recesses are probably innervated. Innervation has been demonstrated in these structures in the lumbar spine.[55,56]

Pain may arise from injury to any innervated part of the motion segment. It may also arise from injury to spinal nerves or dorsal root ganglia, which are closely related to these joints. For example, the dorsal rami of C2 and C3, which form the greater occipital nerve and the third occipital nerve, can be affected by injury. They supply the skin of the medial upper neck and the occipital scalp as far as the vertex. They also supply rostral segments of postvertebral muscles and the posterior capsules of the lateral atlantoaxial joints and the C2-3 and C3-4 zygapophyseal joints. We have observed both perineural and intraneural bruising in our postmortem studies of neck injuries.[50]

PAIN REFERRAL PATTERNS

Pain is often referred to the skin, but pain is also referred through the sensory nerves of muscles. Trapezius, sternomastoid, and levator scapulae are innervated by C3 and C4, the rhomboids by C5, and the short scapulohumeral muscles by C5 and C6; the longer trunk-humeral muscles have multisegmental innervation (C5 to T1). When these muscles are injured or involved in reflex spasm, they may generate patterns of referred pain similar to those of the underlying spinal joints.[57] Explaining cervical headache, Bogduk[53] points to the convergence of afferents from C1-3 with the spinal tract of the trigeminal nerve in the gray matter of the upper cervical cord, in the "trigeminocervical nucleus." The ophthalmic and maxillary divisions of the trigeminal nerve are best represented in this "nucleus."

Two neck sprain syndromes are described: a "cervico-encephalic syndrome" in which trauma to upper cervical motion segments (e.g., discs, facets, muscles, or dura) causes neck pain and headaches, and a "lower cervical syndrome" from traumatic lesions to lower cervical motion segments, in which pain radiates from the neck to the upper limb, shoulder, or scapular region.[58-60]

SUMMARY

The unique anatomy of lower cervical segments gives the cervical spine a wide range of mobility but carries with it the risk of less stability in these mobile joints. The orientation of the cervical zygapophyseal joints at 45 degrees to the long axis of the spine and the childhood growth of uncinate processes lead to the development of uncovertebral clefts, progressing to early transverse fissuring of cervical intervertebral discs in young adults, through the nucleus and posterior annulus fibrosus, with loss of the "encapsulated nucleus" found in lumbar intervertebral discs. This is frequently associated, in middle-aged and elderly adults, with loss of disc height in the midcervical and lower cervical discs and with the development of uncovertebral osteophytes, which pose threats to the cervical spinal nerves. Spontaneous fusion of lower cervical segments makes elderly people susceptible to upper cervical injuries with risk to the spinal cord. In younger individuals, the relative instability of these mobile cervical segments, and the lack of strong anterior protective muscles compared to thoracolumbar segments, increases their vulnerability to extension injury. Tears to the anterior annulus and injuries to the capsule, synovium, and articular cartilages of cervical zygapophyseal joints are common sequelae of severe whiplash.

References

1. Huelke DF, Nusholz GS: Cervical spine biomechanics: a review of the literature, *J Orthopaed Research*, 4:232, 1986.
2. Penning L, Wilmink JT: Rotation of the cervical spine: a CT study in normal subjects, *Spine* 12:732, 1987.
3. Taylor JR, Twomey LT: Sagittal and horizontal plane movement of the lumbar vertebral column in cadavers and in the living, *Rheum Rehab* 19:223, 1980.
4. White AA, Panjabi MM: *Clinical biomechanics of the spine*, ed 2, Philadelphia, 1990, JB Lippincott.
5. Hayashi K, Yakubi T: The origin of the uncus and of Luschka's joint in the cervical spine, *J Bone Joint Surg* 67A:788, 1985.
6. Taylor JR, Twomey LT: Contrasts between cervical and lumbar motion segments, *Critical Reviews in Physical and Rehabilitation Medicine* 12:345, 2000.
7. Tondury G: Anatomie fonctionelle des petites articulations du rachis, *Ann de Med Phys* XV:173, 1972.
8. Brunnstrom S: *Clinical kinesiology*, ed 1, Philadelphia, 1962, FA Davis.
9. Kakulas BA, Taylor JR: Pathology of injuries of the vertebral column. In Frankel GL, editor: *Handbook of clinical neurology*, vol 61, Amsterdam, 1992, Elsevier.
10. Fast A, Zincola DF, Marin EL: Vertebral artery damage complicating cervical manipulation, *Spine* 12:840, 1987.
11. Taylor JR: Growth and development of the human intervertebral disc, PhD thesis, Edinburgh, 1973, University of Edinburgh.

12. Bardeen CR: Early development of cervical vertebrae in man, *Am J Anat* 8:181, 1908.
13. Taylor JR, Twomey LT: The role of the notochord and blood vessels in development of the vertebral column and in the aetiology of Schmorl's nodes. In Grieve GP, editor: *Modern manual therapy of the vertebral column*, Edinburgh, 1986, Churchill Livingstone.
14. Verbout AJ: The development of the vertebral column. In Beck F, Hild W, Ortmann R, editors: *Advances in anatomy, embryology & cell biology*, vol 90, Berlin, 1985, Springer Verlag.
15. Taylor JR, Twomey LT: Factors influencing growth of the vertebral column. In Grieve GP, editor: *Modern manual therapy of the vertebral column*, Edinburgh, 1986, Churchill Livingstone.
16. Tanaka T, Uhthoff HK: The pathogenesis of congenital vertebral malformations, *Acta Orthop Scand* 52:413, 1981.
17. Williams PL, Warwick R, Dyson M, Bannister LH: *Gray's anatomy*, ed 37, Edinburgh, 1989, Churchill Livingstone.
18. Taylor JR, Taylor MM: Cervical spinal injuries: an autopsy study of 109 blunt injuries, *J Musculoskeletal Pain* 4:61, 1996.
19. Taylor JR, Taylor MM, Twomey LT: Posterior cervical dura is much thicker than the anterior cervical dura, *Spine* 21:2300, 1996 (letter).
20. Panjabi M, Dvorak J, Duranceau J et al: Three-dimensional movement of the upper cervical spine, *Spine* 13:727, 1988.
21. Schonstrom N, Twomey LT, Taylor J: The lateral atlantoaxial joints and their synovial folds: an in vitro study of soft tissue injuries and fractures, *J Trauma* 35:886, 1993.
22. Schaffler MB, Alkson MD, Heller JG, Garfin SR: Morphology of the dens: a quantitative study, *Spine* 17:738, 1992.
23. Ellis JH, Martel W, Lillie JH, Aisen AM: Magnetic resonance imaging of the normal craniovertebral junction, *Spine* 16:105, 1991.
24. Yoganandan N, Pintar F, Butler J et al: Dynamic response of human cervical spine ligaments, *Spine* 14:1102, 1989.
25. Pal GP, Sherk HH: The vertical stability of the cervical spine, *Spine* 13:447, 1988.
26. Bogduk N: The rationale for patterns of neck and back pain, *Patient Manage* 8:13, 1984.
27. Bogduk N, Marsland A: The cervical zygapophysial joint as a source of neck pain, *Spine* 13:610, 1988.
28. Dvorak J, Panjabi MM: Functional anatomy of the alar ligaments, *Spine* 12:183, 1987.
29. Panjabi MM, Duranceau J, Geol V et al: Cervical human vertebrae: quantitative three-dimensional anatomy of the middle and lower regions, *Spine* 16:861, 1991.
30. Milne N: Comparative anatomy and function of the uncinate processes of cervical vertebrae in humans and other mammals, PhD thesis, Perth, 1993, University of Western Australia.
31. Dommisse GF: Blood supply of spinal cord, *J Bone Joint Surg* 56B:225, 1974.
32. Tulsi RS, Perrett LV: The anatomy and radiology of the cervical vertebrae and the tortuous vertebral artery, *Aust Radiol* 19:258, 1975.
33. Stopford JSB: The arteries of the pons and medulla oblongata, *J Anat* 50:131, 1916.
34. Kearney D: Asymmetry of the human vertebral arteries, unpublished research project, 1993.
35. Parke WW: The vascular relations of the upper cervical vertebrae, *Orthop Clin North Am* 9:879, 1978.
36. Penning L: Functional pathology of the cervical spine, *Excerpta Medica Foundation*, Baltimore, 1968, Williams & Wilkins.
37. van Mameren H, Drukker J, Sanches H, Beurgsgens J: Cervical spine motions in the sagittal plane. I. Ranges of motion of actually performed movements: an x-ray cine study, *Eur J Morphol* 28:47, 1990.
38. Scott JE, Bosworth T, Cribb A, Taylor JR: The chemical morphology of age related changes in human intervertebral disc glycosaminoglycans from the cervical, thoracic and lumbar nucleus pulposus and annulus fibrosus, *J Anat* 184:73, 1994.

39. Hirsch CF, Schajowicz F, Galante J: Structural changes in the cervical spine, Orstadius Boktryckeri Aktiebolag, 1967, Gothenberg (monograph).
40. Taylor JR, Milne N: The cervical mobile segments. Proceedings of Whiplash Symposium, Aust Physio Assocn (SA Branch: Orthopaedic Special Interest Group), Adelaide, Australia, 1988.
41. Taylor JR, Twomey LT: Acute injuries to cervical joints, *Spine* 18:1115, 1993.
42. Taylor JR, Finch P: Acute injury of the neck: anatomical and pathological basis of pain, *Ann Acad Med* (Singapore) 22:187, 1993.
43. Taylor JR, Gurumoorthy K: A comparison of cervical and thoracic injuries in 45 autopsy spines. Annual scientific meeting of the Spine Society of Australia, Coffs Harbour, New South Wales, 1999 (abstract 20).
44. Bohlman HH, Emory SE: The pathophysiology of cervical spondylosis and myelopathy, *Spine* 13:843, 1988.
45. Clark CC: Cervical spondylitic myelopathy: history and physical findings, *Spine* 13:847, 1988.
46. Lysell E: Motion in the cervical spine: an experimental study on autopsy specimens, *Acta Orthop Scand Suppl* 123:1, 1969.
47. Jones MD (cited by Penning L): *Functional pathology of the cervical spine*, Baltimore, 1968, Williams & Wilkins.
48. Scher AT: Hyperextension trauma in the elderly: an easily overlooked spinal injury, *J Trauma* 23:1066, 1983.
49. Taylor JR, Kakulas BA: Neck injuries, *Lancet* 338:1343, 1991.
50. Taylor JR, Twomey LT, Kakulas BA: Dorsal root ganglion injuries in 109 blunt trauma fatalities, *Injury* 29:335, 1998.
51. Bogduk N, Windson M, Inglis A et al: The innervation of the cervical intervertebral discs, *Spine* 13:2, 1988.
52. Mendel T, Wink CS, Zimny ML: Neural elements in human cervical intervertebral discs, *Spine* 17:132, 1992.
53. Bogduk N: Cervical causes of headache and dizziness. In Grieve GP, editor: *Modern manual therapy of the vertebral column*, Edinburgh, 1986, Churchill Livingstone.
54. Ashton IK, Ashton BA, Gibson SJ et al: Morphological basis for back pain: the demonstration of nerve fibers and neuropeptides in the lumbar facet joint but not in ligamentum flavum, *J Orthop Res* 10:72, 1992.
55. Giles L, Taylor J: Innervation of human lumbar zygapophyseal joint synovial folds, *Acta Orthop Scand* 58:43, 1987.
56. Giles LG, Taylor JR, Cockson A: Human zygapophyseal joint synovial folds, *Acta Anatomica* 126:110, 1986.
57. Travell J, Simons D: *Myofascial pain and dysfunction: the trigger point manual*, Baltimore, 1983, Williams & Wilkins.
58. Cloward RB: Cervical discography: a contribution to the etiology and mechanism of neck, shoulder and arm pain, *Ann Surg* 150:1052, 1959.
59. Dwyer AC, Bogduk N, Aprill C: Cervical zygapophyseal joint pain patterns. I. A study in normal volunteers, *Spine* 15:453, 1990.
60. Radanov BP, Dvorak J, Valac L: Cognitive deficits in patients after soft tissue injury of the cervical spine, *Spine* 17:127, 1992.

CHAPTER

2

Biomechanics of the Cervical Spine

Nikolai Bogduk

Fundamental to the understanding of disorders of an organ is a knowledge of its normal physiology. Such a body of knowledge exists for organs such as the heart, the kidneys, and the lungs. Consequently, the causes and consequences of cardiac failure, renal failure, and respiratory failure can be understood in terms of the normal function of these organs, and subsequently, treatment can be instituted on a rational and valid basis.

Such a body of knowledge does not exist for the musculoskeletal system. Some appreciation has emerged of the physiology of the lower limbs through gait analysis, but there is no information of comparable standard for the vertebral column.

Biomechanics is the first step to determining the physiology of the musculoskeletal system. When the principles of engineering are applied and mathematical analyses are used, the way in which a mechanical system operates can be determined. However, the more complicated the system, the more laborious and difficult is its analysis and the more complicated the result seems.

The first stage of biomechanical analysis is the study of *kinematics*—observing and measuring how the system moves. The second stage is *kinetics*—determining the forces that operate on the system (to produce the observed or observable movements). With respect to the cervical spine, the study of kinetics is subsumed in the field of mathematical modeling. The intricacies and detail involved render mathematical modeling of the cervical spine a complex and difficult field.

The literature is limited and quite demanding. Interested readers are directed to certain seminal[1-3] and comprehensive[4,5] publications. This chapter is restricted to the kinematics of the cervical spine.

ATLANTOOCCIPITAL KINEMATICS

The atlantooccipital joints are designed to allow flexion-extension but to preclude other movements. During flexion, the condyles of the occiput roll forward and glide backward in their atlantial facets; in extension, the converse combination of movements occurs. Axial rotation and lateral flexion of the occiput require one or both oc-

Table 2-1 Reported Results of Studies of Normal Ranges of Motion of the Atlantooccipital Joint

Source	Range of Motion (Degrees) Mean	Range	SD
Brocher[9]	14.3	0-25	
Lewit and Krausova[10]	15		
Markuske[11]	14.5		
Fielding[12]	35		
Kottke and Mundale[13]		0-22	
Lind et al[14]	14		15

SD, Standard deviation.

cipital condyles to rise out of their atlantial sockets, essentially distracting the joint; the resultant tension developed in the joint capsules limits these movements.

Studies of the ranges of these movements in cadavers have found the range of flexion-extension to be about 13 degrees; the range of axial rotation was 0 degrees, but about 8 degrees was possible when the movement was forced.[6] A detailed radiographic study of cadaveric specimens[7,8] found the mean ranges (± standard deviation [SD]) to be flexion-extension, 18.6 degrees (± 0.6); axial rotation, 3.4 degrees (± 0.4); and lateral flexion, 3.9 degrees (± 0.6). It also revealed that when flexion-extension was executed, it was accompanied by negligible movements in the other planes; however, when axial rotation was executed as the primary movement, 1.5 degrees of extension and 2.7 degrees of lateral flexion occurred. Thus axial rotation was achieved artificially through a combination of these other movements.

Radiographic studies of the atlantooccipital joints in vivo have addressed only the range of flexion-extension because axial rotation and lateral flexion are impossible to determine accurately from plain radiographs. Most studies agree that the average range of motion is 14 to 15 degrees (Table 2-1). For some reason, the values reported by Fielding[12] are distinctly out of character. What is conspicuous in Table 2-1 is the enormous variance in range exhibited by normal individuals, which indeed led one group of investigators[13] to refrain from offering either an average or a representative range; and this is reflected formally by the results of Lind et al,[14] in which the coefficient of variation is over 100%.

ATLANTOAXIAL KINEMATICS

The atlantoaxial joints are designed to accommodate axial rotation of the head and atlas as one unit on the remainder of the cervical spine. Accordingly, the atlas exhibits a large range of axial rotation but is also quite mobile in other respects; the atlas is not bound directly to the axis by any substantive ligaments, and few muscles act directly on it to control its position or movements. Consequently, the atlas essentially lies like a passive washer between the skull and C2 and is subject to passive movements in planes other than that of axial rotation. This underlies some of the paradoxical movements exhibited by the atlas.

Paradoxical movements arise because of the location of the joints of the atlas with respect to the line of gravity and the line of action of the flexor and extensor muscles acting on the head. No extensor muscles insert into the atlas; consequently, its extension movements are purely passive, depending on the forces acting on the skull.

Whether the atlas flexes or extends during flexion-extension of the head depends on where the occiput rests on the atlas. If during flexion of the head, the chin is first protruded, the center of gravity of the head will come to lie relatively anterior to the atlantoaxial joints. Consequently, the atlas will be tilted into flexion by the weight of the head, irrespective of any action by the longus cervicis on its anterior tubercle. However, if the chin is tucked backward, the center of gravity of the head will tend to lie behind the atlantoaxial joints, and paradoxically, the atlas will be squeezed into extension by the weight of the head, even though the head and the rest of the neck will move into flexion.

In cadavers the atlantoaxial joints exhibit about 47 degrees of axial rotation and some 10 degrees of flexion-extension.[6] Lateral flexion, such as will occur, is brought about by the atlas sliding sideways; an apparent tilt occurs because the facets of the axis slope downward and laterally; therefore as the atlas slides laterally, it slides down the ipsilateral facet of the axis and up the contralateral facet, thereby incurring an apparent lateral rotation that measures about 5 degrees.[15]

Plain radiography cannot be used to determine accurately the range of axial rotation of the atlas because direct, top views of the moving vertebra cannot be obtained. Consequently, the range of axial rotation can only be inferred from plain film. For this reason, few investigators have hazarded an estimate of the range of axial rotation; most of them have reported only the range of flexion-extension exhibited by the atlas (Table 2-2).

One approach to obtaining values of the range of axial rotation of the atlas has been to use biplanar radiography.[17] The results of such studies reveal that the total range of rotation (from left to right) of the occiput versus C2 is 75.2 degrees ± 11.8 (mean ± SD). Moreover, axial rotation is, on average, accompanied by 14 ± 6 degrees of extension and 2.4 ± 6 degrees of contralateral lateral flexion. Axial rotation of the atlas is thus not a pure movement; it is coupled with a substantial degree of extension or in some cases, flexion. The coupling arises because of the passive behavior of the atlas under axial loads from the head; whether it flexes or extends during axial rotation depends on the shape of the atlantoaxial joints and the exact orientation of any longitudinal forces acting through the atlas from the head.

Another approach to studying the range of axial rotation of the atlas has been to use computed tomographic (CT) scanning. This facility was not available to early in-

Table 2-2 Ranges of Motion of the Atlantoaxial Joints

	Ranges of Motion (Degrees)		
	Axial Rotation		
Source	One Side	Total	Flexion-Extension
Brocher[9]			18 (2-16)
Kottke and Mundale[13]			11
Lewit and Krausova[10]			16
Markuske[11]			21
Lind et al[14]			13 (±5)
Fielding[12]		90	15
Hohl and Baker[16]	30		(10-15)

vestigators of cervical kinematics, and data stemming from its application have appeared only in recent years.

In a rigorous series of studies, Dvorak and colleagues examined first the anatomy of the atlantoaxial ligaments,[18] the movements of the atlas in cadavers,[19-21] and how these could be demonstrated using CT.[22] Subsequently, they applied the same scanning technique to normal subjects and to patients with neck symptoms after motor vehicle trauma in whom atlantoaxial instability was suspected clinically.[23,24]

They confirmed earlier demonstrations[25] that the transverse ligament of the atlas was critical in controlling flexion of the atlas and its anterior displacement.[20] They showed that the alar ligaments were the cardinal structures that limit axial rotation of the atlas,[19,20] although the capsules of the lateral atlantoaxial joints contribute to a small extent.[20] In cadavers, 32 ± 10 degrees (mean ± SD) of axial rotation to either side could be obtained, but if the contralateral alar ligament was transected, the range increased by some 30% (i.e., by about 11 degrees).[22]

In normal individuals, the range of axial rotation, as evident in CT scans, is 43 ± 5.5 degrees (mean ± SD) with an asymmetry of 2.7 ± 2 degrees (mean ± SD).[23] These figures establish 56 degrees as a reliable upper limit of rotation, above which pathological hypermobility can be suspected, with rupture of the contralateral alar ligament being the most likely basis.[23]

In studying a group of patients with suspected hypermobility, Dvorak et al[23,24] found their mean range of rotation to be 58 degrees. Although the number of patients so afflicted is perhaps small, the use of functional CT constitutes a significant breakthrough. Functional CT is the only available means of reliably diagnosing patients with alar ligament damage. Without the application of CT, these patients would continue to remain undiagnosed and their complaint ascribed to unknown or psychogenic causes.

LOWER CERVICAL KINEMATICS

Many studies have been devoted to studying the movements of the lower cervical spine. In literature it has been almost traditional for yet another group each year to add another contribution to issues such as the range of movement of the neck.[26-48]

Early studies examined the range of movement of the entire neck, typically by applying goniometers to the head.[32-34,37,45] Fundamentally, however, such studies describe the range of movement of the head. Although they provide implicit data on the global function of the neck, they do not reveal what actually is happening inside the neck.

Some investigators examined neck movements by studying cadavers.[35,38,44] Such studies are an important first iteration because they establish what might be expected when individual segments come to be studied in vivo and how it might best be measured. However, cadaver studies are relatively artificial; the movement of skeletons without muscles does not accurately reflect how intact, living individuals move.

Investigators recognized that for a proper comprehension of cervical kinematics, radiographic studies of normal individuals were required,[26-31,36,39-42,46-48] and a large number of investigators produced what might be construed as normative data on the range of motion of individual cervical segments and the neck as a whole (Table 2-3).

What is conspicuous about these data, however, is that whereas ranges of values were sometimes reported, SDs were not. It seems that most of these studies were undertaken in an era before the advent of statistical and epidemiological rigour. Two

Table 2-3 Reported Results of Studies of Normal Ranges of Motion of the Cervical Spine in Flexion and Extension

Source	Number	Total Average Range of Motion (Degrees)* C2-3	C3-4	C4-5	C5-6	C6-7
Bakke[26]	15	13 (3-22)	16 (8-23)	17 (11-24)	20 (12-29)	18 (11-26)
De Seze[27]	9	13	16	19	28	18
Buetti-Bauml[28]	30	11 (5-18)	17 (13-23)	21 (16-28)	23 (18-28)	17 (13-25)
Kottke and Mundale[13]	78	11	16	18	21	18
Penning[30]	20	13 (5-16)	18 (13-26)	20 (15-29)	22 (16-29)	16 (6-25)
Zeitler and Markuske[31]	48	16 (4-23)	23 (13-38)	26 (10-39)	25 (10-34)	22 (13-29)
Mestdagh[40]	33	11	12	18	20	16
Johnson et al[41]	44	12	18	20	22	21
Dunsker et al[42]	25	10 (7-16)	13 (8-18)	13 (10-16)	20 (10-30)	12 (6-15)

*With ranges, if reported.

early studies[29,39] provided raw data from which means and SDs could be calculated, and two recent studies[14,46] provided data properly described in statistical terms (Table 2-4).

The early studies of cervical motion were also marred by lack of attention to the reliability of the technique used; interobserver and intraobserver errors were not reported. This leaves unknown the extent to which observer errors and technical errors compromise the accuracy of the data reported. Only those studies conducted in recent years specify the accuracy of their techniques,[14,46] so only their data can be considered acceptable.

The implication of collecting normative data is that somehow it might be used diagnostically to determine abnormality. Unfortunately, without means and SDs and without values for observer errors, normative data are at best illustrative, and cannot be adopted for diagnostic purposes. To declare an individual or a segment to be abnormal, an investigator must clearly be able to calculate the probability of a given observation constituting a normal value and must determine whether or not technical errors have biased the observation.

One study has pursued this application using reliable and well-described data.[46] For active and passive cervical flexion, mean values and SDs were determined for the range of motion of every cervical segment using a method of stated reliability. Furthermore, it was claimed that symptomatic patients could be identified on the basis of hypermobility or hypomobility.[46] However, the normal range adopted in this study was one SD either side of the mean.[46] This range is irregular and illusory.

It is more conventional to adopt the two-SD range as the normal range. This convention establishes a range within which 96% of the asymptomatic population lies; only 2% of the normal population will fall above these limits, and only 2% will fall below. Adopting a one-SD range classifies only 67% of the normal population within the limits, leaving 33% of normal individuals outside the range. This means that any population of putatively abnormal individuals will be "contaminated" with 33% of the normal population. This reduces the specificity of the test and increases its false-positive rate.

Table 2-4 Summary of the Results of Studies of Cervical Flexion and Extension that Reported Both Mean Values and Standard Deviations

Source	Number	Mean Range and Standard Deviation of Motion in Degrees				
		C2-3	C3-4	C4-5	C5-6	C6-7
Aho et al[29]	15	12 ± 5	15 ± 7	22 ± 4	28 ± 4	15 ± 4
Bhalla and Simmons[39]	20	9 ± 1	15 ± 2	23 ± 1	19 ± 1	18 ± 3
Lind et al[14]	70	10 ± 4	14 ± 6	16 ± 6	15 ± 8	11 ± 7
Dvorak et al[46]	28	10 ± 4	15 ± 3	19 ± 4	20 ± 4	19 ± 4

Table 2-5 Mean Values and Ranges of Axial Rotation of Cervical Motion Segments as Determined by CT Scanning

Segment	Range of Motion (Degrees)	
	Mean	Range
Occ-C1	1.0	−2 to 5
C1-C2	40.5	29-46
C2-C3	3.0	0-10
C3-C4	6.5	3-10
C4-C5	6.8	1-12
C5-C6	6.9	2-12
C6-C7	2.1	2-10
C7-T1	2.1	−2 to 7

Data from Penning and Wilmink.[49]

Axial Rotation

Axial rotation of the typical cervical vertebrae is difficult to study. This motion can be viewed directly only under CT scanning, but even CT scanning does not accurately depict the motion. Because of the slope of the zygapophyseal joints, axial rotation of a typical cervical vertebra is inexorably coupled with ipsilateral lateral flexion. Consequently, axial rotation is not executed in a constant plane, and the images seen on CT are confounded by motion out of the plane of view. CT therefore provides only an approximate estimate of the range of axial rotation of the typical cervical vertebrae. One study has provided normative data using this technique[49] (Table 2-5).

More valid measures can obtained from trigonometric reconstructions of movements studied by biplanar radiography. However, the accuracy of this method depends on the accuracy of identifying like points on four separate views of the same vertebra (an anteroposterior and a lateral view in each of two positions). Accuracy in this process is not easy to achieve.[8] Nevertheless, one study[17] has provided normative data using this technique (Table 2-6). What is noticeable from these data is that biplanar radiography reveals a somewhat more generous range of axial rotation than does CT but that this rotation is coupled with a lateral flexion of essentially the same magnitude.

Table 2-6 Normal Ranges of Motion of Cervical Spine in Axial Rotation, and Ranges of Coupled Motions, as Determined by Biplanar Radiography

		Coupled Movement	
	Axial Rotation	Flexion-Extension	Lateral Flexion
Segment	Mean Degrees (SD)	Mean Degrees (SD)	Mean Degrees (SD)
Occ-C2	75 (12)	−14 (6)	−2 (6)
C2-3	7 (6)	0 (3)	−2 (8)
C3-4	6 (5)	−3 (5)	6 (7)
C4-5	4 (6)	−2 (4)	6 (7)
C5-6	5 (4)	2 (3)	4 (8)
C6-7	6 (3)	3 (3)	3 (7)

SD, Standard deviation.
Data from Mimura et al.[17]

Uncinate Processes

One of the long-standing mysteries of the cervical spine has been the function of the uncinate processes. In some interpretations their role has been trivialized as acting as "guide rails" for flexion and extension.[38] However, a fascinating and compelling theory has been enunciated by Penning.[49,50]

By taking CT scans, first parallel to the plane of the cervical zygapophyseal joints and then perpendicular to this plane, Penning[49,50] revealed that the uncinate processes formed a concave cup under the reciprocally curved convex vertebral body above (Figure 2-1). This invites the interpretation that the cervical interbody joints are in fact saddle joints.

In the sagittal plane the upper surface of a vertebral body is gently convex, and the inferior surface of the vertebra above is gently concave. This permits the movements of flexion and extension in the sagittal plane. Meanwhile, in the plane of the zygapophyseal joints, the upper surface of the vertebral body is concave between the uncinate processes, and the reciprocal surface of the vertebra above is convex. This permits side-to-side rotation in the saddle of the joint; but this freedom of motion is not in the conventional coronal plane; it occurs in the plane of the zygapophyseal joints (i.e., some 40 degrees ventrad of the coronal plane).[51]

Viewed in this way, the cervical interbody joints permit only two forms of movement: sagittal rotation and axial rotation in the plane of the zygapophyseal joints (Figure 2-2). This latter movement is tantamount to a modified form of what would have been called *axial rotation*. Side-bending of the cervical vertebra is not possible; movement perpendicular to the plane of the zygapophyseal joints is precluded by impaction of the joints (Figure 2-3).

This model of cervical motion is attractive not only because it explains the function of the uncinate processes but also because it explains the structure of the cervical intervertebral discs. In the cervical spine, the annulus fibrosus is thick and well developed anteriorly but is deficient posteriorly.[52] At an early age, clefts develop in the region of the uncinate processes and progressively extend across the back of the disc, essentially transecting any posterior annulus fibrosus.[50] Such transverse fissures are a normal and ubiquitous feature of adult cervical discs.[53] This morphology of the disc means that the anterior ends of consecutive vertebral bodies are strongly bound to one another by the anterior annulus and their relative positions are fixed. Meanwhile, no

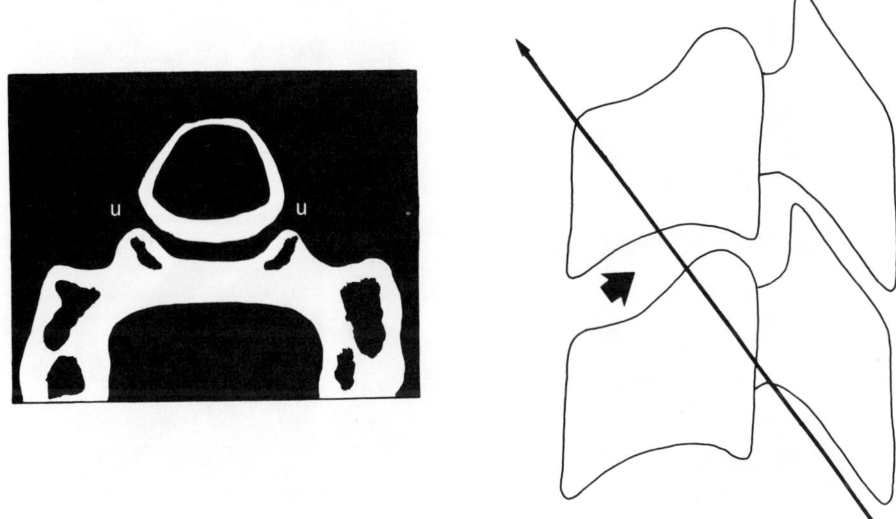

Figure 2-1
The appearance of the uncovertebral region as revealed by CT scans parallel to the plane of the zygapophyseal joints. The long arrow depicts the plane of scan; the short arrow depicts the direction in which the segment is viewed. Note how the uncinate processes *(u)* present a concave cup to the reciprocally curved vertebral body above, thereby constituting the transverse component of a saddle joint between the cervical vertebral bodies.

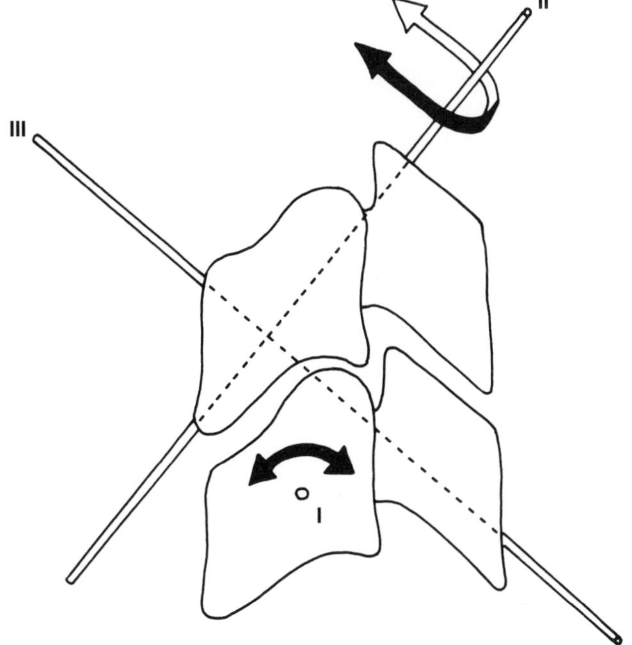

Figure 2-2
The planes of motion of a cervical motion segment. Flexion and extension occur around a transverse axis *(axis I)*. Axial rotation occurs around a modified axis *(axis II)*, passing perpendicular to the plane of the zygapophyseal joints, and this motion is cradled by the uncinate processes. The third axis *(axis III)* lies perpendicular to both of the first two axes, but no motion can occur about this axis (see Figure 2-3).

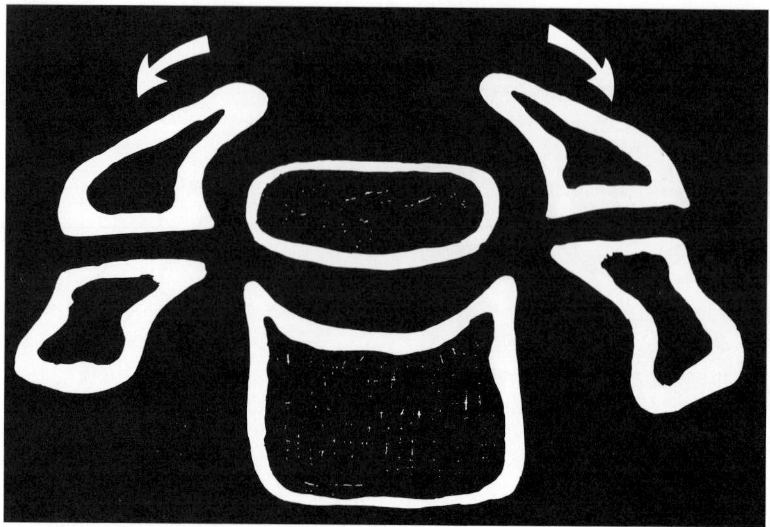

Figure 2-3
A view of a cervical motion segment looking upward and forward along axis III (see Figure 2-2) to demonstrate how rotation around this axis is precluded by impaction of the facets of the zygapophyseal joints.

annulus binds their posterior ends, which are relatively free to swing side to side in the plane of the zygapophyseal joints.

This structure coincides with the mechanics of axial rotation of the cervical vertebrae (Figure 2-2). The axis of rotation passes through or near the anterior ends of the vertebral bodies (i.e., through where the bodies are fixed by the anterior annulus fibrosus). Lying near the axis, the anterior ends of the vertebral bodies do not require freedom to swing side to side. Essentially, the vertebral bodies pivot about the binding anterior annulus. Meanwhile, for axial rotation to occur (in the plane of the zygapophyseal joints), the posterior ends of the vertebral bodies must be able to swing. They are able to do so because of the transverse clefts. In the absence of clefts, a strong posterior annulus would impede or prevent axial rotation. Notionally the posterior longitudinal ligament would also impede axial rotation, but it seems to have sufficient laxity to permit the 6 degrees or so of movement that occurs in axial rotation.

Range of Motion

Regardless of how fashionable it may have been to study ranges of motion of the neck and regardless of how genuine may have been the intent and desire of early investigators to derive data that could be used to detect abnormalities, a definitive study has now appeared that has put paid to all previous studies and renders any further studies of cervical motion using conventional radiographic techniques irrelevant. The tabulated, earlier data (Tables 2-3 and 2-4) are no longer of any use.

Van Mameren et al[54] used an exquisite technique to study cervical motion in flexion and extension in normal volunteers. High-speed cineradiographs were taken in which top-quality images were produced on each frame, allowing accurate biomechanical analyses to be undertaken frame by frame. The subjects undertook flexion from full extension, and also extension from full flexion. A total of 25 exposures were obtained during each sequence. The experiments were repeated 2 weeks and 10 weeks after the first observation. These studies allowed the ranges of motion of individual cervical segments to be studied and correlated against total range of motion of the neck and against the direction in which movement was undertaken. Moreover, the stability of the observations over time could be determined. The results are shattering.

The maximal range of motion of a given cervical segment is not necessarily reflected by the range apparent when the position of the vertebra in full flexion is compared to its position in full extension. Often the maximal range of motion is exhibited at some stage during the excursion but before the neck reaches its final position. In other words, a vertebra may reach its maximal range of flexion, but as the neck continues toward "full flexion," that vertebra actually reverses its motion and extends slightly. This behavior is particularly apparent at upper cervical segments (Occ-C1, C1-2).

A consequence of this behavior is that the total range of motion of the neck is not the arithmetic sum of its intersegmental ranges of motion. Thus what others have observed and quantified as the range of total cervical motion is not even directly related to intersegmental motion. For clinical purposes it is imperative that the range of intersegmental motion be studied explicitly lest abnormal movements be masked within the range of total neck movements; moreover, a single flexion film and a single extension film is not enough to reveal maximal intersegmental motion. That can only be revealed cineradiographically.

A second result is that intersegmental range of motion differs according to whether the motion is executed from flexion to extension or from extension to flexion. At the same sitting, in the same individual, differences of 5 to 15 degrees can be recorded, particularly at Occ-C1 and C6-7. The collective effect of these differences, segment by segment, can result in differences of 10 to 30 degrees in total range of cervical motion.

There is no criterion for deciding which movement strategy should be preferred. It is not a question of standardizing a convention as to which direction of movement should (arbitrarily) be recognized as standard. Rather, the behavior of cervical motion segments simply raises a caveat that no single observation defines a unique range of movement. Since the strategy used can influence the observed range, an uncertainty arises; depending on the segment involved, an observer may record a range of movement that may be 5 or even 15 degrees less or more than the range of which the segment is actually capable. By the same token, claims of therapeutic success in restoring a range of movement must be based on ranges in excess of this range of uncertainty.

The third result is that ranges of movement are not stable with time. A difference in excess of 5 degrees for the same segment in the same individual can be recorded if it is studied by the same technique but on another occasion, particularly at segments Occ-C1, C5-6 and C6-7. Rhetorically, the question becomes—which observation was the true normal? The answer is that normal ranges within an individual do not come in discrete quanta; they vary, and it is this variance (and not a single value) and the range of variation that constitute the normal behavior. The implication is that a single observation of a range must be interpreted and can be used for clinical purposes only with this variation in mind. A lower range today, a higher range tomorrow, or vice versa, could be only the normal, diurnal variation and not something attributable to a disease or to a therapeutic intervention.

CADENCE

Commentators in the past have maintained that as the cervical spine as a whole moves there must a set order in which the individual cervical vertebra move (i.e., there must be a normal pattern of movement, or cadence). Buonocore et al[55] asserted,

> "The spinous processes during flexion separate in a smooth fan-like progression. Flexion motion begins in the upper cervical spine. The occiput separates smoothly from the posterior arch of the atlas, which then separates smoothly from the spine of the axis, and so on down the spine. The interspaces between the spinous processes become generally equal in complete flexion. Most important, the spinous processes separate in orderly progression. In extension the spines rhythmically approximate each other in reverse order to become equidistant in full extension."

This idealized pattern of movement is not what normally occurs. During flexion and extension, the motion of the cervical vertebrae is regular but not simple; it is complex and counterintuitive. The motion is not easy to describe either. Van Mameren[56] undertook a detailed analysis of his cineradiographs of 10 normal individuals performing flexion and extension of the cervical spine. His descriptions are complex, reflecting the intricacies of movement of individual segments. However, a general pattern can be discerned.

Flexion is initiated in the lower cervical spine (C4-7). Within this block, and during this initial phase of motion, the C6-7 segment regularly makes its maximal contribution, before C5-6, followed by C4-5. That initial phase is followed by motion at Occ-C2, and then by C2-3 and C3-4. During this middle phase, the order of contribution of C2-3 and C3-4 is variable. Also during this phase, a reversal of motion (i.e., slight extension) occurs at C6-7 and, in some individuals, at C5-6. The final phase of motion again involves the lower cervical spine (C4-7), and the order of contribution of individual segments is C4-5, C5-6, and C6-7. During this phase, Occ-C2 typically exhibits a reversal of motion (i.e., extension). Flexion is thus initiated and terminated by C6-7. It is never initiated at midcervical levels. Occ-C2, C2-3, and C3-4 contribute maximally during the middle phase of motion but in variable order.

Extension is initiated in the lower cervical spine (C4-7), but the order of contribution of individual segments is variable. This is followed by the start of motion at Occ-C2 and at C2-4. Between C2 and C4 the order of contribution is quite variable. The terminal phase of extension is marked by a second contribution by C4-7, in which the individual segments move in the regular order—C4-5, C5-6, C6-7. During this phase the contribution of Occ-C2 reaches its maximum.

The fact that this pattern of movements is reproducible is remarkable. Studied on separate occasions, individuals consistently show the same pattern with respect to the order of maximal contribution of individual segments. Consistent between individuals is the order of contribution of the lower cervical spine and its component segments during both flexion and extension. Such variation as occurs between individuals applies only to the midcervical levels: C2-4.

INSTANTANEOUS AXES OF ROTATION

Having noted the lack of use of range-of-motion studies, some investigators explored the notion of quality of motion of the cervical vertebrae. They contended that although perhaps not revealed by abnormal ranges of motion, abnormalities of the cervical spine might be revealed by abnormal patterns of motion within individual segments.

When a cervical vertebra moves from full extension to full flexion, its path appears to lie along an arc whose center lies somewhere below the moving vertebra. This center is called the *instantaneous axis of rotation (IAR)* and its location can be determined using simple geometry. If tracings are obtained of lateral radiographs of the cervical spine in flexion and in extension, the pattern of motion of a given vertebra can be revealed by superimposing the tracings of the vertebra below. This reveals the extension position and the flexion position of the moving vertebra in relation to the one below (Figure 2-4). The location of the IAR is determined by drawing the perpendicular bisectors of intervals connecting like points on the two positions of the moving vertebra. The point of intersection of the perpendicular bisectors marks the location of the IAR (Figure 2-4).

The first normative data on the IARs of the cervical spine were provided by Penning.[30,36,50] He found them to be located in different positions for different cervical segments. At lower cervical levels the IARs were located close to the intervertebral disc of the segment in question, but at higher segmental levels the IAR was located substantially lower than this position.

However, a problem emerged, with Penning's data.[30,36,50] Although he displayed the data graphically, he did not provide any statistical parameters such as the mean location and variance; nor did he explain how IARs from different individuals with vertebra of different sizes were plotted onto a single, common silhouette of the cervical spine. This process requires some form of normalization, which Penning[30,36,50] did not describe.

Subsequent studies pursued the accurate determination of the location of the IARs of the cervical spine. First, it was found that the technique used by Penning[36,43,50] to plot IARs was insufficiently accurate; the basic flaw lay in how well the images of the cervical vertebrae could be traced.[57] Subsequently, an improved technique with smaller interobserver errors was developed[58] and used to determine the location of IARs in a sample of 40 normal individuals.[59]

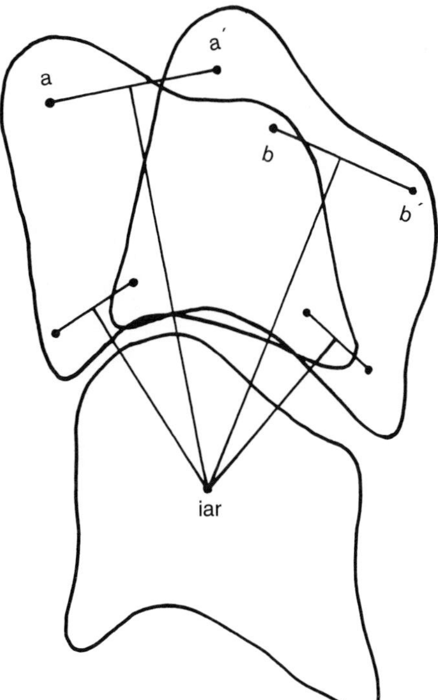

Figure 2-4
A sketch of a cervical motion segment, illustrating how the location of its instantaneous axis of rotation *(iar)* can be determined by geometry.

Accurate maps were developed of the mean location and distribution of the IARs of the cervical motion segments (Figure 2-5) based on raw data normalized for vertebral size and coupled with measure of interobserver errors. The locations and distributions were concordant with those described by Penning,[30,36,50] but the new data offered the advantage that because they were described statistically, they could be used to test accurately hypotheses concerning the normal or abnormal locations of IARs.

Some writers have protested against the validity and reliability of IARs, but the techniques they have used to determine their location have been poorly described and not calibrated for error and accuracy.[60] In contrast, van Mameren et al[61] have rigorously defended IARs. They have shown that a given IAR can be reliably and consistently calculated within a small margin of technical error. Moreover, in contrast to range of motion, the location of the IAR is independent of whether it is calculated on the basis of anteflexion or retroflexion films, and strikingly the IAR is stable over time. No significant differences in location occur if the IAR is recalculated 2 weeks or 10 weeks after the initial observation.[61] Thus the IAR stands as a reliable, stable parameter of the quality of vertebral motion through which abnormalities of motion could be explored.

Abnormal IARs

The first exploration of abnormal quality of cervical motion was undertaken by Dimnet et al,[62] who proposed that abnormal quality of motion would be exhibited by abnormal locations of the IARs of the cervical motion segment. In a small study of six symptomatic patients they found that in patients with neck pain the IARs exhibited a wider scatter than in normal individuals. However, they compared samples of patients and not individual patients; their data did not reveal in a given patient which and how many IARs were normal or abnormal or to what extent.

A similar study was pursued by Mayer et al.[63] They claimed that patients with cervical headache exhibited abnormal IARs of the upper cervical segments. However,

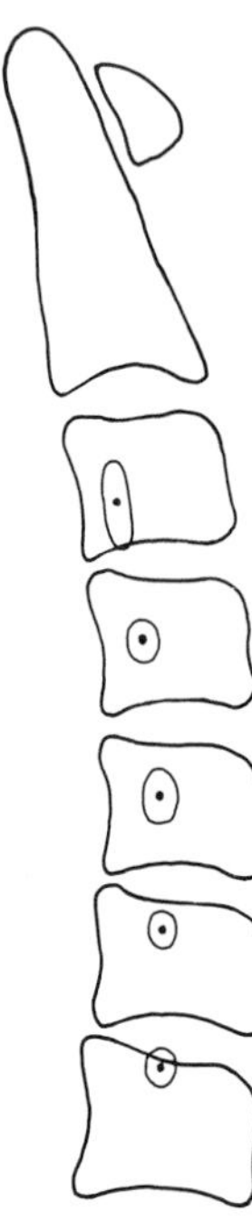

Figure 2-5
A sketch of an idealized cervical vertebral column illustrating the mean location and two-SD range of distribution of the instantaneous axes of rotation of the typical cervical motion segments.

their normative data were poorly described with respect to ranges of distribution, nor was the accuracy of their technique used to determine both normal and abnormal axes described.

Nevertheless, these two studies contended that if reliable and accurate techniques were to be used it was likely that abnormal patterns of motion could be identified in patients with neck pain, in the form of abnormal locations of their IARs. This contention was formally investigated.

Amevo et al[64] studied 109 patients with posttraumatic neck pain. Flexion-extension radiographs were obtained and IARs were determined for all segments from C2-3 to C6-7 when possible. These locations were subsequently compared with previously determined normative data.[59] It emerged that 77% of the patients with neck pain exhibited an abnormally located axis at one segmental level at least. This relationship between axis location and pain was highly significant statistically (Table 2-7); there was clearly a relationship between pain and abnormal patterns of motion.

Further analysis revealed that most abnormal axes were at upper cervical levels, notably at C2-3 and C3-4. However, there was no evident relationship between the segmental level of an abnormally located IAR and the segment found to be symptomatic on the basis of provocation discography or cervical zygapophyseal joint blocks.[64] This suggested that perhaps abnormal IARs were not caused by intrinsic abnormalities of a painful segment but were secondary to some factor such as muscle spasm. However, this contention could not be explored because insufficient numbers of patients had undergone investigation of upper cervical segments with discography or joint blocks.

Biological Basis

Mathematical analysis shows that the location of an IAR is a function of three basic variables: the amplitude of rotation (θ) of a segment, its translation (T), and the location of its center of rotation (CR).[65] In mathematical terms, with respect to any universal coordinate system (X, Y), the location of the IAR is defined by the following equations:

$$X_{IAR} = X_{CR} + T/2$$
$$Y_{IAR} = Y_{CR} - T/[2 \tan (\theta/2)]$$

in which (X_{IAR}, Y_{IAR}) is the location of the IAR, and (X_{CR}, Y_{CR}) is the location of the center of reaction.

In this context, the center of reaction is a point on the inferior end-plate of the moving vertebra in which compression loads on that vertebra are maximal, or the

Table 2-7 Chi-squared Analysis of Relationship Between Presence of Pain and Location of Instantaneous Axes of Rotation

	Instantaneous Axis of Rotation*		
	Normal	Abnormal	
Pain	31	78	109
No Pain†	44	2	46
	75	80	155

*$X^2 = 58.5$; df = 1; $p < 0.001$.
†For patients with no pain, $n = 46$, and by definition 96% of these (44) exhibit normal IARs.[64]

mathematical average point in which compression loads are transmitted from the vertebra to the underlying disc. It is also the pivot point around which the vertebra rocks under compression, or around which the vertebra would rotate in the absence of any shear forces that add translation to the movement.[65]

The equations dictate that the normal location, and any abnormal location, of an IAR is governed by the net effect of compression forces, shear forces, and moments acting on the moving segment. The compression forces exerted by muscles and by gravity and the resistance to compression exerted by the facets and disc of the segment determine the location of the center of reaction. The shear forces exerted by gravity and by muscles and the resistance to these forces exerted by the intervertebral disc and facets determine the magnitude of translation. The moments exerted by gravity and by muscles and the resistance to these exerted by tension in ligaments, joint capsules, and the annulus fibrosus determine the amplitude of rotation.

These relationships allow the location of an IAR to be interpreted in anatomical and pathological terms. Displacement of an IAR from its normal location can occur only if the normal balance of compression loads, shear loads, or moments is disturbed. Moreover, displacements in particular directions can occur only as a result of certain finite combinations of disturbances to these variables. For example, the IAR equations dictate that downward and backward displacement of an IAR can occur only if there is a simultaneous posterior displacement of the center of reaction and a reduction in rotation.[65] Mechanically, this combination of disturbances is most readily achieved by increased posterior muscle tension. On the one hand, this tension eccentrically loads the segment in compression, displacing the center of reaction posteriorly; meanwhile, the increased tension limits forward flexion and reduces angular rotation. An abnormal IAR, displaced downward and backward, is therefore a strong sign of increased posterior muscle tension. Although the tension is not recorded electromyographically or otherwise, its presence can be inferred from mathematical analysis of the behavior of the segment. Although the tension is not "seen," the effects of its force are manifest (just as the presence of an invisible planet can be detected by the gravitational effects it exerts on nearby celestial bodies).

Upward displacement of an IAR can occur only if there is a decrease in translation or an increase in rotation, all other variables being normal. This type of displacement is most readily produced if flexion-extension is produced in the absence of shear forces (i.e., the segment is caused to rotate only by forces acting essentially parallel to the long axis of the cervical spine). How this might occur naturally is explained in the next section.

APPLICATIONS

Recent radiographic studies of normal volunteers undergoing experimental whiplash impacts have provided revealing insights in the mechanisms of whiplash injury.[66] During the first 100 ms or so after impact, the cervical spine is subjected to axial compression. This arises because the trunk and thorax are thrust upward into the neck, toward the head, which initially does not move and whose inertia constitutes a resistance to the upward thrust. As a result, the cervical spine undergoes a sigmoid deformation (Figure 2-6). During this deformation, the upper cervical segments undergo flexion, while the lower segments extend, typically at C5-6. This extension, however, is not normal in quality. It occurs about an abnormal IAR.

The IAR is displaced upward from its normal location, into the bottom of the extending vertebra. The movement occurs about an abnormal axis because no shear

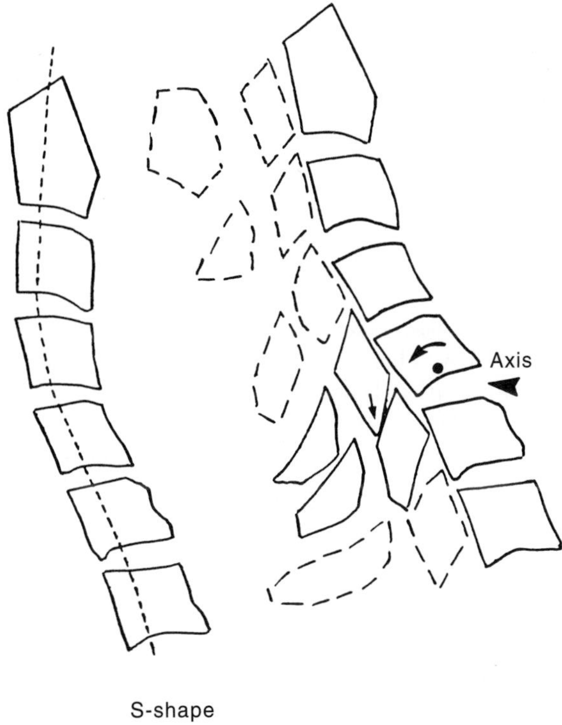

Figure 2-6
Tracings of radiographs of the cervical spine of normal volunteers undergoing a whiplash impact, at 110 ms after impact and shortly before. The cervical spine undergoes a sigmoid deformation during which the lower cervical vertebrae undergo extension *(curved arrow)* around an abnormally high axis of rotation. This results in abnormal separation of the vertebral bodies anteriorly *(arrowhead)* and impaction of the zygapophyseal joints posteriorly *(small arrow)*.
(Based on Kaneoka et al: *Spine* 24:763, 1999.)

forces are exerted on the segment to produce translation. The vertebra is subjected to only an upward thrust. Essentially the vertebra pivots about its center of reaction. In mathematical terms, the value of T is zero, and the IAR equations reduce to the following:

$$X_{IAR} = X_{CR}$$
$$Y_{IAR} = Y_{CR}$$

The effects of this abnormal rotation are that anteriorly, the vertebral bodies separate to an abnormal degree and posteriorly, the articular processes of the zygapophyseal joints impact (Figure 2-6). The facets are forced to impact because in the absence of a posterior shear force, they cannot slide backward. Instead, the inferior edge of the upper articular process chisels into the supporting surface of the lower articular process.

This pattern of (abnormal) motion predicates the possible injuries that can occur. The anterior annulus fibrosus is subject to tension and can be torn or avulsed from the vertebral end-plate. The zygapophyseal joints can suffer an impaction injury, which could involve tearing of intraarticular meniscoids or infractions of the subchondral bone.

A discussion of the mechanics and pathology of whiplash is beyond the scope of this chapter, but this example is raised to illustrate how the principles and details of biomechanics eventually find their way into relevant aspects of clinical practice.

References

1. Deng YC, Goldsmith W: Response of a human head/neck/upper-torso replica to dynamic loading. II. Analytical/numerical model, *J Biomech* 20:487, 1987.
2. De Jager MKJ, Sauren A, Thunnissen J, Wismans J: A three-dimensional head-neck model: validation for frontal and lateral impacts. Proceedings of the 38th Stapp Car Crash Conference, Society for Automotive Engineers, paper no. 942211, Fort Lauderdale, Fla, 1994.
3. Dauvilliers F, Bendjellal F, Weiss M et al: Development of a finite element model of the neck. Proceedings of the 38th Stapp Car Crash Conference, Society for Automotive Engineers paper no. 942210, Fort Lauderdale, Fla, 1994.
4. De Jager MKJ: Mathematical head-neck models for acceleration impacts, thesis, Netherlands, 1996, Technical University of Eindhoven.
5. Yoganandan N, Myklebust JB, Ray G, Sances A: Mathematical and finite element analysis of spine injuries, *CRC Crit Rev Biomed Eng* 15:29, 1987.
6. Werne S: The possibilities of movement in the craniovertebral joints, *Acta Orthop Scand* 28:165, 1958.
7. Worth DR, Selvik G: *Movements of the craniovertebral joints.* In Grieve GP, editor: *Modern manual therapy of the vertebral column,* Edinburgh, 1986, Churchill Livingstone.
8. Worth D: Cervical spine kinematics, PhD thesis, Adelaide, Australia, 1985, Flinders University of South Australia.
9. Brocher JEW: Die occipito-cervical-gegend: eine diagnostische pathogenetische studie, Stuttgart, Germany, 1955, Georg Thieme Verlag (cited by van Mameren et al[54]).
10. Lewit K, Krausova L: Messungen von Vor- and Ruckbeuge in den Kopfgelenken, *Fortsch Rontgenstr* 99:538, 1963.
11. Markuske H: Untersuchungen zur Statik und Dynamik der kindlichen Halswirbelsaule: Der Aussagewert seitlicher Rontgenaufnahmen: Die Wirbelsaule in Forschung und Praxis, 1971 (cited by van Mameren et al[54]).
12. Fielding JW: Cineroentgenography of the normal cervical spine, *J Bone Joint Surg* 39A:1280, 1957.
13. Kottke FJ, Mundale MO: Range of mobility of the cervical spine, *Arch Phys Med Rehab* 40:379, 1959.
14. Lind B, Sihlbom H, Nordwall A, Malchau H: Normal ranges of motion of the cervical spine, *Arch Phys Med Rehab* 70:692, 1989.
15. Dankmeijer J, Rethmeier BJ: The lateral movement in the atlantoaxial joints and its clinical significance, *Acta Radiol* 24:55, 1943.
16. Hohl M, Baker HR: The atlantoaxial joint, *J Bone Joint Surg* 46A:1739, 1964.
17. Mimura M, Moriya H, Watanabe T et al: Three-dimensional motion analysis of the cervical spine with special reference to the axial rotation, *Spine* 14:1135, 1989.
18. Saldinger P, Dvorak J, Rahn BA, Perren SM: Histology of the alar and transverse ligaments, *Spine* 15:257, 1990.
19. Dvorak J, Panjabi MM: Functional anatomy of the alar ligaments, *Spine* 12:183, 1987.
20. Dvorak J, Scheider E, Saldinger P, Rahn B: Biomechanics of the craniocervical region: the alar and transverse ligaments, *J Orthop Res* 6:452, 1988.
21. Crisco JJ, Oda T, Panjabi MM et al: Transections of the C1-C2 joint capsular ligaments in the cadaveric spine, *Spine* 16:S474, 1991.

22. Dvorak J, Panjabi M, Gerber M, Wichmann W: CT-functional diagnostics of the rotatory instability of upper cervical spine. I. An experimental study on cadavers, *Spine* 12:197, 1987.
23. Dvorak J, Hayek J, Zehnder R: CT-functional diagnostics of the rotatory instability of the upper cervical spine. II. An evaluation of healthy adults and patients with suspected instability, *Spine* 12:725, 1987.
24. Dvorak J, Penning L, Hayek J et al: Functional diagnostics of the cervical spine using computer tomography, *Neuroradiology* 30:132, 1988.
25. Fielding JW, Cochran GVB, Lawsing JF, Hohl M: Tears of the transverse ligament of the atlas, *J Bone Joint Surg* 56A:1683, 1974.
26. Bakke SN: Rontgenologischen Beobachtungen uber die Bewegungen der Wirbelsaule, *Acta Radiol Supp* 13:1, 1931.
27. De Seze S: Etude radiologique de la dynamique cervicale dans la plan sagittale, *Rev Rhum Mal Osteoartic* 3:111, 1951.
28. Buetti-Bauml C: Funcktionelle Rontgendiagnsotik der Halswirbelsaule. Stuttgart, Germany, 1954, Georg Thieme Verlag (cited by van Mameren et al,[54] Aho et al,[29] and Dvorak et al[46]).
29. Aho A, Vartianen O, Salo O: Segmentary antero-posterior mobility of the cervical spine, *Ann Med Int Fenn* 44:287, 1955.
30. Penning L: Funktioneel rontgenonderzoek bij degeneratieve en traumatische afwijikingen der laag-cervicale bewingssegmenten, thesis, Groningen, Netherlands, 1960, Reijuniversiteit Groningen.
31. Zeitler E, Markuske H: Rontegenologische Bewegungsanalyse der Halswirbelsaule bei gesunden Kinden, *Forstschr Rontgestr* 96:87, 1962 (cited by van Mameren et al[54]).
32. Ferlic D: The range of motion of the "normal" cervical spine, *Bull Johns Hopkins Hosp* 110:59, 1962.
33. Bennett JG, Bergmanis LE, Carpenter JK, Skowund HV: Range of motion of the neck, *J Am Phys Ther Assn* 43:45, 1963.
34. Schoening HA, Hanna V: Factors related to cervical spine mobility. I. *Arch Phys Med Rehab* 45:602, 1964.
35. Ball J, Meijers KAE: On cervical mobility, *Ann Rheum Dis* 23:429, 1964.
36. Penning L: Nonpathologic and pathologic relationships between the lower cervical vertebrae, *AJR* 91:1036, 1964.
37. Colachis SC, Strohm BR: Radiographic studies of cervical spine motion in normal subjects: flexion and hyperextension, *Arch Phys Med Rehab* 46:753, 1965.
38. Lysell E: Motion in the cervical spine: an experimental study on autopsy specimens, *Acta Orthop Scandinav Suppl* 123:41, 1969.
39. Bhalla SK, Simmons EH: Normal ranges of intervertebral joint motion of the cervical spine, *Can J Surg* 12:181, 1969.
40. Mestdagh H: Morphological aspects and biomechanical properties of the vertebro-axial joint (C2-C3), *Acta Morphol Neerl-Scand* 14:19, 1976.
41. Johnson RM, Hart DL, Simmons EH et al: Cervical orthoses: a study comparing their effectiveness in restricting cervical motion, *J Bone Joint Surg* 59A:332, 1977.
42. Dunsker SB, Coley DP, Mayfield FH: Kinematics of the cervical spine, *Clin Neurosurg* 25:174, 1978.
43. Penning L: Normal movement in the cervical spine, *AJR* 130:317, 1978.
44. Ten Have HA, Eulderink F: Degenerative changes in the cervical spine and their relationship to mobility, *J Pathol* 132:133, 1980.
45. O'Driscoll SL, Tomenson J: The cervical spine, *Clin Rheum Dis* 8:617, 1982.
46. Dvorak J, Froehlich D, Penning L et al: Functional radiographic diagnosis of the cervical spine: flexion/extension, *Spine* 13:748, 1988.
47. Dvorak J, Panjabi MM, Novotny JE, Antinnes JA: In vivo flexion/extension of the normal cervical spine, *J Orthop Res* 9:828, 1991.
48. Dvorak J, Panjabi MM, Grob D et al: Clinical validation of functional flexion/extension radiographs of the cervical spine, *Spine* 18:120, 1993.

49. Penning L, Wilmink JT: Rotation of the cervical spine: a CT study in normal subjects, *Spine* 12:732, 1987.
50. Penning L: Differences in anatomy, motion, development and aging of the upper and lower cervical disk segments, *Clin Biomech* 3:37, 1988.
51. Nowitzke A, Westaway M, Bogduk N: Cervical zygapophyseal joints: geometrical parameters and relationship to cervical kinematics, *Clin Biomech* 9:342, 1994.
52. Mercer S, Bogduk N: The ligaments and annulus fibrosus of human adult cervical intervertebral discs, *Spine* 24:619, 1999.
53. Oda J, Tanaka H, Tsuzuki N: Intervertebral disc changes with aging of human cervical vertebra from the neonate to the eighties, *Spine* 13:1205, 1988.
54. van Mameren H, Drukker J, Sanches H, Beursgens J: Cervical spine motion in the sagittal plane. I. Range of motion of actually performed movements: an x-ray cinematographic study, *Eur J Morphol* 28:47, 1990.
55. Buonocore E, Hartman JT, Nelson CL: Cineradiograms of cervical spine in diagnosis of soft tissue injuries, *JAMA* 198:25, 1966.
56. van Mameren H: Motion patterns in the cervical spine, thesis, Maastricht, Netherlands, 1988, University of Limburg.
57. Amevo B, Macintosh J, Worth D, Bogduk N: Instantaneous axes of rotation of the typical cervical motion segments. I. An empirical study of errors, *Clin Biomech* 6:31, 1991.
58. Amevo B, Worth D, Bogduk N: Instantaneous axes of rotation of the typical cervical motion segments. II. Optimisation of technical errors, *Clin Biomech* 6:38, 1991.
59. Amevo B, Worth D, Bogduk N: Instantaneous axes of rotation of the typical cervical motion segments: a study in normal volunteers, *Clin Biomech* 6:111, 1991.
60. Fuss FK: Sagittal kinematics of the cervical spine: how constant are the motor axes? *Acta Anat* 141:93, 1991.
61. van Mameren H, Sanches H, Beurgsgens J, Drukker J: Cervical spine motion in the sagittal plane. II. Position of segmental averaged instantaneous centers of rotation: a cineradiographic study, *Spine* 17:467, 1992.
62. Dimnet J, Pasquet A, Krag MH, Panjabi MM: Cervical spine motion in the sagittal plane: kinematic and geometric parameters, *J Biomech* 15:959, 1982.
63. Mayer ET, Hermann G, Pfaffenrath V et al: Functional radiographs of the craniovertebral region and the cervical spine, *Cephalalgia* 5:237, 1985.
64. Amevo B, Aprill C, Bogduk N: Abnormal instantaneous axes of rotation in patients with neck pain, *Spine* 17:748, 1992.
65. Kaneoka K, Ono K, Inami S, Hayashi K: Motion analysis of cervical vertebrae during whiplash loading, *Spine* 24:763, 1999.
66. Bogduk N, Amevo B, Pearcy M: A biological basis for instantaneous centres of rotation of the vertebral column, *Proc Instn Mech Engrs* 209:177, 1995.

CHAPTER 3

Biomechanics of the Thorax

Diane Lee

For clinicians who follow a biomechanical approach to the assessment and treatment of musculoskeletal dysfunction, a model of optimal function is required. The biomechanical model of the thorax presented in the second edition of this book was originally proposed by Lee[1] in 1993. The model was derived from clinical observation and influenced primarily by the study of Panjabi et al.[2] Few studies have added to our biomechanical knowledge base since then. In 1996, Willems et al[3] reported on their in vivo findings of coupled motion in the thorax. The results from this study, and the influence it has had on the original model presented in 1993, will be discussed in this chapter.

Models should evolve, and the biomechanical model of the thorax is no exception. Specifically, not much has changed except that the description of how the thorax moves is less specific and allows for individual variance. It remains the basis for the manual therapy techniques presented in Chapter 16. To facilitate the subsequent discussion, the reader is referred to Table 3-1, which outlines certain terms and their definitions used in this chapter.

A landmark study of the biomechanics of the thorax was published by Panjabi et al[2] in 1976. They investigated the primary and coupled motions of the thorax in several cadavers. In the study, 396 load displacement curves were obtained for six degrees of motion: three translations and three rotations along and about the x, y, and z axes (Figure 3-1) for each of the 11 motion segments of the thoracic spine. The specimens ranged from 19 to 59 years of age. The motion segment included the anterior interbody joint, the posterior zygapophyseal joints, and the costovertebral and costotransverse joints. The ribs were cut 3 cm lateral to the costotransverse joints, and the front of the chest was removed. The functional spinal unit was left intact; however, the functional costal unit was not. This work, combined with clinical observation, formed the basis for the original biomechanical model.[1]

Willems et al[3] measured primary and coupled rotations of the thoracic spine in an in vivo study. A total of 60 subjects between 18 and 24 years of age were studied using a 3SPACE FASTRAK System. (The FASTRAK is an electromagnetic system that tracks the motion in three dimensions [3-D] and sends the information to a computer

Table 3-1 Definition of Terminology

Term	Definition
Osteokinematics[4]	Study of the motion of bones regardless of the motion of the joints Angular motions are named according to the axis about which they rotate Coronal axis: flexion-extension Paracoronal axis: anterior-posterior rotation Sagittal axis: side-flexion Vertical axis: axial rotation Linear motions are named according to the axis along which they translate Coronal axis: mediolateral translation Paracoronal axis: anteromedial posterolateral translation Vertical axis: traction-compression Sagittal axis: anteroposterior translation
Arthrokinematics[4]	Study of the motion of joints regardless of the motion of the bones Named according to the direction in which the joint surfaces glide
Coupled motion	Combination of movements that occur as a consequence of an induced motion

whose software interprets the data, "allowing the calculation of the position of each sensor in space."[3]) The subjects were screened and excluded if they had a current or past history of thoracic pain, long-term respiratory disorders, or a significant scoliosis. An examination of the thoracic spine for segmental function was not done before the study. Sensors were attached to one spinous process in each of three regions of the thorax, one between T1 and T4, a second between T4 and T8, and the third between T8 and T12. Each subject was seated, the pelvis and thighs were secured, and the lumbar spine was supported. With arms folded across the chest, each subject was asked to move to maximal range in thoracic flexion, extension, axial rotation, and lateral flexion. Each motion was carefully taught to each subject to ensure the motion desired was actually occurring in the thorax. The methods and results from this study have been carefully considered and will be discussed with respect to the biomechanical model of thoracic motion.

According to mathematical[5-8] and theoretical[1] models, the thorax is capable of 6 degrees of motion (Figure 3-1) along and about the three cardinal axes of the body. However, it is known that no movement occurs in isolation.[2,3] All angular motion (rotation) is coupled with a linear motion (translation) and vice versa. As the thorax moves to meet its biomechanical demands, it must accommodate the requirements of respiration. To do this, it needs flexibility in motion patterning.

The biomechanics of the thorax vary according to the region considered. Two regions will be discussed in this chapter—the midthorax and the lower thorax. The *midthorax* is defined as the region between T3 and T6 and includes the associated vertebral, costal, and sternal components. The *lower thorax* is defined as the region between T7 and T10 and includes the associated vertebral and costal components.

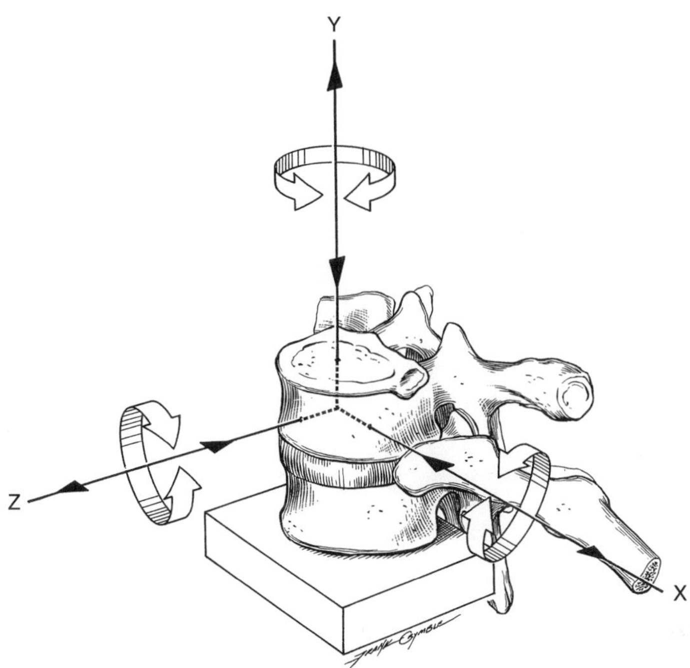

Figure 3-1

In an in vitro study by Panjabi et al,[2] 396 load-displacement curves were obtained for 6 degrees of motion at each thoracic segment. The amplitude of the induced motion as well as the amplitude and direction of any consequential coupled motion was recorded.
(From Lee D: *J Manual Manipulative Ther* 1[1]:14, 1993.)

MIDTHORACIC REGION

FLEXION

Flexion of the thoracic vertebrae occurs during forward bending of the trunk. Panjabi et al[2] found that forward sagittal rotation (flexion) around the x axis was coupled with anterior translation along the z axis (5 mm) and very slight distraction (Figure 3-2). When anterior translation along the z axis (1 mm) was induced in the experimental model, forward sagittal rotation around the x axis and very slight compression also occurred. In the in vivo study of Willems et al,[3] sagittal plane motion was the purest and showed the least incidence of coupled motion. No axial rotation or lateral flexion should occur during sagittal plane motion of the thorax.

The osteokinematic motion of the ribs, which occurs during forward sagittal rotation of the thoracic vertebrae, was not noted by either Panjabi et al[2] or Willems et al.[3] Saumarez[5] noted that there can be considerable independent movement of the sternum and the spine, "thus allowing mobility of the spine without forcing concomitant movements of (the) rib cage." This is supported clinically in that three movement patterns are apparent and depend on the relative flexibility between the spinal column and the rib cage. In the very young (subjects younger than 12 years of age), the head of the rib does not fully articulate with the inferior aspect of the superior vertebra.[9] In other words, the superior costovertebral joint is not completely developed before

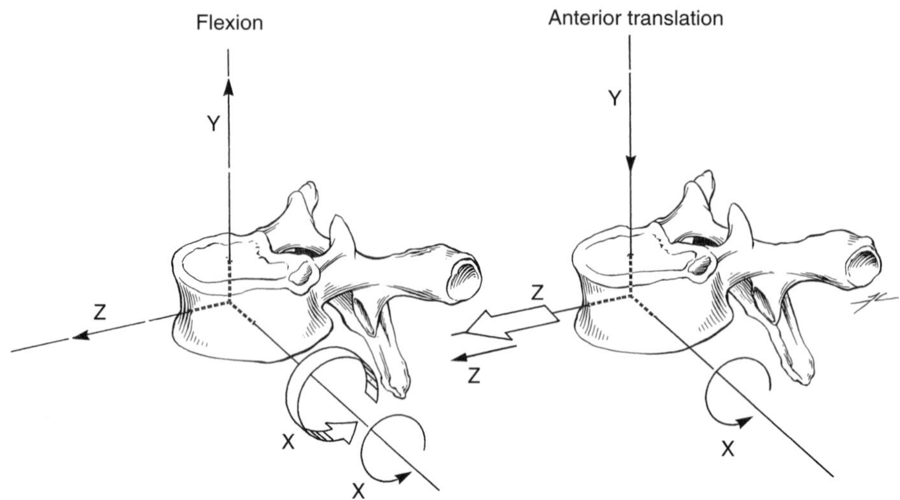

Figure 3-2
Forward sagittal rotation around the *x* axis induced anterior translation along the *z* axis and slight distraction along the *y* axis. Anterior translation along the *z* axis induced forward sagittal rotation around the *x* axis and slight compression along the *y* axis.
(Redrawn from Panjabi et al.[2] From Lee D: *J Manual Manipulative Ther* 1[1]:15, 1993.)

puberty. The secondary ossification centers for the head of the rib do not develop until puberty. Therefore children have a much more mobile chest. In the skeletally mature the superior costovertebral joints limit the degree of rotation possible in all three planes. In old age, the costal cartilages tend to ossify superficially,[9] thereby further decreasing the pliability and relative flexibility of the thorax. This change in relative flexibility is apparent when examining the specific costal osteokinematics during forward-backward bending of the trunk.

1. During flexion of the *mobile thorax*, forward sagittal rotation of the superior vertebra couples with anterior translation. This anterior translation appears to "pull" the superior aspect of the head of the rib forward at the costovertebral joint, inducing an anterior rotation of the rib. The rib rotates about a paracoronal axis along the line of the neck of the rib so that the anterior aspect travels inferiorly and the posterior aspect travels superiorly (Figure 3-3).

   Arthrokinematically, the inferior facets of the superior thoracic vertebrae glide superoanteriorly at the zygapophyseal joints during flexion of the thoracic vertebrae. The superior articular processes of the inferior thoracic vertebrae present a gentle curve convex posterior in both the sagittal and the coronal planes. The superior motion of the inferior articular processes follows the curve of this convexity, and the result is a superoanterior glide. Thus the arthrokinematic motion of the joint surfaces supports the osteokinematic motion of the vertebrae, anterior translation being coupled with forward sagittal rotation. The anterior rotation of the neck of the rib results in a *superior glide* of the tubercle at the costotransverse joint (Figure 3-3). Since the costotransverse joints of the midthoracic vertebrae are concavoconvex (the facet on the transverse process is concave) in both the sagittal and the coronal planes,[9] the superior glide of the tubercle results in an anterior rotation of the neck of the rib. Once again, the arthrokinematic motion at the costotransverse joint supports the osteokinematic motion of the rib during forward bending of the trunk.

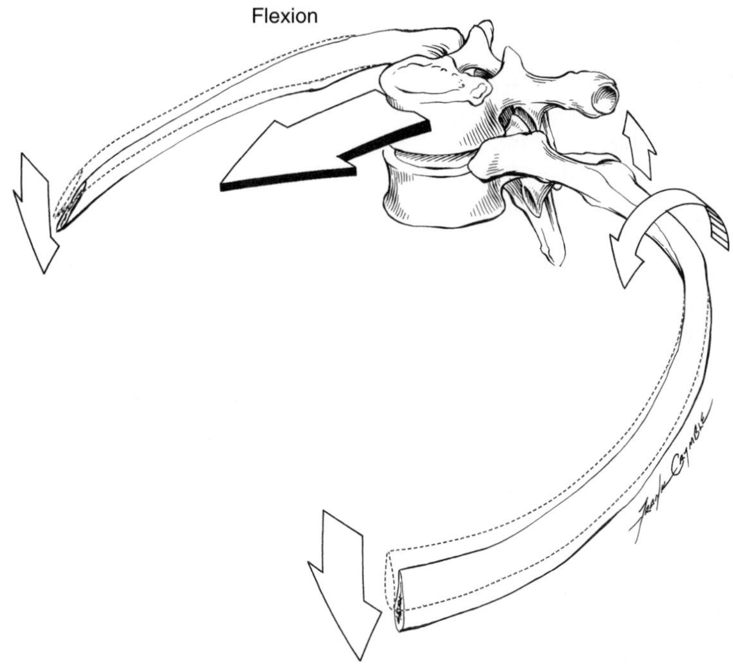

Figure 3-3
The osteokinematic and arthrokinematic motion proposed to occur in the mobile thorax during flexion.
(From Lee D: *J Manual Manipulative Ther* 1[1]:15, 1993.)

2. In the *stiff thorax*, the ribs appear to be less flexible than the spinal column. During flexion, the anterior aspect of the rib travels inferiorly, and the posterior aspect travels superiorly. Once the range of motion of the rib cage is exhausted, the thoracic vertebrae continue to forward flex on the now-stationary ribs. The arthrokinematics of the zygapophyseal joints remain the same as in the first movement pattern described. At the costotransverse joints, the arthrokinematics are different. As the thoracic vertebrae continue to forward flex, the concave facets on the transverse processes travel superiorly relative to the tubercle of the ribs. The result is a relative *inferior glide* of the tubercle of the rib at the costotransverse joint.
3. The third movement pattern occurs when the relative flexibility between the spinal column and the rib cage is the same. During flexion of the thorax, the quantity of movement is reduced, and there is no apparent movement between the thoracic vertebrae and the ribs. Some superoanterior gliding occurs at the zygapophyseal joints; however, very little, if any, anterior translation occurs.

The limiting factors to flexion of the thoracic functional spinal unit (FSU) include all of the ligaments posterior to and including the posterior half of the intervertebral disc. In studies by Panjabi et al,[10,11] the thoracic FSU was loaded to failure in both flexion and extension. *Failure* was defined as a complete separation of the two vertebrae of more than 10 mm of translation or 45degrees of rotation. The ligaments were transected sequentially and the contribution of the various ligaments to the stability of the FSU was noted. They found that the FSU remained stable in flexion until the costovertebral joint was transected. The integrity of the posterior one third of the disc and the costovertebral joints is critical to anterior translation stability in the thorax.

EXTENSION

Extension of the thoracic vertebra occurs during backward bending of the trunk and bilateral elevation of the arms. Panjabi et al[2] found that backward sagittal rotation (extension) around the x axis was coupled with posterior translation along the z axis (1 mm) and very slight distraction (Figure 3-4). When backward translation along the z axis (2.5 mm) was induced in the experimental model, posterior sagittal rotation around the x axis and very slight compression also occurred.

The osteokinematic motion of the ribs that occurs during backward sagittal rotation of the thoracic vertebrae was not noted in studies by Panjabi et al[2] or Willems et al.[3] Clinically, the movement patterns observed appear once again to depend on relative flexibility between the spinal column and the rib cage. The following three patterns have been noted.

1. During extension of the *mobile thorax*, backward sagittal rotation of the superior vertebra couples with the posterior translation and "pushes" the superior aspect of the head of the rib backward at the costovertebral joint, inducing a posterior rotation of the rib (Figure 3-5). The rib rotates about a paracoronal axis along the line of the neck of the rib so that the anterior aspect travels superiorly and the posterior aspect travels inferiorly.

   Arthrokinematically, the inferior facets of the superior thoracic vertebrae glide inferoposteriorly at the zygapophyseal joints during extension of the thoracic vertebrae. The superior articular processes present a gentle curve convex posterior in both the sagittal and the coronal planes. The inferior motion of the inferior articular processes follows the curve of this convexity, and the result is an inferoposterior glide. Thus the arthrokinematic motion of the joint surfaces supports the osteokinematic motion of the vertebrae, posterior translation being coupled with backward sagittal rotation.

   The posterior rotation of the neck of the rib results in an *inferior glide* of the tubercle at the costotransverse joint (Figure 3-5). Since the costotransverse joints

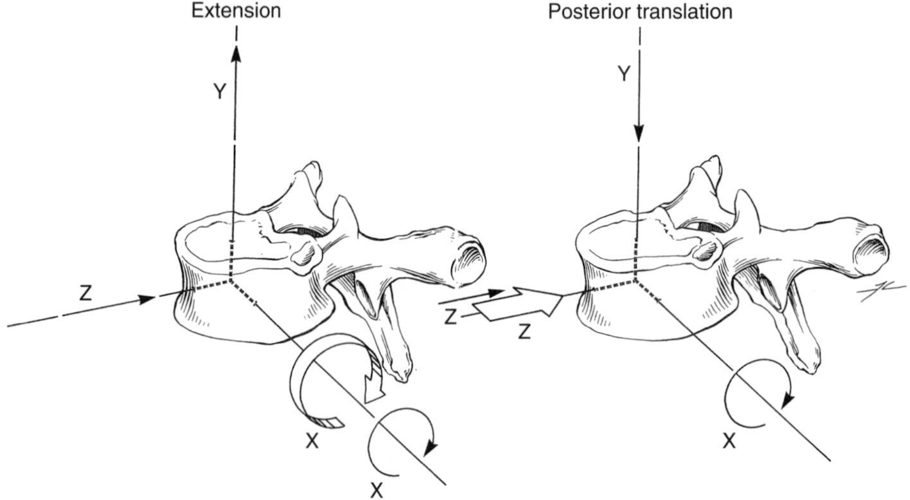

Figure 3-4
Backward sagittal rotation around the x axis induced posterior translation along the z axis and slight distraction along the y axis. Posterior translation along the z axis induced backward sagittal rotation around the x axis and slight compression along the y axis.
(Redrawn from Panjabi et al.[2] From Lee D: *J Manual Manipulative Ther* 1[1]:17, 1993.)

of the midthoracic vertebrae (T2 to T6) are concavoconvex in both the sagittal and the coronal planes, the inferior glide of the tubercle results in a posterior rotation of the neck of the rib. Once again, the arthrokinematic motion supports the osteokinematic motion of the rib during backward sagittal rotation.

2. During extension of the *stiff thorax*, the ribs are less flexible than the spinal column. Initially, the anterior aspect of the rib travels superiorly, whereas the posterior aspect travels inferiorly. Once the range of motion of the rib cage is exhausted, the thoracic vertebrae continue to extend on the now-stationary ribs. The arthrokinematics of the zygapophyseal joints remain the same as in the first movement pattern described. At the costotransverse joints, the arthrokinematics are different. As the thoracic vertebrae continue to extend, the concave facets on the transverse processes travel inferiorly relative to the tubercle of the ribs. The result is a relative *superior glide* of the tubercle of the rib at the costotransverse joint.
3. The third movement pattern occurs when the relative flexibility between the spinal column and the rib cage is the same. During extension of the thorax, the quantity of movement is reduced, and there is no apparent movement between the thoracic vertebrae and the ribs. Some inferoposterior gliding occurs at the zygapophyseal joints only; however, very little, if any, posterior translation occurs.

The limiting factors to extension of the thoracic FSU include all of the ligaments anterior to and including the posterior longitudinal ligament. Panjabi et al[10,11] sequentially transected the anterior longitudinal ligament, the anterior half of the intervertebral disc, the costovertebral joints, and the posterior half of the intervertebral disc and noted the contribution of each to the stability of the FSU in

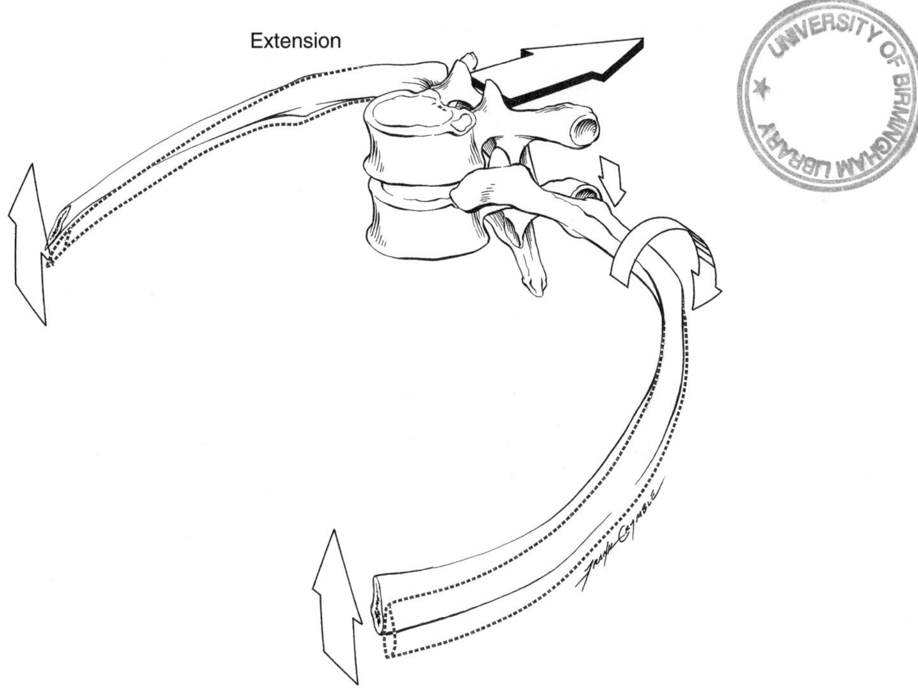

Figure 3-5

The osteokinematic and arthrokinematic motion proposed to occur in the thorax during extension.

(From Lee D: *J Manual Manipulative Ther* 1[1]:17, 1993.)

extension. It was found that the FSU remained stable in extension until the posterior longitudinal ligament was transected.

These are the common patterns noted when sagittal plane motion of the thorax is observed. It is possible for individuals to voluntarily change their pattern of motion. For example, in the mobile thorax the spine can extend inducing a posterior rotation of the ribs *in space*, and then while holding this position, it is possible to anteriorly rotate the ribs. This flexibility allows the thorax to accommodate the demands coming from respiration and from movements of the upper extremities and the head.

LATERAL BENDING

Side-flexion of the thoracic vertebrae occurs during lateral bending of the trunk. Panjabi et al[2] found that side-flexion, or rotation around the *z* axis, was coupled with contralateral rotation around the *y* axis and ipsilateral translation along the *x* axis. Translation along the *x* axis was coupled with ipsilateral side-flexion around the *z* axis and contralateral rotation around the *y* axis (Figure 3-6).

In their in vivo study, Willems et al[3] found that the pattern of coupling during lateral bending was variable, although an ipsilateral relationship predominated. Since the movement of the sensor was compared only to its baseline starting position, the pattern noted in this study can reflect only how the spinous process moved in space, and no comment can be made on segmental motion patterning. In other words, during lateral bending of the trunk, Willems et al[3] noted that the vertebra tended to side-flex and rotate in an ipsilateral direction. Side-flex and rotate compared to what? No comment can be made on what T4 did relative to T5 because this was not measured. This study shows that compared to its starting position, T4 side-flexed and rotated in an ipsilateral direction during lateral bending of the thorax.

It is interesting to postulate on what produces coupled motion in the thorax. In the midcervical spine, it is thought[12,13] that the oblique orientation of the zygapophyseal joints, together with the uncinate processes, directs the ipsilateral rotation and

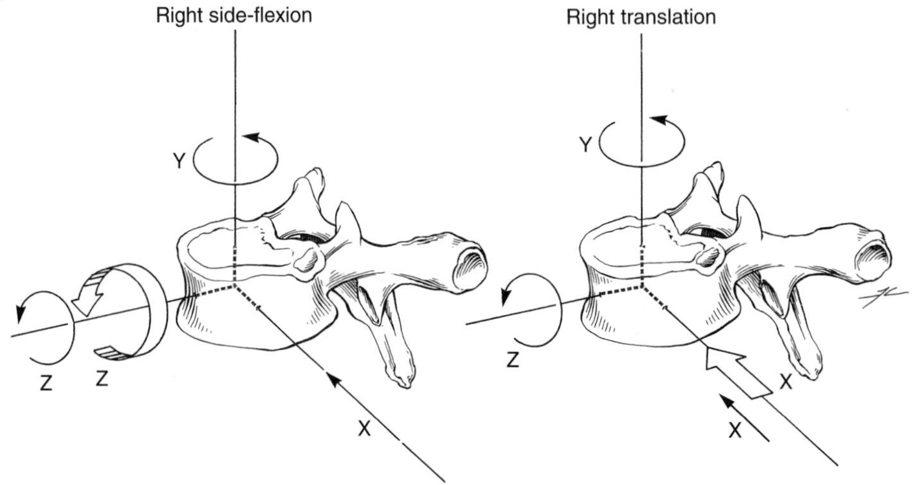

Figure 3-6
Right side-flexion around the *z* axis induces left rotation around the *y* axis and right translation along the *x* axis. Right lateral translation along the *x* axis induces right side-flexion around the *z* axis and left rotation around the *y* axis.
(Redrawn from Panjabi et al.[2] From Lee D: *J Manual Manipulative Ther* 1[1]:17, 1993.)

side-flexion that occurs. In the lumbar spine, the zygapophyseal joints also are known[14] to influence the direction of motion coupling during rotation. However, the facets of the zygapophyseal joints in the thoracic spine lie in a somewhat coronal plane and would not limit pure side-flexion during lateral bending of the trunk. It is difficult to see how they could be responsible for the rotation found to occur during side-flexion.

Clinical Hypothesis

As the trunk bends laterally to the right, a left convex curve is produced. The thoracic vertebrae side-flex to the right, the ribs on the right approximate, and the ribs on the left separate at their lateral margins (Figure 3-7). In both the mobile and the stiff thorax, the ribs appear to stop moving before the thoracic vertebrae. The thoracic vertebrae then continue to side-flex to the right. This motion can be palpated at the costotransverse joint.

This slight increase in right side-flexion of the thoracic vertebrae against the fixed ribs is proposed to cause the following arthrokinematic motion. At the costotransverse joints, a relative superior glide of the tubercle of the right rib and a relative inferior glide of the tubercle of the left rib occurs as the vertebra continues to side-flex to the right against the fixed ribs. Since the costotransverse joint is concavoconvex in a sagittal plane, the superior glide of the right rib produces a *relative* anterior rotation of the neck of the rib with respect to the transverse process (remember though that the rib is stationary and the moving bone is the thoracic vertebra). The inferior glide of the left rib produces a posterior rotation of the neck of the rib *relative* to the transverse process. Again, it is important to note that the moving bone is the thoracic vertebra, not the rib. Since the tubercle of the rib is convex, as the thoracic vertebra side-flexes to the right, it has to move posteriorly and inferiorly on the right and anteriorly and superiorly on the left. Osteokinematically, this produces a right rotation of the tho-

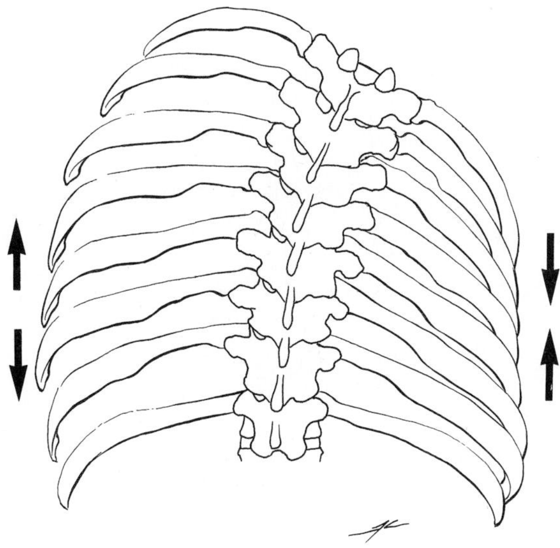

Figure 3-7
As the thorax side-flexes to the right, the ribs on the right approximate, and the ribs on the left separate at their lateral margins. The costal motion appears to stop first; the thoracic vertebrae then continue to side-flex slightly to the right.
(From Lee D: *J Manual Manipulative Ther* 1[1]:18, 1993.)

racic vertebra *relative to its starting position.* This is exactly what Willems et al[3] found in their study. However, consider what happens not just in space but between two thoracic vertebrae. As T5 side-flexes to the right on the fixed fifth ribs, it rotates to the right (necessitated by the shape of the tubercle of the fifth ribs). The T4 vertebra follows this motion; however, the relative anterior rotation of the right fifth rib and posterior rotation of the left fifth rib limit the amplitude of the right rotation of T4 such that it rotates *less to the right* than T5 and is therefore relatively left rotated (Figure 3-8). This only occurs at the limit of lateral bending.

In summary, during lateral bending of the midthorax, the vertebrae side-flex and rotate ipsilaterally relative to their starting position.[3] Relative to one another, the superior vertebra rotates less than the level below and therefore is actually rotated to the left in comparison. This coupling of motion occurs only at the end of the range. In the midposition, either ipsilateral or contralateral coupling can occur.

Panjabi et al[2] found that right lateral translation along the x axis (0.5 to 1 mm) occurred during right side-flexion (Figure 3-6). The effect of this right lateral translation is negated by the left lateral translation that occurs as the superior vertebra rotates to the left. The net effect is minimal, if any, mediolateral translation of the ribs along the line of the neck of the rib at the costotransverse joints. The clinical impression is that no anteromedial or posterolateral slide of the ribs occurs during lateral bending of the trunk.

At the zygapophyseal joints, the left inferior articular process of the superior thoracic vertebra glides superomedially and the right glides inferolaterally to facilitate right side-flexion and left rotation of the superior vertebra. The arthrokinematic motion of the joint surfaces supports the osteokinematic motion of the vertebrae and ribs.

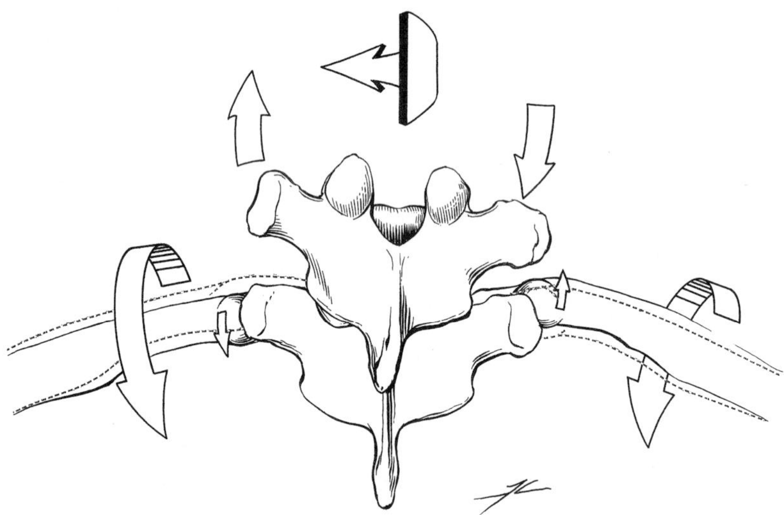

Figure 3-8

The superior glide of the right rib at the costotransverse joint induces anterior rotation of the same rib as a result of the convexoconcavity of the joint surfaces. The inferior glide of the left rib at the costotransverse joint induces posterior rotation of the same rib. This relative costal rotation is proposed to limit the right rotation of the superior vertebra so that the inferior vertebra rotates further to the right. The relative coupling of vertebral motion is therefore right side-flexion and left rotation of the superior vertebra relative to the inferior vertebra.

(From Lee D: *J Manual Manipulative Ther* 1[1]:18, 1993.)

ROTATION

Panjabi et al[2] found that rotation around the *y* axis coupled with *contralateral* rotation around the *z* axis and contralateral translation along the *x* axis (Figure 3-9). This is not consistent with clinical observation (Figure 3-10). In the midthoracic spine, rotation around the *y* axis has been found to be coupled with *ipsilateral* rotation around the *z* axis and contralateral translation along the *x* axis. In other words, when axial rotation is the first motion induced, rotation and side-flexion appear to occur to the same side in the midthoracic spine (Figure 3-10). In their in vivo study, Willems et al[3] found intersubject variation in motion patterning when the primary movement was axial rotation; however, an ipsilateral relationship was predominant. It may be that the thorax must be intact and stable both anteriorly and posteriorly for this in vivo coupling of

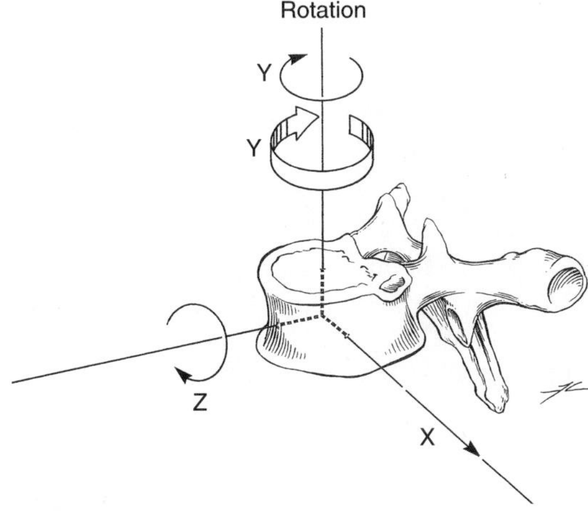

Figure 3-9
Panjabi et al[2] found that right rotation around the *y* axis induced left side-flexion around the *z* axis and left translation along the *x* axis.
(From Lee D: *J Manual Manipulative Ther* 1[1]19, 1993.)

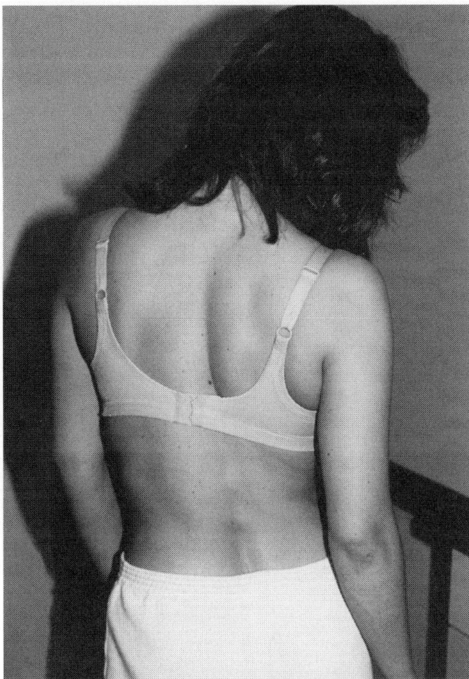

Figure 3-10
Right side-flexion couples with right rotation during right axial rotation of the trunk.

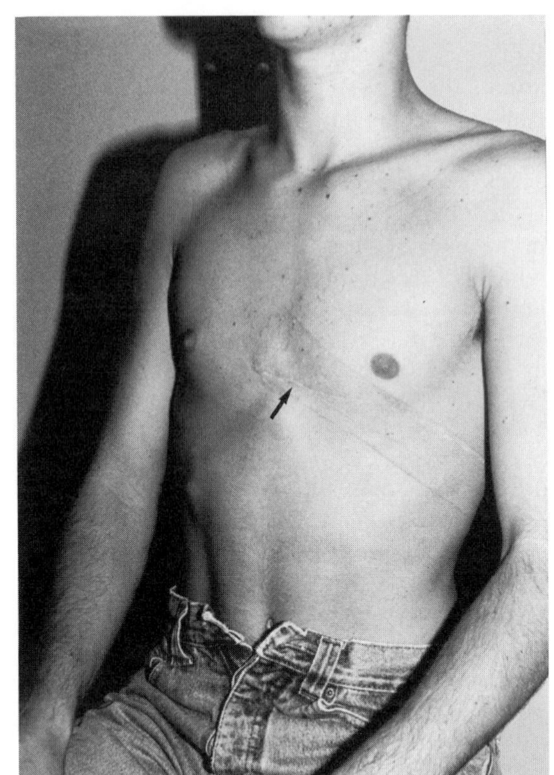

Figure 3-11
This 17-year-old male had the costal cartilage of the left sixth rib removed (note the incision).

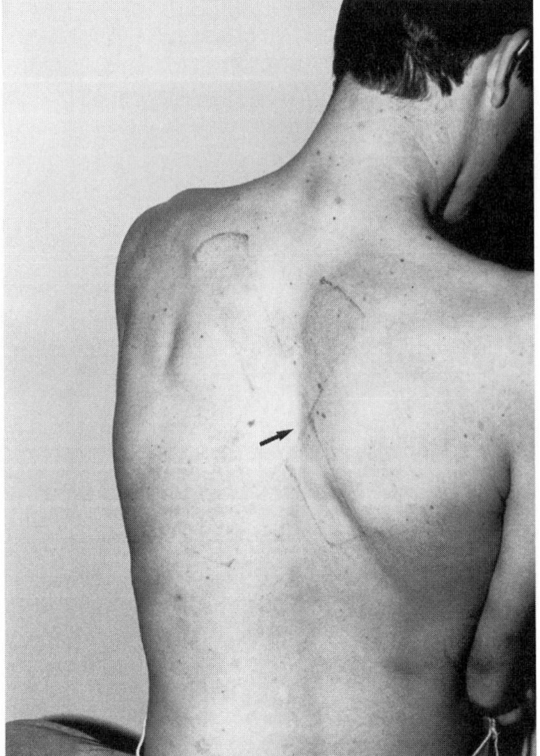

Figure 3-12
Right rotation of the midthorax couples with left side-flexion when the anterior aspect of the chest is unstable.

motion to occur. The anterior elements of the thorax were removed 3 cm lateral to the costotransverse joints in the study by Panjabi et al.[2]

When the anterior elements of the thorax are removed surgically, ipsilateral side-flexion and rotation cannot occur in the midthorax. The 17-year-old male illustrated in Figures 3-11 and 3-12 had the costal cartilage of the left sixth rib removed for cosmetic reasons. He had persistent pain in the midthorax, and on examination of axial rotation, contralateral side-flexion occurred at the sixth segment.

Clinical Hypothesis

During right rotation of the trunk, the following biomechanics appear to occur in the midthorax. The superior vertebra rotates to the right and translates to the left (Figure 3-13). Right rotation of the superior vertebral body "pulls" the superior aspect of the head of the left rib forward at the costovertebral joint (inducing anterior rotation of the neck of the left rib) and "pushes" the superior aspect of the head of the right rib backward (inducing posterior rotation of the neck of the right rib). The left lateral translation of the superior vertebral body "pushes" the left rib posterolaterally along the line of the neck of the rib and causes a posterolateral translation of the rib at the left costotransverse joint. Simultaneously, the left lateral translation "pulls" the right rib anteromedially along the line of the neck of the rib and causes an anteromedial translation of the rib at the right costotransverse joint. An anteromedial posterolateral slide of the ribs relative to the transverse processes to which they attach is thought to occur during axial rotation (Figure 3-13, *inset*).

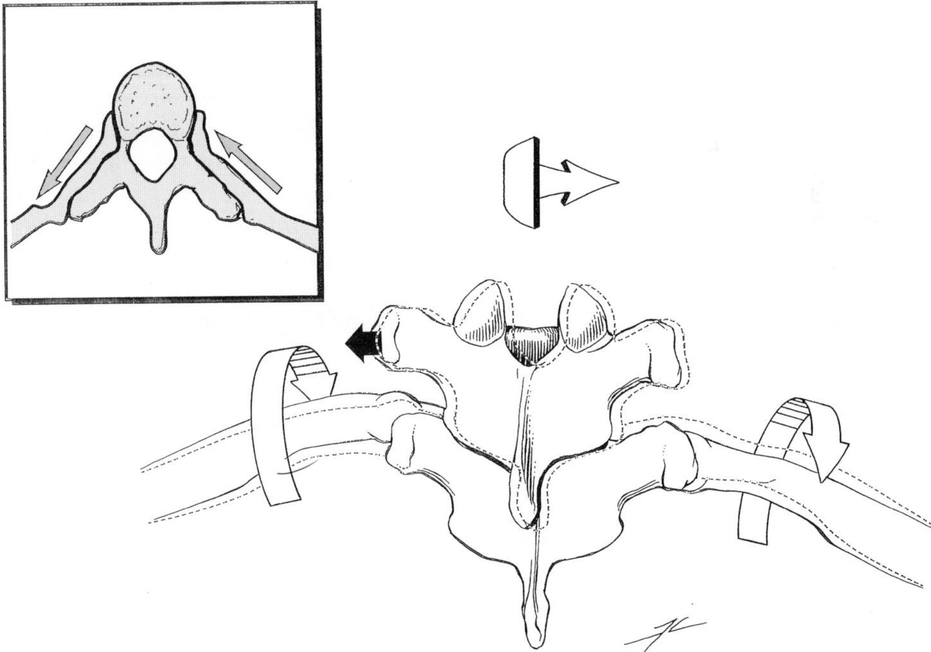

Figure 3-13

As the superior thoracic vertebra rotates to the right it translates to the left. The right rib posteriorly rotates and the left rib anteriorly rotates as a consequence of the vertebral rotation. The left lateral translation pushes the left rib in a posterolateral direction and pulls the right rib anteromedially *(inset)*.

(From Lee D: *J Manual Manipulative Ther* 1[1]:19, 1993.)

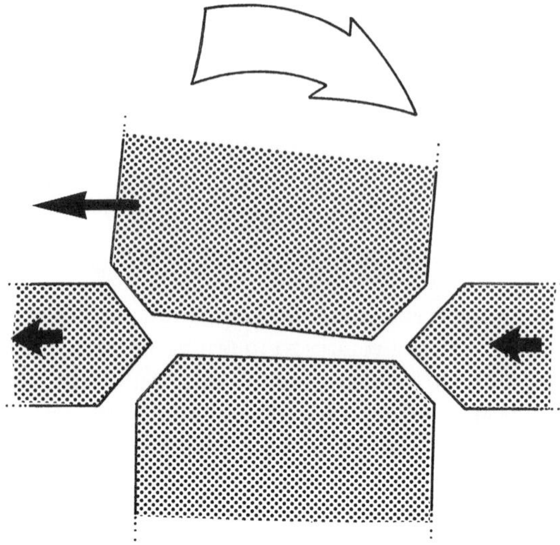

Figure 3-14
At the limit of left lateral translation, the superior vertebra side-flexes to the right along the plane of the pseudo U joint (analogous to the uncovertebral joint of the midcervical spine) formed by the intervertebral disc and the superior costovertebral joints.
(From Lee D: *J Manual Manipulative Ther* 1[1]:20, 1993.)

When the limit of this horizontal translation is reached, both the costovertebral and the costotransverse ligaments are tensed. Stability of the ribs both anteriorly and posteriorly is required for the following motion to occur. Further right rotation of the superior vertebra occurs as the superior vertebral body tilts to the right (i.e., glides superiorly along the left superior costovertebral joint and inferiorly along the right superior costovertebral joint). This tilt causes right side-flexion of the superior vertebra during right rotation of the midthoracic segment (Figure 3-14).

At the zygapophyseal joints, the left inferior articular process of the superior vertebra glides superolaterally and the right inferior articular process glides inferomedially to facilitate right rotation and right side-flexion of the thoracic vertebra. The arthrokinematic motion of the joint surfaces supports the osteokinematic motion of the vertebrae and ribs.

LOWER THORACIC REGION

Significant differences in the anatomy of this region influence the biomechanics. The facets on the transverse processes of the lower thoracic vertebrae are more planar and tend to be oriented in a superolateral direction.[9] A superoinferior glide of the rib will therefore *not necessarily* be associated with the same degree of anteroposterior rotation found in the midthoracic region. The costal cartilages of ribs 7 to 10 are less firmly attached to the sternum.[9] The inferior demifacet on the body of T9 for the tenth rib is small and often absent. The tenth rib articulates with one facet on the body of T10 and often does not attach to the transverse process at all.

FLEXION-EXTENSION

Flexion of the thoracic vertebrae in this region is also accompanied by anterior translation of the superior vertebra.[2] Extension of the lower thorax is accompanied by posterior translation of the superior vertebra.[1] Clinically, it appears that the associated ribs follow the sagittal motion, although minimal articular motion is necessary at the costovertebral joints of ribs 9 and 10 since they do not have a large attachment to the superior vertebra. The zygapophyseal joints glide superiorly during flexion and inferiorly in extension.

Lateral Bending

The biomechanics of the lower thorax during lateral bending of the trunk depends on the apex of the curve produced in side-flexion. For example, if during right lateral bending of the trunk the apex of the side-flexion curve is at the level of the greater trochanter on the left, then all of the thoracic vertebrae will side-flex to the right and the ribs will approximate on the right and separate on the left. As the rib cage is compressed on the right and stops moving, further right side-flexion of the lower thoracic vertebrae will result in a superior slide of the ribs at the costotransverse joints on the right. Given the orientation of the articular surfaces, the glide that occurs is posteromediosuperior on the right and anterolateroinferior on the left with minimal, if any, rotation of the neck of the rib. The ribs do not appear to direct the superior vertebra into contralateral rotation as they do in the midthorax. The vertebrae are then free to follow the rotation that is congruent with the levels above and below.

However, if the apex of the side-flexion curve is within the thorax (i.e., at T8), then the osteokinematics of the lower thoracic vertebrae appear to be very different. The rib cage remains compressed on the right and separated on the left, but the thoracic vertebrae side-flex *to the left* below the apex of the right side-flexion curve (i.e., T9 to T12). Given the orientation of the articular surfaces of the costotransverse joints, the glide that occurs on the right is in an anterolateroinferior direction (posteromediosuperior on the left) with minimal, if any, rotation of the neck of the rib. Once again, the ribs do not appear to direct the superior vertebra to rotate in a sense incongruent to the levels above and below.

Rotation

The same flexibility of motion coupling is apparent in the lower thorax when rotation is considered. In fact, the lower thoracic levels appear to be designed to rotate with minimal restriction from the costal elements. The coupled movement pattern for rotation in this region can be ipsilateral side-flexion or contralateral side-flexion. The coronally oriented facets of the zygapophyseal joints do not dictate a coupling of side-flexion when rotation is induced. The absence of a costotransverse joint and the lack of a direct anterior attachment of the associated ribs facilitates this flexibility in motion patterning.

CONCLUSION

The known biomechanics of the intact thorax continues to be far from complete. Willems et al[3] acknowledge that "altered tension in muscles may change forces on the ribs and vertebrae which could in turn influence the pattern of coupled motion in vivo, particularly in the upper thoracic area." Inclusion criteria for studies such as these should involve a biomechanical examination and not just exclusion by lack of symptoms or history of problems, since "it is not uncommon to find tightness in muscles . . . even in asymptomatic persons."[3] This is an excellent study and with further refinement of the inclusion criteria (biomechanical evaluation) and methodology (sensors on adjacent levels) could yield significant information pertinent to the biomechanical model.

Manual therapy techniques (see Chapter 16) are just one tool used in the treatment of mechanical dysfunction in the thorax. Although the variability and flexibility of motion patterning within the thorax are acknowledged, this biomechanical model is still useful for the selection of manual therapy techniques. Ultimately, the goal is to restore effortless motion of sufficient amplitude performed with the control and strength necessary to meet whatever load is being imposed on the thorax. When used in conjunction with education and exercise, manual therapy following this biomechanical model can be effective in facilitating recovery.

References

1. Lee D: Biomechanics of the thorax: a clinical model of in vivo function, *J Manual Manipulative Ther* 1:13, 1993.
2. Panjabi MM, Brand RA, White AA: Mechanical properties of the human thoracic spine, *J Bone Joint Surg* 58A:642, 1976.
3. Willems JM, Jull GA, Ng JKF: An in vivo study of the primary and coupled rotations of the thoracic spine, *Clin Biomech* 2(6):311, 1996.
4. MacConaill MA, Basmajian JV: *Muscles and movements: a basis for human kinesiology*, ed 2, New York, 1977, Kreiger.
5. Saumarez RC: An analysis of possible movements of the human upper rib cage, *J Appl Physiol* 60:678, 1986.
6. Saumarez RC: An analysis of action of intercostal muscles in human upper rib cage, *J Appl Physiol* 60:690, 1986.
7. Andriacchi T, Schultz A, Belytschko T, Galante J: A model for studies of mechanical interactions between the human spine and rib cage, *J Biomech* 7:497, 1974.
8. Ben-Haim SA, Saidel GM: Mathematical model of chest wall mechanics: a phenomenological approach, *Ann Biomed Eng* 18:37, 1990.
9. Williams P, Warwick R, Dyson M, Bannister LH: *Gray's anatomy*, ed 37, Edinburgh, 1989, Churchill Livingstone.
10. Panjabi MM, Hausfeld JN, White AA: A biomechanical study of the ligamentous stability of the thoracic spine in man, *Acta Orthop Scan* 52:315, 1981.
11. Panjabi MM, Thibodeau LL, Crisco JJ, White AA: What constitutes spinal instability? *Clin Neurosurg* 34:313, 1988.
12. Penning L, Wilmink JT: Rotation of the cervical spine: a CT study in normal subjects, *Spine* 12:732, 1987.
13. Bogduk N: Contemporary biomechanics of the cervical spine. Proceedings of the MPAA seventh biennial conference, Blue Mountains, New South Wales, Australia, 1991.
14. Bogduk N: *Clinical anatomy of the lumbar spine and sacrum*, ed 3, New York, 1997, Churchill Livingstone.

CHAPTER 4

Innervation and Pain Patterns of the Cervical Spine

Nikolai Bogduk

Two types of pain may arise from the cervical spine. One type occurs when nerve endings in the innervated tissues of the cervical spine are stimulated. The pain is felt locally in the neck but may also be referred to distant regions such as the head, the chest wall, and the upper limb girdle and into the upper limb itself. Since it arises from the somatic structures of the cervical spine, this type of pain is called *somatic pain;* when it is referred to other regions, it is known as *somatic referred pain.* The other type of pain occurs when a cervical spinal nerve root is irritated. It is felt not in the neck but in the upper limb or upper limb girdle. To specify its origin and to distinguish it from somatic referred pain, this type of pain is known as *cervical radicular pain.*

SOMATIC PAIN

Neck pain can arise from any structure in the cervical spine that receives a nerve supply. Consequently, an appreciation of the innervation of the cervical spine forms a foundation for interpreting the differential diagnosis of cervical pain syndromes.

The posterior elements of the neck are those structures that lie behind the intervertebral foramina and nerve roots. These structures are all innervated by the dorsal rami of the cervical spine nerves.[1] The lateral branches of the cervical dorsal rami supply the more superficial posterior neck muscles, such as iliocostalis cervicis, longissimus cervicis and capitis, and splenius cervicis and capitis.[1] The medial branches of the cervical dorsal rami supply the deeper and more medial muscles of the neck, such as the semispinalis cervicis and capitis, multifidus, and the interspinales.[1] These nerves also innervate the cervical zygapophyseal joints[1,2] (Figure 4-1). The suboccipital muscles are innervated by the C1 and C2 dorsal rami.[1]

The anterior elements of the neck are in front of the cervical spinal nerves and include the cervical intervertebral discs, the anterior and posterior longitudinal ligaments, the prevertebral muscles, and the atlantooccipital and atlantoaxial joints and their ligaments. The prevertebral muscles of the neck (longus cervicis and capitis) are innervated by the ventral rami of the C1 to C6 spinal nerves.[3] Other muscles in the neck also innervated by the cervical ventral rami are the scalenes, the trapezius, and

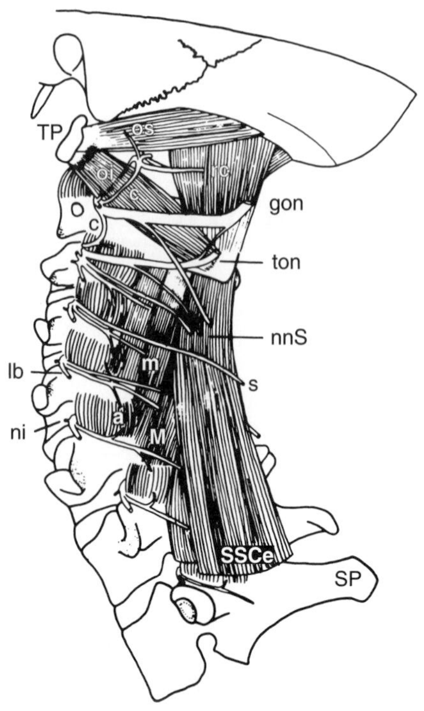

Figure 4-1
Deep dissection of the left cervical dorsal rami. The superficial posterior neck muscles have been resected. The lateral branches *(lb)* of the dorsal rami and the nerves to the intertransversarii *(ni)* have been transected, leaving only the medial branches *(m)* intact. The C1 dorsal ramus supplies the obliquus superior *(os)*, obliquus inferior *(oi)*, and rectus capitis *(rc)* muscles. The medial branches of the C2 and C3 dorsal rami, respectively, form the greater occipital *(gon)* and third occipital *(ton)* nerves. Communicating loops *(c)* connect the C1, C2, and C3 dorsal rami. Three medial branches *(nnS)* of the C2 and C3 dorsal rami innervate the semispinalis capitis, whereas the C3 to C8 medial branches send articular branches *(a)* to the zygapophyseal joints before innervating the multifidus *(M)* and semispinalis cervicis *(SSCe)*, and those at C4 and C5 form superficial cutaneous branches *(s)*. *TP*, transverse process of atlas; *SP*, spinous process of T1.
(From Bogduk N: *Spine* 7:319, 1982.)

the sternocleidomastoid. Although the latter two muscles receive their motor innervation from the accessory nerve, their sensory supply is from the upper two or three cervical ventral rami.[3] The atlantooccipital and lateral atlantoaxial joints are innervated, respectively, by the C1 and C2 ventral rami.[2]

The ligaments of the atlantoaxial region are innervated by the C1 to C3 sinuvertebral nerves, which also innervate the dura mater of the upper spinal cord and the posterior cranial fossa[4] (Figure 4-2). As they cross the back of the median atlantoaxial joint, these nerves furnish branches to that joint.[4] At lower cervical levels (C3 to C8), the dura mater is innervated by an extensive plexus of nerves derived from the cervical sinuvertebral nerves.[5] Fibers within the plexus extend along the dural sac for several segments above and below their segment of origin.

Previous descriptions of the innervation of the cervical intervertebral discs need to be modified in light of recent observations on the structure of these discs. Unlike lumbar discs, the cervical discs lack a uniform, concentric annulus fibrosus.[6] Rather,

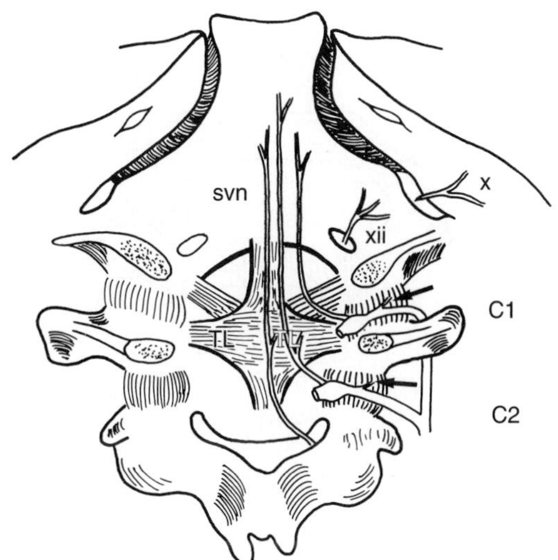

Figure 4-2
Distribution of the upper three cervical sinuvertebral nerves and the innervation of the atlantooccipital and atlantoaxial joints. Articular branches *(arrows)* to the atlantooccipital and atlantoaxial joints arise from the C1 and C2 ventral rami, respectively. The C1 to C3 sinuvertebral nerves *(svn)* pass through the foramen magnum to innervate the dura mater over the clivus. En route, they cross and supply the transverse ligament of the atlas *(TL)*. The dura mater of the more lateral parts of the posterior cranial fossa is innervated by meningeal branches of the hypoglossal *(xii)* and vagus *(x)* nerves.

the annulus is a crescentic structure, thick anteriorly but tapering in thickness laterally on each side toward the anterior edge of the uncinate process. Posteriorly it is represented only by a thin bundle of paramedian fibers. An annulus is lacking at the posterolateral regions of the discs. These regions are simply covered by the alar fibers of the posterior longitudinal ligament that extend laterally to the posterior edge of the uncinate process (Figure 4-3). These differences in structure of the cervical intervertebral disc do not affect the pattern of innervation of the discs, but they do affect the target tissues.

The anterior longitudinal ligament of the cervical spine is accompanied by a plexus of nerves[7] whose components are derived from the cervical sympathetic trunks[7] and from the vertebral nerves that accompany the vertebral arteries[8] (Figure 4-3). Branches of this plexus innervate the anterior longitudinal ligament and also penetrate the ligament to enter the annulus fibrosus anteriorly and laterally. In the anterior and anterolateral regions of the disc, nerve fibers penetrate at least the outer third and up to the outer half of the annulus fibrosus.[7,9,10]

The posterior longitudinal ligament is accompanied by a similar plexus derived from the cervical sinuvertebral nerves.[7] Branches of this plexus supply the posterior longitudinal ligament, but the absence of a substantive annulus posteriorly in the cervical intervertebral discs means that the disc itself receives no posterior innervation. The apparent distribution of sinuvertebral nerves to the discs posteriorly[9] is, perforce, restricted to the posterior longitudinal ligament. Whether the paramedian fibers of the annulus fibrosus receive an innervation has yet to be demonstrated.

In addition to the joints and muscles of the cervical spine, the major arteries of the neck also receive a sensory innervation. The source of innervation of the internal ca-

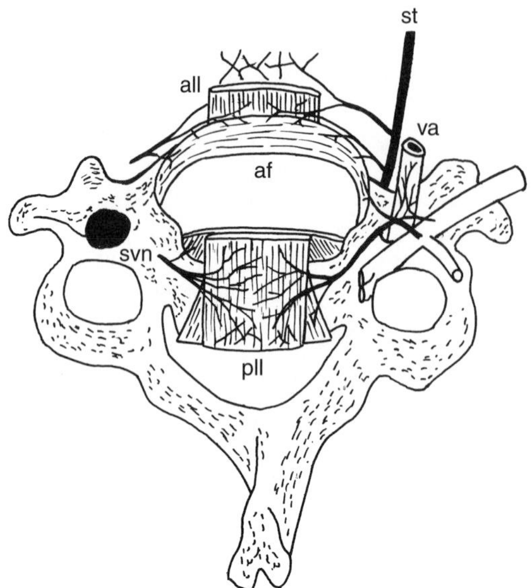

Figure 4-3
The innervation of a cervical intervertebral disc. The anterior longitudinal ligament *(all)* is accompanied by a plexus of nerves derived from the cervical sympathetic trunks *(st)* and the nerves that accompany the vertebral artery *(va)*. Branches of this plexus penetrate the anterior and anterolateral aspects of the annulus fibrosus. The posterior longitudinal ligament *(pll)* is supplied by a plexus derived from the sinuvertebral nerves.

rotid artery has not been established, but that of the vertebral artery is the vertebral nerve,[8] through which afferents return to the cervical dorsal root ganglia.[11]

The somatic structures that receive an innervation and are therefore potential sources of cervical pain are the cervical zygapophyseal joints; the posterior, prevertebral, and anterolateral neck muscles; the atlantooccipital and atlantoaxial joints and their ligaments; the cervical dura mater; and the cervical intervertebral discs and their ligaments. The major arteries of the neck, disorders of which are important in the differential diagnosis of neck pain, should be added to this list.

SOMATIC REFERRED PAIN

Referred pain is pain perceived in a region separate from the location of the primary source of the pain. Strictly and more explicitly, referred pain is pain perceived in a territory innervated by nerves other than the ones that innervate the actual source of pain. As a rule, both sets of nerves usually stem from the same spinal segment, such that the source of pain may be innervated by the dorsal ramus of spinal nerve but the pain is referred into regions innervated by the ventral ramus of the same spinal nerve. In some instances the pain may be referred into regions innervated by spinal nerves adjacent to the one that innervates the source of pain. In such cases it is not clear whether the pattern of referral is due to multisegmental innervation of the source of pain or to multisegmental distribution within the spinal cord of afferents from the primary source.

The term *somatic referred pain* pertains to referred pain that is elicited by stimulation of nociceptive, afferent fibers from somatic tissues, such as joints, ligaments, bones, and muscles. The term is used to distinguish referred pain arising from these tissues from pain arising from viscera. When pain is referred from viscera, the term *visceral referred pain* can be used. Both types of referred pain are generated by similar mechanisms, and the terms simply distinguish the origin of the pain.

The most plausible mechanism of somatic referred pain is convergence, in which primary afferent fibers from a particular structure synapse on second-order neurons in the spinal cord that also happen to receive afferents from another region. Under these conditions pain elicited by the structure can be misperceived as arising from the region whose afferents converge on the second-order neuron. In the case of cervical somatic referred pain, afferents from the cervical spine converge on common neurons with afferents from peripheral regions such as the head, chest wall, and upper limb. Consequently, a nociceptive signal rising from the cervical spine may be perceived as rising from the head, the chest wall, or the upper limb.

In the context of somatic referred pain, convergence has attracted little formal study from physiologists, although the few studies that have been conducted validate the concept. In animal experiments, convergence has been demonstrated between trigeminal afferents and afferents in the C1 spinal nerve[12] and also between afferents from the superior sagittal sinus and afferents in the greater occipital nerve.[13] In the lumbar spinal cord, afferents from spinal structures relay to neurons that subtend large regions of the lower limbs and trunk.[14] Otherwise, the cardinal evidence concerning cervical somatic referred pain stems from clinical experiments.

Stimulation of the cervical interspinous muscles with noxious injections of hypertonic saline produces somatic referred pain in normal volunteers.[15-17] Stimulation of upper cervical levels produces referred pain in the head. Stimulation of lower cervical levels produces pain in the chest wall, shoulder girdle, and upper limb. Distension of the cervical zygapophyseal joints with contrast medium in normal volunteers produces referred pain that is perceived in the head or shoulder girdle, depending on which segmental level is stimulated.[18] Similar patterns are produced when the nerves supplying these joints are stimulated electrically.[19] Earlier studies showed that electrical and mechanical stimulation of the lower cervical intervertebral discs produces pain in the posterior chest wall and scapular region[20] and that pressure on the posterior longitudinal ligament produces pain in the anterior chest.[21] More recent studies have shown that the patterns of referred pain from the cervical intervertebral discs resemble those from the cervical zygapophyseal joints of the same segmental level.[22,23]

All of these experimental and clinical observations indicate that noxious stimuli from the cervical spine are capable of causing pain in the head, upper limb, and chest wall. None of the experiments in normal volunteers and patients involved spinal nerves and nerve roots. Therefore nerve root irritation cannot have been the cause of pain. Convergence in the central nervous system is the only mechanism postulated to date that explains these phenomena.

The capacity of cervical pain to be referred to the head, upper limb, or chest wall can pose diagnostic difficulties. For instance, in patients with pain referred to the head, the presenting complaint could be headache rather than neck pain, and this headache may be misinterpreted as tension headache if the cervical cause is not recognized. Referred pain to the anterior chest wall may mimic angina.[24,25]

PATTERNS OF REFERRED PAIN

The early experiments on somatic referred pain were undertaken to establish charts of referred pain patterns.[16,17] It was noted that referred pain tends to follow a segmental pattern in that stimuli to lower levels in the neck resulted in the referral of pain to more caudal areas in the upper limb or chest wall. The apparent patterns of referred pain differed from those of dermatomes, and to distinguish this different pattern, the concept of sclerotomes was introduced.[26]

The term *sclerotome* was invoked to complement those of *dermatome* and *myotome*. Just as dermatomes represented the segmental innervation of skin and myotomes represented the segmental innervation of muscles, sclerotomes were supposed to represent the segmental innervation of skeletal tissues.[26] This notion, however, is fallacious. Dermatomes and myotomes have an anatomical basis; sclerotomes do not. Dermatomes can be determined by dissection, by tracing areas of numbness after section of segmental nerves, and by mapping the distribution of vesicles in herpes zoster. They have a physical substrate. Similarly, myotomes can be mapped electromyographically by stimulating segmental nerves and by tracing denervation of muscles after section of spinal nerves. Like dermatomes, they can be determined objectively. Sclerotomes were not objectively determined. They were simply based on maps of areas in which volunteers perceived referred pain. As such, they are entirely subjective. Although they may reflect some sort of pattern of innervation of peripheral tissues, this pattern has not been established objectively. Moreover, there is no evidence that referred pain is perceived only in skeletal tissues. Somatic referred pain is perceived also in muscles. Consequently, there are no grounds for segregating sclerotomes from myotomes. Furthermore, referred pain patterns may be based as much on patterns of central nervous connections, or more, as on the segmental distribution of peripheral nerves.

If one consults the literature carefully, it emerges that what have been portrayed as maps of sclerotomes are essentially idealized representations.[26] They were not derived from quantitative analysis of data. Indeed, when one performs such an analysis, variance rather than consistency appears to be the rule. In those studies that provided quantitative data[15-17] different individuals reported different distributions of referred pain, even when exactly the same structures and segmental levels were stimulated. Moreover, the distributions of referred pain reported in different studies differed markedly (Figure 4-4).

Because of these inconsistencies, maps of sclerotomes serve little clinical purpose. They do not allow the segmental location of a source of pain to be determined from the pattern of distribution of pain. Maps of the distribution of referred pain from specific cervical structures have proved more useful.

Distinctive patterns of referred pain occur when the cervical zygapophyseal joints are experimentally stimulated in normal volunteers[18,19] (Figure 4-5); these patterns have been found to be valid in identifying symptomatic zygapophyseal joints in patients with neck pain.[27] However, these pain patterns are not diagnostic of zygapophyseal joint pain; they indicate only the segmental origin of the pain. Recent studies of discography have shown that the pain patterns of the cervical intervertebral discs are essentially the same as those for zygapophyseal joints with the same segmental number as the disc.[22,23] Thus the virtue of pain charts lies not in establishing which structure is the source of somatic referred pain, but only in pinpointing the segment involved. In this regard, pain charts are not infallible. Their utility decreases if patients have widespread pain or unusual patterns of pain.

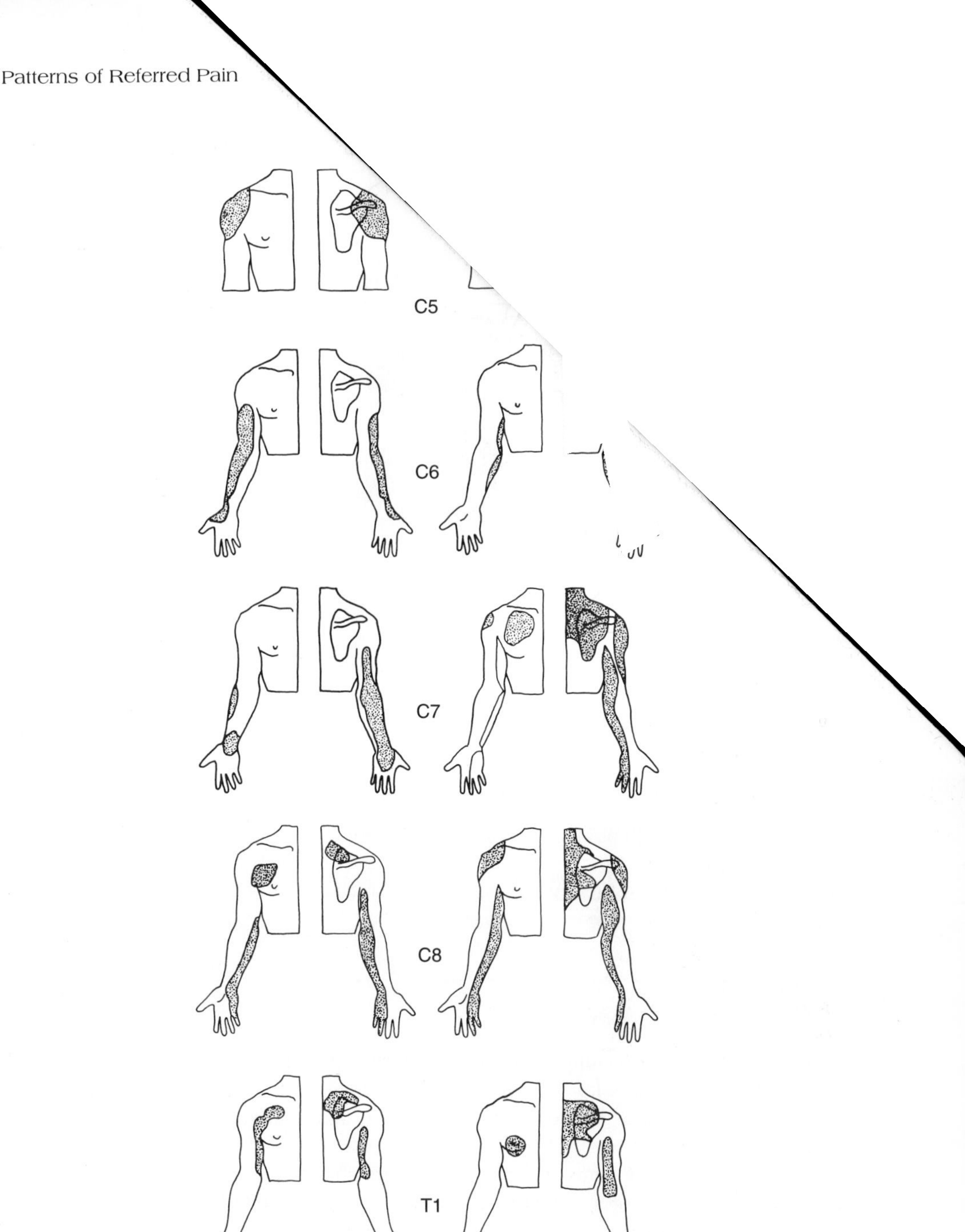

Figure 4-4
Patterns of referred pain induced in normal volunteers by stimulation of the interspinous muscles at the levels indicated. The left-hand figures are based on the studies of Kellgren.[16] The right-hand figures are based on the studies of Feinstein et al.[17] Comparison of the two sets of figures reveals the variation in patterns of referred pain from the same cervical structures and segmental levels.

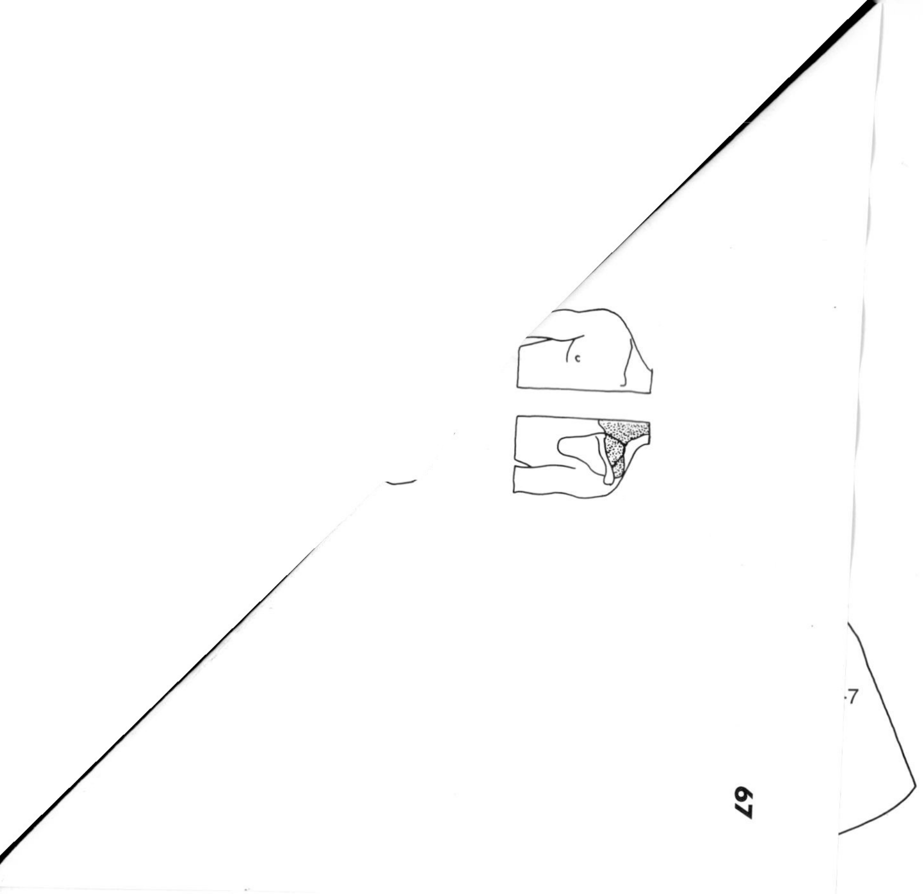

Figure 4-5
Patterns of referred pain produced by stimulating the cervical zygapophyseal joints in normal volunteers.
(Modified from Dwyer A, Aprill C, Bodguk N: *Spine* 14:453, 1990.)

RADICULAR PAIN

There is little scientific information on the nature and mechanism of cervical radicular pain.[28] What is known about radicular pain is based largely on studies of lumbar radicular pain. Moreover, confusion persists between radicular pain and radiculopathy.

Radiculopathy is a neurological condition in which conduction is impaired along fibers of a nerve root or spinal nerve. If conduction is blocked in sensory nerves, the resultant features are numbness and loss of proprioception, depending on which particular afferents are affected. If conduction is blocked in motor nerves, the resultant feature is segmental weakness in the muscles innervated by the affected nerve. Diminished reflexes can occur if either the sensory or motor arm of the reflex is impaired. Paresthesia is a sign of ischemia and occurs when the blood supply to a segmental nerve is impaired.[29]

Radiculopathy, per se, does not cause pain; it results in loss of neurological function. However, radiculopathy can occur in association with pain, and it is for this reason that confusion can arise. The presence of radiculopathy does not imply that the associated pain is radicular in origin.

Radiculopathy can occur in association with somatic referred pain. This combination can arise when one lesion produces somatic pain and another lesion produces radiculopathy, or it can arise when the one lesion is responsible for both but by different mechanisms. For example, an osteoarthritic zygapophyseal joint may produce local and referred somatic pain, but if the joint develops an osteophyte that compresses the adjacent spinal nerve, it will also produce radiculopathy. Resecting the osteophyte will relieve the radiculopathy but will not relieve the somatic pain.

Nevertheless, lesions affecting the cervical spinal nerves or their roots can produce radicular pain. However, the clinical features of this form of pain are poorly defined. The features of lumbar radicular pain are better understood.

Compression of lumbar nerve roots does not cause radicular pain[30]; it produces only paresthesia and numbness. For radicular pain to be produced, either the dorsal root ganglion has to be compressed or the compressed nerve roots must have been previously affected by inflammation.[31-33] In that event, however, radicular pain is distinctive in character. It is a shooting, lancinating pain that travels along the affected limb in a narrow band.[33] In this regard, radicular pain differs from somatic pain because the latter is a dull, deep aching pain perceived in wide areas whose location is relatively static.

The extent to which these features can be transcribed from lumbar radicular pain to cervical radicular pain is not known. The only experiments that have been conducted directly on cervical spinal nerves involved needling these nerves in volunteers.[34] Such acute stimuli did not serve to typify the character of the pain evoked, but they did provide maps of cervical radicular pain.

The distribution of pain from a given cervical spinal nerve varies considerably from individual to individual.[34] The pain can be perceived in various regions across the back of the shoulder girdle and anterior chest wall and into the upper limb. Proximally, there is no distinctive pattern that can be discerned as representative of a given spinal nerve. Such patterns emerge only peripherally but even then with little distinction between segments (Figure 4-6). When the C4 spinal nerve is stimulated, the area where most subjects feel pain is centered over the lateral aspect of the neck and the top of the shoulder girdle. A similar distribution applies to C5, but the area tends to extend further distally into the upper limb, over the deltoid muscle. Pain from C6 extends from the top of the shoulder along the cephalic border of the upper limb and into the index finger and thumb. Pain from C7 is somewhat similar but tends to concentrate more posteriorly along the cephalic border and extend to the middle and ring fingers. Although differences in the average pattern can be discerned (Figure 4-6), these typical regions overlap so much that in a given case, the segmental origin of the pain cannot be confidently determined simply from the distribution of pain.

A further confounding factor is that the distribution of cervical radicular pain is not unlike the distribution of somatic referred pain. Therefore in a patient with pain in the upper limb, the pattern of pain cannot be used to distinguish radicular pain from somatic referred pain.

Unless and until studies are conducted on the nature of pain and its differences in patients with proven radicular pain and patients with proven somatic referred pain, no valid statement can be made concerning their distinction. Although readers might be accustomed to ascribing the pain seen in a patients' radiculopathy to nerve root irritation, they should be circumspect in continuing to do so. They should realize that they can readily diagnose radiculopathy on the basis of the distribution of paresthesia, numbness, weakness, and loss of reflexes, but this action tells them nothing of the origin of the pain. Although they may have been taught to infer that the pain is radicular, this inference is based on traditional teaching and not on experimental data or valid observations.

Although experiments in normal volunteers have produced somatic referred pain to distal regions of the upper limb (Figure 4-4), modern clinical studies have not reported such patterns of distant referral in patients. Somatic referred pain from the

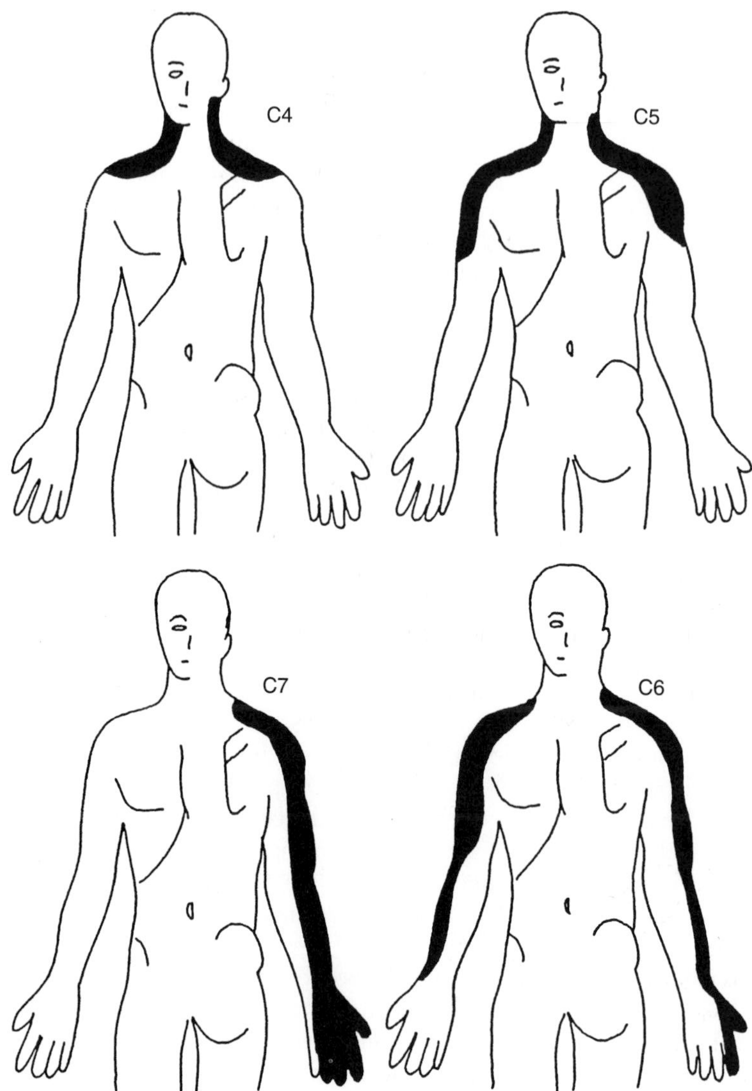

Figure 4-6
Maps of the distribution of pain evoked by mechanical stimulation of the C4, C5, C6, and C7 spinal nerves.
(From Bogduk N: Medical management of acute cervical radicular pain: an evidence-based approach, Newcastle, Australia, 1999, Newcastle Bone and Joint Institute. Based on Slipman CW, Plastaras CT, Palmitier RA et al: *Spine* 23:2235, 1998.)

cervical zygapophyseal joints[18,35,36] and from the cervical intervertebral discs[2,23] is usually located proximally—over the shoulder girdle and into the upper arm. Referred pain into the forearm or hand has not been reported from these structures and would appear to be uncommon. Accordingly, the following two operating rules can be constructed on the basis of available published data:

1. Pain over the shoulder girdle and upper arm could be either somatic referred pain or radicular pain.
2. Pain in the forearm and hand is unlikely to be somatic referred pain and is more likely to be radicular in origin.

These inferences are corroborated by surgeons with experience of operating on patients under local anesthesia. Some have explicitly stated that "the pain in the neck, rhomboid region, and anterior chest was referred pain from the disc itself, while arm pain was usually the result of nerve compression."[37] Others concur that arm pain is caused by nerve root irritation but that more proximal pain is referred from the neck.[38]

Until better data become available, these rules serve to assist practitioners in assessing patients with radiculopathy. The objective is to prevent radicular pain from being overdiagnosed and misdiagnosed. In cases of doubt, it is preferable that the doubt be recorded rather than a misdiagnosis be perpetrated and perpetuated.

References

1. Bogduk N: The clinical anatomy of the cervical dorsal rami, *Spine* 7:319, 1982.
2. Lazorthes G, Gaubert J: L'innervation des articulations interapophysaire vertebrales, *Comptes Rendues de l'Association des Anatomistes*, 43:488, 1956.
3. Williams PL, editor: *Gray's anatomy*, ed 38, Edinburgh, 1995, Churchill Livingstone, p 808.
4. Kimmel DL: Innervation of the spinal dura mater and dura mater of the posterior cranial fossa, *Neurology* 10:800, 1960.
5. Groen GJ, Baljet B, Drukker J: The innervation of the spinal dura mater: anatomy and clinical implications, *Acta Neurochir* 92:39, 1988.
6. Mercer S, Bogduk N: The ligaments and annulus fibrosus of human adult cervical intervertebral discs, *Spine* 24:619, 1999.
7. Groen GJ, Baljet B, Drukker J: Nerves and nerve plexuses of the human vertebral column, *Am J Anat* 188:282, 1990.
8. Bogduk N, Lambert G, Duckworth JW: The anatomy and physiology of the vertebral nerve in relation to cervical migraine, *Cephalalgia* 1:11, 1981.
9. Bogduk N, Windsor M, Inglis A: The innervation of the cervical intervertebral discs, *Spine* 13:2, 1988.
10. Mendel T, Wink CS, Zimny ML: Neural elements in human cervical intervertebral discs, *Spine* 17:132, 1992.
11. Kimmel DL: The cervical sympathetic rami and the vertebral plexus in the human foetus, *J Comp Neurol* 112:141, 1959.
12. Kerr FWL: Structural relation of the trigeminal spinal tract to upper cervical roots and the solitary nucleus in the cat, *Exp Neurol* 4:134, 1961.
13. Angus-Leppan H, Lambert GA, Michalicek J: Convergence of occipital nerve and superior sagittal sinus input in the cervical spinal cord of the cat, *Cephalalgia* 17:625, 1997.
14. Gillette RG, Kramis RC, Roberts WJ: Characterization of spinal somatosensory neurons having receptive fields in lumbar tissues of cats, *Pain* 54:85, 1993.
15. Campbell DG, Parsons CM: Referred head pain and its concomitants, *J Nerv Ment Dis* 99:544, 1944.
16. Kellgren JH: On the distribution of pain arising from deep somatic structures with charts of segmental pain areas, *Clin Sci* 4:35, 1939.
17. Feinstein B, Langton JBK, Jameson RM, Schiller F: Experiments on referred pain from deep somatic tissues, *J Bone Joint Surg* 36A:981, 1954.
18. Dwyer A, Aprill C, Bogduk N: Cervical zygapophyseal joint pain patterns. I. A study in normal volunteers, *Spine* 15:453, 1990.
19. Fukui S, Ohseto K, Shiotani M et al: Referred pain distribution of the cervical zygapophyseal joints and cervical dorsal rami, *Pain* 68:79, 1996.
20. Cloward RB: Cervical diskography: a contribution to the aetiology and mechanism of neck, shoulder and arm pain, *Ann Surg* 130:1052, 1959.
21. Murphey F: Sources and patterns of pain in disc disease, *Clin Neurosurg* 15:343, 1968.
22. Schellhas KP, Smith MD, Gundry CR, Pollei SR: Cervical discogenic pain: prospective correlation of magnetic resonance imaging and discography in asymptomatic subjects and pain sufferers, *Spine* 21:300, 1996.

23. Grubb SA, Kelly CK: Cervical discography: clinical implications from 12 years of experience, *Spine* 25:1382, 2000.
24. Booth RE, Rothman RH: Cervical angina, *Spine* 1:28, 1976.
25. Brodsky AE: Cervical angina: a correlative study with emphasis on the use of coronary arteriography, *Spine* 10:699, 1985.
26. Inman VT, Saunders JBD: Referred pain from skeletal structure, *J Nerv Ment Dis* 99:660, 1944.
27. Aprill C, Dwyer A, Bogduk N: Cervical zygapophyseal joint pain patterns. II. A clinical evaluation, *Spine* 15:458, 1990.
28. Bogduk N: Medical management of acute cervical radicular pain: an evidence-based approach, Newcastle, Australia, 1999, Newcastle Bone and Joint Institute.
29. Ochoa JL, Torebjork HE: Paraesthesiae from ectopic impulse generation in human sensory nerves, *Brain* 103:835, 1980.
30. MacNab I: The mechanism of spondylogenic pain. In Hirsch C, Zotterman Y, editors: *Cervical pain,* Oxford, England, 1972, Pergamon.
31. Howe JF: A neurophysiological basis for the radicular pain of nerve root compression. In Bonica JJ, Liebeskind JC, Albe-Fessard DG, editors: *Advances in pain research and therapy,* vol 3, New York, 1979, Raven Press.
32. Howe JF, Loeser JD, Calvin WH: Mechanosensitivity of dorsal root ganglia and chronically injured axons: a physiological basis for the radicular pain of nerve root compression, *Pain* 3:25, 1977.
33. Smyth MJ, Wright V: Sciatica and the intervertebral disc: an experimental study, *J Bone Joint Surg* 40A:1401, 1959.
34. Slipman CW, Plastaras CT, Palmitier RA et al: Symptom provocation of fluoroscopically guided cervical nerve root stimulation: are dynatomal maps identical to dermatomal maps? *Spine* 23:2235, 1998.
35. Barnsley L, Lord SM, Wallis BJ, Bogduk N: The prevalence of chronic cervical zygapophysial joint pain after whiplash, *Spine* 20:20, 1995.
36. Lord S, Barnsley L, Wallis BJ, Bogduk N: Chronic cervical zygapophysial joint pain after whiplash: a placebo-controlled prevalence study, *Spine* 21:1737, 1996.
37. Murphey F, Simmons JCH, Brunson B: Surgical treatment of laterally ruptured disc: review of 648 cases, 1939 to 1972, *J Neurosurg* 38:679, 1973.
38. Yamano Y: Soft disc herniation of the cervical spine, *Int Orthop* 9:19, 1985.

CHAPTER 5

Innervation and Pain Patterns of the Thoracic Spine

Nikolai Bogduk

During the life of the first two editions of this book, few, if any, definitive studies were published on the nature, origin, diagnosis, or treatment of mechanical, or idiopathic, thoracic spinal pain. This problem remains underserved by the literature. Such information that might be harvested on this topic still stems from seminal studies undertaken more than 40 years ago. There have, however, been certain developments in the modern era. At last, formal studies of the innervation of the thoracic spine have been conducted[1,2]; and modern studies of pain patterns have been undertaken using radiologically controlled techniques.[3]

INNERVATION

The thoracic spine is innervated in a manner similar to that of the cervical and lumbar spines. The posterior elements (those structures that lie behind the intervertebral foramina) are innervated by the thoracic dorsal rami. The anterior elements (which lie anterior to the intervertebral foramina and spinal nerves) are innervated by the sinuvertebral nerves.

Thoracic Dorsal Rami

Each thoracic dorsal ramus arises from its spinal nerve and passes directly posteriorly, entering the back through an osseoligamentous tunnel bounded by a transverse process, the neck of the rib below, the medial border of the superior costotransverse ligament, and the lateral border of a zygapophyseal joint (Figure 5-1). The nerve then runs laterally through the space between the anterior lamella of the superior costotransverse ligament anteriorly, and the costolamellar ligament and the posterior lamella of the superior costotransverse ligament posteriorly (Figure 5-1). It divides in this space, some 5 mm from the lateral margin of the intervertebral foramen, into a medial and a lateral branch.[1]

From its origin the medial branch passes slightly dorsally and inferiorly, but largely laterally, within the intertransverse space. There, it is embedded in areolar tis-

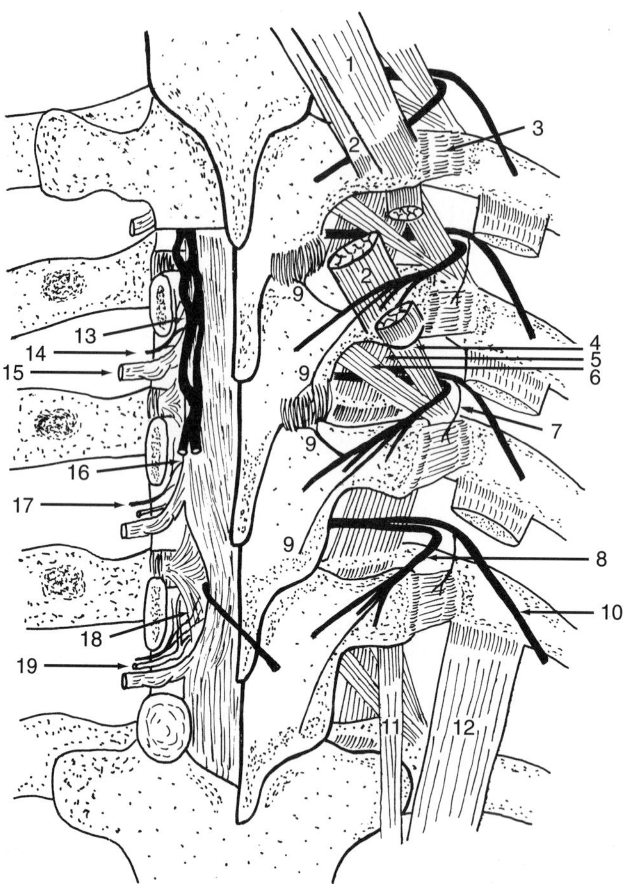

Figure 5-1
The innervation of the thoracic spine as viewed from the rear. On the left, the vertebral laminae have been resected to reveal the contents of the vertebral canal. The dural sac has been retracted to demonstrate the thoracic sinuvertebral nerves. On the right, the courses of the thoracic dorsal rami are shown. For clarity, muscles such as the levatores costarum and iliocostalis have not been depicted. *1*, Semispinalis thoracis; *2*, multifidus; *3*, lateral costotransverse ligament covering costotransverse joint; *4*, posterior lamella of the superior costotransverse ligament; *5*, costolamellar ligament; *6*, anterior lamella of the superior costotransverse ligament; 7, nerve to costotransverse joint; *8*, medial branch of dorsal ramus; *9*, articular branches to zygapophyseal joints; *10*, lateral branch of dorsal ramus; *11* and *12*, medial and lateral slips of longissimus thoracis; *13*, branches of sinuvertebral nerves to epidural vessels; *14*, sinuvertebral nerve; *15*, spinal nerve; *16*, branches of sinuvertebral nerve to dura mater; *17*, sinuvertebral nerve; *18*, branches to posterior longitudinal ligament; *19*, radicular artery.

sue and accompanied by small arteries and veins. Opposite the tip of the transverse process, the medial branch curves dorsally around the lateral border of the posterior lamella of the superior costotransverse ligament and aims inferiorly for the superolateral corner of the transverse process. It enters the posterior compartment of the back by crossing this corner and running caudally along the posterior surface of the tip of the transverse process, through the cleavage plane, between the origin of multifidus medially and that of the semispinalis laterally.[1] Covered by the semispinalis, the medial branch curves inferiorly and medially over the dorsal aspect of the fascicles of multifidus, to which it supplies multiple filaments. Other branches supply the semispinalis. At upper thoracic levels, a long branch continues over the dorsal surface of the multifidus toward the midline, where it penetrates the fascicles of spinalis thoracis, splenius cervicis, rhomboids, and trapezius to become cutaneous.[4] At lower thoracic levels, the medial branches of the dorsal rami retain an exclusively muscular distribution.

Each medial branch furnishes ascending and descending articular branches to the zygapophyseal joints.[1] Ascending branches arise from the medial branch as it passes caudal to the zygapophyseal joint above. These branches are short and ramify in the inferior aspect of the joint capsule. Slender, descending branches arise from the medial branch as it crosses the superolateral corner of the transverse process. They follow a sinuous course between the fascicles of multifidus to reach the superior aspect of the capsule of the zygapophyseal joint below.[1] The capsules of the joints are endowed with free nerve endings and mechanoreceptors, although the latter are more sparse than in the cervical and lumbar zygapophyseal joints.[2]

The lateral branches of the thoracic dorsal rami continue the projection of the dorsal ramus in the intertransverse space, initially running parallel to the medial branches before they enter the posterior compartment of the back. Beyond the tip of the transverse process, each lateral branch descends caudally and laterally, weaving between the fascicles of the longissimus thoracic muscle (Figure 5-1). As a rule, each nerve supplies the fascicles of longissimus that attach to the transverse process and rib above the level of origin of the nerve and sometimes the fascicle from the rib next above.[5] Continuing caudally and laterally, the lateral branches enter and supply the iliocostalis muscles. The lateral branches of the lower thoracic (T7 to T12) dorsal rami eventually emerge from the iliocostalis lumborum to become cutaneous.[4] Those from higher levels have an entirely muscular distribution. Articular branches to the costotransverse joints arise from the lateral branch just above each joint where the medial branch leaves the lateral branch[6] (Figure 5-1).

Thoracic Sinuvertebral Nerves

The thoracic sinuvertebral nerves are recurrent branches of the thoracic spinal nerves. Each nerve arises from two roots—a somatic root and an autonomic root. The somatic root arises from the anterior surface or superior border of the spinal nerve just outside the intervertebral foramen. It passes into the intervertebral foramen, running in front of or sometimes above the spinal nerve, and joins with the autonomic root after a course of about 2 to 3 mm.[5,7] The autonomic root arises from the grey ramus communicans at each segmental level or, in some cases, from the sympathetic ganglion nearest the spinal nerve.[5,7] Having been formed, each sinuvertebral nerve passes through the intervertebral foramen and enters the vertebral canal, embedded amongst the branches of the segmental spinal artery and the tributaries of the spinal vein, anterior to the spinal nerve. In the intervertebral foramen the nerve gives rise to filaments that supply the vertebral lamina and a branch that crosses the upper border of the neck of the nearby rib to supply the periosteum of the neck.[5,7] Other branches are distributed to the vessels within the vertebral canal. Terminal branches ramify in the anterior surface of the vertebral laminae, the dural sac, and the posterior longitudinal ligament.[5,7]

As in the cervical and lumbar spine, the thoracic spine is innervated by dense microscopic plexuses that accompany the posterior and anterior longitudinal ligaments[8] (Figure 5-2). The posterior plexus is derived from the thoracic sinuvertebral nerves;

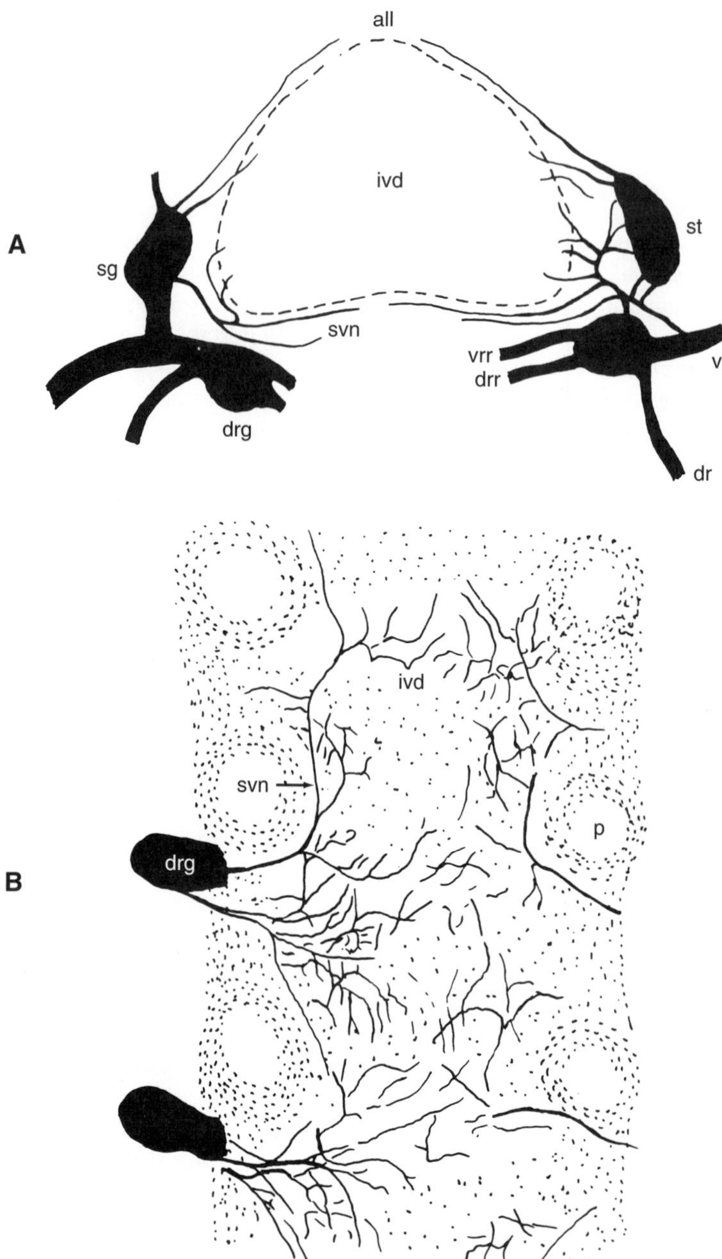

Figure 5-2

The pattern of innervation of the thoracic vertebral bodies and intervertebral discs, as seen in human fetuses. **A,** Transverse section. Branches to the anterior longitudinal ligament *(all)* emanate from the sympathetic trunks *(st)* and sympathetic ganglia *(sg)*. Branches to the posterolateral and posterior aspects of the intervertebral disc *(ivd)* stem from the sympathetic trunk and from the sinuvertebral nerves *(svn)* that are directed to the posterior longitudinal ligament. *drg,* Dorsal root ganglion; *dr,* dorsal ramus; *vr,* ventral ramus; *drr,* dorsal root; *vrr,* ventral root. **B,** Longitudinal view showing the posterior longitudinal plexus. The sinuvertebral nerves *(svn)* form a dense plexus that ramifies over the back of the intervertebral discs *(ivd)*. *p,* Location of pedicles; *drg,* dorsal root ganglion.

(Based on Groen GJ, Baljet B, Drukker J: *Am J Anat* 188:282, 1990.)

the anterior plexus from the thoracic sympathetic trunks and rami communicantes. Each plexus furnishes branches that supply the longitudinal ligaments and branches that penetrate the vertebral bodies and intervertebral discs. Branches from the posterior plexus innervate the ventral aspect of the dural sac.[8]

SOURCES OF PAIN

The structures that receive an innervation, and therefore are possible sources of pain in the thoracic region, are the thoracic vertebrae, the dura mater, the intervertebral discs and longitudinal ligaments, the posterior thoracic muscles, the costotransverse joints, and the thoracic zygapophyseal joints. Of these structures, studies have demonstrated the ability of the thoracic muscles, the thoracic discs, and the zygapophyseal joints to produce thoracic spinal pain.

When injected with hypertonic saline in normal volunteers, the thoracic interspinous muscles and ligaments produce local and referred pain across the posterior chest wall.[9,10] When provoked by discography, the thoracic discs produce posterior thoracic pain in normal volunteers and reproduce pain in patients with posterior thoracic pain.[11] In normal volunteers, distending the thoracic zygapophyseal joints with injections of contrast medium produces posterior thoracic pain.[3] Thoracic spinal pain can be relieved by intraarticular injections of bupivacaine and triamcinolone into the zygapophyseal joints.[12]

PATTERNS OF PAIN

In the thoracic region the phenomenon of referred pain poses more diagnostic difficulties than in any other region of the vertebral column. Of foremost importance is the diagnosis of visceral pain referred to the chest wall. Chest pain can be caused by cardiac, pulmonary, and pleural disease, as well as diseases of the mediastinum, esophagus, and diaphragm. Because many of these diseases are potentially life threatening, they must be recognized and managed or specifically excluded. Specialist consultation may be required for this purpose. However, preoccupation with visceral disease has led to the neglect and even denial of the possibility that chest wall pain may be somatic or skeletal in origin.

Experiments in normal volunteers have shown that noxious stimulation of the interspinous structures at thoracic levels can produce somatic referred pain to both the posterior and anterior chest wall.[9,10] This pain follows somewhat of a segmental pattern (Figure 5-3), insomuch as stimulation of higher levels causes referred pain at higher levels in the chest wall. However, there is no consistent location for referred pain from a particular segment. The locations ascribed to different segments differ in different studies, and the segmental pattern is not always strictly sequential. Stimulation of a particular segment may cause referred pain at a higher level than stimulation of the segment below (Figure 5-3). Because of these variations and irregularities, the location of any referred pain cannot be used to deduce the exact segmental location of its source.

Similar patterns of pain arise from the thoracic zygapophyseal joints[3] (Figure 5-4). The pattern is again quasisegmental; the higher the source, the higher the location of the referred pain; but again, the patterns overlap. In principle, however, it would appear that the segmental location of a patch of posterior thoracic spinal pain might be identified from the distribution of pain with an accuracy of perhaps plus or minus one or two segments.

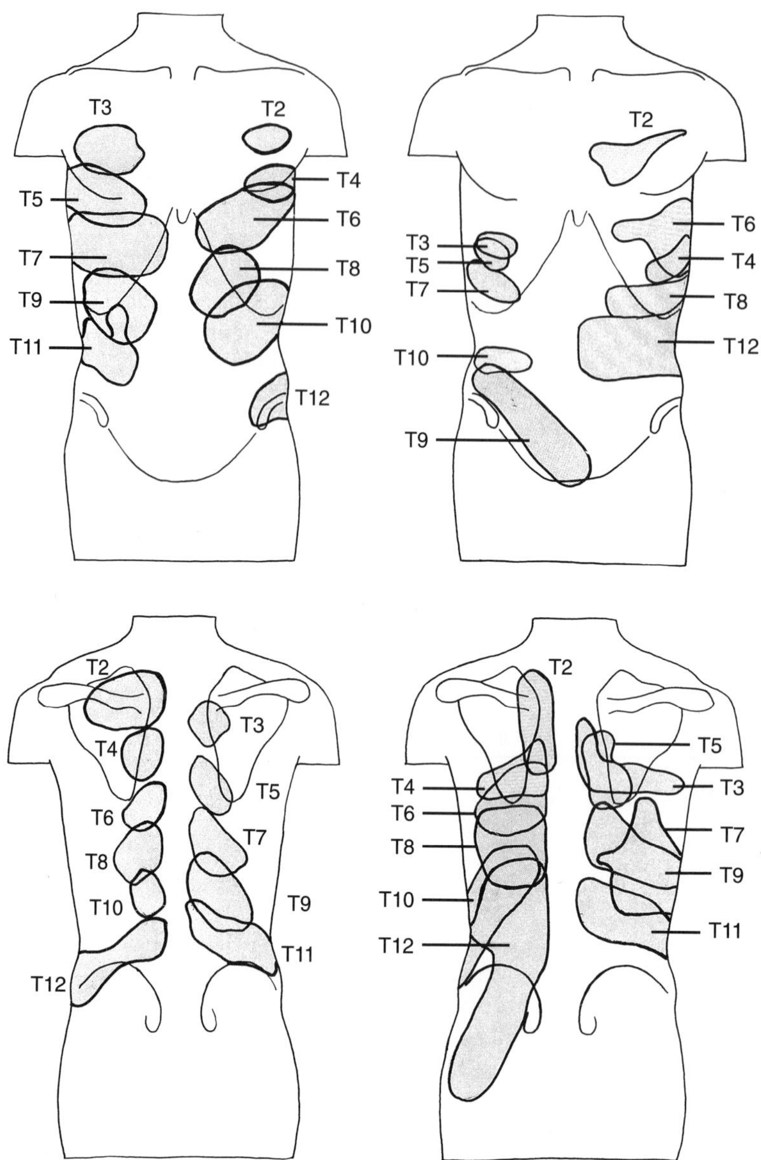

Figure 5-3
Referred pain patterns in the chest. The shaded areas illustrate the distribution of referred pain reported by normal volunteers after stimulation of interspinous structures at the segmental levels indicated. The figures on the left are based on the data of Kellgren.[9] Those on the right are based on Feinstein et al.[10] Note the differences in the distribution of pain in the two sets of figures, and the extensive overlap in distribution shown in the figures on the right.

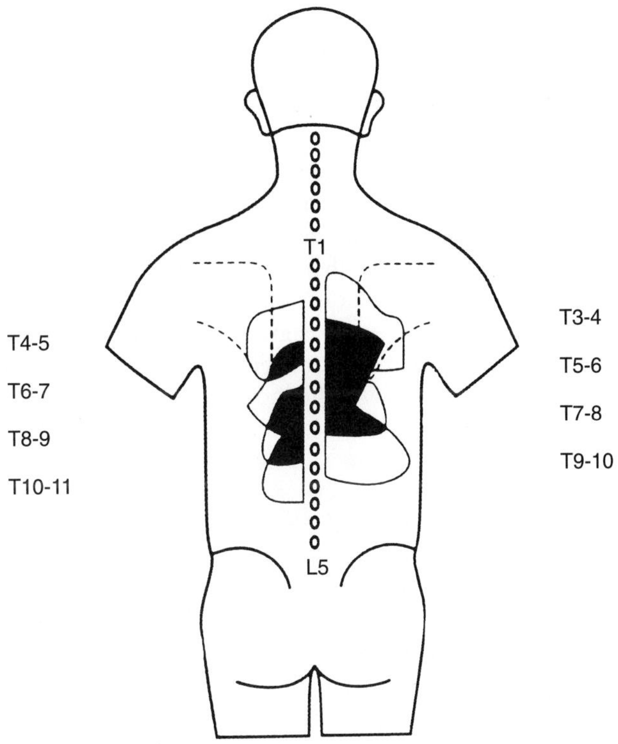

Figure 5-4
Referred pain patterns of the thoracic zygapophyseal joints.
(From Dreyfuss P, Tibiletti C, Dreyer SJ: *Spine* 19:807, 1994.)

PATHOLOGY

There is an absence of any pathological data, or even circumstantial evidence, to explain why thoracic discs, muscles, zygapophyseal joints, or costovertebral joints might be a source of thoracic pain. It is therefore difficult to state with any certainty what disorders might afflict these various structures to produce pain.

Infective and neoplastic diseases of the bone can affect the thoracic vertebrae, but such conditions are usually evident on radiological investigations and are not likely causes of idiopathic thoracic pain. Neoplastic disorders of the thoracic dura or epidural blood vessels typically manifest themselves by causing symptoms of spinal cord compression and have not been described as causing pain without neurological signs. Herniation of thoracic intervertebral discs is an uncommon disorder but is usually attended by signs of nerve root irritation or spinal cord compression.[13] Furthermore, thoracic disc herniations most commonly occur at lower thoracic levels (T9 to T10) and are associated with pain in the lumbar region and abdominal wall rather than in the chest.[13]

Very few pathological conditions have been described as affecting the posterior thoracic muscles and the synovial joints of the thoracic spine. The costotransverse and thoracic zygapophyseal joint can be involved in ankylosing spondylitis, but it would be unusual for this condition to be the source of thoracic pain in the absence of signs of concomitant involvement of the sacroiliac joints or other features of ankylosing spondylitis. Rheumatoid arthritis can affect the costotransverse joints[14,15] and may spread from these sites to involve the adjacent intervertebral discs.[15] Rheumatoid arthritis is also recognized as affecting the thoracic zygapophyseal joints, although not as severely as the costotransverse joints.[15] The German literature[16] describes degenerative joint disease of the thoracic zygapophyseal and costotransverse joints, but there is no physiological evidence of whether or not all joints so affected become painful.

A notion attractive to manual therapists is that either thoracic zygapophyseal joints or the costotransverse joints can be affected by mechanical disorders that cause pain and are amenable to manipulative therapy. However, the pathology of these putative disorders is not known. Further study of these conditions depends critically on the development and implementation of diagnostic blocks of these joints.

The issue of muscular pain is even more speculative. The thoracic spine is abundantly covered by posterior muscles, and the thoracic transverse processes and ribs are virtually riddled with muscle attachments. Moreover, much of the posterior thoracic musculature is formed by lumbar muscles inserting into thoracic levels or cervical muscles arising from thoracic levels. This arrangement invites the suggestion that thoracic pain arising from muscles could be caused by cervical or lumbar disorders that disturb the normal function of these overlapping muscles. Spasm of these muscles as a result of cervical or lumbar pain or excessive tension in them as a result of abnormal lumbar or cervical mechanics could be perceived as straining their thoracic attachments and thereby causing pain. However, clinical or physiological evidence substantiating any of these concepts is lacking. No studies have shown that anesthetizing certain muscle insertions relieves thoracic pain secondary to cervical or lumbar diseases, nor have any controlled studies verified that correction of abnormal cervical or lumbar postures relieves thoracic muscular pain.

These various reservations and seemingly negative conclusions should not be interpreted as denials of the possibility that idiopathic thoracic pain can be caused by disorders of the thoracic synovial joints or muscles. Indeed, the analogy with the lumbar and cervical regions makes it likely that at least the zygapophyseal and costotransverse joints would be potent sources of otherwise undiagnosed thoracic pain. However, what is emphasized is the absence, to date, of any definitive clinical, experimental, or pathological data that permits endorsement of this notion.

DISCUSSION

In a sense this chapter may not seem helpful for readers hoping to find explanations and answers to thoracic pain problems, because the conclusions made are so diluted with reservations. However, this accurately reflects the state of the art with respect to idiopathic thoracic pain. In the absence of appropriate anatomical, experimental, and clinical data, one cannot make legitimate conclusions. There is a dire need for basic data in this field.

References

1. Chua WH, Bogduk N: The surgical anatomy of thoracic facet denervation, *Acta Neurochir* 136:140, 1995.
2. McLain RF, Pickar JG: Mechanoreceptor endings in human thoracic and lumbar facet joints, *Spine* 23:168, 1998.
3. Dreyfuss P, Tibiletti C, Dreyer SJ: Thoracic zygapophyseal joint pain patterns: a study in normal volunteers, *Spine* 19:807, 1994.

4. Johnston HM: The cutaneous branches of the posterior primary divisions of the spinal nerves, and their distribution in the skin, *J Anat Physiol* 43:80, 1908.
5. Hovelacque A: *Anatomie des nerfs Craniens et Rachidiens et du System Grand Sympathique*, Paris, 1927, Doin.
6. Wyke BD: Morphological and functional features of the innervation of the costovertebral joints, *Folia Morphol Praha* 23:286, 1975.
7. Hovelacque A: Le nerf sinu-vertebral, *Ann Anat Path Medico-Chir* 2:435, 1925.
8. Groen GJ, Baljet B, Drukker J: Nerves and nerve plexuses of the human vertebral column, *Am J Anat* 188:282, 1990.
9. Kellgren JH: On the distribution of pain arising from deep somatic structures with charts of segmental pain areas, *Clin Sci* 4:35, 1939.
10. Feinstein B, Langton JBK, Jameson RM, Schiller F: Experiments on referred pain from deep somatic tissues, *J Bone Joint Surg* 36A:981, 1954.
11. Wood KB, Schellhas KP, Garvey TA, Aeppli D: Thoracic discography in healthy individuals: a controlled prospective study of magnetic resonance imaging and discography in asymptomatic and symptomatic individuals, *Spine* 24:1548, 1999.
12. Wilson PR: Thoracic facet joint syndrome—clinical entity? *Pain Supp* 4:S87, 1987.
13. Taylor TKF: Thoracic disc lesions, *J Bone Joint Surg* 46B:788, 1964.
14. Weinberg H, Nathan H, Magora F et al: Arthritis of the first costovertebral joint as a cause of thoracic outlet syndrome, *Clin Orthop* 86:159, 1972.
15. Bywaters EGL: Rheumatoid discitis in the thoracic region due to spread from costovertebral joints, *Ann Rheum* Dis 33:408, 1974.
16. Hohmann P: Degenerative changes in the costotransverse joints, *Zeitshr fur Orthop* 105:217, 1968.

PART II

Examination and Assessment

CHAPTER 6

Clinical Reasoning in Orthopedic Manual Therapy

Nicole Christensen, Mark A. Jones, and Judi Carr

In varying ways and with varying degrees of success, physical therapists address daily the examination, evaluation, and management of patient problems. The challenges associated with clinical practice today can in part be attributed to the complex, highly integrated decision making required of physical therapists to provide individualized, efficient, and effective evidence-based intervention, often while operating within significant time and economic constraints. Clinical reasoning in physical therapy and characteristics of successful and efficient clinical practice, typified by the performance of expert physical therapists, have been focused on in recent literature in the field of physical therapy.[1-15] This has been in part, a result of the ongoing struggle by physical therapists to advance the growth and validation of their profession. A recognized need to define and promote those characteristics that lead to superior clinical performance exists within the profession in order to firmly establish physical therapists as autonomous, competent healthcare professionals, capable of sound clinical decision making and effective patient management.

Concern for the development of expert clinical performance by physical therapists has led to the rapidly growing interest in the topic of clinical reasoning. *Clinical reasoning* can be defined as the cognitive processes, or thinking, used in the evaluation and management of patients.[7] Because this cognitive processing guides the clinician in the decision making that dictates his or her course of action, proficiency in clinical reasoning is likely to contribute to greater clinical success and efficiency in overall patient management. However, further research is required to substantiate this belief. Cognitive processing and expert-novice differences have been studied extensively in the medical education field, under the subject of medical problem solving. However, relatively little formal research about those aspects of clinical reasoning that might help differentiate expert from less-expert levels of performance among physical therapists has been published.[1,3-6,11] The research that has been conducted provides some evidence that expert physical therapists possess a multitude of personal and professional attributes that characterize their expertise.[4] Experts also appear to use a number of diagnostic and nondiagnostic clinical-reasoning strategies to understand, effectively work with, and manage patients and their problems.[2]

This chapter attempts both to act as a reference point for related chapters and to assist readers in recognizing and analyzing their own clinical-reasoning skills. As such, the chapter will present a model of clinical reasoning for physical therapy and will relate this model to relevant findings of research in physical therapy and medicine. A structure for the organization of clinical knowledge in manual therapy is proposed, and a clinical example illustrates the clinical-reasoning process facilitated by this type of organization of knowledge.

CLINICAL REASONING IN PHYSICAL THERAPY

Research specific to clinical reasoning among physical therapists suggests that the process they use is comparable to that used by medical clinicians.[3,6,11,12,14] To foster these traits in novice practitioners, much of the early medical-education research emphasized identification and understanding of the process of problem solving used by expert physicians.[16-18] The conclusions of this research included the identification of the clinical-reasoning process of physicians as hypothetico-deductive reasoning, wherein hypotheses are generated, tested, and modified as necessary, based on the outcome of testing.[16,18,19] The goal of this process within medicine is to arrive at an accurate diagnosis so that an appropriate therapeutic intervention can be prescribed.

The model presented in the medical-education literature by Barrows and Tamblyn[20] was adapted by Jones[7] to describe the clinical-reasoning process in physical therapy. Barrows and Tamblyn described the steps in the clinical-reasoning process as the following[20]:

1. Information perception and interpretation
2. Hypothesis generation
3. Inquiry strategy and clinical skills
4. Problem formulation
5. Diagnostic and therapeutic decisions

The early model by Jones,[7] like the one proposed by Barrows and Tamblyn,[20] emphasizes the cyclical and interactive nature of each step in the reasoning process. This model emphasizes the relationship between memory and all stages of the process and explains that the process of clinical reasoning itself enhances memory and adds to the existing knowledge base. Clinical reasoning of physical therapists working in manual therapy has been shown to be consistent with this proposed model.[10,12] Clinical expertise that results in more effective patient outcomes develops in part through the use of clinical reasoning in patient interactions.[21] Jones[8] has expanded on his original model and now includes the collaborative component of clinical reasoning: the patient plays a key role, acting as a partner with the physical therapist in the clinical-reasoning process. This model is illustrated in Figure 6-1.

Each physical therapist is unique, with a personal history of experiences that have contributed to the development of his or her knowledge base, belief system, and cultural and social values. Likewise, every patient enters into the clinical environment with his or her own internal frame of reference and perceptions based on life experiences. The collaborative component of the clinical-reasoning process highlights the interaction between the individuals inhabiting the clinical roles of physical therapist and patient, rather than between a generic "care-giver" and "care-receiver." This interaction is a powerful factor influencing the clinical outcome. The emphasis on the role of the patient within the clinical-reasoning process is reflected in some of the more recent literature in physical therapy and pain sciences.[2-4,22-27]

It should be noted that the clinical-reasoning process itself is goal oriented. These goals describe projected outcomes and involve a shared vision of the potential out-

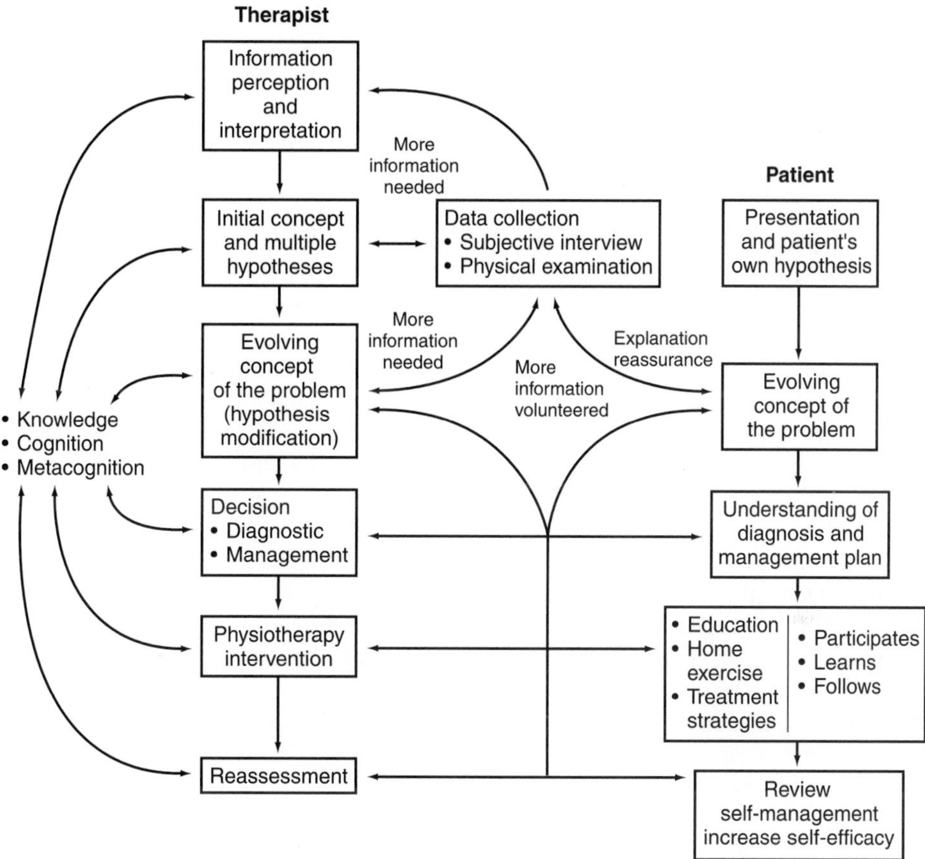

Figure 6-1
Collaborative reasoning in physical therapy.
(Redrawn from Jones MA: *Man Ther* 1:17, 1995.)

come of physical therapy intervention negotiated between the physical therapist and patient.[22,23] The goal of the clinical-reasoning process for physical therapists is not only to come to a diagnostic decision but also to work with each patient in making the best management decisions within that patient's life context.[21]

Information Perception, Interpretation, and the Development of Initial Hypotheses

The first component of the process as described by Jones[8] is the perception and subsequent interpretation of initial relevant information. Even while greeting a patient, a therapist can observe specific cues such as age, facial statement, introductory communication style, appearance, resting posture, and movement patterns. Much valuable information can be gained by consciously taking a moment to process this available information before beginning formal interview of the patient. Researchers in medical education have noted that experts make more extensive use of such initial information from patient encounters than do novices.[28] This fact seems to support the notion that expert clinicians use this information—developed over time through experience with similar patients—to identify clinical patterns stored in memory.[29] Such information can be used in more effective development of an initial concept of the patient's problem and in the generation of early multiple hypotheses.

General conclusions drawn from the early research on information processing in medical clinical reasoning included the nearly universal use of the hypothetico-deductive process of generating and testing hypotheses by clinicians, regardless of their specialty or level of experience.[17-19] Later researchers[30-32] have suggested that novices rely solely on this deductive, backward reasoning ("hypothesis-driven") process, whereas expert reasoning is more accurately described by an inductive, forward reasoning ("data-driven") process that directly involves the recognition of clinical patterns. It seems reasonable that this may indeed occur. Since expert clinicians have vast knowledge bases of clinical patterns and variations on the basic patterns, a process of matching a patient problem to one already stored in memory might be a more efficient way of arriving at a diagnosis. This view is supported by the categorization research conducted in psychology and medicine.[33] However, while using the techniques of forward reasoning and pattern recognition that are characteristic of successful expert performance, even expert clinicians must rely on backward reasoning when they lack sufficient knowledge to arrive at a diagnosis from the data alone.[31,34-36] In fact, experts seldom miss subtle clues indicating that a patient's problem is not as it first appears, indicating that they entertain alternate hypotheses as well.[35]

Thus, the clinical-reasoning process might be best represented by a combination of pattern recognition and hypothesis testing throughout the clinical-reasoning process. Regardless of whether a clinician uses a hypothetico-deductive or pattern-recognition process, success in reasoning has been linked to the speed with which hypotheses are generated and the quality of these early hypotheses.[18,19,35] A superior knowledge base from which to quickly generate quality hypotheses seems to be central in determining outcome because these hypotheses coordinate and guide all subsequent activity in the data-gathering process.

DATA COLLECTION

Data collection is tailored to the working hypotheses, and to develop an evolving concept of the problem, the therapist interprets the data by reference to his or her knowledge base. That is, the subjective and physical examination data prove or disprove previously generated hypotheses. The initial hypotheses are refined and reranked, and ultimately the list of possibilities is narrowed throughout the subjective and physical examination. Both the subjective and physical examination benefit from the adoption of what Barrows and Tamblyn[20] referred to as "search and scan" strategies. Search strategies are the main reasoning strategies in an examination and are aimed at identifying the temporal features of a patient's symptoms, the factors that aggravate and improve them, and their relationship to other symptoms. Search strategies in physical therapy include those previously described, which tend to provide information useful in supporting, refining, and reranking hypotheses. Scan inquiries, on the other hand, are routine data-gathering procedures unrelated to specific hypotheses. They provide background information, safety information, and quick checks of other regions less likely to be involved in a patient's condition.

Each new item of data should be evaluated in light of the multiple hypotheses being considered. An important principle, as proposed by Maitland,[37] is described by the phrase "making the features fit." This implies that when the collected information does not support current hypotheses, more information should be obtained to clarify the interpretation of the data. Research has demonstrated that superior clinical reasoning results when multiple quality hypotheses are generated.[32] Data are then interpreted as confirming the appropriate hypotheses through backward reasoning with disconfirming strategies to eliminate alternate hypotheses. This process of "imposing coherence"[32] on the data will also enable the clinician to build previously unrecognized variations into the existing knowledge of clinical patterns stored in memory.

The physical therapist also begins to integrate information gained from the patient to develop an understanding of how the patient's "whole self" affects and is affected by his or her presenting problem. The exchange between physical therapist and patient during data collection shapes both the physical therapist's and the patient's concepts of the problem. This raises the importance of superior communication skills and effective inquiry strategies in the data-collection process—decisions are based on the data or information that is gathered from the subjective examination of the patient. Means by which to enhance communication with patients include the following:

- Attention to nonverbal communication
- Provision of opportunity for the patient to offer spontaneous information related to his or her symptoms or life situation
- Use of the patient's own words when communicating about the problem
- Avoidance of assumptions by clarification of all information given

Examples of inquiry strategies include the following:

- Asking open-ended questions
- Forcing choices
- Repeating a patient's story
- Using silence when appropriate

Although good communication is a key to quality data collection in the subjective and physical examination, superior manual skills are also invaluable in gathering accurate data that will support or negate hypotheses about the structures at fault in a particular clinical disorder. The physical examination is not performed as a routine series of tests. Rather, it is a direct extension of the data collection and hypothesis testing performed throughout the subjective examination. If data collected at any stage of the data-collection process are faulty (e.g., incomplete, inaccurate, unreliable), clinical decisions based on this data are at risk.

Diagnostic and Management Decisions

When enough information has been gathered from both the subjective and physical examinations, the therapist is able to make a diagnostic and management decision. It must be emphasized that the goal of the clinical-reasoning process to this point is not only to arrive at a diagnosis but also to use clinical reasoning to incorporate data about the patient as a person into the management plan. Physical therapists must collaborate with the patient throughout the process; this necessitates the understanding of who the patient is, the patient's understanding of his or her problems and management, and how the patient's life has been impacted by his or her problems.

Physical therapy research has demonstrated that clinical reasoning of expert clinicians is characterized in part by these areas outside of diagnosis.[2-4,6] Jones et al[21] propose that various clinical-reasoning strategies are used by physical therapists to apply and organize clinical-reasoning principles to both diagnostic and nondiagnostic activities necessary for a holistic approach to clinical practice. These clinical-reasoning strategies[21] include the following:

- *Diagnostic reasoning:* identification of the functional limitations and associated impairments, underlying pain mechanisms, tissue structures involved, and factors related to development and maintenance of the patient's problem
- *Procedural reasoning:* choices of appropriate treatment technique, dosage, and progression

- *Interactive reasoning:* communication, in the form of socialization, which builds rapport and provides the physical therapist with a means to develop understanding of the context of the patient's problem
- *Collaborative reasoning:* shared decision making between the therapist and patient, which fosters in the patient a sense of self-responsibility and involvement in physical therapy management
- *Teaching as reasoning:* provision of appropriate physical or conceptual education of the patient by the therapist (e.g., explanation of the problem and management recommended, movement reeducation, work or leisure activity modifications) to promote patient understanding and maintain or enhance effectiveness of physical therapy intervention and prevention of reinjury
- *Predictive reasoning:* developing and communicating a prognosis that reflects the realistic anticipated outcome of physical therapy intervention within the context of the relevant contributing physical, psychological, social, work, and recreational factors for a particular patient presentation
- *Ethical/pragmatic reasoning:* strategies used to resolve external ethical, practical and nonideal circumstances that affect clinical practice and thus impact the clinical reasoning within an individual patient's treatment intervention
- *Narrative reasoning:* the attempt to understand patients' "stories" beyond the mere chronological sequence of events. Here the cognitive and affective/social aspects of patients' problem(s) are sought to more fully understand the context in which the problems exist and the effects those problems are having on their lives. In addition, therapists may tactically use the telling of "stories" regarding other patients as a means of building rapport, educating and communicating prognostic outcomes

Thus various clinical-reasoning strategies are used throughout the clinical-reasoning process to enable the clinician to address all components of a patient problem in a comprehensive, integrated, holistic manner.

In addition to making a diagnosis and establishing a treatment-intervention strategy based on his or her evaluation, the physical therapist must facilitate the patient's understanding of this diagnosis and management decision to set mutually inclusive treatment outcome goals at this stage. Management decisions at this stage also address whether it is appropriate to treat the patient, to refer the patient to a specialist physical therapist, or to refer him or her to another health care provider outside of physical therapy.

Physical Therapy Intervention and Reassessment

Intervention in physical therapy includes direct manual techniques, exercise instruction, and patient education.[23] Any direct treatment intervention must be followed by continuous reassessment to ensure efficacy. Even treatment is viewed as a form of hypothesis testing, because the results of treatment modify or reform hypotheses, which then contribute further to the therapist's evolving concept of the patient's problem. Often reassessment can reveal unexpected or ineffective results of selected treatments, which in turn lead to valuable expansion of the knowledge base with regard to variations in the presentation and responses to treatment of various clinical patterns. Reassessment by the physical therapist occurs within and between treatment sessions. To facilitate the rehabilitation process, a desired outcome of patient education is the patient's empowerment to assess his or her own symptoms as well. Physical therapy intervention also involves indirect treatment components, including case management/coordination of care with other involved persons and written documentation.[23] These services are necessary components that contribute to the provision of comprehensive patient-centered care.

The collaboration of the physical therapist with the patient throughout the clinical-reasoning process will result in significant learning by both the patient and physical therapist.[21] A principal aim of physical therapy is to promote patient learning (e.g., altered understanding, beliefs, attitudes, and health behaviors). A patient's full understanding of and participation in the management of his or her problem, resulting in an increase in understanding and, in turn, self-efficacy is thought to have a significant positive impact on treatment outcomes.[21,24-27,38] In addition, the physical therapist can build on clinical knowledge by learning how multiple factors in addition to the physical structures involved in a patient's problem interact and produce variations on classic clinical patterns.[21]

Physical therapy in the twenty-first century will require therapists to approach health care in the broader context of life, with greater emphasis on prevention of illness and dysfunction and promotion of good health. In support of the nondiagnostic reasoning strategies recommended, Higgs and Hunt[39] and Higgs et al[40] highlight the need for therapists to expand their interactional and teaching skills to better deliver this more holistic level of health care.

Knowledge, Cognition, and Metacognition

It can be seen from the proposed model that a physical therapist's knowledge base affects and is affected by every phase of the clinical-reasoning process. Closely linked to the clinician's knowledge in the reasoning process are his or her skills of cognition and metacognition.

Cognitive skills include analysis and synthesis of data and inquiry skills. Many common errors in clinical reasoning are linked to errors in cognition. Examples cited in related literature include the following:

- Blindly following recipes or protocols
- Considering too few hypotheses
- Attending only to those features of a presentation that support a favorite hypothesis and either neglecting the negating features, or not testing competing hypotheses
- Making assumptions without clarifying
- Overemphasis on biomedical or clinical knowledge[7,17]

In addition to reflecting on clinical cases, the physical therapist can reflect on his or her own reasoning process throughout each component of managing a patient case. This awareness and monitoring of one's own thinking process is called *metacognition.* Cognitive skills such as data analysis and synthesis allow the clinical-reasoning process to continue, whereas the metacognitive skills provide a critical review of this cognitive performance. In essence, this requires the clinician to think or process information on two planes simultaneously. By reflecting on clinical cases, the therapist's knowledge of clinical presentations and their treatment will expand; by reflecting on his or her own performance, the therapist's knowledge of how to function efficiently and effectively will expand. Such metacognitive reflection should include the quality of data obtained, the breadth and depth of reasoning used, and limitations in one's own knowledge. Expert physical therapists not only know a great deal but they also are well aware of what they do not know and readily question the basis of their beliefs. With accumulated experience in clinical reasoning, which includes reflecting on patient encounters and outcomes, a physical therapist's knowledge base has the potential to grow rapidly to a point at which pattern recognition becomes very rapid and the clinician can function intuitively in a large proportion of cases.

KNOWLEDGE BASE CONTENT AND ORGANIZATION

As depicted in the model of clinical reasoning presented on page 87, a physical therapist's knowledge base affects and is affected by every phase of the clinical-reasoning process. Within the more recent medical-education literature, researchers have emphasized that the organization, or structure, of a clinician's knowledge base—more than the content of that knowledge base—results in effective, accurate diagnosis.[34,38,41-46] When the knowledge is there but cannot be easily accessed by the clinician in a clinical situation because of a lack of organization, the clinical-reasoning process suffers.

Knowledge has been described in the literature of cognitive psychology as a record of the processing and reprocessing of information within human memory. This processing produces knowledge that is structured into networks of interrelationships.[44,47] Problem-solving studies in areas such as chess and physics have demonstrated that the memory of experts is characterized by possession of highly organized and interrelated patterns of meaningful information.[48-50] These patterns, or schemata, are modifiable information structures that represent generalized concepts underlying an object, situation, event, sequence of events, action, or sequence of actions.[51] They are prototypes in memory of frequently experienced situations that individuals use to recognize and interpret other situations.[33]

Physical therapists may call on various types of knowledge in varying degrees when going through a process of clinical reasoning. These types of knowledge include basic science and biomedical knowledge, clinically acquired knowledge (often in the form of recognized clinical patterns and "if/then" rules of action), everyday knowledge about life and social situations, and tacit knowledge. *Tacit knowledge* is a term that connotes the habitual knowledge gained through experience, which is difficult to translate into words yet greatly influences the way clinicians see and gather information from patients.[52]

A physical therapist's organization of knowledge may include schemata for facts, procedures, concepts, principles, and clinical pattern presentations. Relevant facts in the clinical-reasoning process include anatomical information, pathophysiological mechanisms, and the physical properties of modalities used by physical therapists. Procedures might include examination and treatment strategies, manual techniques, and exercise progressions.

Examples of concepts represented by discrete schemata in memory are neural pathomechanics and irritability. Neural pathomechanics signifies some form of pathology in the physiology and mechanics, or mobility of the continuous tissue tract of the nervous system, and the influences of physiology and mechanics on each other. Involvement of neural pathomechanics in a patient's symptoms necessitates attention to this aspect of the problem through the ongoing management and reassessment of the patient's condition. Irritability is a measure of how easily and to what extent the patient's symptoms are provoked by daily activities. Judgment about the irritability component of the patient's disorder is then used to guide the extent of the physical examination and treatment intervention that can be performed at the first evaluation without risk of aggravating the patient's disorder.

Principles represented in memory by schemata are the underlying rationales that guide the physical therapist in the application of specific knowledge from any other schema. Examples include the principles that guide the selection of techniques and grade of passive-movement treatment appropriate for a particular combination of signs and symptoms.[37,53]

A clinical pattern presentation is represented in memory by a schema that may contain information typical of that particular patient's problem—data relating to predisposing or contributing factors, the sites and nature of symptoms, history, the behavior of symptoms, and physical signs that are present when such a pattern is seen clinically. These "sub-schemas" are linked so that the identification of one item of data enables the clinician to easily recall other information related to that clinical pattern.

It is evident that the content of knowledge varies among individuals. In addition, some medical-education literature suggests that there may be a different structure to the knowledge of clinicians at varying levels of expertise (i.e., at different stages between novice and expert).[29,54-57] Schmidt and Boshuizen[57] have proposed that the development of expertise in medicine progresses through stages in which clinical reasoning and knowledge acquisition are interdependent. The first stage involves the accumulation of biomedical, basic scientific knowledge. This knowledge is linked in a network as presented through formal education. As more knowledge is added to the network, connections between concepts are formed, facilitating the development of clusters of related concepts. Clinical reasoning in this early stage is largely based on biomedical concepts, and students have difficulty in differentiating relevant from irrelevant patient findings, thus leading to excessive numbers of hypotheses. Schmidt and Boshuizen refer to the development of clusters of related concepts as *knowledge encapsulation.*

The second stage in the development of medical expertise involves the integration of biomedical knowledge into clinical knowledge. This occurs with students' increasing experience with patients. The knowledge structures used in clinical reasoning at this stage contain little in the way of direct biomedical concepts. Rather, links are formed between patient findings and clinical concepts, enabling clinicians to form hypotheses and make diagnoses. Schmidt and Boshuizen[57] describe only examples of diagnostic concept clusters. Within physical therapy, diagnostic concept clusters—such as zygapophyseal joint arthralgia and variations of disc disorders—can be identified, but nondiagnostic clusters such as physical and psychosocial predisposing factors also exist. These factors are discussed later in the section on hypothesis categories. As students begin to recognize clinical patterns, their ability to differentiate relevant from irrelevant cues improves, and shortcuts in reasoning become evident for typical cases.

The third stage in developing expertise is characterized by the development in the clinician's memory of stereotypical "illness scripts." These are analogous to the clinical patterns recognized by physical therapists and include information about predisposing conditions (e.g., personal, social, or medical hereditary conditions that influence the patients' presentations), the pathophysiological process taking place, and the presenting signs and symptoms typical of the condition. Not mentioned by Schmidt and Boshuizen[57] but also included in the clinical patterns recognized by physical therapists are the probable prognostic outcomes associated with different problems. These illness scripts, or patterns, are activated as a whole in the clinician's memory, which increases the efficiency of the knowledge network as the amount of searching necessary to locate related information is decreased.[57]

According to Schmidt and Boshuizen,[57] the final stage in the development of expert knowledge content and structure involves the storage of real clinical encounters as "instance scripts" in memory. These memories of patient encounters are stored as discrete units in memory and are not merged with the stereotypical illness script or clinical pattern in memory. They include the individual physical and psychosocial presentations of particular patients and how their problems were successfully or unsuccessfully managed. Experts are believed to possess a rich memory of such patient "stories."[58] The more experience a clinician gathers, the better he or she is able to recognize the variations (stored as instance scripts) of basic clinical patterns seen in daily practice.

Schmidt and Boshuizen[57] suggest that to improve clinical reasoning, education must focus on the development of adequate knowledge structures. This requires further understanding of the knowledge structures that physical therapists use when reasoning through clinical cases. The notion that biomedical knowledge is encapsulated in clinical knowledge is particularly relevant to education in physical therapy, which often has a similar structure of basic science subjects preceding clinical experience. This suggests that students of physical therapy are also likely to develop biomedical schema that must then be encapsulated into clinical patterns as the students gain clinical experience. Patel and Kaufman[59] cite a series of studies consistent with Schmidt and Boshuizen's theory that the use of biomedical concepts in clinical reasoning decreases with expertise. Although this has not yet been demonstrated with physical therapists, it can be hypothesized that a similar phenomenon occurs as "textbook" information becomes altered or superseded by clinical experience.

Patel and Kaufman[59] see the key role of knowledge in biomedical science as facilitating explanation and coherent communication. This is typically not activated in the context of familiar conditions.[31,60] In the context of complex, unfamiliar cases, biomedical knowledge is used to understand and provide causal explanations for patient data.[60,61] As such, this knowledge assists in the organization of disjointed facts. Patel and Kaufman[59] purport that since well-organized, coherent information is easier to remember than disjointed facts, this use of biomedical knowledge should facilitate further clinical learning.

ORGANIZATION OF CLINICAL KNOWLEDGE WITH HYPOTHESIS CATEGORIES

Because the knowledge required in the practice of physical therapy is vast and diverse, the importance of a good organizational system is increased. Clinical experience in reasoning through a patient problem, as demonstrated by the clinical reasoning model, has the potential to expand, modify, and enhance the knowledge base of the physical therapist. However, this opportunity is lost if the new knowledge gained in the clinical encounter is stored in a disorganized fashion, for this knowledge will not then be easily accessible to the clinician in future experiences. The following discussion proposes an example of a way to organize information obtained from clinical encounters for immediate use and for storing it accessibly in memory. In this system, originally proposed by Jones[7] and built on by others,[24,25] clinical reasoning is characterized by the adoption of several discrete but related hypothesis categories. Hypothesis categories are clusters of related concepts—in this case particularly relevant to the practice of orthopedic manual therapy. These categories include the following:

- Functional limitation and disability (physical or psychological limitations in functional activities and the associated social consequences)
- Pathobiological mechanisms
- Source of symptoms or dysfunction (often equated with diagnosis or impairment)
- Contributing factors
- Precautions and contraindications
- Prognosis
- Management

Rivett and Higgs[12] and Mildonis et al[10] have explored the clinical-reasoning process and how clinicians structure generation of hypotheses throughout the process; the system of hypothesis categories has been shown to be used in the clinical reasoning of physical therapists working in manual therapy.[12] The following case presentation illustrates the use of these hypothesis categories.

Clinical Case Example

A 28-year-old computer graphic designer complains of a medial scapular ache on the right side at about the level of the spine of her scapula. Preliminary questioning reveals that she is single, has no children, and works full time. Outside of work she is fairly active, regularly walks 30 to 40 minutes per day for exercise, and states that about 3 months ago she took up rock climbing to strengthen her upper body. The patient describes her ache as deep and intermittent. Before investigating the details of the patient's symptoms, the physical therapist notices that she appears fit and healthy but has assumed a very slumped sitting posture, with her head thrust forward and shoulders rounded.

The patient experiences her ache after prolonged periods of working at her computer (e.g., 2 hours) and then notes difficulty ("stiffness") in lifting her head up out of what she demonstrates to be a slightly flexed and right-rotated typing posture. Her ache resolves immediately when she is out of this posture during the morning but occurs more quickly (i.e., within 10 minutes) toward the end of her working day. By the time she leaves work she experiences a constant ache that takes several hours to resolve. She has given up her evening walks since the onset of this problem. Although turning her neck does not hurt, she notes that it feels stiff to turn in either direction as the day progresses. At the end of the day her head feels heavy to hold up. Thoracic and arm movements have no effect on her ache. The stiffness and heaviness continue through the evening but resolve after a night's sleep. Sleeping has never been a problem for the patient, and in the mornings she has no discomfort but complains of some general neck stiffness that lasts between 10 and 15 minutes on waking. She is not sure whether looking up is a problem since she never really needs to, except when rock climbing; she has avoided rock climbing since the onset of this problem because she thought it might aggravate her symptoms.

The patient reports that her ache began spontaneously about 3 weeks ago while she was working at the computer. She is unaware of what might have caused it but recalls gardening for several hours the previous day, something she rarely does for more than half an hour at a time. The ache has gradually worsened in intensity over the 3 weeks since it began. The patient has never had a similar problem but reports that she had a car accident about 6 months ago and had some generalized soreness and stiffness across the base of her neck for about 2 months after the accident. At that time, she received physical therapy, consisting of mobilization and heat to the affected part of her neck and instructions in home exercises. The treatment helped to relieve those symptoms, but she has not continued with the exercise program that was given to her. When this episode of neck pain occurred, she was hesitant to resume her exercise program without first checking that the exercises were appropriate for this problem. Other than this current medial scapular ache, the patient has no health problems or relevant past history.

In response to questioning, the patient states she is concerned that this episode of neck pain might be a reoccurrence of the problem she had after her car accident and possibly related to discontinuing her prescribed exercise program. She states that since she had such positive resolution of her symptoms with physical therapy treatment the last time, she expects that her outcome from physical therapy treatment this time will also be very positive.

Dysfunction, Functional Limitation, and Disability

As described by Gifford and Butler,[25] *dysfunction* refers to general or specific limitations with activities or physical functions. Psychosocial dysfunction exists when maladaptive thoughts, beliefs, and emotions and the associated social consequences affect the patient's behavior. Other terms have been used to describe these problems within the context of the disablement model.[23] These terms, which describe components of this hypothesis category, include the following[23]:

- *Impairments:* loss or abnormality of physiological, psychological, or anatomical structure or function
- *Functional limitations:* restrictions of the ability to perform—at the level of the whole person—a physical action, activity, or task in an efficient, typically expected, or competent manner
- *Disability:* limitations of function within particular social contexts and physical environments

The patient described in the case presentation on page 96 has impaired static postural alignment and active cervical spine mobility. Data collected throughout the physical examination would no doubt reveal additional specific impairments related to the function of the tissues producing or contributing to symptoms. The patient could be considered functionally limited in her ability to perform her work activities without symptoms. There is no information indicating that this patient's problem has reached the level of disability yet. Examples of disability within this patient case scenario might include the inability to carry out the tasks required of a computer graphic designer.

Although fear of exacerbating her condition has limited performance of her routine fitness (walking) and recreational (rock climbing) activities, there is no suspicion of psychosocial dysfunction at this point in the patient-therapist interaction. Caution in performing these activities does not appear to be maladaptive within the context of the recent onset and limited intervention for the problem thus far. The patient is demonstrating a reasonable understanding of her problem and a positive attitude toward physical therapy intervention thus far.

Pathobiological Mechanisms

This hypothesis category is comprised of data about tissue mechanisms and pain mechanisms. It was designed to facilitate the physical therapist in expanding his or her clinical-reasoning process to include consideration of the mechanisms by which the patient's symptoms are being initiated and maintained by the nervous system. Tissue mechanisms relate to issues of tissue health and stages of tissue healing. How well the patient's presentation "fits" with what would be expected during the corresponding stage of the normal tissue-healing process is integral in developing a hypothesis of the pain mechanism at work. Gifford and Butler[25] and Gifford[62-64] divide the category of pain mechanisms into the following subcategories:

1. Input mechanisms: nociceptive and peripheral neurogenic
2. Processing mechanisms: central neurogenic
3. Output mechanisms: somatic motor, autonomic, neuroendocrine and neuroimmune

Pain mechanisms relate to particular physiological/pathophysiological processes that can give rise to pain in sensory, cognitive, emotional and behavioral dimensions.[25,62-64] A brief description of each is given next. The reader should refer to literature by Gifford and Butler[24-26,62-64] for a more comprehensive explanation of these processes and systems.

Input Mechanisms

Nociceptive Pain. Nociceptive pain originates from target tissues of nerves, such as muscle, ligament, bone, and tendon. This pain mechanism is characterized by symptoms that present in clear neuroanatomical patterns and behave "normally." Symptoms are linked to the occurrence of injury, inflammation, and repair. This pain is clearly identified as a normal response to stimulus of injured tissue, and thus the physical examination provides a relatively accurate means of identifying the source.

Peripheral Neurogenic Pain. Peripheral neurogenic pain originates in neural tissue "outside" the dorsal horn, such as spinal nerves and peripheral nerves. The epineurium, perineurium, and endoneurium of peripheral neural tissues are highly innervated and thus capable of generating ectopic pain symptoms. Symptoms fall within a corresponding innervation field and may consist of aching, cramping, and burning, as well as paresthesia. This pain mechanism may also be viewed as a "normal" response to injury to the peripheral nervous system tissues. As such, the physical testing of neural function and mechanics will assist in localizing the nerves involved.

Processing Mechanism

Central Pain. Central pain connotes pain and increased sensitivity resulting from and maintained by altered structure and processing within the central nervous system (CNS) (e.g., increased excitability of wide dynamic ranging interneuron cells within the dorsal horn). Pain resulting from central sensitization of the nervous system is ongoing after tissues have had time to heal. Symptoms are atypical, often poorly localized, and often unstable. Although all pain can be exacerbated chemically by emotional or general physical stress, in a central pain state both physical and psychosocial stress are thought to be significant contributing factors in maintaining the pain. Hence, a patient's cognition (i.e., understanding of the problem and intervention required) and affect (i.e., feelings about the problem, management, and effects on his/her life) are important dimensions of all pain states but are particularly involved in central pain. Special care is needed in the interpretation of physical examination findings in cases in which a central pain mechanism is dominant. The sensitization resulting from the CNS dysfunction will create many "false positives" in the physical examination (e.g., tender tissues, painful movements) that can easily lead to incorrect conclusions regarding the source of the symptoms (i.e., that the dysfunction is primarily in the painful tissues). If these "false positives" are interpreted in a central pain state as implicating peripheral target tissues as a local source of symptoms, intervention strategies are often inappropriately applied to these target tissues and result in poor physical therapy outcomes.

Output Mechanisms

Somatic Motor. The somatic motor mechanism involves altered motor activity (increased or decreased) and movement patterns in response to pathology, and also learning. Although pathology and pain can inhibit muscle function and lead to altered movement patterns, many posture and movement abnormalities are associated with problems of motor learning as well as motor control. These faulty movement patterns may be acquired through habitual postures and activities of life or as the consequences of maintained pain.

Autonomic. The autonomic mechanism is a controversial output system in which features of abnormal sympathetic activity are common in some chronic pain states, although the underlying pathology is unclear. Although the sympathetic nervous system (SNS) is normally active in all pain states, it can be pathologically active in some. This pathological activity contributes to dysfunction and maintained pain.

Neuroendocrine. The neuroendocrine system is an output system responsible for the regulation of energy through the body to meet the immediate demands of a situation. Like the SNS, the neuroendocrine system is responsive to our thoughts and feelings. Stress, for example, triggers a chain of events from the hypothalamus to the adrenal cortex that enables the appropriate channeling of energy for an individual to escape the perceived threat. However, maintained stress, as is common in so many chronic pain states, can result in maladaptive neuroendocrine activity that is detrimental to tissue health and impedes tissue recovery.

Neuroimmune. The neuroimmune system is an output system with close links to the brain, the SNS, and the endocrine system. Chronic pain and psychological dysfunction can interfere with normal immune and healing processes via this system.

The pathobiological mechanisms hypothesis category is invaluable in focusing physical therapists on developing hypotheses about where symptoms are produced and maintained within the nervous system, and what other systems might be affected. If a patient has a "normal," adaptive pain mechanism, wherein symptoms are the result of pathology in the implicated local tissues, it is appropriate to then determine the precise diagnosis and to identify a specific site to direct manual treatment. However, when pain symptoms are the result of "abnormal," maladaptive pain states resulting from and maintained by altered CNS processing, physical therapists must steer away from a "tissue-based" paradigm and instead use more holistic, less tissue-specific treatment intervention strategies.[24-26,62-64]

The pain mechanism dominant in the patient in the case presentation can be classified as nociceptive pain. Her symptoms behave mechanically and appear to originate from stress to local tissues close to or in the area of symptoms. There is a recognizable mechanism of injury in her history, which offers a plausible explanation for the initiation and progression of her symptoms thus far. She appears to have a reasonable understanding of and an appropriate response to her problem. She has not revealed any maladaptive feelings, beliefs, or behaviors that might be contributing to her problem. Also, her symptoms appear to fit with what would be expected from peripheral tissues undergoing healing within 3 weeks of onset, considering that the stress to the injured tissues has not been alleviated since the time of injury.

Source of Symptoms or Dysfunction

The *source of symptoms* refers to the structure from which the symptoms are emanating. Information contributing to the formation of hypotheses about the source of a patient's symptoms or dysfunction is available from each of the major aspects of the patient's presentation. For example, from the patient information described before, a physical therapist might begin to generate hypotheses about the source of the patient's symptoms based on their site(s) because different structures are associated with different patterns of symptoms. In this patient with a medial scapular ache, the therapist might consider the source of the ache to possibly include cervical spinal structures, thoracic spinal structures, and local soft tissues in the interscapular region.

The behavior of the symptoms (e.g., aggravating factors, irritability, easing factors, 24-hour pattern) can also help to implicate certain structures. The therapist considers which structures are most involved or compromised by a certain aggravating activity, or conversely, what stresses on what structures are reduced by a particular easing activity. For the patient in the case presentation, the lower cervical intervertebral discs and neural structures are the structures most implicated by the behavior of symptoms. Examples in this case include symptoms aggravated by computer work in a sustained forward head posture and slumped sitting, difficulty in returning the head to neutral, symmetrical stiffness in turning the neck right and left, and heaviness of the head as the day progresses. Since thoracic and arm movements have no effect on the ache, the thoracic joints and local muscles and soft tissues are less implicated, although specific physical tests of these structures are still required for confirmation of the source of the patient's condition. Structures more likely to be implicated by symptoms of spontaneous, gradual onset and the history of a car accident and cervical spine injury are cervical and neural. No information in the behavior of symptoms or history of the problem indicates the presence of an abnormal pain mechanism; thus symptoms can be hypothesized to be originating in local tissues. For this hypothesis category, as for all of the others, each new item of information must be seen in the light of the information already obtained, and hypotheses in the category must be weighed accordingly, with those supported by most of the information heading the list of possibilities.

The generation of hypotheses about the source of symptoms is important in that it ensures treatment will be directed to the appropriate area. However, in reality, it is often not possible to clinically confirm which specific tissues are at fault. Even with the assistance of advanced diagnostic or imaging procedures, by which pathology can be demonstrated, confirmation of those tissues as being the true source of the symptoms is impossible. Many degenerative changes evident on the various imaging procedures are asymptomatic and thus may be minimally relevant or even completely unrelated to the patient's problem at hand. It is not unusual for even the most skillful and experienced physical therapist to achieve only a relative localization of the area from which the symptoms are emanating (e.g., cervical spine versus thoracic spine, in the present example), even with a detailed evaluation and meticulous reassessments of chosen interventions. Therefore a balance in the specificity of hypotheses generated regarding the source of the symptoms is required.

Attempting to hypothesize about specific structures such as contractile tissues, specific joints, or neurogenic pain is still important—and sometimes even critical—to ensure safety (e.g., vertebrobasilar insufficiency, spinal cord pathology, or instability). However, the therapist must recognize the limitations of such clinical diagnoses and take care to avoid limiting management only to theoretically based or evidence-based procedures directed to a single tissue. This relates directly to the value of the disablement model of clinical practice, in which treatment is guided by identified impairments and functional limitations and not solely by diagnostic labels.[23,37] The application of thorough assessment and balanced reasoning, wherein identified impairments are considered in conjunction with known and hypothesized pathology, will enable therapists to deliver effective treatments while continuing to better understand, expand, and eventually validate clinical impressions.

Contributing Factors

Contributing factors are any predisposing or associated factors involved in the development or maintenance of the patient's problem. These include environmental, psychosocial, physical, and biomechanical factors. Hypotheses about contributing factors should be considered separately from the source of a patient's symptoms and evaluated specifically through physical testing and treatment to assess their involvement in the patient's symptoms.

In the case of the patient described in the example, contributing factors may include her poor posture and the nature of her job, which requires long periods in an activity that accentuates this posture. Her posture itself may be antalgic or related to joint and neural hypomobility, muscle imbalance, or poor muscle endurance, which in turn may be the result of learned habitual posture and movement patterns. Her past history of injury to the same area in a car accident is also likely a factor here, as is the relatively recent introduction of strenuous rock-climbing activity, which requires upper extremity work and extended periods of time looking up. Both of these factors involve past and more recently accumulated stress in tissues involved in her previous symptomatic condition and may have contributed to development of her current symptoms.

It is quite probable that the onset of the patient's symptoms is related to her gardening activities the day before onset of the problem; thus her previously nonaggravating work posture now causes her difficulty. Also, any correlation between the onset of her symptoms and the time at which the patient gave up doing her home exercises might implicate a lack of specific therapeutic exercise as a factor contributing to the symptoms.

Precautions and Contraindications to Physical Therapy

Hypotheses about precautions and contraindications to physical examination and treatment determine the extent of physical examination that may safely be undertaken (i.e., how many physical tests are performed and whether provocation of symptoms is to be avoided). In addition, these hypotheses help determine whether physical treatment is indicated and, if so, whether there are constraints to treatment (e.g., techniques carried out short of pain provocation versus techniques performed with the intent of reproducing a patient's pain). Factors taken into consideration include the dominance of pain mechanisms, severity, irritability, and stability of the disorder; stage of tissue healing; rate of impairment; patient's general health; and other special screening questions, such as those relating to unexplained weight loss or any steroid use. In the context of the case example, the dominant pain mechanism appears to be nociceptive, and the presentation is not so severe that reproduction of the patient's symptoms would have to be avoided (i.e., the patient can continue working despite her ache). Likewise, the irritability and stability of the symptoms do not necessitate observation of any specific precautions in examination or treatment intervention.

Prognosis

Hypotheses about the prognosis for a patient enable the physical therapist to convey to the patient an estimate of the extent to which the patient's disorder appears amenable to physical therapy and of the time frame in which recovery can be expected. Many individual factors are considered and weighed as either "negative" (unfavorable) or "positive" (favorable) with respect to how the problem is likely to respond to physical therapy intervention. Such factors include the mechanical (usually more positive) versus inflammatory (usually more negative) balance of the disorder; irritability of the disorder; presence of normal (adaptive) or abnormal (maladaptive) pain mechanism; degree of damage or injury (often reflected in the forces involved and immediate signs and symptoms of the disorder); the length of history and progression of the disorder; preexisting disorders; the patient's expectations, personality and lifestyle; and current stage of tissue healing and healing potential. The overall picture of a favorable or unfavorable prognosis is obtained by the combination of all of these factors.

The case example presented in this chapter demonstrates positive factors in that the patient is young and her condition does not appear to be predominantly inflammatory but rather mechanical and nociceptive. Her symptoms are not irritable; the history is recent; and the progression is gradual, all of which point to a more positive prognosis. Also positive is her history of a favorable response to physical therapy and her lack of psychosocial dysfunction. Her history of a car accident and the nature of her job are relatively negative factors that must be weighed against the positive factors in the prognosis in this patient's case.

Management

The formation of physical therapy intervention hypotheses is facilitated by clues gained in analysis of many factors considered throughout the patient-therapist interaction. These include the patient's main complaint, site of symptoms, behavior of symptoms, precautionary questions, onset and progression of symptoms, mechanism of injury, stage of tissue healing, pain mechanism, past treatment, pain threshold, personality, physical examination, ongoing management, and goals negotiated between the physical therapist and patient.

During each clinical encounter, hypothesis categories such as those described above should be pursued concurrently as information is elicited about a patient's problem. The hypothesis categories can be used both as a means by which to organize this information and also to facilitate access to the required relevant knowledge stored in the therapist's memory. Each new clue obtained while examining a patient should be considered in the light of relevant hypothesis categories; this will result in the building of a comprehensive clinical picture through the refinement of working hypotheses in each category.

CONCLUSION

Clinical reasoning in physical therapy involves the process of pattern recognition, which facilitates hypothesis generation and testing of hypotheses. The extent to which either is used is largely related to a clinician's level of experience and in particular to the clinician's organization of knowledge. A model of the clinical-reasoning process used by physical therapists is proposed to assist clinicians in conceptualizing this important skill. A structure for the organization of knowledge is put forward in the form of "hypothesis categories." Although these categories will not necessarily be appropriate for all clinicians in all clinical settings, physical therapists are strongly encouraged to consider the reasoning behind their inquiries, tests, and management interventions; this will help to identify categories of hypotheses that reflect the clinical judgments typically encountered in the different areas of practice. Therapists can then critically analyze their own reasoning, with consideration given to the *breadth* of the hypotheses they consider, the *means* by which hypotheses will be tested, *whether* supporting and negating data are sought, and whether established clinical patterns are substantiated. This form of personal reflection and assessment should lead to more effective management for each patient and a more rapid acquisition of expertise for the physical therapist.

References

1. Beeston S, Simons H: Physiotherapy practice: practitioners' perspectives, *Phys Theory Practice* 12:231, 1996.
2. Jones MA, Edwards I, Gifford L: Conceptual models for implementing biopsychosocial theory in clinical practice, *Man Ther* 7:2, 2002.
3. Embrey DG, Guthrie MR, White OR et al: Clinical decision making by experienced and inexperienced pediatric physical therapists for children with diplegic cerebral palsy, *Phys Ther* 76:20, 1996.
4. Jensen GM, Gwyer J, Shepard KF et al: *Expertise in physical therapy practice*, Boston, 1999, Butterworth Heinemann.
5. Jensen GM, Shepard KF, Hack LM: The novice versus the experienced clinician: insights into the work of the physical therapist, *Phys Ther* 70:314, 1990.
6. Jensen GM, Shepard KF, Hack LM: Attribute dimensions that distinguish master and novice physical therapy clinicians in orthopedic settings, *Phys Ther* 72:711, 1992.
7. Jones MA: Clinical reasoning in manual therapy, *Phys Ther* 72:875, 1992.
8. Jones MA: Clinical reasoning and pain, *Man Ther* 1:17, 1995.
9. May BJ, Dennis JK: Expert decision making in physical therapy: a survey of practitioners, *Phys Ther* 71:190, 1992.
10. Mildonis MK, Godges JJ, Jensen GM: Nature of clinical practice for specialists in orthopaedic physical therapy, *JOSPT* 29(4):240, 1999.
11. Payton OD: Clinical-reasoning process in physical therapy, *Phys Ther* 65:924, 1985.
12. Rivett D, Higgs J: Hypothesis generation in the clinical reasoning behavior of manual therapists, *Phys Ther Educ* 11(1):40, 1997.
13. Rothstein JM, Echternach JL: Hypothesis oriented algorithms for clinicians: a method for evaluation and treatment planning, *Phys Ther* 66:1388, 1986.
14. Thomas-Edding D: Clinical problem solving in physical therapy and its implications for curriculum development. Proceedings of the Tenth International Congress of the World Confederation for Physical Therapy, Sydney, Australia, May 17-22, 1987.
15. Zimny NJ: Clinical reasoning in the evaluation and management of undiagnosed chronic hip pain in a young adult, *Phys Ther* 78(1):62, 1998.
16. Barrows HS, Feightner JW, Neufeld VR, Norman GR: *Analysis of the clinical methods of medical students and physicians*, Final Report, Ontario Department of Health, Hamilton, Ontario, Canada, 1978.
17. Elstein AS, Shulman LS, Sprafka SS: *Medical problem solving: an analysis of clinical reasoning*, Cambridge, Mass, 1978, Harvard University Press.
18. Neufeld VR, Norman GR, Feightner JW et al: Clinical problem-solving by medical students: a cross-sectional and longitudinal analysis, *Med Educ* 15:315, 1981.
19. Barrows HS, Norman GR, Neufeld VR, Feightner JW: The clinical reasoning of randomly selected physicians in general medical practice, *Clin Invest Med* 5:49, 1982.
20. Barrows HS, Tamblyn RM: *Problem-based learning: an approach to medical education*, New York, 1980, Springer.
21. Jones M, Jensen G, Edwards I: Clinical reasoning in physiotherapy. In Higgs J, Jones MA, editors: *Clinical reasoning in the health professions*, ed 2, Oxford, England, 2000, Butterworth-Heinemann.
22. Dutton R: *Clinical reasoning in physical disabilities*, Baltimore, 1995, Williams & Wilkins.
23. American Physical Therapy Association: Guide to physical therapist practice, *Phys Ther* 77(11):1160, 1997.
24. Gifford LS: Pain. In *Rehabilitation of movement: theoretical basis of clinical practice*, London, 1997, Saunders.
25. Gifford LS, Butler D: The integration of pain sciences into clinical practice, *Hand Ther* 10:86, 1997.
26. Gifford L: Pain, the tissues and the nervous system: a conceptual model, *Physiother* 84:27, 1998.
27. Gifford LS: The mature organism model. In Gifford LS, editor: *Topical issues in pain*: physiotherapy pain association yearbook, Falmouth, United Kingdom, 1998, NOI Press.

28. Hobus PPM, Schmidt HG, Boshuizen HPA, Patel VL: Contextual factors in the activation of first diagnostic hypotheses: expert-novice differences, *Med Educ* 21:471, 1987.
29. Boshuizen HPA, Schmidt HG: On the role of biomedical knowledge in clinical reasoning by experts, intermediates and novices, *Cogn Sci* 16:153, 1992.
30. Groen GJ, Patel VL: Medical problem-solving: some questionable assumptions, *J Med Ed* 19:95, 1985.
31. Patel VL, Groen GJ: Knowledge-based solution strategies in medical reasoning, *Cogn Sci* 10:91, 1986.
32. Arocha JF, Patel VL, Patel YC: Hypothesis generation and the coordination of theory and evidence in novice diagnostic reasoning, *Med Decision Making* 13(3):198, 1993.
33. Hayes B, Adams R: Parallels between clinical reasoning and categorization. In Higgs J, Jones MA, editors: *Clinical reasoning in the health professions*, ed 2, Oxford, England, 2000, Butterworth-Heinemann.
34. Feltovich PJ, Barrows HS: *Issues of generality in medical problem solving*. In Schmidt HG, DeVolder ML, editors: *Tutorials in problem-based learning*. Assen/Maastricht, Netherlands, 1984, Van Gorcum.
35. Barrows HS, Feltovich PJ: The clinical-reasoning process, *Med Educ* 12:86, 1987.
36. Elstein AS, Shulman LS, Sprafka SA: Medical problem solving: a ten year retrospective review, *Health Prof* 13:5, 1990.
37. Maitland GD: *Vertebral manipulation*, ed 5, London, 1986, Butterworths.
38. Bordage G, Grant J, Marsden P: Quantitative assessment of diagnostic ability, *Med Educ* 24:413, 1990.
39. Higgs J, Hunt A: Rethinking the beginning practitioner: introducing the "interactional professional." In Higgs J, Edwards H, editors: *Educating beginning practitioners: challenges for health professional education*, Oxford, England, 1999, Butterworth-Heinemann.
40. Higgs C, Neubauer D, Higgs J: The changing health care context: globalization and social ecology. In Higgs J, Edwards H, editors: *Educating beginning practitioners: challenges for health professional education*, Oxford, England, 1999, Butterworth-Heinemann.
41. Bordage G, Lemieux M: Semantic structures and diagnostic thinking of experts and novices, *Acad Med Suppl* 66:70, 1991.
42. Bordage G, Zacks R: The structure of medical knowledge in the memories of medical students and general practitioners: categories and prototypes, *Med Educ* 18:406, 1984.
43. Ericsson A, Smith J editors: *Toward a general theory of expertise: prospects and limits*, New York, 1991, Cambridge University Press.
44. Grant J, Marsden P: The structure of memorized knowledge in students and clinicians: an explanation for medical expertise, *Med Educ* 21:92, 1987.
45. Grant J, Marsden P: Primary knowledge, medical education and consultant expertise, *Med Educ* 22:173, 1988.
46. Patel VL, Groen GJ, Frederiksen CH: Differences between medical students and doctors in memory for clinical cases, *Med Educ* 20:3, 1986.
47. Anderson JR: *Cognitive psychology and its implications*, ed 3, New York, 1990, Freeman.
48. DeGroot AD: *Thought and choice in chess*, New York, 1965, Basic Books.
49. Chase WG, Simon HA: Perception in chess, *Cogn Psychol* 4:55, 1973.
50. Chi MTH, Feltovich PJ, Glaser R: Categorization and representation of physics problems by experts and novices, *Cogn Sci* 5:121, 1981.
51. Rumelhart DE, Ortony E: The representation of knowledge in memory. In Anderson RC, Spiro RJ, Montague WE, editors: *Schooling and the acquisition of knowledge*, Hillsdale, NJ, 1977, Lawrence Erlbaum.
52. Mattingly C: What is clinical reasoning? *Am J Occup Ther* 45:979, 1991.
53. Maitland GD: The Maitland concept: assessment, examination, and treatment by passive movement. In Twomey LT, Taylor JR, editors: *Physical therapy of the low back*, ed 2, New York, 1994, Churchill Livingstone.

54. Boshiuzen HPA, Schmidt HG, Coughlin LD: On the application of medical basic science in clinical reasoning: implications for structural knowledge differences between experts and novices. In Patel VL, Groen GJ, editors: *Proceedings of the Tenth Annual Conference of the Cognitive Science Society,* August 17-19, 1988, Montreal, vol 59, Hillsdale, NJ, 1988, Lawrence Erlbaum Associates.
55. Boshuizen HPA, Schmidt HG: The development of clinical reasoning expertise: implications for teaching. In Higgs J, Jones MA, editors: *Clinical reasoning in the health professions,* ed 2, Oxford, England, 2000, Butterworth-Heinemann.
56. Schmidt HG, Boshuizen HPA, Norman GR: *Reflections on the nature of expertise in medicine.* In Keravnou E, editor: *Deep models for medical knowledge engineering,* Amsterdam, 1992, Elsevier Science Publishers.
57. Schmidt HG, Boshuizen HPA: On acquiring expertise in medicine, *Educ Psychol Rev* 5:205, 1993.
58. Fleming MH, Mattingly C: Action and narrative: two dynamics of clinical reasoning. In Higgs J, Jones MA, editors: *Clinical reasoning in the health professions,* ed 2, Oxford, England, 2000, Butterworth-Heinemann.
59. Patel VL, Kaufman DR: Clinical reasoning and biomedical knowledge: implications for teaching. In Higgs J, Jones MA, editors: *Clinical reasoning in the health professions,* ed 2, Oxford, England, 2000, Butterworth-Heinemann.
60. Patel VL, Groen GJ, Arocha JF: Medical expertise as a function of task difficulty, *Mem Cogn* 18:394, 1990.
61. Joseph GM, Patel VL: Domain knowledge and hypothesis generation in diagnostic reasoning, *Med Decision Making* 10:31, 1990.
62. Gifford LS: Tissue and input-related mechanisms. In: Gifford LS, editor: *Topical issues in pain, physiotherapy pain association yearbook,* Falmouth, United Kingdom, 1998, NOI Press.
63. Gifford LS: The "central" mechanisms. In: Gifford LS, editor: *Topical issues in pain, physiotherapy pain association yearbook,* Falmouth, United Kingdom, 1998, NOI Press.
64. Gifford LS: Output mechanisms. In: Gifford LS, editor: *Topical issues in pain, physiotherapy pain association yearbook,* Falmouth, United Kingdom, 1998, NOI Press.

CHAPTER 7

Examination of the Cervical and Thoracic Spine

Mary E. Magarey

Physical therapy examination of a patient with a cervical or thoracic spine disorder will have optimal benefit if based on an impairment approach rather than one related to specific structural diagnosis. Recent advances in the pain sciences have demonstrated that knowledge of the source of symptoms in many neuroorthopedic disorders is less definite than previously thought.[1] Therefore, in this chapter, an approach that allows detailed examination of the potential neural, muscular, skeletal, and soft tissue sources of symptoms, within the context of a broader consideration of patient dysfunction or disability, is presented. Interpretation of results of examination must be made in the context of the whole clinical picture, not simply that of the specific structures addressed. The rationale behind this approach is further outlined in Chapters 6 and 11 of this text and in the chapter "Clinical Reasoning in the Use of Manual Therapy Techniques for the Shoulder Girdle" from the text *Evaluation and Rehabilitation of the Shoulder*.[2]

The cervical and thoracic sections of the vertebral column are closely related functionally and anatomically and, in most instances, should be examined as a single unit. However, neuroorthopedic problems may present with a principal component in one section of the spine only, with possible predisposing factors in the other section. For ease of presentation, physical examination of the cervical and thoracic areas is approached separately, with reference when appropriate to the situations in which combined examination is indicated.

Clinical reasoning is the foundation of patient examination and management espoused in this text. This chapter should therefore be read in conjunction with Chapter 6. Perusal of the second edition of *Clinical Reasoning in the Health Professions* (Higgs and Jones, 2000)[3] is recommended for a broad review of clinical reasoning across the health professions and Chapter 12 of that text[4] for specific discussion on clinical reasoning in physical therapy.

Clinical reasoning is characterized by the adoption of several discrete but related hypothesis categories. These are clusters of related concepts. These hypothesis categories are further explained in Chapter 6 and include the following:

- Dysfunction-disability (physical or psychological and the associated social consequences)
- Pathobiological mechanisms

- Source of symptoms or dysfunction (often equated with diagnosis or impairment)
- Contributing factors
- Management
- Prognosis

The examination of any patient with symptoms of neuroorthopedic dysfunction has two main parts: (1) a questioning/interview section, in which hypotheses in the aforementioned categories are developed in the context of both physical and psychosocial aspects of the patient's presenting problem, and (2) a physical examination section, in which hypotheses developed during the interview are further examined. Both aspects of the evaluation are of equal importance in establishing a global picture of the patient's problems and therefore the most appropriate direction of management. The specific clinical decisions regarding structural examination of the cervicothoracic spine must be made in the broader context of understanding the patient's functional problems, the dominant pathobiological mechanisms, the source of the symptoms, factors contributing to the development and maintenance of the problem, precautions to physical therapy examination and management, and prognosis.

SUBJECTIVE EXAMINATION

The aim of the interview, or subjective examination, is to determine the problems from the patient's perspective, interpreted in a way that allows an appropriate physical examination within the context of the whole clinical picture. Although the interview is individualized to enable the therapist to form hypotheses in the categories mentioned, some standard scanning questions are essential, and for the sake of efficiency, some basic routine in the interview process is advisable. However, spontaneity of response, with its provision of valuable information, may be lost if the interview becomes too structured. The skilled examiner is able to allow more freedom in the interview, thereby providing opportunity for such spontaneity.

To place the patient's problems into an appropriate context, the initial part of the interview should consist of inquiry about the patient's personal profile. Such a profile includes information about the person's age; the status in terms of long-term relationships; the family situation in which the patient lives; the patient's occupation, interests, and hobbies; and any issues of particular concern to the patient or that might influence a painful presentation. The patient may consider some of this information personal and irrelevant to the neck problem. However, the context in which the patient's problem occurs has an influence on the way in which that patient will respond to the problem and therefore is of considerable interest to the examining therapist. This should be explained to the patient. Some of the more personal information may not be elicited until later in the examination process, however, by which time the patient has had the opportunity to develop a rapport with the therapist.

In most situations an early priority is to establish the patient's functional limitations and/or disability (dysfunction), allowing the patient to report his or her problems, including the patient's understanding of and feeling about those problems and the effect they are having on the patient's life. Inquiry in this direction provides the opportunity for good communication between therapist and patient. This early information also provides a keen opportunity to form initial hypotheses related to pathobiological mechanisms, source of symptoms or dysfunction, and potentially, management and prognosis. It also allows the therapist to recognize so-called yellow flags, or psychosocial features, often associated with development or perpetuation of long-term disability.[5]

SITE, CHARACTER, DEPTH, AND SEVERITY OF THE SYMPTOMS

The significance placed on the site of symptoms and the precision with which that site should be identified depends on the pathobiological mechanism hypothesized.[1] The precise site of symptoms is of less significance in a central neural processing problem than in an input dominant presentation. However, the site of symptoms should indicate a number of possible initial hypotheses in relation to a source that can then be further developed as additional information is gained. Therefore, in most situations, a detailed analysis of the site of a patient's symptoms should be obtained. This information is best represented pictorially on a body chart, which also can be used to indicate the character, depth, constancy, and severity of the symptoms (Figure 7-1). These additional factors further assist in developing hypotheses because predictable patterns associated with particular disorders are common. All symptoms are recorded on the body chart, even when apparently unrelated to the principal problem. Such symptoms may provide indications of neural processing disorders or biomechanically

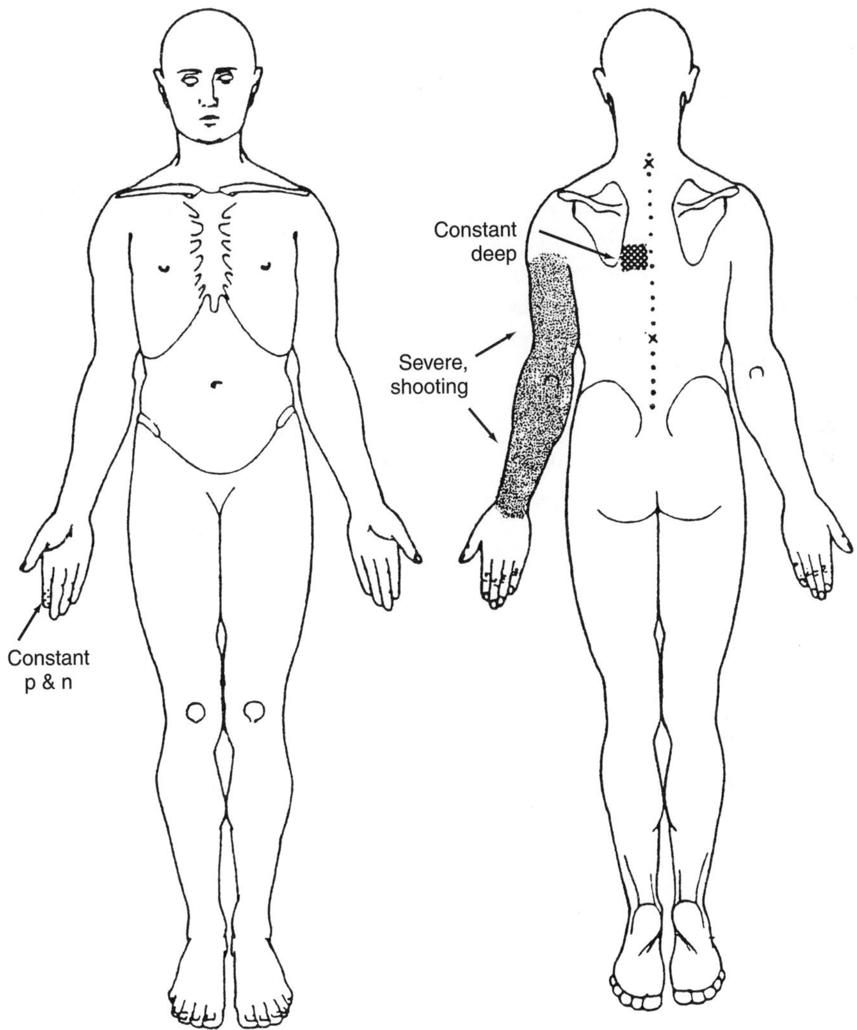

Figure 7-1
Body chart illustrating symptoms typical of a C7 disc lesion with nerve root compression.

linked input and output disorders with no somatic connection. Absence of symptoms in other areas also should be indicated on the body chart; such recording is important medicolegally.

In the example given in Figure 7-1, constant deep pain near the medial border of the scapula adjacent to the T7 spinous process may implicate the C6 to C7 intervertebral disc[6]; severe, shooting pain on the posterior aspect of the arm and forearm with constant paresthesia of the tip of the index finger might implicate the C7 nerve root. The severity of the pain coupled with its constancy would indicate an acute disorder. Similarly, some factor responsible for the symptoms is unrelenting despite the mechanical variations in position and stress from the day's activities, thus providing supporting evidence for the presence of an inflammatory process. The physical therapist viewing the body chart should immediately consider an acute C6 to C7 disc disorder causing compression or irritation of the C7 nerve root as the most likely source of this patient's symptoms and should direct further questioning toward confirming or disproving this hypothesis. Innervation and pain patterns of the cervical and thoracic spine (see Chapters 4 and 5) should be read in conjunction with this section.

The character of symptoms, particularly pain, may help to identify their source because specific structures and systems often appear to produce typical types of pain. For example, the pain from an acute nerve root irritation tends to be severe, burning, shooting, and unrelenting, whereas chronic nerve root pain often is described as "annoying, nagging, of nuisance value." The same kind of words tend to be used by different patients to describe pain that appears to be from a similar source.

A similar situation arises with depth. Although the patient's estimation of the depth of symptoms need bear no relation to the actual depth of their source, the descriptions given again tend to be consistent between patients. Pain appearing to arise from the intervertebral disc is described as deep, whereas local zygapophyseal joint pain tends to be more superficial—"I can put my finger right on it."

The severity of the symptoms can be a guide to the state of the disorder, but because many factors are responsible for an individual's perception of pain, severity is most useful as an indicator of the degree of functional restriction imposed by the symptoms. The perceived severity and that assessed by the physical therapist during the interview may not correlate, thereby providing valuable information in the hypothesis category of pathobiological mechanisms, possibly giving a clue to the presence of an affective component. Knowledge of the severity of the symptoms, coupled with information regarding the patient's behavior, helps determine the detail in which the patient can safely be examined at the first visit.

Behavior of Symptoms

The way in which symptoms behave during the day and their response to activity provides the physical therapist with information related to all hypothesis categories.

Mechanical Stimuli. Symptoms that respond to mechanical stimuli in a predictable manner usually are considered to have a mechanical cause. For example, if pain is provoked each time the patient turns and is relieved by returning to a neutral position, the pain can be assumed to be a result of mechanical stress related to turning. Zusman[1] warned of the danger of placing too much emphasis on attribution of structural sources to symptoms that are mechanically evoked, as a result of the intricate and complex interconnections and potential for altered responses in the spinal and supraspinal neuron pools. Consequently, the therapist should always be aware of the potential for a clinical reasoning error in this regard.

Symptoms that show no predictable response to mechanical stimuli are unlikely to be mechanical in origin, and their presence should alert the therapist to the possibility of a more sinister disorder or one with a central processing component. For example, constant cervical pain unaltered by rest or activity may be inflammatory in origin. Such information should strongly influence further assessment and management of the patient.

Night Pain. Symptoms of mechanical origin may worsen initially on retiring but usually are relieved by rest and therefore will be less severe on waking in the morning. The exceptions are those mechanical disorders aggravated by postures adopted or movements taking place during sleep. If sleeping posture or movement is a problem, the patient may waken with pain, eased quickly with a change of position. Symptoms of inflammatory origin are unrelieved and in fact are frequently worsened by rest, so the patient has difficulty sleeping and often needs to get out of bed and move around to gain relief. Rising in the morning is difficult because of stiffness, usually with associated discomfort, and both symptoms may take several hours to ease.

24-Hour Pattern. Establishing the pattern followed by the symptoms during a 24-hour period provides information about the functional limitations imposed by the disorder, the response to mechanical stimuli, and the presence of different components of the problem, in particular, any inflammatory component, in addition to any other factors contributing to production or continuation of the symptoms. It also provides an indication of the predictability of symptoms, thereby assisting formation of hypotheses about mechanisms and approach to examination and management. The severity and irritability of the disorder also can be established, providing additional information related to precautions and contraindications, management, and prognosis. Knowing the type of activities or postures that aggravate and ease the symptoms provides information related to the source and may identify possible management strategies. A zygapophyseal joint pattern, for example, may be compressive, with symptoms provoked on extension or ipsilateral flexion movements, or distractive, with flexion and contralateral flexion implicated.

Routine Screening Questions. A number of activities or postures can provide useful information about potential sources of symptoms within the cervicothoracic region, and therefore screening to cover these should be included routinely if the patient does not identify the activities spontaneously. For the cervical region, these include the following:

- Activities involving sustained flexion, such as reading, computer work, driving, and handcrafts
- Return from a flexed position, particularly after sustained flexion
- Effect of different speeds of movement
- Effect of the weight of the head—particularly relevant in acute injuries, when a patient often will describe a sensation of the head feeling too heavy and relief of symptoms only when supine
- Activities involving cervical extension, such as hanging clothes, shaving, and hair washing in a hairdresser's washbasin
- Activities involving rotation, such as turning the body when driving the car in reverse
- Use of the upper limb, such as reaching, and pushing or pulling
- Effect of thoracic or lumbar and lower limb posture (e.g., a long-sitting position)
- Effect of carrying loads in the arms or of carrying a bag over the shoulder

For the upper cervical spine, other particularly useful features that should be routinely screened for include the following:
- Headache or earache
- Tinnitus
- Symptoms in the face, jaw, or mouth
- Any symptoms associated with dysfunction of the vertebrobasilar system (see Chapter 8)

In the thoracic spine, other features that should be routinely screened for include the following:
- Effect of breathing, particularly of taking a deep breath, and the effect of sneezing, coughing, or wheezing
- Presence and behavior of any upper-limb dysfunction or pain
- Activities involving trunk rotation, such as reaching for the drawer in a desk and reaching into the back of the car
- Activities involving sustained trunk flexion, such as computer work, desk work, and driving
- Sympathetic function, such as altered sweating, temperature control of the limbs, palpitations, heaviness in the arms, or sensations of swelling in the limbs
- Symptoms related to visceral disorders, such as duodenal ulcer or gastric reflux (The excellent text by Boissonnault[7] on screening for medical disease is recommended to provide further information on this important aspect of examination.)

PRECAUTIONS AND CONTRAINDICATIONS TO TREATMENT BY PHYSICAL MODALITIES

Scanning questions related to precautions and contraindications to examination or treatment by physical modalities should be asked routinely with every patient. The specific relevant information is outlined here. Adequate recording of the responses to the individual questions is important medicolegally, in addition to its significance to patient safety.

Structural Stability of the Source of the Symptoms or Adjacent Structures.

Any indication of structural instability, such as may be present after a rear-end motor vehicle collision, clearly indicates a need for caution in examination and management because stress placed on an unstable segment may lead to compromise to adjacent neural or vascular structures. Hypermobility of the craniovertebral junction has been described by Aspinall.[8] The subjective complaints and clinical signs potentially indicating the presence of craniovertebral hypermobility or instability were identified as follows:
- Occipital numbness or paraesthesia, which may indicate trespass on the second cervical nerve root
- Symptoms of vertebrobasilar insufficiency (VBI) (see Chapter 8)
- Signs of spinal cord compromise:
  - —Delayed myelopathy ranging from paraparesis to Brown-Séquard's syndrome
  - —Dysesthesia in the hands, with clumsiness and weakness of the lower limbs or spastic weakness of the lower limbs with slight general wasting and hyperreflexia
  - —Ankle clonus and extensor plantar reflexes
  - —Difficulty with walking and possible effects on sphincter control
  - —History of recent upper cervical or cranial trauma, or unguarded movement
  - —Marked inability to resist upper cervical flexion or extension
  - —Increased range of contralateral rotation after a traumatic injury involving flexion and rotation, in which the alar ligaments may be stretched

Because cardiac and respiratory centers lie at the level of the atlas, craniovertebral instability is potentially life-threatening. Consequently, inquiry about these symptoms or historical features is an important component of the interview. Instability also may occur at the C4-5 or C5-6 levels often associated with hypomobility of the cervicothoracic junction and a forward head posture, particularly if trauma such as rear-end motor vehicle collision is superimposed.[9]

Evidence of structural instability may be seen on diagnostic imaging, indicating the need for caution. Plain radiographs, however, may not demonstrate craniovertebral hypermobility, with computed tomography (CT) or magnetic resonance imaging (MRI) the more reliable assessment.

Integrity of Vital Structures. Determining the integrity of vital structures in the area (in particular, the vertebrobasilar and carotid arterial systems and the spinal cord) is vital. The vertebrobasilar system is covered in Chapter 8, which should be read in conjunction with this chapter. Insufficiency of the carotid system may be indicated by symptoms related to its area of supply, which is greater and more diversified than that of the vertebrobasilar system. There is even less potential for compromise to the carotid system than the vertebrobasilar system in management of the cervical spine, but symptoms indicating its involvement should still be considered a potential for caution, particularly in relation to anterior cervical examination.

Loss of integrity of the spinal cord is likely to be manifested initially by the presence of bilateral paresthesia or anesthesia of the hands or feet, with the altered sensation presenting in a glove or stocking distribution. Hypertonicity may lead to unsteadiness or clumsiness of gait or other physical tasks.

General Health of the Subject. General health questions provide information about the status of the cardiopulmonary system and the presence or absence of systemic diseases or illness (e.g., diabetes mellitus or cancer). Smoking and alcohol or other recreational drug history can provide an indication of general tissue health, important because of its impact on the neuroendocrine system (see Chapter 15). Past medical history may be relevant, particularly in the cervical area, where juvenile rheumatoid arthritis or rheumatic fever may lead to weakening of upper cervical ligaments. A history of previous cancer may alert the therapist to the possibility of secondary deposits in bone. Previous radiotherapy, for the treatment of carcinoma of the breast, for example, may result in localized sternal and costal osteoporosis. Systemic diseases such as ankylosing spondylitis also may lead to ligamentous weakening in the upper cervical spine. In women, inquiry as to menstrual status is relevant because of the reduction in bone mineral density associated with menopause.

Pharmacological Status. The pharmacological status of the patient should be determined, particularly in relation to the following medications:

- *Oral steroids*—prolonged use of corticosteroids may lead to a decrease in bone density. Even use of corticosteroids many years in the past can lead to long-term bone density loss, the significance of which depends on the pretreatment density level.
- *Anticoagulant medication*—the use of anticoagulants will lead to a reduction in clotting ability. Consequently, firm techniques may cause bruising or hemarthrosis.
- *Aspirin*—even small doses of aspirin in the 2 weeks before examination create a degree of anticoagulant effect. Therefore care should be taken with any firm technique.
- *Analgesics*—analgesic agents may mask potentially harmful effects of physical examination and management by reducing perception of pain. Conversely, if a patient is

in considerable pain, appropriate use of these drugs may enhance treatment, allowing more rapid progression than would otherwise be possible.

- *Nonsteroidal antiinflammatory drugs (NSAIDs)*—the antiinflammatory effect of NSAIDs may mask harmful effects of physical evaluation and management in a manner similar to that possible with analgesics. However, the response to NSAIDs also provides an indication of the degree of inflammation associated with the disorder and therefore also provides some indication of appropriate management and prognosis. In contrast, some disorders can tolerate and benefit from physical treatment only if it is undertaken with a cover of NSAIDs or analgesics.
- *Hormone replacement therapy*—the use of hormones will affect bone mineral density in postmenopausal women and may have other neuroendocrine effects.
- *Recreational drug use*—because many recreational drugs have central nervous system effects, they may lead to altered pain perception.

Medical Evaluation of the Patient. Knowledge of the degree of medical evaluation undertaken is of value to the therapist. The results of diagnostic imaging may provide indications of structural problems requiring caution. With the advent of sophisticated methods of diagnostic imaging, inquiry simply about plain radiographs is inadequate. Scanning questions should include CT, MRI, or bone scans and the films and radiological reports viewed if possible. Blood tests, nerve function tests, Doppler studies, and myelograms and their results provide an indication of the significance placed on the symptoms by the medical practitioner, and favorable results of such tests strengthen the confidence with which the physical therapist can approach examination and management.

Information from the subjective examination provides an evolving clinical picture in which supporting and negating evidence leads to continuing modification of the initial and subsequent hypotheses.

HISTORY

The timing of history taking can be crucial to the understanding of a problem and to efficient time management. If a disorder is of recent or sudden onset and the symptoms are severe, taking the history immediately after establishing the patient's main problem is beneficial, whereas knowledge of behavior and area of symptoms in a patient with a chronic condition makes history taking more succinct. Having gained some insight into the problem, the examiner is better able to recognize the significant information in the history. Similarly, in most instances, taking the history of the current problem before that of previous episodes also is advisable because irrelevant information from the past history then can be sifted. The detail in which the intervening period is investigated depends on the type of problem and the relationship between the initial episode and the present symptoms.

In addition to the history of symptoms related to the present problem, inquiry into previous symptoms and traumatic episodes may be relevant, particularly if there are indications of altered central processing. The presenting symptoms may be part of a multiple crush phenomenon,[10] in which the history, characteristics, behavior, and response to treatment of previous problems may provide useful clues to the potential cause of the current problem.

The history should be taken in considerable detail, determining both the mechanism of injury, if traumatic, and the presence of any possible predisposing factors. The relationship between local and referred or radicular symptoms, or two different areas or types of symptoms, and the severity and nature of the patient's pathological condition may be determined in part by the history of each symptom relative to the others. The skill and importance of history taking have been discussed comprehensively by Maitland.[11]

PLANNING THE PHYSICAL EXAMINATION

On completion of the subjective examination, the therapist has reached a series of working hypotheses related to the various categories indicating the structures requiring examination. In addition, the need for specific testing related to precautionary factors, such as VBI, is identified and a decision made about the extent of examination that can be performed without exacerbation of the patient's disorder.

LIMITED EXAMINATION

A decision to limit the physical examination is made on the basis of any subjective features that indicate the need for caution. These features include the following:

- Severity or "irritability" of the disorder
- Symptoms that are worsening
- History of recent traumatic onset of symptoms
- Subjective evidence of potential involvement of vital structures, such as the vertebrobasilar system, the spinal cord, or nerve roots
- History of systemic disorders or general health considerations that may lead to alteration in integrity of the structures to be examined (e.g., underlying rheumatoid arthritis)
- History of corticosteroid use and current use of aspirin or anticoagulant medication
- Indications that the symptoms do not behave in a predictable pattern, and therefore response to examination procedures is likely to be unpredictable
- Indication of a significant affective component to the disorder, in which case extensive physical examination may exacerbate both the physical and affective components of the problem
- Indications of potential structural instability

The concept of irritability is one related to the ease of exacerbation of symptoms, the severity of symptoms provoked, and the time taken for them to subside. Irritability presents as a continuum, from the very irritable condition in which minimal movement provokes severe pain that takes a long time to settle to minor discomfort that is aggravated only by prolonged activity and that settles within minutes of cessation of the activity. Limiting examination to prevent exacerbation of highly irritable symptoms allows the possibility of treatment successfully directed at reducing pain within the first visit.

If provocation of symptoms is the reason for limiting evaluation, examination procedures should be limited to the point of onset of symptoms or initial exacerbation of resting symptoms (termed P_1). In addition, return to the resting level of symptoms should be ensured before proceeding to the next examination procedure. If symptoms do not settle, further examination should be omitted. A movement found to relieve symptoms may be further examined with the addition of other movements in different combinations to determine whether a particular combination may be useful as a treatment technique (see Chapter 9).

All examination procedures should be limited using these same principles. For example, if muscle contraction increases pain, that aspect of a neurological examination should be omitted. Similarly, if indications were present of potential VBI but full range of active rotation was not possible, full VBI evaluation should be deferred until the range of movement is increased and levels of symptoms reduced. Passive examination also should be modified, perhaps performed only with the patient supine and with additional support to ensure a pain-free resting position. The depth and extent of such an examination should follow the same principles as those that apply to active examination procedures.

When examination is limited by potential structural or general health considerations, a movement should not be taken to full range and overpressure applied, even if that movement provokes no symptoms. Consequently, examination may be limited not by the onset of symptoms but by the onset of tissue resistance or its absence when it should be present. If pain were also a significant factor, the onset of either pain or tissue resistance would determine the extent of each examination procedure. All aspects of the examination need to be limited in the same way.

Similarly, examination limited on the basis of symptoms related to the spinal cord or vascular systems should not go further than the initial onset of the specific symptoms. In this situation, full examination in certain directions may be safe and appropriate if symptoms are not reproduced, whereas movements in other directions must be limited either by the onset of symptoms or soft tissue resistance. An example is a patient who experiences severe dizziness only when looking upward. Examination of cervical extension in isolation or when combined with other movements should be performed with extreme care not to provoke dizziness, whereas other nonprovocative movements may be examined fully.

Although limited examination does not provide the physical therapist with knowledge about the behavior of pain, tissue resistance, or muscle spasm beyond the point at which the examination procedure was abandoned, information can still be gained about the relative involvement of the joint, muscular, neural, or vascular systems without aggravation of the symptoms. Therefore initiation of treatment is possible in a symptom-free, safe environment at the first consultation—a major priority. The additional information can be obtained as the symptoms settle and examination can be taken further. However, when examination is limited as a result of structural or health-related issues, treatment must continue to be restricted to those procedures that can be performed safely within the limitations of the relevant features.

Full Examination

All examination procedures may be taken to their fullest extent. If routine procedures are inadequate to provide the necessary information, examination may be taken further (e.g., with the addition of compression to movement, movements performed at speed, movements sustained at the limit, or combinations of movements). Such an evaluation is possible if the subjective examination has indicated that no exacerbation of symptoms is likely because the condition is not irritable or severe, the nature and progression are stable and predictable, and no other precautionary factors are present. With optimal information about the mechanisms, source of the symptoms, and predisposing or contributing factors, the choice of treatment and priority of each factor in management can be made with considerable confidence.

During examination, the relative significance of symptoms provoked at the limit of range and their relationship to soft tissue resistance (i.e., the degree of stiffness) can be determined by comparison with the physical therapist's knowledge of normal and comparison with the contralateral movement. For a movement of the spine to be considered normal, full gross and intersegmental range must be present, with overpressure provoking the same amount of discomfort and demonstrating the same pattern of ligamentous tightening as the corresponding contralateral movement or as would be expected for the patient's age and somatotype.

Despite the freedom to examine all components fully, some priorities must be set, because one consultation often does not provide enough time for such a detailed assessment. Consequently, the physical therapist must decide on which features are to be examined as high priority and which can be left until the following consultations. The decision on the direction of examination is determined by the balance of information gained during the subjective examination. Often those features related to the hypothesis category of source are likely to receive highest priority, whereas examination of those related to contributing or predisposing factors may be delayed. Features related to treatment safety should always be examined at the first consultation.

However, in some situations the evidence is strong that the contributing factors, such as poor dynamic control and posture, are the key features of the presenting problem. In this case the examination would be more appropriately directed at muscle function and patient awareness of posture rather than at the specific structures likely to be responsible for production of pain. Equally, if the psychosocial elements of a problem appear dominant, addressing those before the physical components also would be appropriate.

Although two distinct categories have been described for clarity, the decision as to the extent of examination is based on the reasoning process undertaken throughout the subjective examination and may involve a combination of these categories, in which some test procedures may be examined fully and others are restricted or omitted—in reality, this is a continuum rather than separate categories.

PHYSICAL EXAMINATION

The physical examination should be a continuation of the clinical reasoning process undertaken during the subjective examination rather than an indiscriminate application of a standardized set of procedures. Although core examination procedures are undertaken with most patients, within the limitations of appropriate examination, the physical examination should be individualized, thus providing an assessment specific for each patient. The physical therapist should continue the process of hypothesis testing of all categories, with the examination findings either confirming or negating the hypotheses and providing useful clues to appropriate management.

Jones and Jones[12] provided an excellent presentation on the principles of the physical examination, and this should be read in conjunction with this chapter. Here the particular examination procedures relevant to the cervical and thoracic spine are presented. However, those structures and systems extrinsic to the local area that could contribute to the disorder in the cervicothoracic region also must be considered and examined in sufficient depth to determine their involvement.

If physical examination is to fulfill its aim of determining an appropriate management decision, the physical therapist must be aware of the clinical patterns commonly seen in patients with symptoms in the cervical or thoracic area or those to which these spinal regions can refer, either somatically or autonomically. However, maintenance of an open mind and use of reflective reasoning in addition to recognition of clinical patterns allows recognition of new patterns and variations of those already known.

Consideration of systems (e.g., the muscular or neural systems) and their influence on presentation rather than simply on particular structures is important with all patients but is particularly relevant to those in whom a central processing abnormality is suspected. In these situations, such consideration takes a higher priority than it does in an acute nociceptive presentation.[9,13] With every patient, extensive detail of examination is necessary if subtle variations in clinical patterns and new patterns are to be recognized.[12]

Structures to be Examined

In the cervical and thoracic areas, all potential sources implicated during the subjective examination should be tested during the physical examination. These include the following:

- All structures underlying the area of symptoms
- All structures that can refer to the area of symptoms
- All structures that could potentially be implicated in the production of the symptoms

All potential contributing factors implicated during the subjective examination also should be tested. These include the following:

- All structures that can mechanically affect other structures, thereby contributing to symptom production (e.g., weakness of upper cervical flexors and tightness of upper cervical extensors leading to a forward head posture and development of symptoms in the cervicothoracic junction)
- All structures that can affect symptom production either chemically or nutritionally from sites remote from the symptomatic area (e.g., vascular compromise or chemical effects in the nervous system, such as the double crush phenomenon)[10]

Consequently, although the focus of this chapter is on the cervical and thoracic portions of the spine, potentially, the entire body may need to be assessed to determine other factors possibly contributing to cervical or thoracic symptoms. Among these possible factors are altered pelvic and lower limb biomechanics that could potentially lead to the development of abnormal cervical posture with associated abnormal neural, biomechanical or chemical responses.

To reach a confident differential physical diagnosis, evaluation of those structures less likely to be involved is as important as that of the most likely sources. Accordingly, knowledge of lack of involvement is as important in the decision-making process as knowledge of involvement. However, the examination still should be directed as appropriate for the individual patient rather than follow a recipe-type approach.

Physical Signs of Potential Involvement

Many physical signs, interpreted in relation to the patient's age and somatotype, may alert the physical therapist to the involvement of the structure in the production of symptoms. These include the following:

- Abnormal appearance (e.g., bony asymmetry, muscle contours, and trophic changes)
- Abnormal movement (functional, active, passive, and resistive)
- Abnormal feel on palpation (e.g., temperature, swelling, thickening, and tightness)

The potential involvement of a structure is strengthened if any of the following occur:

- Alteration of the abnormality (e.g., asymmetry or pattern of movement) affects the patient's symptoms.
- Direct or indirect stress on a structure reproduces the patient's symptoms.
- Direct or indirect stress on a structure capable of referring symptoms, either somatically or autonomically, to the symptomatic area demonstrates abnormality of that structure (e.g., hypomobility and local pain on stress of the Occ to C1 joint in a patient with unilateral headaches).

- Direct or indirect stress on a structure capable of contributing to the predisposition of symptom development demonstrates abnormality of that structure (e.g., tightness of upper trapezius in a patient complaining of cervical pain).

Reproduction of symptoms by direct or indirect stress of structures implicated is not essential and in many cases, unlikely. Demonstration of an abnormality in the implicated structure is sufficient, and the relevance of that abnormality to the disorder will be determined during management. Understanding the relationship between posture, movement, and symptoms and their association with pathophysiology and pathomechanics assists in determining the relative importance of physical abnormalities. Consequently, continual assessment of these relationships during examination is essential, and their interpretation in relation to the hypotheses is a significant clinical skill.

Components of the Physical Examination

The components of the physical examination of the cervical or thoracic spine include observation of the patient, both during the subjective examination and, more formally, during the physical examination, and analysis of the following:

- Posture
- Patient's most symptom-provoking activity from a functional perspective
- Physiological movements, both active and passive
- Passive accessory movements
- Soft tissue texture and extensibility
- Conduction in and mobility of the nervous system
- Muscle performance
- Conduction in the vascular system
- Upper extremities
- Viscera

Assessment of the lumbar spine, pelvis, and lower extremities may be necessary as part of an evaluation of factors contributing to the production of symptoms in the neck or thoracic region.

Each component of the physical examination offers opportunities to test the hypotheses developed during the subjective examination; the information gained will lead to modification of existing hypotheses or the development of new ones.

Observation and Posture. The patient's cervical and thoracic posture and willingness to move should be observed while the patient is undressing and during the subjective examination. The patient should be undressed sufficiently that the spine, shoulder girdles, upper limbs, and trunk are readily visible; preferably the lower extremities also are visible while an evaluation of posture is undertaken. If a patient is uncomfortable with such physical exposure, a gown that allows limited exposure without causing the sense of compromise of personal comfort should be available. For an initial assessment of posture, the patient should be viewed in the standing position so that an indication of the total body posture can be gained, including the potential involvement of abnormal lower body posture as a predisposing factor to the development of cervical or thoracic symptoms.

Posture should be viewed from in front, behind, and laterally. The position of the head on neck, neck on thorax, scapular position, and thoracic kyphosis may be observed in the frontal plane, making sure that the patient's hair does not obscure the contour of the neck. The degree of lumbar lordosis, particularly relative to the thoracic kyphosis, general contour of abdomen and buttocks, pelvic posture, and the degree of hyperextension of the knees also can be assessed. In the sagittal plane posteriorly, the symmetry of the head, the position of the spinous processes and shoulder girdles, the symmetry and degree of development or tightness of the posterior muscle groups, and the amount of rotation of the arms can be seen. Anteriorly, the symmetry of the head and neck position; the bony symmetry of the chest; the symmetry of development; the tone and tightness of anterior muscle groups; the height of the nipples and the position of the umbilicus may be assessed.

Assessment of the patient's posture in sitting also is relevant because many functional activities are undertaken in the sitting position and the therapist can start to develop an impression of habitual functional postures and movements. For example, a patient may stand well during formal assessment of posture, such that little abnormality is detected, but immediately may adopt a slumped, flexed posture in sitting. If the patient's occupation involves extended periods of sitting at a computer, for instance, such an habitual flexed posture could be highly relevant to the provocation of cervicothoracic symptoms.

Although technically a component of active examination, evaluation of the patient while walking allows identification of the patient's general movement patterns, providing valuable information about involvement of movement of the cervicothoracic region in the function. An example of when this is useful is the patient with a severe headache who holds the head, cervical spine, and to a lesser extent, the thoracic spine rigid during walking in an attempt to not aggravate the head pain. Such an antalgic movement pattern becomes a valuable reassessment tool as the severity of the headache is reduced. A further example is the patient who appears to lead with the head during gait, demonstrating excessive upper cervical extensor activity that is often associated with overactive levator scapulae and apparently lengthened underactive trapezii. Viewing this movement pattern provides useful clues to factors contributing to the patient's cervicothoracic symptoms.

ACTIVE EXAMINATION

Analysis of the Functional Provoking Activity and Differentiation of Movements

If the patient can reproduce the symptoms with a particular movement, activity, or posture, that factor should be analyzed. Functional activities consist of combinations of different movements that can be examined initially in isolation and then in different combinations in an attempt to determine the principal provocative component. An example is a tennis player with midthoracic pain at late cocking and early acceleration of a serve. At this point in the swing, the player's thoracic spine is likely to be in a position of extension with rotation toward and lateral flexion away from the serving arm. Either limitation of any components or a combination of those components may be the cause of the pain. With the patient adopting the position of discomfort, the therapist increases each component of the provoking activity individually while assessing any alteration of symptoms. Thoracic rotation in neutral position may be pain free, but when performed with the spine already in extension and lateral flexion, it may provoke pain. Further analysis related to the potential involvement of the nervous system in the production of symptoms during the serve may be tested by placing the arm in the serving position of late cocking (i.e., shoulder abduction, extension, and lateral rotation) and altering the position either of the wrist and hand or the elbow to determine whether these maneuvers alter the thoracic symptoms. Once the patient is in a position that provokes pain, very little alteration of a component, if relevant, is likely to alter the symptoms.

Similar principles of differentiation may be applied to any movement that provokes symptoms and involves more than one structure or system that may be implicated. Differentiation may take several forms, including the following:

- Taking the combined movement to the point of production of symptoms, maintaining one component and altering the other such that the stress on one is increased with a corresponding decrease in the other. For example, if combined cervical and thoracic rotation provokes pain, the movement can be held at a point in range where pain is produced. The trunk is then rotated slightly further, increasing the stress on thoracic rotation but decreasing stress on cervical rotation. The response to this procedure may be confirmed by derotating the shoulder girdle, leading to a decrease in stress on thoracic rotation and a corresponding increase on cervical rotation.
- Examining one of the implicated movements while the other is maintained in a neutral position and comparing the symptom response with that from similar examination of the other implicated movement. For example, if combined cervical and thoracic rotation is painful, the symptom response to thoracic rotation can be compared with that to cervical rotation. This procedure and the one above are often used together, with one procedure confirming the response found in the other.
- Moving of a noninvolved structure, which may be added to a painful position or movement to determine the involvement of other systems, particularly the nervous system, in the production of symptoms. The example of addition of wrist and finger extension to the arm position during the act of serving in tennis falls into this category.
- If a joint is implicated, differentiating an intraarticular or periarticular source by examining of a movement both with and without the application of compression across the joint surfaces. If pain on movement is exacerbated by the addition of minor joint compression, intraarticular structures are implicated. The specific structures involved are not yet known, but possible explanations have been proposed.[14]

Analysis of a provoking factor and differentiation of movement in this way can assist in determining the source of the symptoms and in directing the remainder of the examination appropriately. If the symptoms can be reproduced, the movements most significant to the patient's problem are determined, and further examination can be directed in more detail toward them rather than toward other less significant aspects of evaluation. The information gained also can be useful in the selection of management strategies, and the provoking factor then becomes a valuable reassessment test. However, if the condition is severe or irritable, examination of the provoking factor may be omitted or assessed taking each component only to the onset of symptoms.

Active Physiological Movements

The standard movements to be examined in the cervical or thoracic region are flexion, extension, lateral flexion, and rotation. If the examination is to be limited, particularly by the onset of pain, the procedure must be explained to the patient beforehand because cooperation is necessary to avoid the exacerbation of symptoms. Determination of gross range of physiological movement and the provocation, or lack of provocation, of symptoms is inadequate during either a limited or full examination. Details of symptoms at rest, the quality of active movement, and the relationship between changes in symptoms and quality and range of movement provide useful information. If a movement is limited by pain (or other symptoms), the therapist should note the range and quality of movement, return the spine to a neutral position, and clarify the site and character of the symptoms produced. If a movement is full range and pain free or restricted but pain free, overpressure should be applied. Overpressure may stress the whole cervical or thoracic spine or different portions separately, depending on which is relevant to the particular patient. The relationship between symptoms and soft tissue resistance is assessed during application of passive overpressure. To simplify the text that follows, all test movements are described assuming that they can be taken to the end of range and that overpressure can be applied.

Cervical Spine. When examining routine active cervical movements, the patient should be sitting with the thighs fully supported, arms resting comfortably on the thighs, and shoulders relaxed. The lumbar and thoracic spine should be in a relatively neutral but comfortable position for a routine assessment. The benefits of this standard positioning for examination are consistency for later reevaluation and stability and comfort for the patient. All movements should be observed from in front of the patient to note any deviation that occurs with the movement (e.g., any lateral flexion or rotation associated with flexion or extension), as well as from the side to note the gross range and intersegmental movement, particularly that of the upper (head on neck) and lower (neck on thorax) cervical regions. Movement of the whole cervical spine should be examined first, with movement isolated to the upper or lower portions later if indicated. Overpressure also may isolate the upper or lower portion depending on its relevance to a particular patient (Figure 7-2).

Thoracic Spine. Movements of the thoracic spine should be observed both from behind the patient to note any deviation that occurs with the movement and to observe intersegmental movement and from the side to observe gross and intersegmental range of movement.

Upper Thoracic Spine (T1 to T4). The upper thoracic area is examined in the same way as the low cervical spine, with overpressure localizing the movement. If the patient's problem is one that is difficult to reproduce and overpressure to low cervical movements alone demonstrates no abnormality, these movements may need to be combined with those of the thoracic spine to put sufficient stress on the joint at fault to reproduce symptoms.

Midthoracic Spine (T4 to T8). The midthoracic area is examined with the patient sitting, thighs fully supported. Flexion and extension are examined with the patient's hands clasped behind the cervicothoracic junction and elbows together. *Flexion* involves approximation of elbows to groin, creating a bowing effect that is further emphasized by the direction of overpressure (Figure 7-3). Lumbar extension should be kept to a minimum during examination of thoracic *extension*, which is then easier to localize. Overpressure should localize the movement to individual intervertebral levels (Figure 7-4).

Lateral flexion also is examined with the hands linked behind the cervicothoracic junction, this time with elbows in the frontal plane. Again, lumbar movement should be minimized so that thoracic lateral flexion is emphasized. Overpressure on the angle of each rib further localizes the movement (Figure 7-5).

Rotation of the midthoracic spine is maximal with the spine in flexion. Rotation with the spine in neutral occurs more in the low thoracic area. Therefore midthoracic rotation is examined by asking the patient to rotate while in flexion; for example, "Bend under my arm" while the therapist holds the patient's shoulders. This movement is best performed with the patient's arms folded across the chest. Overpressure is applied through the shoulders (Figure 7-6).

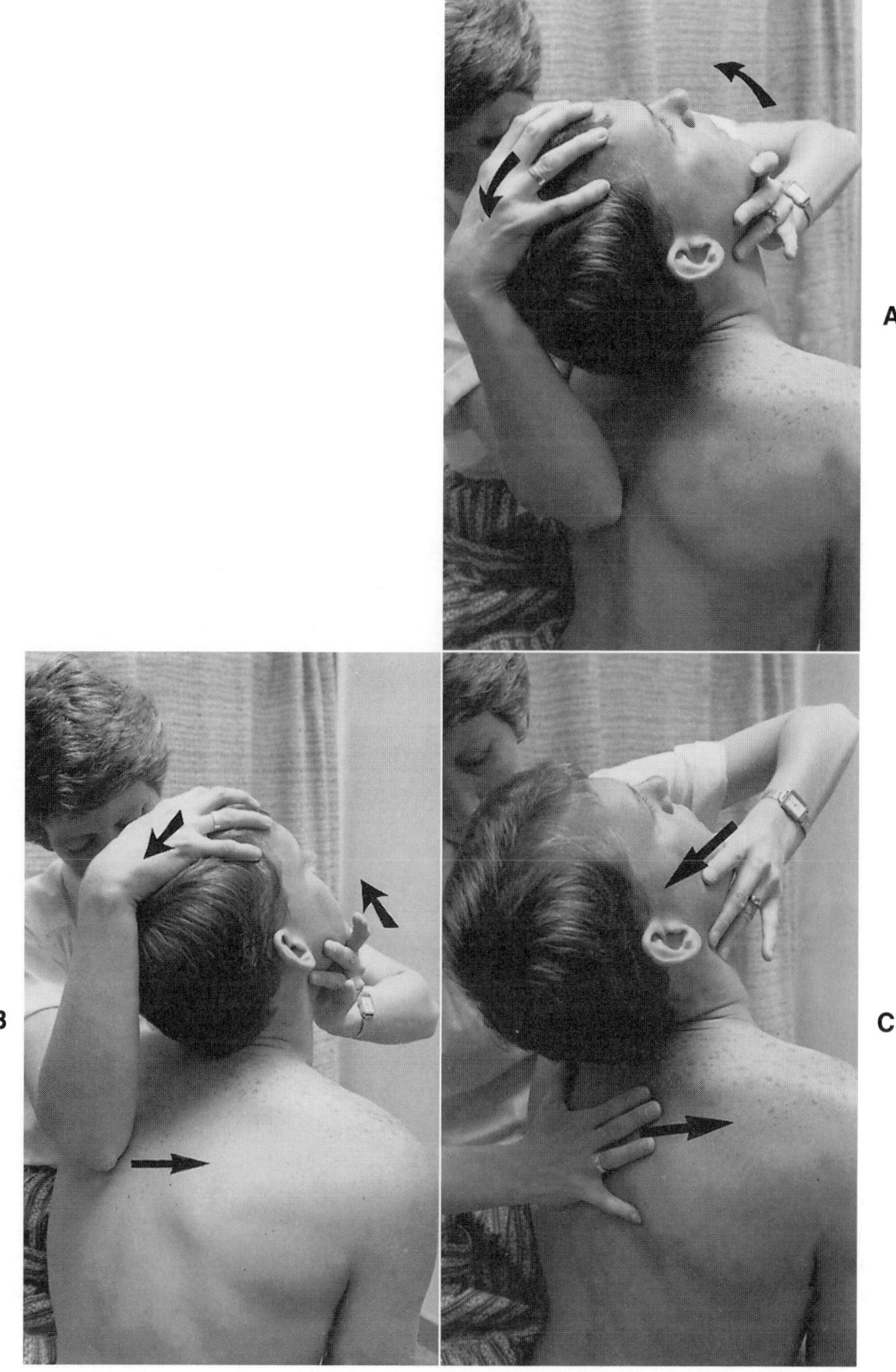

Figure 7-2
Cervical extension. **A,** General cervical extension. **B,** Upper cervical extension. **C,** Lower cervical extension.

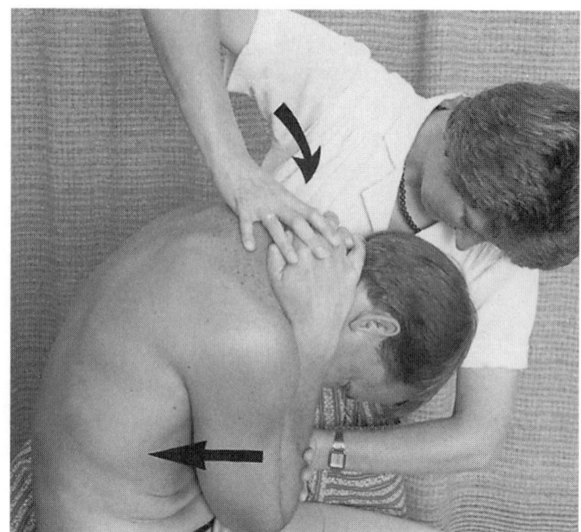

Figure 7-3
Thoracic flexion illustrating the direction of overpressure.

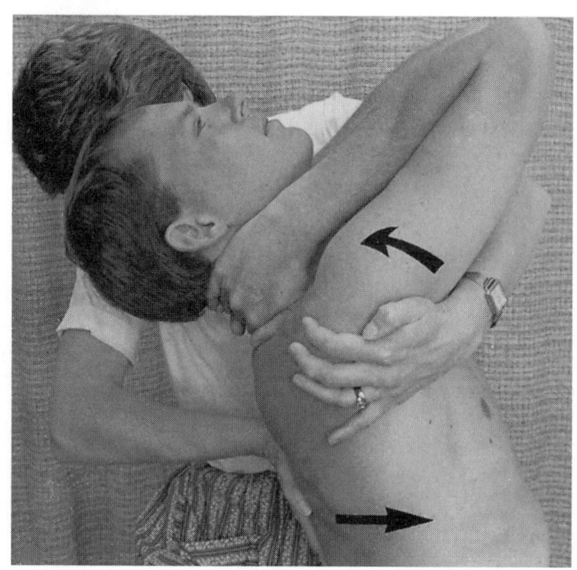

Figure 7-4
Thoracic extension with localized overpressure.

Low Thoracic Spine (T8 to T12). The low thoracic spine is examined with the patient standing with feet together and arms by the sides. The standard active movements scanned are flexion, extension, and lateral flexion, and these are examined in the same way as for the lumbar spine, the direction of overpressure emphasizing movement in the low thoracic area. Rotation is examined with the patient in the sitting position with the thighs fully supported and arms folded across the chest. Overpressure is applied through the shoulders. More detail and pictorial representation of these movements may be found elsewhere.[11,15]

Additional Movement Tests

Provided the examination is not limited by precautionary factors, additional movement tests may be appropriate if any of the following apply:

- Local symptoms have not been reproduced with standard test movements, in an attempt to find a source of those symptoms.

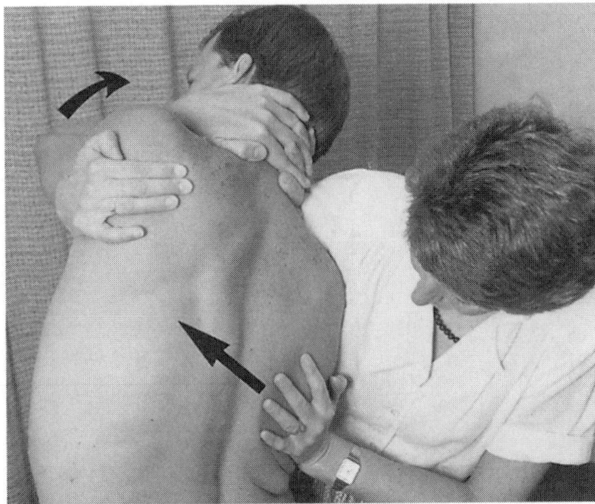

Figure 7-5
Thoracic lateral flexion with localized overpressure.

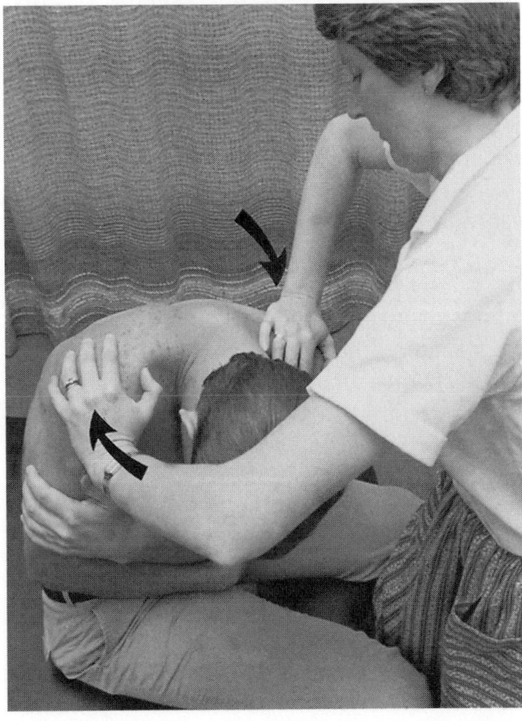

Figure 7-6
Midthoracic rotation with overpressure.

- Symptoms remote to a hypothesized local source have not been reproduced, in an attempt to confirm the local site as the source of the remote symptoms (e.g., headache or supraspinous pain with a potential local cervical source).
- Abnormal movement, either gross or intersegmental, has been detected, but its relevance to the presenting disorder is unclear.
- Standard scanning movement tests have not revealed sufficient information about any of the hypothesis categories.

These additional movement tests may take any form, depending on the subjective indications, but some test procedures are indicated and used often.

Combined Movements. Most natural movements occur in combinations of pure anatomical movement, and any combination of movements can be responsible for the

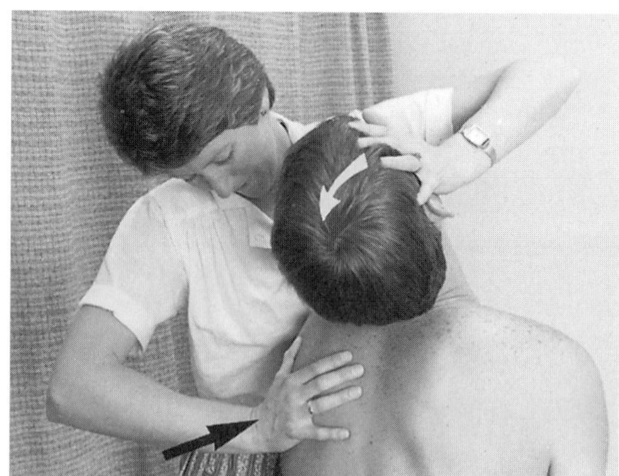

Figure 7-7
A combination of low cervical extension, rotation, and lateral flexion to the same side.

production of symptoms. In the cervical and thoracic spine, those combinations that either stretch or compress one side of the spine often become symptomatic, particularly when the condition is spontaneous in onset rather than traumatic. Movement combinations that compress the articular surfaces and narrow the intervertebral foramina are useful in reproducing referred symptoms, in particular, the combinations of extension with ipsilateral lateral flexion and rotation. The rotation and lateral flexion should be localized to the area implicated (Figure 7-7). Examination of combined movements in the cervical spine is covered in detail in Chapter 9.

Addition of Neurodynamic Procedures. The addition of neurodynamic procedures to movements that demonstrate abnormalities can provide an indication of the involvement in the abnormal movement of altered neural mobility (see slump test, pages 127-129). For example, if supraspinous pain is provoked during cervical flexion, this pain may be associated with a somatic referral from a local zygapophyseal joint. Equally possible is an association with limited movement of the neural structures. Such involvement could be determined by the addition of minimal ankle dorsiflexion or knee extension to the position of painful cervical flexion. Such movement of the ankles or knees alters the tension in and movement of the nervous system with no alteration of local musculoskeletal structures. Consequently, if a change in symptoms is observed, the nervous system is implicated.

Sustained Positions. Sustaining a movement at its limit may be useful, particularly if the subjective indications are that symptoms are provoked either in this way or after return from a sustained position, when a latent response to the examination procedure may be anticipated.

Headaches are often reproduced by upper cervical extension or this movement's combination with ipsilateral lateral flexion and rotation (Figure 7-8), if the position is sustained. Similarly, arm or medial scapular pain may be reproduced with sustained ipsilateral rotation, extension, or the combination of low cervical extension with ipsilateral rotation and lateral flexion.

The movement examined should be held at its limit with overpressure applied as small oscillations for whatever length of time is appropriate for the individual patient and conditions or for sufficient time to allow alteration of viscous tissues in such a way that they might lead to provocation of symptoms. Once the position is released, a similar time span should elapse before the next test procedure is performed to allow for the possibility of a latent response to the movement.

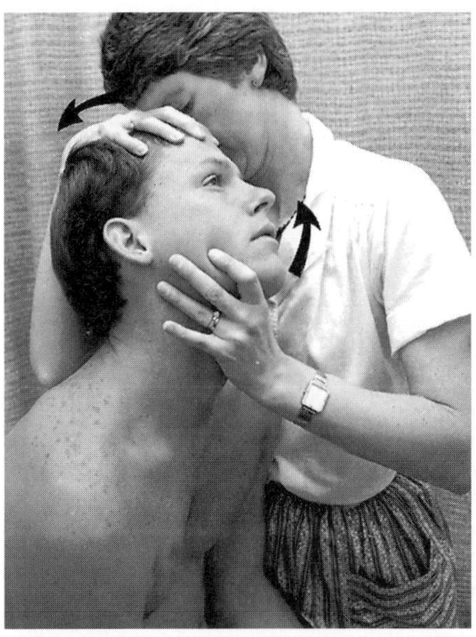

Figure 7-8
A combination of upper cervical extension, rotation, and lateral flexion to the same side.

Speed of Movements. Often, a movement is performed during examination more slowly than during the usual aggravating activity, in which case symptoms are not necessarily provoked. If the movement is repeated at greater speed, the symptoms often will appear.

Repeated Movements. A patient's symptoms may be provoked only with repetition of a movement. By examining movement a number of times, the examiner can accurately determine the number of repetitions required to provoke the symptoms, a fact that may be valuable in reassessment.

Examination after Provocation. Occasionally no amount of examination can reproduce the patient's symptoms because the clinical assessment is unable to stress the affected structures sufficiently. When this occurs, the patient should be requested to report again for examination, this time just after provocation has occurred. While the symptoms are present, examination should reveal some abnormality of movement or position. For example, examination of a computer operator with upper thoracic pain only provoked at the end of a working day may be negative if undertaken on a nonworking day. The patient should be advised to return for reassessment after work, when the symptoms should be easy to reproduce.

Compression/Distraction. In the cervical spine, particularly the upper cervical area, symptoms often are reproduced by compression and, somewhat less often, eased by distraction. Consequently, compression and distraction should be considered as high-priority additional examination procedures for the cervical spine.

Compression may be applied to the cervical spine so that it affects each intervertebral segment equally on both sides or affects one side more than the other. To affect the neck symmetrically, pressure is applied with the spine in neutral, whereas for a more unilateral effect, the neck is laterally flexed to the level being tested before compression is added. The compression is then transmitted through the articular pillar on the concave side of the neck. Compression and distraction of the thoracic spine are usually added so that their effect is symmetrical.

Movements with Compression or Distraction. If compression or distraction alone is unhelpful and the subjective examination indicates that they may be a component of the problem, movements performed with compression or distraction forces added may be helpful. Headaches of upper cervical origin commonly are reproduced by cervical rotation or lateral flexion under compression, whereas medial scapular pain is often provoked by adding compression to a combined position of low cervical extension and lateral flexion.

EXAMINATION OF THE NERVOUS SYSTEM

Involvement of the nervous system may be manifested by impairment of conduction, demonstrated by alteration in sensation, muscle power, and reflexes, and by signs of abnormal movement, demonstrated by abnormal responses to neurodynamic tests, such as the upper limb tension tests (ULTTs) and the slump test.

EXAMINATION FOR IMPAIRMENT OF NEURAL CONDUCTION

Descriptions of the tests for impairment of conduction are presented in detail elsewhere.[11,15,16] Tests for upper motor neuron, lower motor neuron, and peripheral nerve function should be included. Neurological assessment should be included in the following situations:

- When patient has symptoms that are neural in character
- When symptoms are present in the limbs
- When any disorder has a history of trauma or the condition is worsening

The cervical and thoracic spinal segments and their dermatomes, representative muscles, joint action, and reflexes may be found in most anatomical textbooks and are presented precisely by Butler in *Mobilisation of the Nervous System.*[16] They are not presented here. However, a few clinically helpful hints to ensure a sensitive and consistent method of examination are presented.

Recently a system of interpretation of findings related to muscle power and sensory changes has been adopted from that used commonly by clinical neurologists. With this system, the following approach is applied. As an aid to memory, recall that the cervical vertebra with the longest spinous process (vertebrae prominens) is C7, and the longest (middle) finger also is supplied by C7. With the arm in the anatomical position, four quadrants can be formed on the arm, with the long finger as the dividing point. The quadrants are innervated as follows:

- Lateral arm—C5
- Lateral forearm, thumb, and index finger—C6
- Middle finger—C7
- Medial forearm, medial hand, ring finger, and little finger—C8
- Medial arm—T1

When sensation with light touch or pinprick is tested, normal sensation on the unaffected side should be established first, and then sensation on the affected limb should be compared to the normal. A consistent pattern of assessment should be undertaken, starting distally and working in a circular fashion proximally around the limb, moving in the same direction at each level. Care should be taken with assessment of sensation of the fingers and thumb that all surfaces of each finger are tested, as is each phalanx. Decreased or absent sensation commonly is found only over the distal phalanx of the pad of a finger. If care is not taken to ensure that each pad is assessed specifically, such minor sensation loss may not be detected. Similarly, if only the dorsal surface of a finger is tested, the sensation loss could be missed.

Light touch should be tested with a free edge of a tissue to ensure that the touch is truly light, whereas a disposable pin or toothpick is an appropriate tool with which to test pinprick sensation. If the toothpick is held loosely between the index and middle fingers on one side and the thumb on the other and allowed to slip slightly in the grip with each pinprick applied, the intensity of each application will tend to be more consistent than if the toothpick is held rigidly. This will allow more confidence in interpretation of variations in response to testing.

In relation to power, at the shoulder the muscles are innervated by four nerve root levels (C5 to C8) but in an asymmetrical pattern around the shoulder. Muscles associated with abduction are innervated by C5, whereas those associated with adduction are innervated by C6, C7, and C8. At the elbow, the muscles are innervated by the same four nerve roots but in a symmetrical fashion—flexion by C5 and C6 and extension by C7 and C8. With movement distally down the arm, innervation moves down one nerve root (C5 to C8) level; at the wrist both flexors and extensors are innervated by C6 and C7, at the metacarpophalangeal joints flexors and extensors are innervated by C7 and C8, and in the hand the small muscles are innervated by T1. The muscles commonly tested for a routine upper limb neurological examination include the following:

- C4—scapular elevators
- C5—deltoid
- C6—biceps
- C7—triceps
- C8—long finger flexors, extensor pollicis longus
- T1—intrinsics, lumbricals

Tests of nerve conduction must be done with finesse to detect minimal differences that may indicate the early stages of loss of integrity of nervous tissue. Pressure is gradually built to a maximum, at which point the patient's hold can be broken with just a gentle, short controlled overpressure. A muscle with normal innervation tends to "give" to overpressure with a sharp springy recoil, whereas one with a loss of normal innervation tends to give with a sluggish recoil, much like a worn-out spring. However, this subtle difference, which may be the first detectable sign of neurological dysfunction, will be detected only if the overpressure is applied with finesse.

The reflexes routinely tested include the biceps and brachioradialis reflexes (C6) and the triceps reflex (C7). The reflex hammer should be dropped onto the tendon consistently each time to ensure a consistent response, and reflexes must be assessed bilaterally on each occasion they are tested because they are strongly influenced by the general muscle tone on the day of testing. Whenever possible, the therapist must try to adapt positioning from one side of the patient to the other to assess reflexes so that the tendon hammer is manipulated with the same hand. This will ensure as consistent a test as possible so that differences related to handedness of the therapist are not interpreted as differences within the patient.

Neurodynamic Testing for the Upper Quarter

As a result of the potential involvement of central or peripheral nervous system structures in a significant number of nociceptive disorders and the apparent relationship between altered neurodynamics and nociceptive symptoms, assessment of movement of the nervous system should form a routine part of examination of all patients who have symptoms in or related to the cervicothoracic region. Such assessment should involve testing the neuraxis by the slump test[17] and its derivatives and the upper limbs by the upper limb neurodynamic tests.[16] Potential involvement of the autonomic nervous system may be assessed by modifications to the traditional neurodynamic tests such that emphasis is placed on the sympathetic trunk.

Those tests appropriate to the individual are determined by clues from the subjective examination and previous physical examination. In addition to testing the mobility of and tension in the nervous system, neurodynamic testing evaluates movement of the nervous system in its nerve bed (i.e., in relation to its interfacing tissues). These are the tissues that lie adjacent to the nervous system and that are capable of movement independent of the nervous system. The skull and spinal canal make up the bed of the central nervous system. Therefore tissues that need to be considered include bone (skull, vertebral bodies, pedicles, and laminae), discs, ligaments (posterior longitudinal ligament and ligament flavum), fascia, and blood vessels, all of which are innervated to some extent by the sinuvertebral nerve, posterior primary rami, or spinal nerve. In the peripheral nervous system, the nerve bed may consist of muscle, tendon, bony tunnels, fascia, or joint capsules.

Neurodynamic testing is discussed in detail in Butler.[16] Those specific step-by-step details are not repeated here. Butler suggested that a system of easily repeatable base tests with known normative responses should be used as routine starting points, with further examination dependent on the specific presentation of the patient. The most sensitive of these base tests, whose principal effect is on the neuraxis, is the slump test.[17]

Examination of neural mobility with any neurodynamic test should be approached with caution in the following cases:

- Irritable or progressive disorders
- Presentation that indicates an unstable discogenic disorder
- Presence of recent progressive neurological changes
- Recent onset of spinal cord or cauda equina symptoms
- Inflammatory diseases, particularly polyneuropathies

With all neurodynamic testing, movement is taken to the onset of symptoms or to the comfortable limit of movement, if no symptoms are provoked. If symptoms are provoked, the movement is released until those symptoms have dissipated, before the next component is added. This step is omitted from the descriptions of the tests that follow.

Neurodynamic tests are considered relevant or positive for neurogenic involvement under the following circumstances:

- Local and referred symptoms are reproduced that can be altered by changing a component of the test that implicates a neural source.
- Restriction of movement is asymmetrical and not caused by local restriction and can be altered by changing a component of the test that can be neural only (or at least a continuous tissue tract).

The test is considered significant if any of the following occur:

- Symptoms are reproduced.
- There is an asymmetrical restriction of movement.
- There is a symptom response different either from normal or from the other side.

Slump Test. The base slump test involves maximal spinal flexion combined with knee extension and ankle and foot dorsiflexion. The confirming procedure of release of cervical flexion is used commonly, with other sensitizing and confirmatory movements used as indicated.

Slater et al[18] state the addition of thoracic lateral flexion or rotation, particularly to the long-sitting slump position, may place further stress on the sympathetic chain, thereby provoking symptoms of sympathetic origin. These authors also suggested that, as a result of the close association between the thoracic spine and the sympathetic trunk, potential sympathetic involvement should lead to the assessment of movement of skeletal structures in positions of neural tension (e.g., posteroanterior pressures over the costotransverse joints with the arm in a ULTT position or long-sit slump position).

When assessing slump in a patient with cervical pain on flexion, it is often difficult to determine whether that pain is associated with local tissue dysfunction or lack of neural mobility. To distinguish between the two, the cervical movement may be taken to P_1, sustained carefully in that position while knee extension is added. Any change in neck pain is noted. If there is already pain with cervical flexion, the addition of another neurodynamic component, such as knee extension, is likely to increase the symptoms related to altered neural mobility. Only a small amount of movement of the distal component should be required to alter symptoms because they have already been provoked by cervical flexion. The trunk flexion component of the slump is omitted in the first instance because many of the soft tissues in the posterior aspect of the neck also traverse the upper thoracic area and an increase in pain associated with thoracic flexion could be associated with increased tension in those structures rather than altered neural mobility. Hence trunk flexion added to symptomatic cervical flexion is not a useful discriminatory procedure.

Upper Limb Tension Tests. Testing of neurodynamic function in the upper limbs is undertaken by means of the ULTTs.[16] Four base ULTTs have been developed, all testing neurodynamics primarily through the middle trunk of the brachial plexus, each with a bias toward a particular nerve. They include the following:

- ULTT1—median nerve dominant, using shoulder abduction, lateral rotation, forearm supination, wrist and finger extension, and elbow extension.
- ULTT2a—median nerve dominant, using shoulder girdle depression, elbow extension, lateral rotation of the shoulder, forearm supination, and wrist and finger extension. This test may be indicated when the subjective examination indicates a component of depression and protraction in the patient's presentation or when the abduction component of ULTT1 is not possible, as with shoulder pathology.
- ULTT2b—radial nerve dominant, using shoulder girdle depression, elbow extension, forearm pronation, and medial rotation of the shoulder, with wrist and finger flexion. This test is indicated when the subjective examination indicates symptoms in a radial nerve distribution, such as lateral elbow pain or de Quervain's disease.
- ULTT3—ulnar nerve dominant, using shoulder abduction and lateral rotation, elbow flexion, forearm pronation, and wrist and finger extension. This variation is useful when the subjective examination indicates symptoms with an ulnar nerve bias, such as medial elbow pain, symptoms on the ulnar border of the hand, low cervical disorders, or C8 nerve root symptoms.

Sensitizing procedures for all ULTTs include cervical contralateral and ipsilateral flexion and upper cervical flexion. Other movements can be added to each test as appropriate for the individual patient's problem and should reflect the anatomical pathway of the nerve(s) implicated in the symptoms. Cervical side glide and retraction also may be used and are often very powerful sensitizers, although they need to be added by a second operator rather than actively by the patient. The contralateral ULTT can be added, either before or after movement of the test arm into position, as can bilateral straight leg raise.

In addition to assessment of altered mobility, Butler[16] also advocated palpation of nerves where they are accessible. A normal nerve should feel hard and round and should be moveable transversely. This movement may be reduced if the nerve is under tension or adherent to adjacent interface tissues. Swelling or thickening may be detected, indicating abnormality of the nerve. The symptomatic response to palpation also could assist in localization of the site of altered mobility, with specific types of responses apparently related to specific types of involvement of the nerve. However, nerves are not accessible for palpation through their whole course, so palpation evaluation may not demonstrate an abnormality at a site remote from the accessible point.

MUSCLE PERFORMANCE

The cervical and thoracic muscles may be a source of symptoms in conjunction with or independent of underlying vertebral disorders. However, structures within each vertebral segment are capable of referring pain into the adjacent muscles, establishing areas of local tenderness and even tissue changes with no intrinsic muscle disorder. Static contraction of the paraspinal muscles is impossible without some stress on the adjacent noncontractile structures. Therefore differentiation of contractile tissue as a source is difficult and often can be made only in retrospect when the effect on one structure of treating another can be assessed.

Clues to the involvement of muscle as a contributing factor can be found in the subjective examination. For example, a cervicothoracic ache that comes on only toward the end of a day spent working at a computer may indicate a "postural" component in which poor muscular endurance leads to fatigue, resulting in increasingly poor posture and excessive stress on underlying structures. The hypothesis of muscle involvement is further tested during the physical examination.

Chronic disorders of the cervicothoracic region commonly develop typical patterns of muscle imbalance. These can be seen initially during an assessment of posture. The characteristic forward head posture with downwardly rotated and protracted scapulae is typically associated with tightness or overactivity in upper cervical extensors, sternocleidomastoid, scalenes, levator scapulae, rhomboids, pectorals, and shoulder medial rotators and with weakness of deep cervical flexors, long cervical extensors, upper trapezius, lower scapular stabilizers, and shoulder lateral rotators.

The hypothesis of muscle imbalance should be tested with specific assessment of length, strength, and endurance and recruitment during functional activity. In addition, muscles should be recruited in correct movement patterns, which if disturbed, create altered axes of movement with the potential for development of symptoms. Muscle imbalance, its effects, and the tests used to establish it are presented in differing ways in Chapters 10, 13, and 17.

PRECAUTIONARY PROCEDURES

The integrity of vital structures must be established before initiation of management of the cervical or thoracic area. The systems and structures that need to be tested include the nervous system, already discussed; the vascular system, including testing for VBI; and involvement of peripheral vascular tissue either locally or in the thoracic outlet. Testing for instability of the upper cervical spine is a further consideration. These tests need be performed only if there are clues in the subjective examination or early part of the physical examination that indicate a need for their inclusion.

VASCULAR SYSTEM

Testing for Vertebrobasilar Insufficiency. Musculoskeletal Physiotherapy Australia (formerly The Manipulative Physiotherapists Association of Australia), in conjunction with the Australian Physiotherapy Association, has recently revised its recommended protocol for evaluation of the cervical spine with particular reference to symptoms associated with the vertebrobasilar system on the basis of results of recent research and a survey of members.[19,20] In this document a clinical standard is outlined for examination for symptoms suggestive of involvement of the vertebrobasilar system as a component of routine upper quarter examination and before any end-range rotation treatment technique or high-velocity thrust technique (manipulation). The steps involved and the reasoning behind the protocol are covered in Chapter 8.

Thoracic Outlet. The thoracic outlet syndrome may affect neural structures, particularly the C8 or T1 nerve roots, or vascular structures such as the subclavian artery. Symptoms related to the C8 or T1 nerve roots may be provoked by sustained shoulder girdle elevation or one of the ULTTs, whereas subclavian involvement may be tested by palpating the radial pulse in a number of positions.[15]

If the subclavian artery is affected, the radial pulse will be reduced or obliterated with the tests discussed, and symptoms may be provoked. Manual compression of the subclavian artery against the first rib, such that the radial pulse is obliterated, also may provoke symptoms. Anteroposterior pressures and posteroanterior pressures over the first rib are likely to reveal restriction and local pain and may reproduce symptoms of vascular or neurogenic origin.

The thoracic outlet may need to be examined by one of the many tests described in orthopedic textbooks. Edgelow[21] has described appropriate and clinically relevant testing and management of thoracic outlet disorders.

Peripheral Pulses. If evidence of poor circulation, such as ulcerated skin, blanching of the skin, peripheral coldness, or numbness or slow healing of minor skin blemishes is present, the autonomic nervous system or vascular system itself may be implicated. As part of the assessment, examination of the peripheral pulses should be performed. The pulses in the affected area should be checked and compared with those of the other arm to determine the integrity of blood flow through the arm. This assessment should be performed both in the resting position and in aggravating positions in which flow may be compromised. If significant vascular compromise is suspected after such an examination, the patient should be referred to a medical practitioner for further vascular investigation.

TESTS FOR CRANIOVERTEBRAL HYPERMOBILITY

Aspinall[8] described a set of tests for craniovertebral hypermobility. Detailed descriptions of method and the underlying applied anatomy and biomechanics can be found in her paper and are not repeated here. The tests described include the following:

- Sharp-Purser test
- Alar ligament test
- Transverse ligament test
- Alar ligament and dens/atlas osseous stability test
- Tectorial membrane test

No validity studies have been performed on these ligamentous tests. They are potent tests that have led to the provocation of nausea, fainting, and a general sense of apprehension when performed on asymptomatic individuals during class demonstrations. Such symptom provocation may have been partly the result of inappropriately heavy handling by inexperienced practitioners, but it highlights the need to undertake the tests with care, continually asking the patient about provocation of symptoms. However, subjective or historical indications of upper cervical hypermobility or instability should alert the therapist to the need for assessment, and therefore if used appropriately, fatal or significant vascular or neurological compromise from inappropriate management should be avoided.

EXAMINATION OF ASSOCIATED STRUCTURES

Peripheral Joints

Symptoms that spread from the neck or thoracic spine into the upper limb or head and face may have a source that is entirely within the spine or has some component from one or more of the peripheral structures, including the joints over which they pass. Examination of all joints within the area of symptoms will determine the degree of contribution of each to the overall problem. Detailed examination of the peripheral joints is unnecessary because signs are likely to be minimal. The protocol for brief examination of the peripheral joints has been described.[11]

The degree of involvement of the peripheral joint and the spine should be assessed by examination of passive movements of both structures. If abnormalities are found in both structures, treatment of one (usually the spine first) and assessment of alteration in the other will determine the relative contribution of each.

For comparative evaluation to be most effective, appropriate interpretation of passive movement testing is essential. The relationship between soft tissue resistance to passive movement and symptoms during the movement is fundamental in such interpretation. For example, if a high degree of tissue resistance is encountered before the onset of symptoms when testing a peripheral joint, even though pain is provoked early in range with little or no tissue resistance detected in the cervical spine, the neck is the more likely source of the patient's symptoms. A passive movement is more likely to be stressing the source of the symptoms if pain is the dominant feature throughout the movement with or without abnormal resistance. However, care should be taken with such interpretations, particularly with chronic patients who may have a component of centrally initiated nociception.[1]

Viscera

Indications of potential involvement of the thoracic or abdominal viscera will be found in the subjective examination, with clues related to visceral function. The text by Boissonnault[7] should be reviewed for specific differentiating features of visceral pathology. Differentiation of intrinsic visceral pain and that from overlying contractile tissue or referral from the thoracic spine is possible. If palpation of the abdominal wall reproduces the patient's pain, palpation should be repeated with the abdominal muscles contracted, thereby removing the pressure from the viscera. If the pain is unchanged, it is unlikely to be visceral in origin but probably arises from the abdominal wall or thoracic spine. If the pain originates in the abdominal wall, resisted contraction should be painful, with local tenderness accompanied by palpable alterations in tissue texture. If the pain is referred from the spine, changes in the soft tissues and joint movement in the appropriate segment will be evident.

PASSIVE EXAMINATION

Passive examination has the advantage of correlation between range, symptoms, and feel of tissue resistance and texture. As mentioned earlier, interpretation of the relationship between tissue resistance to movement and symptoms is fundamental. The abnormalities that can be detected with passive movement include the following:

- Altered range of movement (either hypermobility or hypomobility)
- Abnormal quality of resistance to passive movement (e.g., the early and rapidly developing resistance associated with gross restriction of movement; lack of normal resistance, or "empty end-feel" of instability; the subtle difference in behavior of resistance in joints often associated with minor symptoms; and "the almost unyielding quality of muscle spasm")
- Provocation of symptoms (local or remote)—if symptoms are reproduced, the direct involvement of the structure being moved can be assumed, with the reservations outlined previously (That these symptoms are abnormal can be determined by comparison with those produced by movement of other related structures. Provocation of local symptoms different from the presenting problem still may be relevant. If intersegmental movement at a level capable of referring to the symptomatic area is locally painful, a spinal source or component may be implicated.)

The relationship between soft tissue resistance to movement and symptom response is of most significance. A structure may demonstrate abnormal movement of no relevance to the presenting problem. Similarly, a structure may be painful when moved or pressed with no intrinsic abnormality present. Abnormality of movement associated with abnormal symptom response in structures capable of producing the presenting symptoms indicates significance. When these related abnormalities also are associated with changes in texture of related soft tissue, their relevance is stronger.

PASSIVE PHYSIOLOGICAL INTERVERTEBRAL MOVEMENTS

The physiological movements available in the vertebral column (i.e., flexion, extension, lateral flexion and rotation) and their combinations can all be examined at each intervertebral level. Intersegmental evaluation of the combined coupled movements[22] is also performed. Passive physiological intervertebral movements (PPIVMs) may be used to do the following:

- Confirm restriction of movement seen on gross active testing (The amount of restriction, the level[s] involved, and the direction of restriction can be confirmed and therefore localized.)
- Detect restriction of physiological movement not obvious on gross testing
- Detect increases, either hypermobility or instability, or decreases in physiological movement and associated joint play (For example, in the cervical spine, the addition of a lateral glide may demonstrate a loss of movement that is not obvious on lateral flexion but that may be significant in production of symptoms.)

The range of movement available and the quality of movement through range and end-feel must be determined and compared with those of adjacent vertebrae and the expected norm for the patient. As with all passive movement examination, the ability to interpret the relationship between soft tissue resistance to movement and symptoms during movement is important. Movements in the coronal plane also must be compared with those of the opposite side. The basic movements of flexion, extension, lateral flexion, and rotation are routinely assessed in addition to the coupled movement combinations.

Description of individual techniques for examining PPIVMs is beyond the scope of this chapter, but detailed descriptions can be found elsewhere.[11,15,22]

Palpation Examination

Palpation examination is extremely informative and therefore an essential aspect of evaluation. An inflammatory disorder may cause a local increase in skin temperature and sweating, both of which may be detected by palpation. The nonbony tissues should be palpated to detect thickening, swelling, muscle spasm, tightness, fibrous bands, or nodules. The vertebral position and the presence of any bony anomalies also should be assessed because alteration in position may result in significant biomechanical changes, which in time may generate sufficient stress to provoke symptoms. Alterations in vertebral position are observed often in the thoracic area.

Soft Tissues. The following areas are of particular significance because changes in tissue texture often are found there. These changes alter with treatment and therefore would appear to be related to the symptoms.

Upper cervical (occiput to C3):

- Capsule of the atlantooccipital joint
- Occipital soft tissues from medial to lateral
- Suboccipital tissues overlying the atlas and between the atlas and occiput
- Tissues immediately adjacent to the spinous process of the axis
- Interlaminar space of C1 to C2 and C2 to C3 zygapophyseal joints
- Tissues overlying and immediately anterior to the transverse processes of atlas and axis

Midcervical (C3 to C5):

- Tissues immediately adjacent to the spinous process
- Laterally between the spinous processes
- Interlaminar spaces and capsules of the midcervical zygapophyseal joints
- Laterally, overlying and anterior to the transverse processes

Low cervical (C5 to T1):

- C7 to T1 area where changes associated with a dowager's hump may be found

Thoracic spine:

- Immediately adjacent to the spinous processes
- Laterally between spinous processes
- Further laterally, over the transverse processes and costotransverse joints
- Angle of the ribs
- Intercostally, depending on the area of symptoms

Vertebral Position and Bony Anomalies. The following abnormalities are found often, although interpretation has never been scientifically validated. Positional abnormalities are relevant to the patient's symptoms if they change with treatment.

Upper cervical:

- Slight rotation or displacement of the atlas relative to the occiput, as shown by asymmetry of depth and prominence of the atlantal transverse processes
- Absence or asymmetry of the bifid processes of the axial spinous process
- Exostoses at the C2 to C3 zygapophyseal joints

Midcervical:

- Prominence of C3 spinous process, frequently associated with chronic headaches
- Prominence of C4 spinous process, usually associated with midcervical pain
- Exostoses at the midcervical zygapophyseal joints

Low cervical:
- Spinous process of C6, often very close to that of C7 and therefore a long way from that of C5, giving the impression of prominence of C5 spinous process

Thoracic:
- One spinous process deviated laterally, either as a result of vertebral rotation or bony asymmetry
- Two spinous processes very close together, creating a large interspinous space at the level below
- One or more spinous processes set deep, with those on either side appearing prominent, the symptoms usually arising predominantly from the deep-set level

Passive Accessory Intervertebral Movements

The earliest detectable changes in movement that occur with aging are changes in the quality of the passive accessory intervertebral movements (PAIVMs).[23-25] Therefore accessory movements are the most sensitive indicators of abnormality of movement in a joint. However, the interpretation of abnormalities in accessory movement of the spine is based predominantly on clinical experience and reflective reasoning, rather than any formal validation.

Accessory movements are routinely examined throughout the spine by using the following methods:
- Posteroanterior oscillatory pressures (PAs) on the spinous process of each vertebra
- PAs over the laminae on each side of the spinous process and over the transverse processes where they are palpable (unilateral PAs)
- Transverse oscillatory pressures against the lateral aspect of the spinous process (not commonly assessed in the cervical spine)

In addition, in the cervical area the following movements are routinely examined:
- Transverse pressures against the transverse process and the laminae
- Anteroposterior oscillatory pressures (APs) unilaterally over the area of the anterior and posterior tubercles

In the thoracic area, unilateral PAs and APs on the ribs and APs on the sternum, sternocostal joints, or costochondral junctions may be indicated in particular patients.

Central movement at any level should be compared with the movement at the level above and below and the expected norm for the patient's age and somatotype; unilateral movements also should be compared with the corresponding movement on the opposite side.

The variations of the basic movements are endless, each providing information that may be useful in confirming the source of symptoms, in contributing to symptom production, and in directing treatment. Indications for the use of variations come from a number of sources, including the aggravating movements, particular movements found to be significant during the active examination, abnormalities found with PPIVMs and interpretation of the basic PAIVMs. If a particular spinal level is suspected as a source or contributing factor and routine movements are normal, the examination should be taken further with variations in direction of movement and assessment of PAIVMs in positions other than neutral.

Abnormalities detected should be relevant to the presenting symptoms. For example, a C2-3 zygapophyseal source may be suspected for unilateral headaches, but PAIVMs do not demonstrate abnormalities proportional to the degree of symptoms. Unilateral PAs over the most lateral available aspect of the zygapophyseal joint with a bias in a cephalad direction, performed with the head in ipsilateral rotation, may demonstrate significant difference in quality of movement and symptom production, both relevant to the headache, when compared with the response to the same movement on the other side. With an irritable or severe disorder in which a limited examination is indicated, examination of PAIVMs may be modified to avoid provocation of symptoms. Indications for appropriate positions will be gained from positions that ease symptoms. Common examples of modifications include posterior examination performed in supine, posterior examination performed in prone but with the neck in slight flexion, and unilateral PAs performed in slight contralateral rotation.

Palpation and PAIVMs can help to differentiate between an intervertebral source of symptoms, a contributing factor, and irrelevant findings. Soft tissue thickening adjacent to a zygapophyseal joint with a feel similar to old leather, combined with painless restriction as evidenced by unilateral PAs, indicates chronic abnormality that is unlikely to be the direct source of symptoms. If the soft tissue at an adjacent level is soft and feels swollen and unilateral PAs demonstrate hypermobility with pain through range, this joint is likely to be the source of the pain. However, the adjacent stiff joint could be hypothesized to be a contributing factor. Abnormalities found in levels more remote from the symptomatic area or in areas that cannot be somatically connected may still be relevant, either as contributing factors or as indicators of underlying neural involvement, particularly if the abnormality is in the midthoracic region. However, their relevance can be determined only in retrospect after appropriate treatment and reassessment of all presenting signs and symptoms.

ASSESSMENT

The process of clinical reasoning is not complete with completion of the physical examination but, instead, is a continual process throughout the course of management. Continuing assessment during and after the physical examination and subsequent treatment sessions allows development and modification of the hypotheses formed during the initial evaluation. Because complete examination is not always possible during the initial evaluation, aspects omitted should be addressed during the following one or two sessions.

In addition to the ongoing reasoning process, continuous assessment minimizes the chances of exacerbation of symptoms after examination with the concomitant harmful effects. Continuous assessment also helps develop the patient's confidence in the physical therapist, a factor that greatly enhances the chance of successful treatment.

This approach of ongoing clinical reasoning, combined with an understanding of clinical patterns, good examination skills, and a mind sufficiently open to recognize subtle variations in familiar patterns and any new patterns that may emerge and open enough to challenge and question assumed knowledge to enhance understanding of underlying pathophysiology, allows physical therapists the opportunity for constant professional growth. If also combined with a degree of reflective thinking and good treatment skills, this approach provides the patient with optimal management.

References

1. Zusman M: Central nervous system contribution to mechanically produced motor and sensory responses, *Aust J Physiother* 38:245, 1992.
2. Jones M, Magarey M: Clinical reasoning in the use of manual therapy techniques for the shoulder girdle. In Tovin B, Greenfield B, editors: *Evaluation and rehabilitation of the shoulder: an impairment based approach*, Philadelphia, 2001, FA Davis.

3. Higgs J, Jones M: *Clinical reasoning in the health professions*, ed 2, Oxford, England, 2000, Butterworth-Heinemann.
4. Jones M, Jensen G, Edwards I: Clinical reasoning in physiotherapy. In: Higgs J, Jones M, editors: *Clinical reasoning for the health professions*, ed 2, Oxford, England, 2000, Butterworth-Heinemann.
5. ACC and the National Health Committee: *New Zealand acute low back pain guide*, Wellington, New Zealand, 1997.
6. Cloward RB: Cervical discography: a contribution to the etiology and mechanism of neck, shoulder, and arm pain, *Ann Surg* 150:1052, 1959.
7. Boissonnault WG: *Examination in physical therapy practice: screening for medical disease*, ed 2, New York, 1995, Churchill Livingstone.
8. Aspinall W: Clinical testing for the craniovertebral hypermobility syndrome, *J Orthoped Sports Phys Therapy* 12:47, 1990.
9. Gifford L, editor: Topical issues in pain: whiplash: science and management; fear: avoidance, beliefs, and behaviour. In *Physiotherapy Pain Association yearbook 1998-1999*, Falmouth, United Kingdom, 1998, NOI Press.
10. Mackinnon SE: Double and multiple "crush" syndromes, *Hand Clin* 8:369, 1992.
11. Maitland GD: *Vertebral manipulation*, ed 6, London, 1986, Butterworths.
12. Jones MA, Jones HM: Principles of the physical examination. In Boyling JD, Palastanga N, editors: *Modern manual therapy: the vertebral column*, ed 2, Edinburgh, 1993, Churchill Livingstone.
13. Harding V: Cognitive-behavioural approach to fear and avoidance. In Gifford L, editor: *Topical issues in pain: whiplash: science and management; fear: avoidance, beliefs, and behaviour: Physiotherapy Pain Association yearbook 1998-1999*, Falmouth, United Kingdom, 1998, NOI Press.
14. Austin L, Maitland GD, Magarey ME: Manual therapy: what, when, and why? In Zuluaga M et al, editors: *Sports physiotherapy: applied science and practice*, Melbourne, 1996, Churchill Livingstone.
15. Grieve GP: *Common vertebral joint problems*, Edinburgh, 1981, Churchill Livingstone.
16. Butler DS: *Mobilisation of the nervous system*, Melbourne, 1991, Churchill Livingstone.
17. Maitland GD: Negative disc exploration: positive canal signs, *Aust J Physiother* 25:129, 1979.
18. Slater H, Vicenzino B, Wright A: "Sympathetic slump": the effects of a novel manual therapy technique on peripheral sympathetic nervous system function, *J Man Manipulative Therapeutics* 2:2:66, 1994.
19. Magarey ME et al: APA pre-manipulative testing protocol: researched and renewed. I. Research Conference of the International Federation of Orthopaedic Manipulative Therapists, Perth, Australia, 2000 (abstract).
20. Magarey ME, Rebbeck T, Coughlan B: APA pre-manipulative testing protocol: researched and renewed. II. Revised clinical guidelines. Conference of the International Federation of Orthopaedic Manipulative Therapists, Perth, Australia, 2000 (abstract).
21. Edgelow P: Thoracic outlet syndrome: a patient-centered treatment approach. In Shacklock M, editor: *Moving in on pain*, Melbourne, 1995, Butterworth-Heinemann.
22. Monaghan M: *Spinal manipulation: a manual for physiotherapists*, Nelson, New Zealand, 2001, Aesculapius.
23. Johnstone PA: Normal temporomandibular joint movement: a pilot study. Proceedings of the Fourth Biennial Conference of Manipulative Therapists Association of Australia, Brisbane, 1985.
24. Milde MR: Accessory movements of the glenohumeral joint: a pilot study of accessory movements in asymptomatic shoulders and the changes related to ageing and hand dominance, thesis, 1981, School of Physiotherapy, South Australian Institute of Technology, Adelaide.
25. Trott PH: Mobility study of the trapezio-metacarpal joint. Proceedings of the second biennial conference of the Manipulative Therapists Association of Australia, Adelaide, 1980.

CHAPTER 8

Premanipulative Testing of the Cervical Spine—Reappraisal and Update

Ruth Grant

Premanipulative testing of the cervical spine has been part of patient screening by manipulative physical therapists for many years. Testing was first described by Maitland in 1968.[1] At that time, the testing procedure comprised specific questioning of the patient for symptoms suggestive of vertebrobasilar insufficiency (VBI)—in particular, dizziness. Physical testing comprised sustained cervical rotation to both sides. The onset of dizziness with these movements was deemed a contraindication to using a passive rotation technique in treatment or to using manipulative techniques in the cervical spine.

This chapter will illustrate how the premanipulative screening protocol for the cervical spine has developed and been formalized, reevaluated, and changed. It will illustrate as well that despite evaluation and redevelopment of premanipulative testing procedures and considerably more research undertaken on the effects of cervical spine movements on vertebral artery (VA) blood flow, evidence of the sensitivity and specificity of these test procedures in detecting the patient at risk of complication after cervical manipulation, still eludes us.

APA PROTOCOL FOR PREMANIPULATIVE TESTING OF THE CERVICAL SPINE

ESTABLISHMENT

Work by Grant[2,3] highlighted for the Australian Physiotherapy Association (APA) the desirability of formalizing a Protocol for Premanipulative Testing of the Cervical Spine and encouraging its use with all patients before cervical manipulation. In January 1988, the Biennial Conference of Manipulative Physiotherapy Teachers of Australia drew up the protocol. The APA approved the protocol in March 1988, and the APA Protocol was published in September of that year.[4] A full description of that Protocol and a detailed literature review underpinning it formed the major part of the chapter entitled "Vertebral Artery Concerns: Premanipulative Testing of the Cervical Spine" in the second edition of this book.[5]

At that time, the APA was the first professional group of any using manipulative techniques in patient treatment in Australia (and as far as was known, worldwide) to have formalized such a protocol. Since that time, other countries' physical therapy associations or special interest groups have formalized similar protocols, including those of Canada, the Netherlands, New Zealand, South Africa, and the United Kingdom. The formalization of a protocol was an initiative that sought to reduce untoward outcomes of cervical manipulative treatment by the use of screening tests and to identify what reasonably could be expected of a prudent, careful practitioner.

The Premanipulative Testing Protocol of the APA was formulated based on the following:

- A knowledge of what was already being undertaken in clinical practice, by way of screening tests
- A knowledge of what movements reduced the lumen of the VA and therefore might alert the practitioner to those patients in whom the vertebrobasilar circulation might be insufficient
- Extensive reviews of case studies of incidents and accidents involving the VA after cervical manipulation
- The knowledge that the screening tests themselves could have a morbid effect on the VA
- The knowledge that in some patients, previous cervical manipulation may have been carried out without incident, yet a (major) complication followed a subsequent manipulative treatment, thus the need to test before every treatment session involving manipulation

It is instructive at this point to very briefly summarize the key features of the APA Protocol[4,5] to remind the reader of them:

1. In any patient for whom treatment of the cervical spine is to be undertaken, the presence or development of dizziness or other symptoms of VBI is carefully assessed.
2. In every patient with upper quarter dysfunction, the subjective examination must specifically ascertain the presence of dizziness or other symptoms suggestive of VBI. Should such symptoms be present, a detailed profile of each must be obtained.
3. The physical examination is divided into the following categories:
    a. Tests undertaken on patients with no history of dizziness or other symptoms of VBI but in whom cervical manipulation is the treatment of choice
        (1) Tests are undertaken with patients sitting or supine as deemed appropriate.
        (2) Tests comprise sustained extension, sustained rotation to left and right, sustained rotation with extension to left and right, and a simulated manipulation position in which the patient's head and neck are held in the position of the manipulative technique that the physical therapist proposes to use in treatment.
        (3) Each test is maintained with overpressure for a minimum of 10 seconds (or less if symptoms are evoked), and on release, a period of 10 seconds should elapse to allow for any latent response to the sustained position.
        (4) The patient is questioned about dizziness during each test, and after each test position has been released, the physical therapist also observes the patient's eyes for nystagmus.
        (5) If any tests are positive, cervical manipulation is not undertaken.
        (6) If tests are negative and no contraindications to manipulation have been elicited on overall clinical evaluation, informed consent is obtained, and cervical manipulation is carried out.

b. Tests undertaken in patients in whom dizziness is a presenting symptom
   (1) Tests are undertaken with the patient in sitting position—if these tests are negative, the physical therapist may decide to repeat these with the patient in supine position.
   (2) Tests comprise those outlined in 3a (with the exception of the simulated manipulation position [SMP]).
   (3) Additional tests that are undertaken comprise testing the position or movement that provokes dizziness as described by the patient (if different from those in 3a) and rapid movement of the head through the available range of relevant movement—for example, rotation. (This latter test is done only if the patient relates dizziness in response to rapid movements.)
   (4) If dizziness is evoked on any of those tests (with the exception of sustained extension), the physical therapist should seek to differentiate dizziness arising from the vestibular apparatus of the inner ear from that elicited by neck movement. Tests are undertaken with the head held still and the trunk rotated.
   (5) Sustaining positions for 10 seconds (or less if symptoms are evoked) and waiting for any latent symptoms as described in 3a.

In summary, if during the physical examination any test is positive—producing or reproducing dizziness and/or associated symptoms suggestive of VBI—then cervical manipulation is contraindicated. The protocol goes on to specify the following:

- The contraindication of cervical manipulation also as a treatment of choice if symptoms are evoked during or after treatment procedures
- Choice of treatment technique and method of application when dizziness or other VBI-like symptoms are present
- The need for informed consent and how it should be gained and recorded
- Avoidance of specific types of manipulative techniques and why
- Use of a single manipulation at the first treatment session and why
- Recommendation that dizziness testing in the SMP should be performed at all subsequent visits by the patient in which cervical manipulation is to be used

Importantly too, the APA Protocol incorporated the following counsel[4] (drawn from Grant[3]):

"However it must be remembered that:

i. an element of unpredictability remains, and incidents do occur even when all premanipulative tests are negative and even when the patient has responded favorably to manipulative treatment in the past
ii. the test procedures themselves hold certain risks
iii. there is a need to carefully and accurately record all dizziness tests and premanipulative testing procedures undertaken and the responses to them on the part of the patient
iv. even when the patient is made aware of the risks attached to a manipulative procedure—that is, informed consent is obtained—the physiotherapist may still remain legally liable if reasonable care—that is, the care expected of the average, competent, and prudent practitioner—is not employed."[4]

Evaluation

Formalizing testing procedures to be carried out before cervical manipulation is all very well, but would physical therapists comply? What was their attitude toward a protocol and toward the issues of informed consent as part of such a protocol?

Three years after the formalization of the APA Protocol, its publication and the recommendations as to its use, Grant and Trott[6] undertook a survey of APA members across Australia. A total of 10% of the APA membership was selected by systematic, stratified random sampling, and a response rate of 63% (455) was obtained.

The questionnaire established the fields in which the members practiced, their genders, their knowledge of the APA Protocol, their attitudinal responses to statements commonly made about the protocol, whether they used manipulative techniques in treatment, their compliance with the subjective and physical examination components of the protocol, whether informed consent was obtained before cervical manipulation, whether screening tests undertaken and informed consent gained were recorded, and whether the format for such recording as suggested in the protocol was used.

A detailed analysis of this survey has been reported elsewhere, including in the second edition of this book.[5,7,8] Key results are presented here.

A total of 89% of the sample knew there was an APA Protocol. Of these, 19% (or 84 physiotherapists) used manipulative techniques in the treatment of upper-quarter disorders. The responses of these 84 physiotherapists are now considered in greater detail. A total of 98% of them knew there was a protocol, and 92% had read it.

The survey contained statements commonly made about the protocol and all respondents used a Likert scale to register their responses. (The common statements that the respondents considered are in italics within the following three points.) Briefly, responses revealed the following:

- Two thirds of these 84 respondents agreed that the APA Protocol for Premanipulative Testing of the Cervical Spine *placed appropriate medicolegal restrictions on the physiotherapy practitioner, and at least two thirds agreed that the protocol was an important initiative and should be retained.*
- However, 41% considered *that the APA Protocol was too time-consuming to be undertaken with every patient before cervical manipulation,* even though the survey revealed that there was a 100% compliance with the subjective examination component of the protocol and that 64% of respondents carried out all the tests routinely.
- A total of 44% agreed that the *requirement for informed consent on the part of the patient before undergoing cervical manipulation would mean that fewer patients would agree to manipulation as a form of treatment, and as a consequence, a valuable method of treatment would be used less frequently.* Despite this response, informed consent was reported as being obtained from patients by 93% of those physiotherapists using manipulative techniques in treatment. Of the 93%, only 58% gained informed consent in every case, and only 50% recorded that such consent had been obtained.
- When informed consent was recorded, 33% of the respondents used the wording suggested in the APA Protocol, whereas 67% either did not use this wording or did not know whether the wording they used was the same as that in the protocol. Before subsequent treatments using cervical manipulation, 89% of respondents performed screening tests, with 91% of these using the simulated manipulation position.

It should be noted that although this initiative was a comprehensive representative survey of *all* APA members, it did not target manipulative physical therapists specifically. Anecdotal evidence appeared to be growing that Australian physical therapists who used manipulative techniques regularly in patient treatment were feeling increasingly constrained by the APA Protocol and were opting not to use cervical manipulation as a treatment of choice on that account. Under the auspices of the National Committee of the Manipulative Physiotherapists Association of Australia

(MPAA), a survey of MPAA members was carried out. The aims of this survey were to determine from MPAA members the following:

- Rate of compliance with the APA Protocol
- Number of members using cervical manipulation
- Risk associated with use of cervical manipulation
- Whether particular techniques were more associated with risk than others, what those risks were, and the frequency of adverse incidents related to the use of cervical manipulation or other cervical techniques
- Rate of compliance of provision of information to and consent from a patient prior to cervical manipulation

A full analysis of this MPAA survey has not been published at the time of this writing. It is instructive, however, to compare responses to this survey as gleaned from preliminary publication[9] with those of the first survey.[5,7,8] Acceptable rates of responses were evident for both (67% for MPAA, 63% for the earlier survey). In both surveys, 98% of respondents who used cervical manipulation in treatment were familiar with the APA Protocol, and 85% and 92%, respectively, had read it. In the MPAA survey, 66% reported using the full protocol before the first use of cervical manipulation in treatment, compared with 64% in the earlier survey. It may be deduced that 63% of respondents in the MPAA survey used the SMP at subsequent visits before a decision to carry out cervical manipulation. This compares with 91% reporting this in the earlier survey. Also, important, 33% of respondents in the MPAA survey actually carried out the full APA Protocol prior to subsequent cervical manipulation, despite the requirement under the protocol for only the SMP to be performed.

Interestingly, given the anecdotal evidence of growing resistance to the protocol by clinicians, two thirds (67%) of respondents to the MPAA survey valued the protocol as part of their clinical practice, with 65% of the view that the MPAA and APA should continue to endorse the use of the protocol. Only 12% were strongly of the view that endorsement should not continue. Indeed, 70% of respondents were reported as identifying that they would continue to use the protocol, even if it were no longer endorsed by the APA. By comparison, in the earlier survey 67% and 66% respectively, considered that the APA Protocol placed appropriate medicolegal restrictions on the practitioner and that the protocol was an important initiative and should be retained.

On these comparisons alone, the reports of anecdotal evidence of a growing lack of compliance with the protocol seem unsubstantiated. However, the gaining of informed consent has undoubtedly been an issue as evidenced by the following comparisons. In the first survey,[5,7,8] 93% of physiotherapists using manipulative techniques in treatment reported that informed consent was gained. Of this 93%, however, only 58% gained informed consent in every case. This compares with 37% in the MPAA survey who obtained informed consent before the use of cervical manipulation with their patients. To what extent, if any, the view of the respondents in the first survey is any guide here is unknown, but 44% of them agreed that the requirement for informed consent on the part of the patient before undergoing cervical manipulation would mean that fewer patients would agree to manipulation as a form of treatment, and as a consequence, a valuable method of treatment would be used less frequently.

The MPAA survey[9] sought information about any incidents the responding manipulative physical therapists considered to be complications of examination and treatment. The survey results indicated an average of one complication per therapist over 2 years. The most common reaction or complication was the inducement of "VBI symptoms" (63%). A total of 57% of these resolved spontaneously, and there were no reported deaths or cerebrovascular accidents. The rate of VBI effects that were described as "minor only" was one per 50,000 manipulations. Given that there were no major sequelae, this represents a very low incidence of any form of adverse reaction to cervical manipulation.

The common denominator in most techniques associated with the incidents reported was a rotatory component. Passive mobilizing techniques accounted for 27.5% of incidents; examination techniques, including protocol procedures, 20%; and cervical manipulation; 16%. A total of 70% of respondents indicated that they could not identify any factor before the incident that would have alerted them to the potential for an adverse effect. Significantly, 60% identified that the APA Protocol had not been carried out before the incident occurring, and in 45% of these cases, the APA Protocol was recommended with the technique undertaken. When asked to identify the number of occasions in which cervical manipulation had not been used as a result of the patient's response to the protocol, 80% indicated more than two occasions because of positive findings on the subjective examination and 68% as a result of positive findings on the physical components of the procedure. The most frequent positive findings were provocation of dizziness (47%) and nausea (18%).

The MPAA used the results of the survey along with widespread consultation with key stakeholders (MPAA membership, APA, State Registration Boards, the legal profession, teaching faculty, and key researchers) and a targeted review of relevant literature to develop clinical guidelines to replace the APA Protocol. These guidelines, "The Australian Physiotherapy Association Clinical Guidelines for Premanipulative Procedures for the Cervical Spine," were endorsed by the APA Board of Directors in April 2000.[10]

Evolution—From Protocol to Clinical Guidelines

Premanipulative testing of the cervical spine after evaluation has gone from a rather prescriptive protocol to a set of clinical guidelines that rely more on the physical therapist's clinical reasoning and clinical judgment. The rationale for this evolution is that in all other aspects of manipulative physical therapy, clinical reasoning is strongly emphasized and it had been curiously absent in the APA Protocol. In addition, a set of clinical guidelines rather than a formal protocol more appropriately reflected the current practice of manipulative physical therapy in Australia.[11]

What are the key differences between the APA Protocol and the APA Clinical Guidelines, and what are the bases for these? The next section delineates key differences.

APA Clinical Guidelines for Premanipulative Procedures for the Cervical Spine

This section will outline the key differences between the APA Protocol for Premanipulative Testing of the Cervical Spine and the new APA Clinical Guidelines for Premanipulative Procedures for the Cervical Spine. It will also provide for the reader the essential details of the Clinical Guidelines, which are as yet unpublished (but available from the Australian Physiotherapy Association, PO Box 6465, St. Kilda Road Central, Victoria, Australia 8008).

Purpose

The APA Protocol was intended for use with all patients before cervical manipulation; however, the Clinical Guidelines have been extended to include all patients before cervical manipulation *and* before the use of techniques involving end-range cervical rotation (e.g., unilateral posteroanterior pressures undertaken in cervical rotation).

PREAMBLE

The preamble to the Clinical Guidelines is expanded beyond its predecessor in the protocol. Both documents identify that the test procedures themselves hold certain risks and recognize that the screening tests will not identify all patients at risk of suffering an adverse reaction to cervical manipulation. The guidelines, which are strengthened by references throughout, include the acknowledgment that the test procedures themselves have somewhat conflicting effects on selected blood flow parameters and that in any event, there is disagreement on what constitutes a clinically meaningful change in blood flow on cervical movement. The guidelines also add trauma and neurological changes as indicative factors for possible effects from manipulation and reiterate that there is no known method for testing the intrinsic anatomy of the VA.

The Guidelines also identify, with appropriate references,[12-19] that as rotation and rotation with extension "are equally sensitive in testing the change in flow velocity or volume flow rate in the VA, it is recommended that only one rotation be used." This remains (as with the protocol before it) a somewhat arbitrary decision as to which cervical movements to include and which to exclude. This is particularly relevant here, because the blood flow studies (using duplex Doppler ultrasound) have all been published since the earlier APA Protocol was formulated. These studies,[12-19,56-59] as this chapter will illustrate, show conflicting results with respect to the effects of both rotation and rotation with extension on blood flow, to the extent that they might be described more accurately as being equally *insensitive* in testing changes in blood flow.

Much like the protocol before it, the Clinical Guidelines outline the examination for the presence of symptoms suggestive of VBI at four stages in the management of a patient with an upper quarter disorder, namely the following:

- Subjective examination
- Physical examination
- Assessment of symptoms provoked *during* treatment of the cervical spine
- Assessment of symptoms *following* treatment

SUBJECTIVE EXAMINATION

Although the subjective examination is essentially the same in structure as the protocol before it, it is expanded in the Clinical Guidelines, to draw the therapist's attention to symptoms associated with dissection of the VA, as well as symptoms potentially of VBI origin. The symptoms identified as possibly associated with VBI include, as before, the five Ds—dizziness, diplopia, dysarthria, dysphagia, drop attacks—with the addition of nausea. All require specific questioning. The symptoms that may also be described by the patient and may have a link with VBI or VA dissection comprise the following:

- Light-headedness
- Strange feelings in the head
- Blackouts/fainting
- Blurriness of vision/transient hemianopia
- Tinnitus
- Vomiting

- Pins and needles in the tongue
- Pallor and sweating
- Other neurological symptoms
- History of cervical trauma

The new emphasis on VA dissection is valuable. Neck pain and headache have been reported in association with VA dissection, as has a history of cervical trauma.[20,21] This section of the Clinical Guidelines also provides useful pointers that differentiate VBI-related symptoms from those related to vestibular disorders, or benign paroxysmal positional vertigo,[22,23] and identifies background conditions that may be present with vestibular diseases.[23,24]

Physical Examination

The physical examination section of the APA Clinical Guidelines has the following three components:

1. Routine screening for *all* patients with upper quarter dysfunction for symptoms possibly associated with VBI
2. Testing for patients who, during the subjective examination, indicate the presence of symptoms potentially associated with VBI
3. Examination before the performance of a technique, which includes not only cervical manipulation but also end-range rotation of the cervical spine

Taken broadly, the physical examination may seem very similar to the APA Protocol, but there are important differences in procedure and in the emphasis on the clinical reasoning and clinical judgment of the therapist. The physical examination is presented in the point form that follows:

- In *every* patient for whom treatment of the cervical spine is to be performed, routine questioning about the provocation of VBI-related symptoms (presumably—but not specifically identified as—the five Ds and nausea) is undertaken during standard physical testing of the cervical spine.
- When patients indicate the presence of potential VBI symptoms during the subjective examination, the mandatory testing procedure under the new Clinical Guidelines is greatly reduced in comparison to the old protocol.
- Mandatory minimal testing recommended includes the following:
  —Sustained end-range cervical rotation to left and right
  —The position or movement that provokes symptoms as described by the patient
- The therapist determines whether cervical rotation is performed in the sitting or supine position, based on clinical reasoning from the patient's history and the subjective presentation. If, however, dizziness or other potential VBI symptoms are evoked, then cervical rotation should be performed in both positions. This assists the therapist in differentiating symptoms that have their origin in the vestibular system and are therefore affected by change in gravity.[23] If symptoms are evoked on rotation, further differentiation should be undertaken in the standing position as well, with the head held still and the trunk rotated (as per the protocol).[4,10]
- In these Clinical Guidelines, the therapist must make the clinical judgment as to whether to perform additional tests. These are not mandatory and could include sustained cervical extension, sustained cervical rotation with extension, simulated manipulation position, and—when the patient relates symptoms specifically to quick movements—quick movements of the head through available range.

- On every occasion in which a cervical manipulation or end-range rotation technique is to be performed, the Clinical Guidelines recommend that mandatory minimal testing is carried out. This is an improvement over the protocol, in which the simulated manipulation position was the only requirement.

Assessment During and After Treatment

The Clinical Guidelines outline more explicitly, and in more detail than the protocol, the situations in which specific questioning about the production of symptoms suggestive of VBI is essential and include the following:

- Immediately before and after a cervical manipulation
- During and immediately after a technique involving end-range rotation
- During and immediately after any treatment in a patient with symptoms suggestive of VBI on subjective examination or in a patient in whom such symptoms are evoked during the physical examination

From the point of view that the tests themselves can hold certain risks, perhaps the most contentious aspect of the guidelines is the advice that "if symptoms are provoked during treatment, the examination protocol . . . should be administered prior to continuation with treatment."[10] This appears to mean the minimal mandatory screening procedure should be performed for further differentiation before continuing with treatment. If this is indeed so, then the procedure would include not only sustained rotation but also, if rotation is positive, repeating it again in either supine or sitting and possibly repeating it again in standing (as trunk rotation), all in the name of differentiation. Thereby potentially increasing any morbidity associated with the tests themselves.

Interpreting the Results of the Examination Procedures

Commendably, under the Clinical Guidelines, the therapist is described as making the decision as to whether to consider cervical manipulation or an end-range rotation technique as treatment options, based on "clinical and biomedical knowledge and the strength of the subjective and physical evidence presented in any particular clinical situation."[10] However, the guidelines do specifically guide the therapist in recommending the following:

- When there is evidence of potential VBI symptoms from *both* the subjective and physical components of the patient examination, neither cervical manipulation nor an end-range rotation technique should be undertaken.
- When at any time there is evidence that symptoms are clearly VBI-related, neither cervical manipulation nor an end-range rotation technique should be used in treatment.

Providing of Information and Obtaining Consent for Cervical Manipulation

The Clinical Guidelines include a substantially revised and considerably more detailed section on providing information to the patient, informed consent, and gaining consent than formed part of the APA Protocol. This is to be commended. Although it is not spelled out in the Clinical Guidelines, the formal requirement to inform the patient about the risk of death, which was part of the protocol, has been removed, based on legal advice that "the risk was sufficiently low (none reported in the MPAA survey) that it did not constitute greater risk than everyday activities and therefore was not required to be reported."[11] The guidelines outline the differences in types of consent as recognized in law so as to assist the therapist in making decisions for gaining consent and recording consent. The recommended method of recording consent is outlined in some detail and includes the following:

Express consent: An individual's explicit indication of agreement either orally or in writing, which should be obtained each time a cervical manipulation is performed. However, it is not necessary to obtain written consent for this or any other procedure.

Implied consent: A situation in which an individual does not specifically indicate agreement but performs some action suggesting consent. Implied consent is sufficient when a patient can stop a treatment technique during its performance. This is sufficient for an end-range rotation technique for example.

Clinical guidelines, like protocols, need regular evaluation. Evaluation has already commenced, as is evidenced by the AJP Forum on Premanipulative Testing of the Cervical Spine.[25]

The remainder of this chapter overviews the underpinnings of the Clinical Guidelines and the earlier protocol.

INCIDENTS AND ACCIDENTS INVOLVING THE VERTEBRAL ARTERY AFTER CERVICAL MANIPULATION

The recent MPAA survey of manipulative physical therapists in Australia gave an incident rate of minor complications of 1 per 50,000 cervical manipulations.[9] Respondents were asked to report any incidents that could be considered complications. The complications, described as "VBI symptoms," on the whole, were deemed minor on analysis, with the majority of these resolving spontaneously. No deaths or cerebrovascular accidents were reported. Rivett and Reid[26] reported the risk of stroke after cervical manipulation in a New Zealand study as varying from 1 in 163,000 to 1 million. Given that the MPAA survey identified that those manipulative physical therapists who responded carried out 3 to 4 cervical manipulations per week on average, Reid and Hing[27] deduced that these therapists were unlikely to perform 163,000 cervical manipulations in a working lifetime. These authors questioned whether premanipulative procedures (such as the Clinical Guidelines and the protocol before them) might, by their very existence, exaggerate the risks of manipulation.

Using an incident rate of one serious vascular accident per million manipulations and a typical course of chiropractic treatment for patients with neck pain or tension headache as 10 to 15 sessions of cervical manipulation over the course of a year, Dabbs and Lauretti[28] calculated that there would be one serious vascular complication per 100,000 patients. They deduced that these complications would be such that one third of patients would recover with mild or no residual effects and approximately 25% would die, yielding a risk of one death per 400,000 patients treated.

There is no way to judge the number of patients who receive manipulative treatment nor the overall number of manipulations performed. Eisenberg et al[29] estimated that approximately 250 million spinal manipulations were performed annually in the United States. It can be deduced that tens of thousands of manipulative techniques are performed across the world on a single day. Many authors have estimated the incidence of serious consequences after cervical manipulative treatment. These include 1 in 200,000 manipulations,[30] 1 in 400,000,[31] 1 in approximately 500,000,[32,33] 0.5 to 2 per million,[28] and 1 in 1.3 million treatment sessions.[34]

Although the precise incidence of vascular accidents after cervical manipulation is unknown, it is clear that serious complications go unreported in the literature, and many transient deficits and/or instances of exacerbations of patients' symptoms after manipulation do occur.[35-39] Two prospective studies are worthy of note. Rivett and Milburn,[38] in their study of manipulative physical therapists in New Zealand, identified a 0.21% incidence rate for minor exacerbations of patients' symptoms after cervical manipulation—namely, 1 in 476 manipulations. Surveying chiropractors in Norway in their prospective study, Senstad et al[39] found 11% of those surveyed identified responses to manipulation that prevented patients from performing their activities of daily living. (However, this 11% included lumbar manipulation as well.) No permanent complications after manipulation were reported in either study.

How might estimates of serious complications after cervical manipulation be put into perspective? Dabbs and Lauretti[28] have drawn comparisons with complications after the use of nonsteroidal antiinflammatory drugs (NSAIDs), which are commonly prescribed for neck pain.[40] NSAIDs are among the most prescribed drugs in the United States and Australia and also account for millions of dollars in annual sales of over-the-counter forms that do not require prescriptions. The authors of this paper reviewed studies that had estimated the probability of serious gastrointestinal ulcers or death from ulcers caused by the use of NSAIDs for conditions that were likely to be also treated by cervical manipulation (e.g., osteoarthritis, cervical spondylosis). The authors estimated that the risk of serious complications or death was 100 to 400 times greater after the use of NSAIDs than after cervical manipulation. Hurwitz et al[41] also drew comparisons between NSAID use and cervical manipulation. They reported the incidence of a "serious gastrointestinal event" as 1 in 1,000 patients, whereas they estimated 5 to 10 complications per 10 million cervical manipulations. It is instructive to note, by way of comparison, that the study reported 15.6 cases of complications per 1,000 patients undergoing surgery to the cervical spine.[41]

WHAT CAN BE LEARNED FROM THESE INCIDENTS AND ACCIDENTS?

What can be deduced from published case reports of serious complications or death after cervical manipulation?[3,20,31,36,37] Complications were experienced predominantly by young adults in their late 30s (mean 39.6 years, range 4 months to 87 years[36]; mean 37.3 years, range 7 to 63 years[3]). Even when practitioners could be correctly identified,[42] the majority of injuries were attributed to manipulation by chiropractors;[3,36] less than 2% of the cases involved physical therapists.[3,36] When a direction of manipulation could be ascertained, the most frequent description was of a rotational thrust.[3,20,36,37] Haldeman et al[20] have stated that rotation is the most common cervical spinal manipulation procedure in use (by chiropractors), and Curtis and Bove[43] report that rotary adjustments of the cervical spine were part of about 30% of visits made to chiropractors. The preponderance of such manipulations undertaken by physical therapists is not known. Just what is meant by a *rotation manipulation* is important, as the APA Protocol recommends that long lever rotatory thrusts should never be used in the cervical spine.

Also the reviews of case reports revealed that only 10% of patients were identified as undergoing their first cervical manipulation when the incident occurred. In analyzing 177 case reports published between 1925 and 1997, Di Fabio[36] stated that "cervical manipulation was not a new treatment for nearly half of the patients." Presumably these patients had previously experienced cervical manipulation without serious incident. Grant[3] and Terrett[37] have recommended testing be undertaken at each patient visit before cervical manipulation. This is clearly delineated both in the APA Protocol and in the APA Clinical Guidelines.

Case reports described multiple manipulations at the treatment session. The APA Protocol[4] proposed that when cervical manipulation is chosen as the method of treatment, a single localized manipulation should be undertaken and its effect assessed. Grant[5] stated, "it is well to consider whether multiple cervical manipulations at a single treatment session are ever necessary in view of the potential cumulative effect on the VA." By contrast, a single cervical manipulation at a treatment session for chronic neck pain was described by Dabbs and Lauretti[28] as having "clear irrelevance to [chiropractic] clinical practice." The APA Clinical Guidelines leave such decisions (namely, the number of cervical manipulations at a treatment session) quite rightly to the clinical judgment of the manipulative physical therapist.

MECHANISM OF INJURY TO THE VERTEBRAL ARTERY

Stretching and momentary occlusion of the VA occur in normal daily activities and are asymptomatic. Indeed, the extracranial portion of the VA (Figure 8-1) appears to be designed for movement and, in some parts, to compensate for lack of support. This extracranial section has a well-developed external elastic lamina and media.[44-46] Interestingly, after the artery penetrates the dura (in its fourth part) and joins with its contralateral fellow to form the basilar artery, the adventitia becomes much reduced; external elastic lamina disappears, and the elastic fibrils in the media become very rare.

The VAs contribute about 11% of the total cerebral blood flow; the remaining 89% is supplied by the carotid system.[48] Asymmetry in the size of the two VAs is exceedingly common.[49,50] Indeed, complete interruption of blood flow in one VA, such as follows its ligation,[51] may be asymptomatic as long as there is a normal configura-

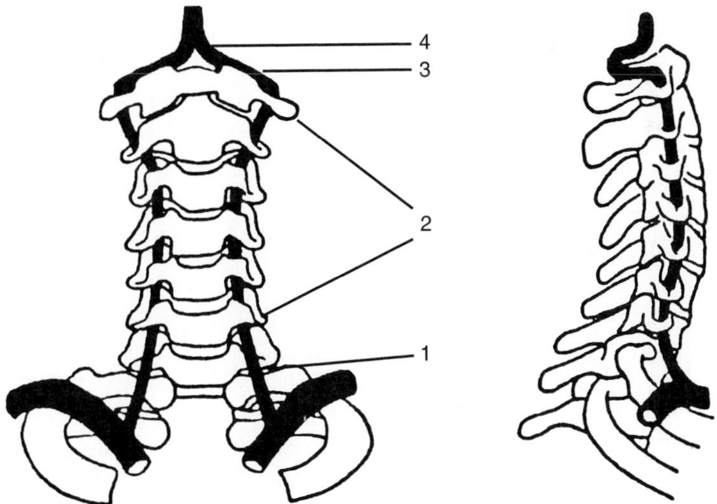

Figure 8-1

Anterior and lateral views of the vertebral artery. The course of the vertebral artery may be described in four parts. The first part *(1)* extends from the subclavian artery to the C6 foramen transversarium. The second part *(2)* runs vertically through the foramina transversaria of the upper six cervical vertebrae. The third part *(3)* passes through the foramen transversarium of the C1 vertebra and turns horizontally across it. The fourth part *(4)* enters the foramen magnum to join the opposite artery to form the basilar artery.

(From Bogduk N: In *The Cervical Spine and Headache Symposium*, Brisbane, 1981, Manipulative Therapists Association of Australia.)

tion of the circle of Willis and adequate flow through the other VA. Thus, although blood flow may be affected by a variety of circumstances, both intrinsic (e.g., atherosclerosis) and extrinsic (e.g., osteophyte impingement), the mere presence of a stenotic or occlusive lesion does not necessarily imply the presence of symptoms. Symptoms will occur when the blood supply to an area is critically reduced. This will depend ultimately on a balance between compromising and compensatory factors.

The major vascular complications after cervical manipulation occurred predominantly in young adults, as was identified previously.[3,36,37] This finding suggests that neither cervical spondylitic and osteoarthrotic changes nor atheroma of the vertebrobasilar system would be pathognomonic in the majority of these cases. Bony changes, when present, are most likely to compromise the VA in its second part (Figure 8-1). Compromise of the VA in the vertical portion through the foramina tranversaria of the upper six cervical vertebrae was infrequently reported in the case studies reviewed. Trauma to the VA after cervical manipulation occurred predominantly in its third part, the atlantoaxial component (Figure 8-2), and in most cases was related to a manipulative thrust technique with a strong rotary component. This part of the artery is subject to stretching as a result of the large range of rotation that occurs at the C1-2 level. As early as 1884, Gerlach[52] recognized from his cadaver studies that rotation of the neck resulted in stretching of the contralateral VA at this level, and many other authors have since confirmed this.

It can be deduced that the extent of the trauma to the VA after a strong rotary manipulation would be greater in the more mobile neck of the young adult than in the older person in whom spondylitic, osteoarthritic, or normal degenerative changes would limit the extent to which the neck could be rotated, thereby according some protection to the atlantoaxial segment of the artery.

The nature of the arterial insult may be such that spasm of the artery ensues. This may be transient, or it may persist and result in brainstem ischemia. If it is transient, it may render the affected artery irritable, so that a manipulation done later may result in a major sequela. The trauma of the manipulation may actually damage the artery

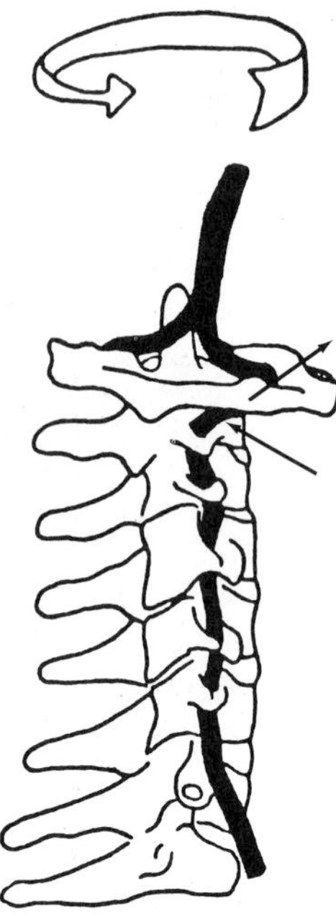

Figure 8-2

A sketch of the right vertebral artery, demonstrating how the atlantoaxial segment *(arrow)* is stretched forward by left rotation of the atlas.

(From Bogduk N: In *The Cervical Spine and Headache Symposium*, Brisbane, 1981, Manipulative Therapists Association of Australia.)

wall, resulting in subintimal tearing, arterial dissection, hematoma, perivascular hemorrhage, thrombosis, or embolus formation. The extent of the damage may well determine the extent of the resulting brainstem ischemia. An understanding of the mechanism of injury highlights the degree of concern raised by the case histories in which practitioners continued to manipulate, in part to relieve the additional symptoms that were created. Indeed, Terrett's recounting of some of these case reports makes chilling reading.[53]

The most frequently reported injury in the large series of case studies delineated by Di Fabio[36] was indeed arterial dissection or spasm, followed by brainstem injury and Wallenberg's syndrome, respectively. Vertebrobasilar arterial dissection and occlusion leading to brainstem and cerebellar ischemia and infarction are rare but often devastating and unexpected causes of stroke. Haldeman et al[20] noted that this type of stroke can occur in otherwise healthy young people, "often with a close temporal relation to common neck movement, cervical spine manipulation or trauma."

RISK FACTORS FOR VERTEBROBASILAR ARTERY DISSECTION

To ascertain the risk factors and precipitating neck movements causing vertebrobasilar arterial dissection after cervical trauma and spinal manipulation, Haldeman et al[20] undertook an extensive review and analysis of the English-language literature before 1993. The 367 case reports included in the study were broken down into four categories: cases of spontaneous onset (160), cases after spinal manipulation (115), cases associated with trivial trauma (58), and cases with major trauma (37). Three cases were classified in two categories.

In their extensive literature review, Haldeman et al[20] found the four most commonly discussed risk factors for vertebrobasilar arterial dissection to be migraine, hypertension, oral contraceptive use, and smoking. They analyzed the case studies for the presence of these risk factors and found the incidence to be equal to or often less than their incidence in the U.S. population at large. Interestingly, the most frequent reporting of migraine, hypertension, and contraceptive use was in the spontaneous dissection group. The next most frequent were migraine and hypertension in the trivial trauma group, followed by the manipulation group. The authors acknowledged the limitations in analysis of retrospective cases—for example, accepting a causal link of trauma in cervical manipulation and looking no further, searching more assiduously to find a cause, or identifying risk factors when reporting cases of spontaneous dissection or trivial trauma. Prospective studies clearly are needed. Migraine appears the most contentious risk factor vis á vis an association with vertebrobasilar arterial dissection. In a consideration of patients who had dissections of vertebral or carotid arteries, D'anglejan-Chatillon et al[54] found migraine sufferers to be more frequently represented (40%) than in a control group (24%). Other authors who considered only VA dissections did not find a greater prevalence of migraine than in the population at large.[20,55,56] Again, however, most studies have been retrospective reviews.

Regardless of the precipitating factor or risk factor, it is very difficult to ignore the close temporal association between trauma and the number of cases of VA dissection, whether it be manipulation, trivial trauma, motor vehicle accidents, or strenuous activities. Significantly, the symptoms of VA dissection are acute neck pain and headache—that is, precisely the symptoms for which patients seek treatment and for which they not uncommonly receive cervical manipulation by way of treatment. Although there appears to be no clear-cut risk factor for VA dissection (other than a relationship with trauma), clinicians need to be on the alert. Clinicians should particularly beware of acute neck pain and headache after sporting activities, strenuous activities, awkward postures, or rapid jerking movements and should remember the temporal association of VA dissection with trauma.[20,21,55,56] Although it was infrequent (9 of 160 cases), a history of nonrecent trauma (i.e., greater than 2 or more months) was the most common factor in Haldeman's retrospective review of spontaneous vertebrobasilar arterial dissection or occlusion.[20]

On behalf of the Canadian Stroke Consortium, Norris et al[21] have been prospectively collecting detailed information on cases of dissection of the vertebral and carotid arteries. A total of 74 patients have been studied to date. A total of 81% of the dissections, which were predominantly vertebrobasilar in origin, were associated with either cervical manipulation (28%), sudden head movement as in a bout of coughing, or dental examination. Norris et al state that "sudden and often severe neck or occipital pain is the hallmark of dissection (74% in our cases) and its onset is a useful index of the actual moment of dissection."[21] They also identified that in 25% of cases of dissection involving the carotid artery, ipsilateral Horner's syndrome was present and was sometimes the only sign that dissection had occurred. Norris et al[21] conclude that neck manipulation should probably be avoided in patients with recent acute onset neck pain, especially if it closely follows an accidental injury.

The emphasis in the new APA Clinical Guidelines on symptoms associated with VA dissection and linkage with a history of cervical trauma (which may be relatively minor) is commendable.

HOW SENSITIVE ARE SCREENING TESTS IN DETECTING PATIENTS AT RISK?

Premanipulative screening tests have been chosen on the basis that these cervical movements (most commonly but not exclusively rotation and rotation combined with extension) narrow the VA, thereby reducing VA blood flow to the brain. When symptoms and signs of VBI are elicited, the deduction is that collateral circulation may be inadequate, and the patient's neck should not be manipulated.

Premanipulative testing however, is much more than simply applying the physical screening tests component. The eliciting of symptoms or signs associated with VBI when using the APA Clinical Guidelines or other premanipulative protocols, does cause the therapist to determine on the weight of clinical evidence, whether manipulation can be safely used, or whether another treatment approach should be chosen.

The therapist must remember, too, that premanipulative testing does not simulate the forces forming part of a cervical manipulation. Should those forces result in damage to the VA (or, for instance, progress an impending VA dissection from previous minor cervical trauma) in the presence of negative findings on screening tests, even excellent collateral circulation would not protect the patient against an incident or accident associated with cervical manipulation.

Nonetheless, the question of the screening tests' sensitivity in detecting the at-risk patient still needs to be answered.

A number of researchers have used diagnostic ultrasound in vivo to assess change in VA blood flow when the head is placed in sustained rotation and/or rotation combined with extension.[12-19,57-60] In the last 6 to 8 years, the advent of duplex Doppler ultrasound with color enhancement has made for greater accuracy in visualizing the VA in both patients and asymptomatic controls and in investigating the effects of screening tests on VA blood flow. Overall, however, the results of these studies are conflicting at best and do not lend support to the sensitivity of the screening tests in detecting patients at risk.

It can be argued that a number of methodological factors contribute to these inconclusive results.[19,61] These include whether the method of assessing VA blood flow had established reliability, which blood flow parameters were used, at what levels of the VA blood flow was measured, which cervical movements or combinations thereof were investigated, whether one or both VAs were measured, whether subjects were in sitting or supine positions, whether subjects were patients with VBI symptoms or asymptomatic volunteers, and the level of expertise of the sonographer.

To date, only three groups of researchers[12,17,19,57-59] have used duplex Doppler ultrasound to investigate the effects of cervical movements that form part of premanipulative testing on VA blood flow in patients with VBI symptoms. These researchers also have compared the effects with those in an asymptomatic control group. All researchers measured the effects of sustained rotation and sustained rotation combined with extension on VA blood flow parameters. All used duplex Doppler ultrasound but measured the VA at different levels and used different blood flow parameters. Despite this variation, no study demonstrated a significant difference in blood flow between patients with clinical signs of VBI and a control group. The expectation based on the rationale for the use of premanipulative testing might well be otherwise—that is, if the tests measured what they were purported to measure, or in other words, if they were to be considered valid.

The sites at which Thiel et al[19] and Licht et al[14,15,57,58] measured blood flow in the VA were at a considerable distance from the site of greatest narrowing and of greatest vulnerability in the VA with premanipulative testing—that is, the atlantoaxial level (C1-2). These researchers used C3-5[19] and "a point midway between the origin of the VA from the . . . subclavian artery and its disappearance into the foramen of the sixth transverse cervical process,"[15] respectively, thereby limiting both the sensitivity and applicability of their findings. The study by Thiel et al[19] had several other limitations. The authors used the systolic/diastolic ratio (S/D ratio) to determine the effect of sustained combined extension/rotation (Wallenberg test) on VA blood flow. This is an impedance ratio and as such is a crude quantification of vessel narrowing with questionable clinical meaning[61-63] that may be useful only in detecting severe stenoses.[64] Furthermore, no reliability studies were reported, and (as mentioned previously) the S/D ratio at C3-5 is an indirect (upstream) measure from the site of greatest VA narrowing (C1-2). The study by Cote et al[12] subjected the data of Thiel et al[19] to further statistical analysis with no new subjects added; thus the same limitations hold. Licht's work,[14,15,57,58] although ground-breaking, suffers too from the use of an indirect (upstream) measure—namely, flow velocity below C6 to investigate the effect of sustained rotation and sustained extension with rotation (de Kleyn's test) on VA blood flow.

The first blood flow parameter to alter with artery narrowing is velocity within the narrowed section itself. The atlantoaxial (C1-2) segment of the VA is the most common site of narrowing secondary to cervical movement as well as the most frequent site of pathological change in incidents and accidents of cervical manipulation, as was outlined earlier. Therefore measurements of blood flow velocity at C1-2 should be undertaken whenever possible. Surprisingly, very few studies using duplex Doppler ultrasound have measured VA blood flow at this site,[59-61] and in only one were patients with VBI symptoms measured.[59] In part, this paucity of studies is caused by the difficulty (even with color enhancement) of measuring reliably at C1-2, yet this level is the most sensitive indicator of low-grade VA narrowing. Rivett et al[59] investigated the effects of screening tests (sustained extension, sustained rotation, sustained rotation with extension) on blood flow in the contralateral VA at C1-2 in 100 patients. A total of 51 of these patients were positive on premanipulative testing, and 49 were negative. A number of hemodynamic parameters were used, including three velocity measures, lumen diameter, and flow rate. Significant changes in most of the hemodynamic parameters were found in both VAs in the test positions. However, differences between the two groups were "clinically minor and generally not statistically significant."[59] A total of 20 patients exhibited partial or total occlusion of the contralateral VA during testing in end-range rotation and combined rotation with extension. Only two of these had VBI symptoms or signs on occlusion. Rivett et al found the sensitivity and specificity of the premanipulative tests to be poor in detecting a patient with a totally or partially occluded VA at C1-2 and, as they deduced thereby, inadequately sensitive and specific to consistently identify patients at potential risk of VA injury and consequent stroke after manipulation.

Thus to date there is no evidence from a hemodynamic perspective that the screening tests are able to detect patients at risk of an incident or accident after cervical manipulation. Furthermore, there is no conclusive evidence that cervical rotation is more or less sensitive in effecting changes in VA blood flow than rotation combined with extension. There is need, however, to undertake more comprehensive hemodynamic evaluations of the effects of premanipulative tests in symptomatic patients than has been done to date before these tests are dismissed on hemodynamic grounds. As mentioned previously, the first blood flow parameter to alter with artery narrowing is velocity within the narrowed section itself. Not only is flow velocity affected at the site of narrowing, but volume of blood flow will also be affected—however, only after critical narrowing levels are reached. Measurement of volume flow rate (as well as blood velocity) is necessary to interpret whether blood velocity is actually increasing, as is the case when there is low-grade narrowing, or whether blood velocity is decreasing because critical levels of narrowing have been reached. Volume flow rate should be measured at a distance from the site of narrowing to avoid turbulent flood flow, therefore not at C1-2. This is because the volume flow calculation assumes uniform blood velocity; hence volume flow rate is frequently measured at C5-6. For a comprehensive hemodynamic evaluation, measures at C1-2 (velocity) and at C5-6 (volume flow) in the VA should be undertaken.

To date, the writer's research laboratory appears to be the only one using this comprehensive approach,[60,61,65] but no evaluations of patients testing positive on premanipulative testing have been assessed to date. The reliability of the hemodynamic measures—namely, peak flow velocity at C1-2 and volume flow rate at C5-6—has been established,[61] and Zaina et al[60] have demonstrated no significant changes in these measures in the contralateral VA with cervical rotation in a young asymptomatic group. The interesting finding that has emerged from this study[60] is that of a pattern for peak flow velocity in the VA at C1-2 on return from sustained end-range rotation to be less than at end-range (significantly so in the case of the neutral head position measurement on return from right rotation in the left VA). Although this preliminary finding needs to be corroborated with a larger sample and tested in patients with clinical signs of VBI, it is the first time this has been reported. Furthermore, it gives some support to the rest period that occurs on return of the patient's head and neck to the neutral position after the application of a screening test, to allow for any latent effect of that test as described in the APA Clinical Guidelines and the APA Protocol.

Schmidt et al[65] also used this comprehensive hemodynamic test procedure to determine the effects of the screening tests in the APA Protocol taken together on VA blood flow in an asymptomatic group. (The simulated manipulation position was not included; only the cervical movements of extension, rotation, and rotation with extension were included.) No significant differences in VA peak velocity at C1-2 or volume flow rate at C5-6 before and after the application of the protocol tests were found in either VA, thereby lending support to a lack of a cumulative effect of these tests on the VAs in a young asymptomatic group. Further analysis of the data revealed an order effect such that the postprotocol VA flow rate at C5-6 measured first differed significantly from that measured second (namely, in the other VA). Which VA was measured first after the application of the protocol tests was randomly determined. The significant difference noted ($p = 0.015$) revealed that the posttest VA volume flow rate measurements sampled first increased, whereas the measurements taken in the remaining VA decreased. These differences remained for up to 20 minutes after application of the protocol tests, after return of head and neck to the neutral position. These findings[59,64] suggest that researchers should put equal emphasis on delineating what happens after the administration of screening tests or immediately on return of the head to the neutral position and thereafter. This assumes greater relevance when consideration is given to what effect the treatment techniques that follow such tests may have on further changing the VA blood flow.

CONCLUSION

Evidence of the sensitivity and specificity of the physical screening tests in detecting the patient at risk of potential complication after cervical manipulation still eludes manual therapists. These tests do not appear to alter blood flow parameters in clinically significant ways in patients with VBI symptoms when compared with controls. Rivett[59] argues that the predictive value of the Clinical Guidelines is largely contingent on the validity of these physical screening tests—in particular, sustained end-range cervical rotation. (The same was no less true of the APA Protocol before them.)

However, what has not been called into question is the ability of the physical therapist to produce, reproduce, and/or independently replicate patients' symptoms that may suggest VBI—that is, to reliably categorize patients as positive or negative on clinical testing.[17,58,67] Such clinical judgment incorporates more than simply the patient's response to the physical screening tests, important though this is. The subjective examination, the history, and the symptom behavior all play key roles in the physical therapist's decision whether to proceed with the use of cervical manipulation in treatment.

Physical therapists are in the excellent position of having a number of treatment approaches at their disposal in the management of patients with upper quarter dysfunction. This is of considerable value if and when there is uncertainty regarding the use of cervical manipulation in treatment.

References

1. Maitland GD: *Vertebral manipulation*, ed 2, London, 1968, Butterworths.
2. Grant R: Clinical testing before cervical manipulation—can we recognise the patient at risk? Proceedings of the tenth international Congress of the World Confederation for Physical Therapy, Sydney, Australia, 1987.
3. Grant R: Dizziness testing and manipulation of the cervical spine. In Grant R, editor: *Physical therapy of the cervical and thoracic spine*, ed 1, New York, 1988, Churchill Livingstone.
4. Protocol for premanipulative testing of the cervical spine, *Aust J Physiother* 34:927, 1988.
5. Grant R: Vertebral artery concerns: premanipulative testing of the cervical spine. In Grant R, editor: *Physical therapy of the cervical and thoracic spine*, ed 2, New York, 1994, Churchill Livingstone.

6. Grant R, Trott PH: Premanipulative testing of the cervical spine—the APA Protocol and its aftermath. Proceedings of the Eleventh International Congress of the World Confederation for Physical Therapy, London, 1991.
7. Grant R: Vertebral artery insufficiency: a clinical protocol for premanipulative testing of the cervical spine. In Boyling JD, Palastanga A, editors: *Grieve's modern manual therapy*, ed 2, Edinburgh, 1994, Churchill Livingstone.
8. Grant R: Vertebral artery testing—the Australian Physiotherapy Association Protocol after 6 years, *Manual Therapy* 1(3):149, 1996.
9. Magarey M, Rebbeck T, Coughlan B et al: APA premanipulative testing protocol for the cervical spine: researched and renewed. I. Research. In Singer KP, editor: Proceedings of the Seventh Scientific conference of the IFOMT in conjunction with the MPAA, Perth, Australia, 2000.
10. Australian Physiotherapy Association: Clinical guidelines for premanipulative procedures for the cervical spine, PO Box 6465, St Kilda Rd Central, Victoria, Australia 8008.
11. Magarey M, Coughlan B, Rebbeck T: APA premanipulative testing protocol for the cervical spine: researched and renewed. II. Revised clinical guidelines. In Singer KP, editor: Proceedings of the Seventh Scientific Conference of the IFOMT in conjunction with the MPAA, Perth, Australia, 2000.
12. Cote P, Kreitz BG, Cassidy JD et al: The validity of the extension-rotation test as a clinical screening procedure before neck manipulation: secondary analysis, *J Manipulative Physio Ther* 19:159, 1996.
13. Li YK, Zhang YK, Lu CM et al: Changes and implications of blood flow velocity of the vertebral artery during rotation and extension of the head, *J Manipulative Physio Ther* 22(2):91, 1999.
14. Licht PB, Christensen HW, Hollund-Carlsen PF: Vertebral artery volume flow in human beings, *J Manipulative Physio Ther* 22(6):363, 1999.
15. Licht PB, Christensen HW, Hojgaard P et al: Triplex ultrasound of vertebral artery flow during cervical rotation, *J Manipulative Physiol Ther* 21(1):27, 1998.
16. Refshauge KM: Rotation: a valid premanipulative dizziness test? Does it predict safe manipulation? *J Manipulative Physio Ther* 17:15, 1994.
17. Rivett D, Sharples KJ, Milburn PD: Effect of premanipulative tests on vertebral artery and internal carotid artery blood flow: a pilot study, *J Manipulative Physiol Ther* 22(6):368, 1999.
18. Stevens A: Functional Doppler sonography of the vertebral artery and some considerations about manual techniques, *J Manual Med* 6:102, 1991.
19. Thiel H, Wallace K, Donat J et al: Effect of various head and neck positions on vertebral artery blood flow, *Clinical Biomechanics* 9:105, 1994.
20. Haldeman S, Kohlbeck FJ, McGregor M: Risk factors and precipitating neck movements causing vertebrobasilar artery dissection after cervical trauma and spinal manipulation, *Spine* 24(8):785, 1999.
21. Norris JW, Beletsky V, Nadareishvili ZG: Sudden neck movement and cervical artery dissection, *Can Med Assoc J* 163(1):38, 2000.
22. Davies RA: Disorders of balance. In Luxon LM, Davies RA, editors: *Handbook of vestibular rehabilitation*, San Diego, 1997, Singular Publishing Group.
23. van de Velde GM: Benign paroxysmal positional vertigo. I Background and clinical presentation, *J Can Chiropract Assoc* 43(1):31, 1999.
24. Baloh RW, Holmaggi GM, editors: *Disorders of the vestibular system*, New York, 1996, Oxford University Press.
25. AJP Forum: Premanipulative testing of the cervical spine, *Aust J Physiother* 47:163, 2001.
26. Rivett D, Reid D: Risk of stroke for cervical manipulation in New Zealand, *NZ J Physiother* 26:14, 1998.
27. Reid D, Hing W: Are we on the right track? AJP Forum: premanipulative testing of the cervical spine, *Aust J Physiother* 47:165, 2001.
28. Dabbs V, Lauretti WJ: A risk assessment of cervical manipulation vs NSAIDs for the treatment of neck pain, *J Manipulative Physiol Ther* 18(8):530, 1995.

29. Eisenberg DM, Kessler RC, Foster C et al: Unconventional medicine in the United States: prevalence, costs and patterns of use, *N Engl J Med* 328:246, 1993.
30. Haynes MJ: Stroke following cervical manipulation in Perth, *J Aust Chirop Assoc* 24(2):42, 1994.
31. Dvorak J, Orelli FW: How dangerous is manipulation to the cervical spine? Case report and results of a survey, *Manual Mede* 2:1, 1985.
32. Patjin J: Complications in manual medicine: a review of the literature, *J Manual Med* 6:89, 1991.
33. Lee KP, Carlini WG, McCormick GF et al: Neurologic complications following chiropractic manipulation: a survey of California neurologists, *Neurology* 45:1213, 1995.
34. Klougart N, Lebouef-Yde C, Rasmussen LR: Safety in chiropractic practice. I. The occurrence of cerebrovascular accidents after manipulation to the neck in Denmark from 1978-1988, *J Manipulative Physiol Ther* 19:371, 1996.
35. Michaeli A: Reported occurrence and nature of complications following manipulative physiotherapy in South Africa, *Aust J Physiother* 39:309, 1993.
36. Di Fabio R: Manipulation of the cervical spine: risks and benefits, *Phys Ther* 75(1):50, 1999.
37. Terrett AGJ: Vascular accidents from cervical spine manipulation: report on 107 cases, *J Aust Chirop Assoc* 17(1):15, 1987.
38. Rivett DA, Milburn P: A prospective study of complications of cervical spine manipulation, *J Manipulative Physiol Ther* 4:166, 1996.
39. Senstad O, Leboeuf-Yde C, Borchgrevink C: Frequency and characteristics of side effects of spinal and manipulative therapy, *Spine* 22:435, 1997.
40. Dillin W, Uppal GS: Analysis of medications used in the treatment of cervical disc degeneration, *Orthop Clin North Am* 23:421, 1992.
41. Hurwitz EL, Aker PD, Adams AH et al: Manipulation and mobilization of the cervical spine: a systematic review of the literature, *Spine* 21:1746, 1996.
42. Terrett AGJ: Misuse of the literature by medical authors in discussing spinal manipulative therapy injury, *J Manipulative Physiol Ther* 18:203, 1995.
43. Curtis P, Bove G: Family physicians, chiropractors and back pain, *J Fam Pract* 35:551, 1992.
44. Wilkinson IMS: The vertebral artery: extracranial and intracranial structure, *Arch Neurol* 27:392, 1972.
45. Winkler G: Remarques sur la structure de l'artere vertebrale, *Quad Anat Prac* 28:105, 1972.
46. George B, Laurian C: *The vertebral artery, pathology and surgery*, Vienna, 1987, Springer Verlag.
47. Bogduk N: Dizziness and the vertebral artery. In *The Cervical Spine and Headache Symposium*, Brisbane, 1981, Manipulative Therapists Association of Australia.
48. Hardesty WH, Whitacre WB, Toole JF et al: Studies on vertebral artery blood flow in man, *Surg Gyn Obstet* 11:662, 1963.
49. Frank JP, Dimarina V, Pannier M et al: Les arteres vertebrales. Segments atlanto-axoidiens V3 et intra-cranien V4 collaterales, *Anat Clin* 2:229, 1980.
50. Cavdar S, Arisan E: Variations in extracranial origin of human vertebral artery, *Acta Anat* 135:236, 1989.
51. Shintani A, Zervas NT: Consequence of ligation of the vertebral artery, *J Neurosurg* 36:447, 1972.
52. Gerlach L: Ueber die bewegungen in den atlasgelenken und deren beziehungen zu der blutstromung in den vertebralarterien. *Beitr Morphol* 1:104, 1884; cited by George B, Laurian C, *The vertebral artery, pathology and surgery*, Vienna, 1987, Springer Verlag.
53. Terrett AGJ: Vascular accidents from cervical manipulation: the mechanisms, *J Aust Chirop Assoc* 25:59, 1988.
54. D'anglejan-Chatillon J, Ribeiro V, Mas JL et al: Migraine—a risk factor for dissection of cervical arteries, *Headache* 29:560, 1989.
55. Silbert PL, Mokri B, Schievink WL: Headache and neck pain in spontaneous internal carotid and vertebral artery dissections, *Neurology* 45:1517, 1995.

56. Sturzenegger M: Headache and neck pain: the warning symptoms of vertebral artery dissection, *Headache* 34:187, 1994.
57. Licht PB, Christensen HW, Hojgaard P et al: Vertebral artery flow and spinal manipulation: a randomized controlled and observer-blinded study, *J Manipulative Physiol Ther* 21(3):141, 1998.
58. Licht PB, Christensen HW, Hoilund-Carlsen PF: Is there a role for premanipulative testing before cervical manipulation? *J Manipulative Physiol Ther* 23(3):175, 2000.
59. Rivett D, Sharples K, Milburn P: Vertebral artery blood flow during pre-manipulative testing of the cervical spine. In Singer KP, editor: Proceedings of the seventh scientific conference of the IFOMT in conjunction with the MPAA, Perth, Australia, 2000.
60. Zaina C, Grant R, Johnson C et al: The effect of cervical rotation on blood flow in the contralateral vertebral artery, (in press).
61. Johnson C, Grant R, Dansie B et al: Measurement of blood flow in the vertebral artery using colour duplex Doppler ultrasound: establishment of the reliability of selected parameters, *Manual Therapy* 5(1):21, 2000.
62. Taylor KJW, Holland S: Doppler ultrasound. I. Basic principles, instrumentation and pitfalls, *Radiology* 174:297, 1990.
63. Polak JF: Peripheral arterial disease: evaluation with colour flow and duplex sonography, *Radiol Clin North Am* 31:71, 1995.
64. Saarinen O, Salmela K, Edgren J: Doppler ultrasound in the diagnosis of renal transplant artery stenosis—value of resistive index, *Acta Radiologica,* 35:586, 1994.
65. Schmidt SG, Grant R, Dansie B et al: The APA Protocol for Premanipulative Testing of the Cervical Spine: is there a change in vertebral artery blood flow following its application? (in press). Submitted to *Manual Therapy.*
66. Grant R: Influence of vertebral artery blood flow research outcomes on clinical judgment. AJP Forum: premanipulative testing of the cervical spine, *Aust J Physiother* 47:167, 2001.
67. Gross AR, Kay TM: Guidelines for pre-manipulative testing of the cervical spine—an appraisal. AJP Forum: premanipulative testing of the cervical spine, *Aust J Physiother* 47:166, 2001.

Combined Movements of the Cervical Spine in Examination and Treatment

CHAPTER 9

Brian C. Edwards

The shape of the articular surfaces and the symptoms associated with joint dysfunction vary quite distinctly at different levels in the cervical spine. Therefore the examination of the cervical spine needs to be divided into the following different compartments:

- High cervical—Occ to C2
- Middle cervical—C3-5
- Low cervical—C6-T1

HIGH CERVICAL SPINE (OCCIPUT TO C2)

The occiput to C2 is an area of the vertebral column that does not lend itself easily to physical examination yet is subject to a variety of mechanical disorders. Hence a considerable portion of this chapter will be developed to the examination of the high cervical spine.

Headaches of cervical origin commonly arise from these levels.[1-3] These types of headaches are presented in detail in Chapter 13.

The anatomy of the high cervical spine is unique and to some degree more complicated than the rest of the vertebral column. The shapes of the bones and their articulations are quite distinctly different in occiput and atlas, atlas and axis, axis and C3, respectively. Such marked changes in anatomical configuration in such close proximity occur nowhere else in the vertebral column.

It is interesting to note that the articulations of the occipitoatlantal and atlantoaxial joints are situated approximately 1 cm anterior to the articulations of the second and third cervical vertebrae. Although the articular surfaces of the occipitoatlantal and atlantoaxial joints vary somewhat, as a general rule, those between the occiput and atlas are concavoconvex and those between atlas and axis are slightly biconvex (excluding the articulation between the odontoid peg and the anterior arch of the atlas).

The main movements that occur between the occiput and atlas are flexion and extension. Although there is some dispute as to whether any rotation occurs between occiput and atlas, a small amount of rotation may be felt between the mastoid process and the transverse process of C1 on passive testing. Lateral flexion of the occiput on the atlas causes the condyles of the occiput to move in a direction opposite to that in which the head is laterally flexed.

Braakman and Penning[4] and Mimura et al[5] suggest that lateral flexion is combined with rotation to the opposite side. When examining the occipitoatlantal complex with combined movements, flexion or extension in combination with rotation—rather than lateral flexion—is more effective in increasing or decreasing stretch or compressive effects.

It has been suggested that the occiput and axis, rather than the atlas and axis,[6] should be considered as a segment because of the ligamentous attachments from axis to occiput—namely, the superior longitudinal band of the cruciform ligament, the apical ligament, and the alar ligaments. Although this is a useful concept, the examination of the high cervical spine is not complete without the testing of movements between the atlas and axis, both singly and in combination.

Examination by Combined Movements

The combining of movements in examination of the cervical and lumbar spine has been presented previously.[7-11] The principle underlying the use of combined movements in the high cervical spine—that is, the effecting of stretch or compression of specific joints and surrounding structures—is the same as for the rest of the vertebral column. It is rare for headache symptoms to be reproduced by standard physiological movements of the high cervical spine alone; commonly, it is only by combining these movements that sufficient tension can be placed on high cervical structures to produce the patient's symptoms.

Occipitoatlantal Complex

Testing in Flexion and Right Rotation. On flexion, the condyles of the occiput move backward in relation to the articular surface of the atlas. When this is combined with rotation to the right, an increased stretch is placed on the posterior aspect of the capsule of the right occipitoatlantal joint (Figure 9-1).

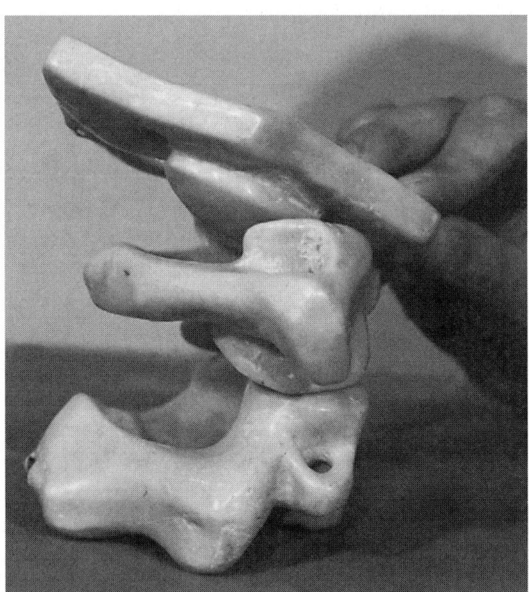

Figure 9-1
Flexion and right rotation: occipitoatlantal complex.
(From Edwards BC: In Grieve GP, editor: *Modern manual therapy of the vertebral column,* Edinburgh, 1986, Churchill Livingstone.)

Method of Testing. The therapist supinates the left forearm and extends the left wrist. The web between the left index finger and left thumb is placed over the symphysis menti. The right hand is placed over the crown of the head, with the fingertips extending down to grasp the skull below the external occipital protuberance. The head is flexed on the cervical spine. Right rotation is added in such a manner as to increase the stretch on the right posterior atlantooccipital membrane (Figure 9-2).

Testing in Extension and Right Rotation. On extension, the condyles of the occiput, move forward in relation to the articular surface of the atlas. When combined with rotation to the right, an increase in the stretch on the anterior capsule of the left occipitoatlantal joint is obtained (Figure 9-3).

Method of Testing. The left hand is placed over the crown of the head, and the right hand under the chin. The head is then extended on the neck, and right rotation of the head is added to increase the stretch of the anterior part of the capsule of the left occipitoatlantal joint (Figure 9-4).

Atlas-Axis Complex

Testing in Right Rotation and Flexion. On right rotation of the atlas on the axis, the left inferior articular surface of the atlas moves forward on the left superior articular surface of the axis, with the opposite movement occurring on the right-hand side. If flexion is then added, an increased stretch of the posterior aspect of the left and right atlantoaxial joints is obtained (Figure 9-5).

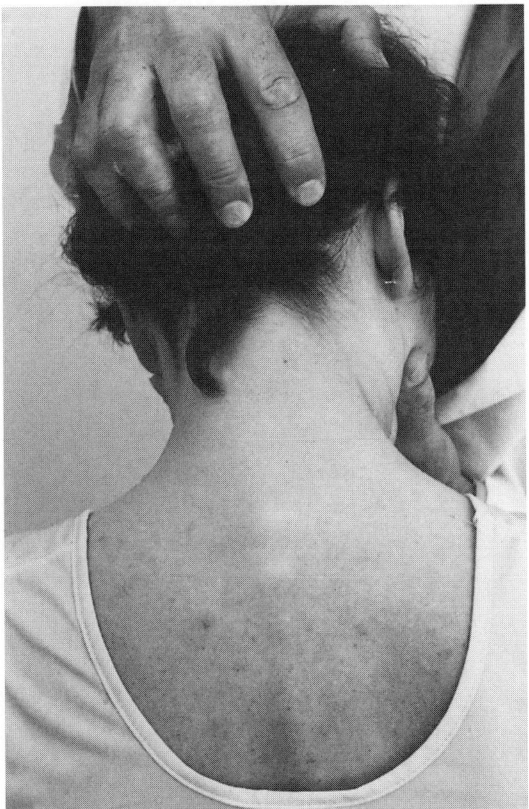

Figure 9-2
Testing flexion and right rotation: occipitoatlantal complex.

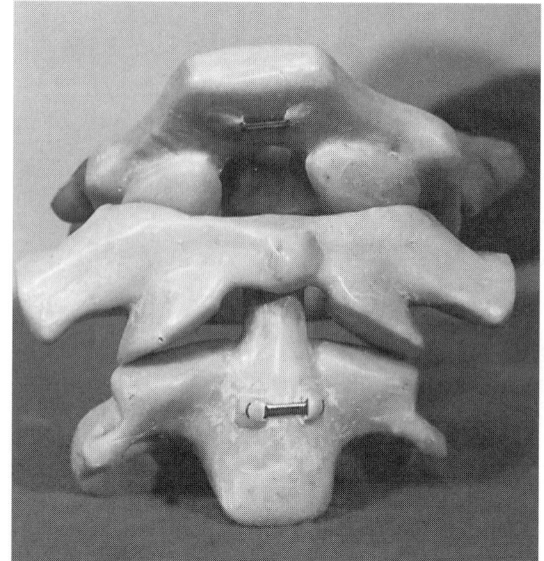

Figure 9-3
Extension and right rotation: occipitoatlantal complex.
(From Edwards BC: In Grieve GP, editor: *Modern manual therapy of the vertebral column,* Edinburgh, 1986, Churchill Livingstone.)

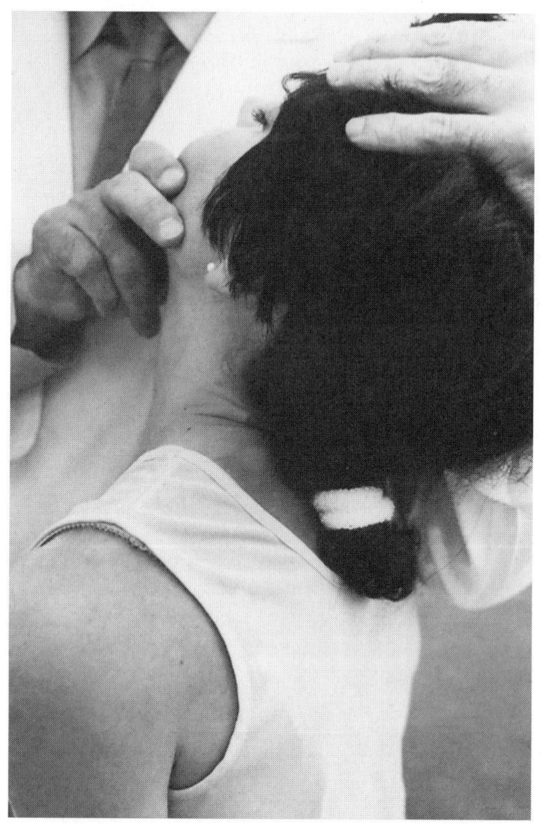

Figure 9-4
Testing extension and right rotation: occipitoatlantal complex.

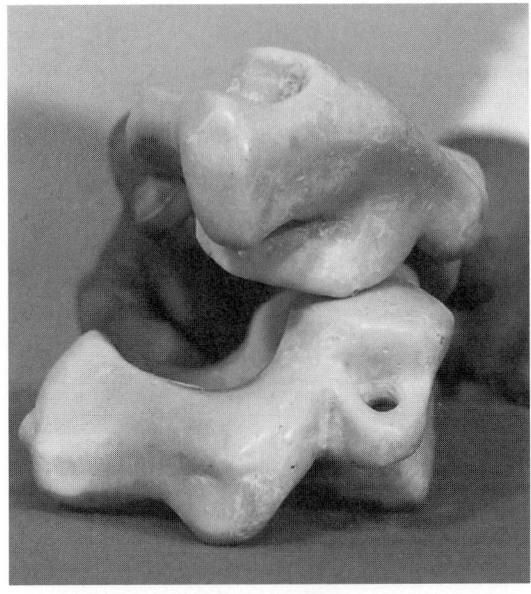

Figure 9-5
Right rotation and flexion: atlas-axis complex.
(From Edwards BC: In Grieve GP, editor: *Modern manual therapy of the vertebral column*, Edinburgh, 1986, Churchill Livingstone.)

Method of Testing. The left hand is placed over the posterior aspect of C2 so that the left middle finger is over the anterior aspect of the left transverse process of C2. The left index finger is placed on the left-hand side of the spine of C2, and the left thumb is placed over the posterior aspect of the superior articulation of C2. The right hand and arm take hold of the patient's head so that the right little finger comes around the arch of C1. The head is then rotated to the right until C2 just starts to rotate. Flexion of the occiput and C1 is then added, thereby increasing the stretch on the posterior aspects of both atlantoaxial joints (Figure 9-6).

Testing in Right Rotation and Extension. On rotation to the right of the atlas on the axis, the left inferior articular surface of the atlas moves forward on the left superior articular surface of the axis, and the opposite occurs on the right side. If extension is added, there is an increase in the stretch on the anterior part of the capsule of the right and left atlantoaxial joint (Figure 9-7).

Method of Testing. The same hand positions as in Figure 9-6 are adopted; however, extension is added so that there is an increased stretch of the anterior capsule of both atlantoaxial joints (Figure 9-8).

Confirmation of Findings by Palpation

The passive testing procedures described before will elicit signs related more to restriction than reproduction of pain. Thus after the examination of physiological movements, the next step is to either confirm the findings by palpation or, when the appropriate symptoms have not been reproduced by combined movements, to identify them by palpation. Very often, specific signs and symptoms will be more easily isolated by palpation.

When performing palpation, the therapist must pay close attention to placing the joint to be examined in the appropriate combined position. This position must be strongly maintained while the palpation procedure is performed.

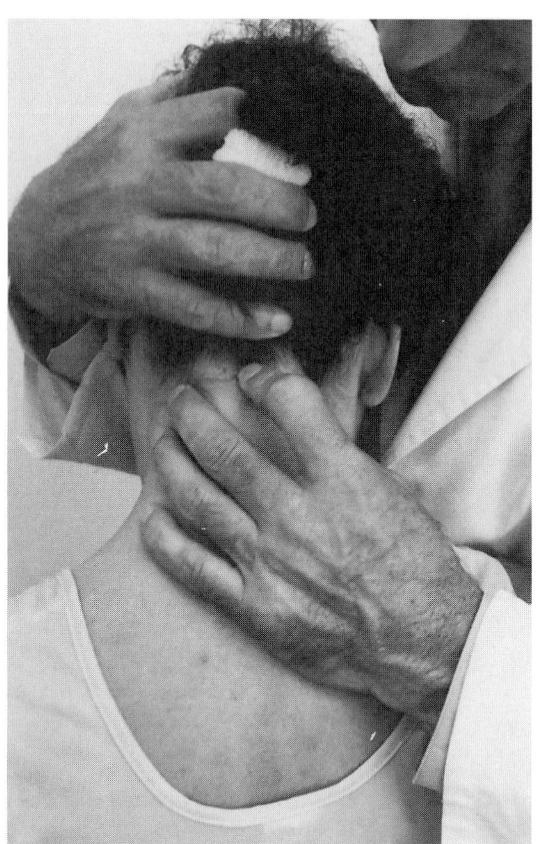

Figure 9-6
Testing right rotation and flexion: atlas-axis complex.

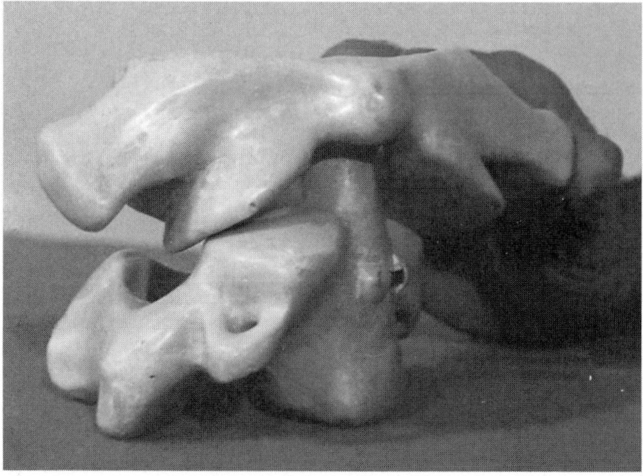

Figure 9-7
Right rotation and extension: atlas-axis complex.
(From Edwards BC: In Grieve GP, editor: *Modern manual therapy of the vertebral column,* Edinburgh, 1986, Churchill Livingstone.)

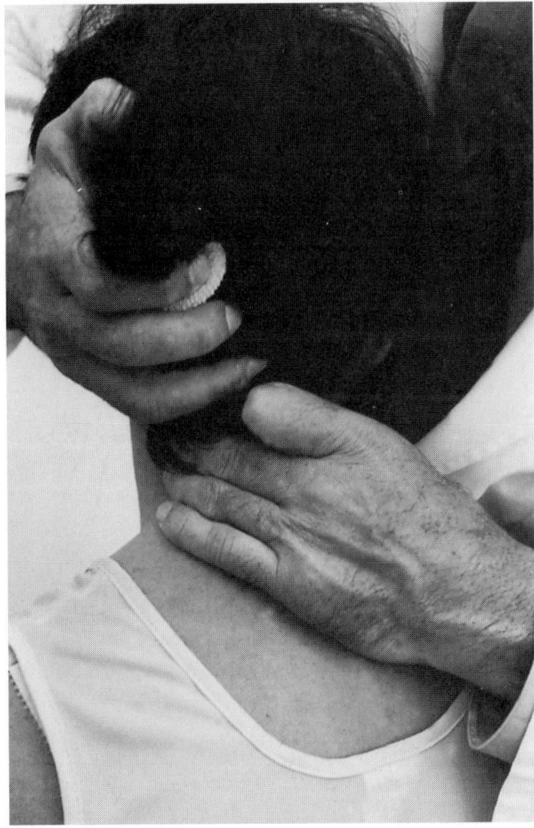

Figure 9-8
Testing right rotation and extension: atlas-axis complex.

Occipitoatlantal Complex

Flexion and Right Rotation. Stressing the posterior aspect of the right atlantooccipital joint by manual palpation is illustrated in Figure 9-9. With the patient in the prone position, his or her head is flexed and rotated to the right. The therapist's thumbtips, placed over the right posterior arch of C1, apply oscillatory pressures to increase the stretch on the right occipitoatlantal articulation (Figure 9-9). Palpation over the anterior aspect of the right transverse process of C1 with the patient's head in flexion and right rotation will decrease the stretch on the right occipitoatlantal joint (Figure 9-10).

Extension and Right Rotation. The stretch on the anterior aspect of the left occipitoatlantal joint will decrease when oscillatory pressures are applied over the left posterior arch of C1 with the patient's head in extension and right rotation, as illustrated in Figure 9-11.

Palpation over the anterior aspect of the left transverse process of C1 with the patient's head in extension and right rotation will increase the stretch on the anterior aspect of the left occipitoatlantal joint (Figure 9-12).

Atlas-Axis Complex

Left Rotation and Flexion. With C1-2 in left rotation and flexion, palpation over the anterior aspect of the right transverse process of C1 will decrease rotation between

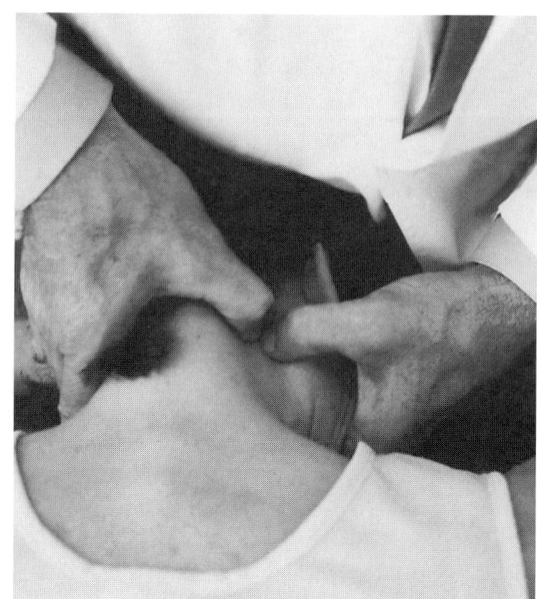

Figure 9-9
Posterior palpation on the right of C1 in flexion and right rotation.

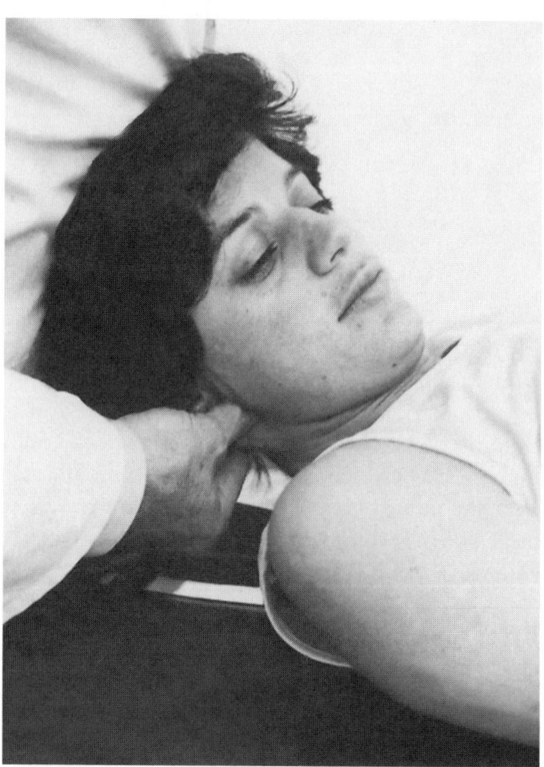

Figure 9-10
Anterior palpation on the right of C1 in flexion and right rotation.

atlas and axis and therefore decrease the stretch on the posterior aspect of the left and right atlantoaxial articulations (Figure 9-13).

With the patient in the same position as illustrated in Figure 9-13, palpation over the anterior aspect of the right transverse process of C2 will increase the stretch on the posterior aspects of the left and right atlantoaxial articulations (Figure 9-14).

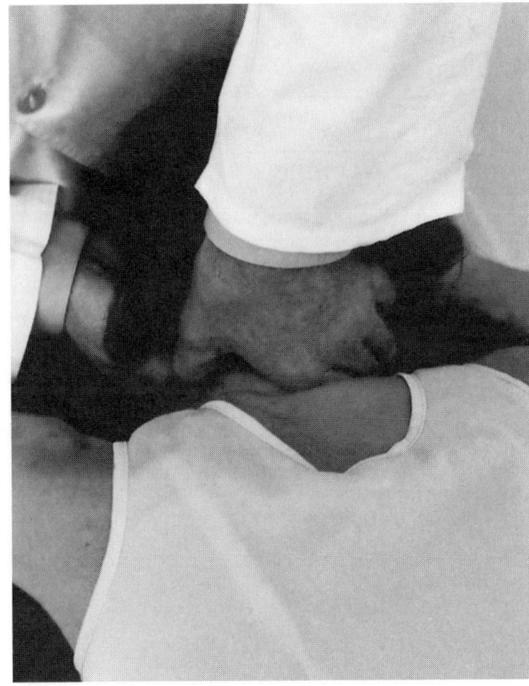

Figure 9-11
Posterior palpation on the left of C1 in extension and right rotation.

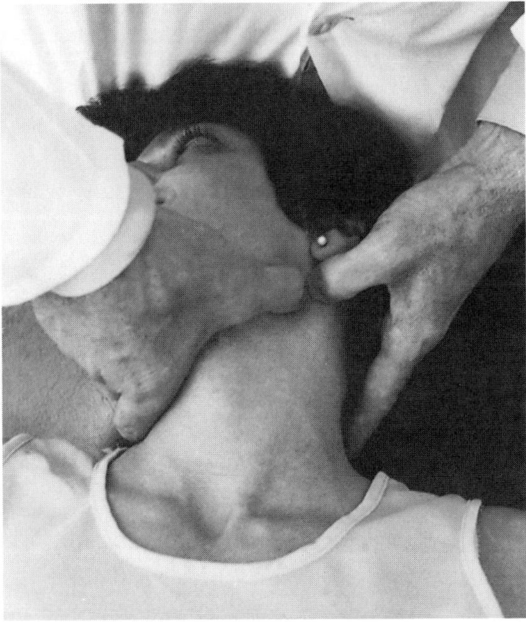

Figure 9-12
Anterior palpation on the left of C1 in extension and right rotation.

When oscillatory pressures are applied over the right posterior aspect of C1, the stretch on the posterior aspect of the atlantoaxial articulations is increased. The palpation position is illustrated in Figure 9-15.

Palpation over the right posterior aspect of C2 by decreasing right rotation also decreases the stretch on the posterior aspect of the atlantoaxial articulations (Figure 9-16).

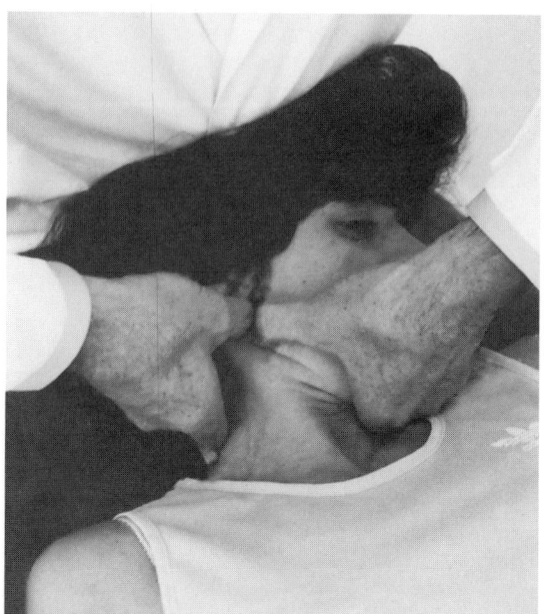

Figure 9-13
Anterior palpation on the right of C1 in left rotation and flexion.

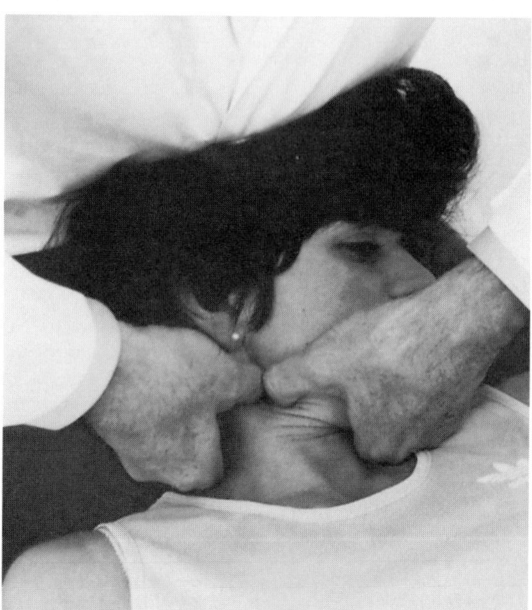

Figure 9-14
Anterior palpation on the right transverse process of C2 in left rotation and flexion.

Right Rotation and Extension. In right rotation and extension, palpation over the anterior aspect of the right transverse process of C1 will increase the rotation of C1 on C2, thereby increasing the stretch on the anterior aspect of the right and left atlantoaxial joints, as illustrated in Figure 9-17.

Palpation over the anterior aspect of the right transverse process of C2 decreases right rotation and decreases the stretch of the anterior aspect of both atlantoaxial joints (Figure 9-18). Palpation over the posterior aspect of the right transverse process of C1 with the head in right rotation and extension will decrease the rotation of C1

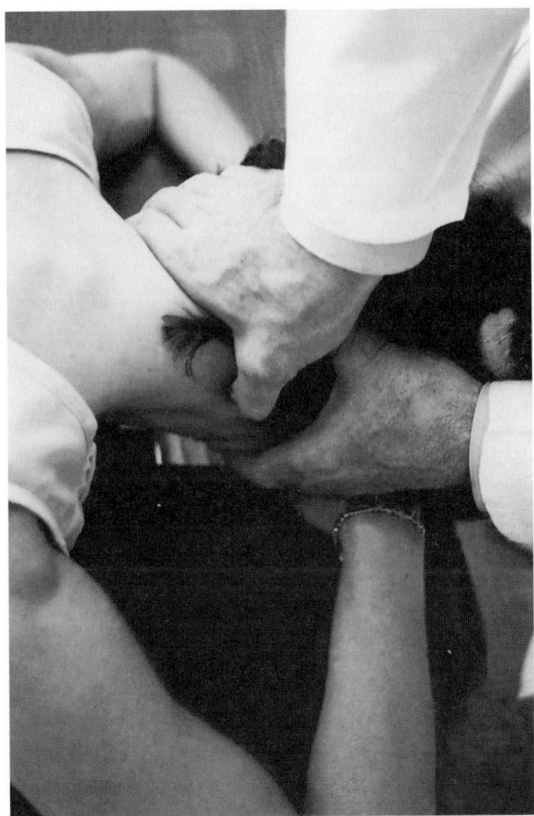

Figure 9-15
Posterior palpation on the right of C1 in left rotation and flexion.

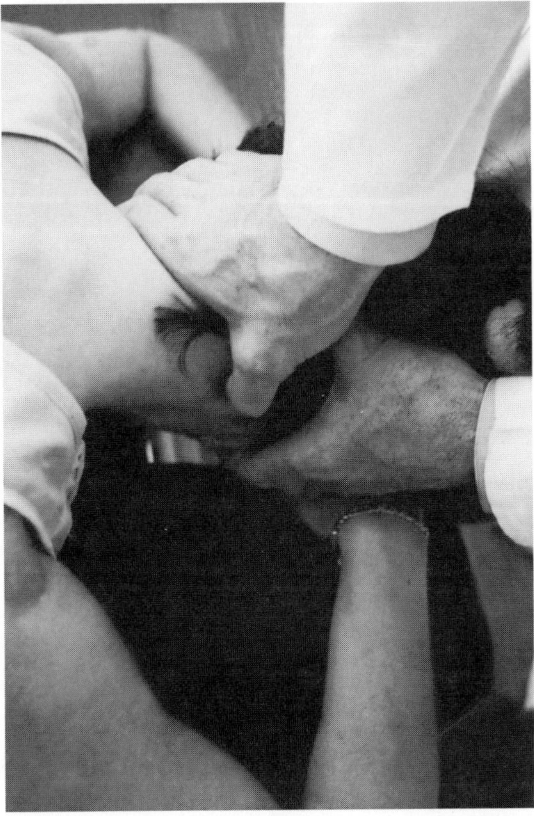

Figure 9-16
Posterior palpation on the right of C2 in right rotation and flexion.

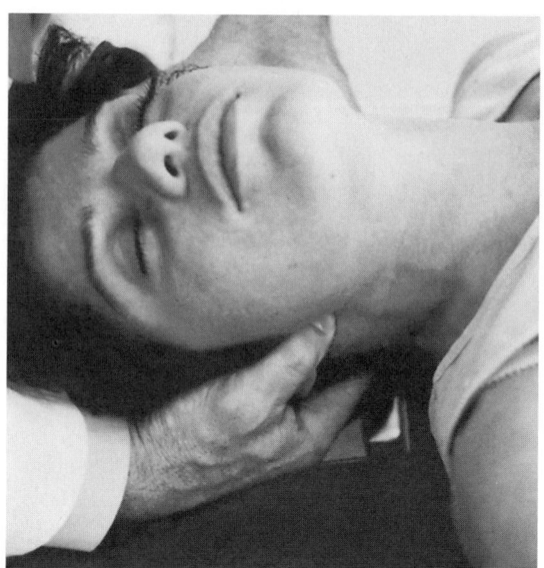

Figure 9-17
Anterior palpation on the right of C1 in right rotation and extension.

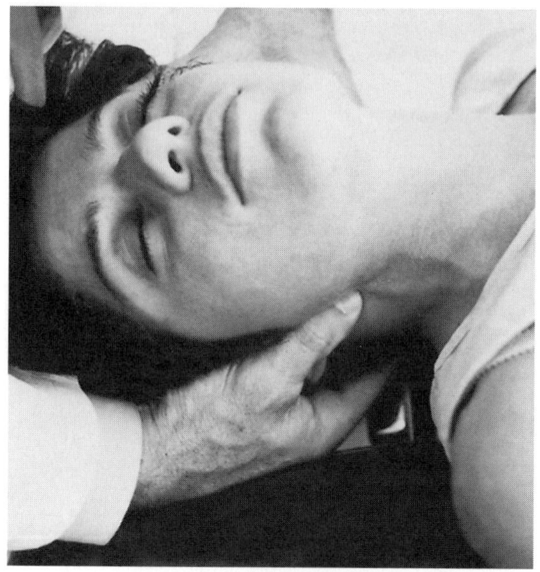

Figure 9-18
Anterior palpation on the right transverse process of C2 in right rotation and extension.

on C2, thereby decreasing the stretch on the anterior aspect of both right and left atlantoaxial joints (Figure 9-19).

Palpatory pressure over the posterior aspect of the right transverse process of C2 increases right rotation and increases the stretch on the anterior aspect of the atlantoaxial articulations (Figure 9-20).

TREATMENT

The examination procedures described are primarily for headaches of cervical origin. One of the essentials of the physical examination for cervical headaches is the repro-

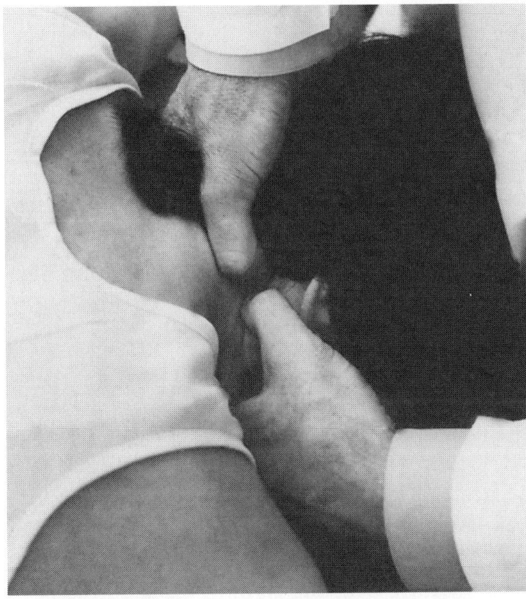

Figure 9-19
Posterior palpation on the right of C1 in right rotation and extension.

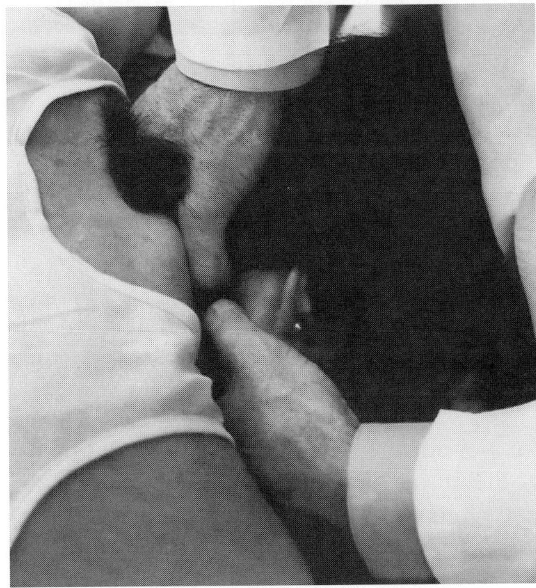

Figure 9-20
Posterior palpation on the right of C2 in right rotation and extension.

duction with physiological movement, palpation, or a combination of both or part, or all, of the headache symptoms.

In the case of unilateral headache symptoms, the palpation procedure should be performed on the side of the symptoms. If tenderness is the main sign elicited, the response of the symptomatic side must be compared with that of the unaffected side by using the same oscillatory pressure. If the headache symptoms are reproduced, the technique chosen for treatment is the reciprocal or opposite movement to the painful direction found on examination; alternatively, the head and neck are placed in the neutral position with movement in the painful direction used. Examples of this approach for the occipitoatlantal and the atlas-axis complex follow.

Occipitoatlantal Complex

Flexion and right rotation of the occiput on the atlas reproduces the patient's right-sided headache symptoms. Posterior pressure over the right transverse process of the atlas with the head in flexion and right rotation in relation to the atlas also reproduces the symptoms.

Anterior pressure over the right transverse process of the atlas with the head in flexion and right rotation, is the first choice of technique, with progression to posterior pressure as the symptoms improve. An alternative treatment approach is to use posterior pressure over the right transverse process of the atlas with the head in neutral and progress the position of the head to right rotation and flexion as the symptoms improve.

Atlas-Axis Complex

Right rotation and flexion reproduces the headache on the right. Anterior pressure over the transverse process of C1 on the right, with the head in the same position as previously described, also produces the headache. The first choice of technique may be anterior pressure over the right transverse process of C1 with the head in the neutral position, progressing to the position of right rotation and flexion as the symptoms improve. Another choice may be anterior pressure over the right of C2 with the head in right rotation and flexion, progressing to anterior pressure over C1 in this position.

There are a number of different choices for localizing the source of the headache by movement and palpation of the cervical spine; however, care must be taken to relate the choice of technique to the position in relation to physiological movements as well as reproduction of symptoms by palpation.

This treatment progression relates to improvement of symptoms. However, if symptoms do not improve, the same progression is made. If finally there is no improvement with this progression, then the position that most strongly reproduces the symptoms is combined with the treatment techniques that also increase the symptoms. If still no improvement is forthcoming, then passive movement procedures will not help the patient's symptoms.

MIDDLE CERVICAL SPINE (C3-5)

In the middle cervical spine (C3-5), the movements of rotation and lateral flexion occur together. It seems most likely that the movements of lateral flexion and rotation occur in the same direction—that is, lateral flexion to the right is combined with rotation to the right.[1] This is at least partly a result of the shape of the joint surfaces but is also affected by the soft tissue structures between the bony articulations and the structures between the neural foramina and vertebral canal. Different movements of the cervical spine, such as flexion with lateral flexion in one direction and rotation in the same direction, can cause stretching or compressing effects of the intervertebral joints on either side. When flexion is performed in the sagittal plane, the articular surfaces of the zygapophyseal joint slide on one another, with the inferior articular facet of the superior vertebra sliding cephalad on the superior articular facet of the inferior vertebra. At the same time the interbody space is narrowed anteriorly and widened posteriorly. Rotation to the left and left lateral flexion cause the right zygapophyseal facet joint to open. Although these movements of lateral flexion and rotation result in a similar upward motion of the superior on the inferior facet, they are not identical movements to those that occur with flexion.

Consider the movements of the cervical spine in relation to the facet joints. With the movement of lateral flexion and rotation to the right (e.g., the fourth cervical vertebra [C4] on the fifth [C5]), the right inferior facet of C4 slides down the right superior facet of C5. A similar movement on the right side occurs in extension. Therefore there is some similarity in terms of direction of movement of the right facet joint in movements of extension, right lateral flexion, and right rotation. The facet joint on the opposite side moves upward during each movement (except with extension).

Examination by Combined Movements

Because of the combination of movements that occur in the cervical spine, the examination of a patient's movements must be expanded to incorporate these principles. At times it is inadequate to examine the basic movements of flexion, extension, lateral flexion, and rotation, and other movements that combine these basic movements must be examined. Aspects of this concept have been described previously.[8,11] The symptoms and signs produced by examining movements involving rotation or lateral flexion performed while the spine is maintained in the neutral position in relation to other movements can be quite different from the signs and symptoms produced when the same movements are performed with the spine in flexion or extension. Testing movements while the spine is maintained in flexion or extension may accentuate or reduce symptoms or may even change local spinal pain to referred pain.[8,11]

The range of movement possible in the neutral position will be different from that obtained when movements are done in combined positions. For example, the range of rotation or lateral flexion may be greater when these movements are performed in the neutral position than when they are being performed in the fully flexed position. In addition to differences in range of movement, there also is much greater stretching or compression of structures on either side.

Examining the cervical spine by combining movements will assist in the treatment program[8,11] in the following ways:

1. By establishing the type of movement response that is present
2. By assisting in the selection of treatment technique, the direction of the technique, and the position of the joint in which the technique is to be performed
3. By predicting the response of the patient's symptoms to a treatment technique

Movement Responses

There are two types of movement responses—regular and irregular.

Regular Movement Responses

Regular movement responses occur when similar movements at the intervertebral joint produce the same symptoms whenever they are performed, although the symptoms may differ in quality or severity. Regular movement responses can further be subdivided into compressing or stretching ones. If the patient's symptoms are produced on the side to which the movement is directed, then the pattern is a compressing movement response. That is, the compressing movements produce the symptoms. If the symptoms are produced on the side opposite to which the movement is directed, then the pattern can be considered a stretching movement response. Examples of regular compressing movement responses include the following:

1. Right cervical rotation produces right suprascapular pain, and this pain is worsened when the same movement is performed in extension and eased when performed in flexion.
2. Cervical extension produces right suprascapular pain, and this pain is worsened when right rotation is added to the extension and increased further when right lateral flexion is added.

Examples of regular stretching movement responses include the following:

1. Right lateral flexion of the cervical spine produces left suprascapular pain, and this pain is accentuated when the same movement is performed in flexion and eased when performed in extension.
2. Flexion of the cervical spine produces left suprascapular pain, and this pain is worsened when right lateral flexion is added and increased further when right rotation is added.

Because the biomechanics of spinal movement are complex and have yet to be fully described, this simple explanation cannot be universally applied. Influences such as the changing instantaneous axes of rotation complicate the situation. The explanation conveyed in this chapter refers to simple physiological patterns of movement and to those patterns in association with accessory movements—for example, pain and restriction of movement on extension of the lower cervical spine being matched by similar restriction with posteroanterior pressure over the spinous process of C5.

Irregular Movement Responses

All movement responses that are not regular fall into the category of irregular movement responses. Irregular movement responses lack the same consistency of symptoms as regular movement responses, and stretching and compressing movements do not follow any recognizable pattern. There does not appear to be a regular relationship between the examination findings obtained when combining movements with either the compressing or stretching components of the movements. Rather, there is an apparent random reproduction of symptoms despite the combining of movements that have similar stretching and compressing effects on the structure on either side of the spine. An example of an irregular movement response is an instance in which right rotation of the cervical spine produces right suprascapular pain (a compressing test movement) that is worsened when right rotation is performed in flexion (a stretching movement) and eased when the movement is performed in extension (a compressing movement).

There are many examples of irregular movement responses commonly indicating that there is more than one component to the disorder—for example, the zygapophyseal joint, the interbody joint, and the canal and foraminal structures may all contribute to the symptoms. Traumatic injuries—for example, whiplash and other traumatic causes of pain—generally do not exhibit regular movement responses. Nontraumatic zygapophyseal and interbody joint disorders, on the other hand, tend to have regular movement responses.

Confirmation of Findings by Palpation

As with the high cervical spine, signs found on physiological movements can be confirmed by palpation. If, for example, right-sided middle cervical pain occurs with right rotation and this pain is accentuated when right rotation is performed in extension, these findings may be confirmed by comparing responses to anterior and posterior palpation. Using this example and assuming an articular problem between C4 and C5, anterior pressure on the right, directed caudally over the anterior tubercle of C4, will increase the symptoms, whereas anterior pressure on the right directed caudally over C5 will decrease the symptoms. A comparison of these findings with those found by posterior palpation is useful. Posterior palpation directed caudally over the right inferior articulation of C4 will increase the symptoms, whereas posterior pressure directed caudally over the right superior articulation of C5 will decrease the symptoms.

TREATMENT

The use of combined movements assists in selection of the technique of treatment by indicating to the therapist how the symptoms vary when similar movements are performed in similar positions.

Regular Movement Responses

When a patient has a regular movement response, the chosen treatment technique is usually the one that is found on examination to involve the most painful direction of movement but is performed in the least painful way. For example, in a patient with right suprascapular pain, right lateral flexion of the cervical spine will reproduce the pain, and the pain will be further increased when the movement of right lateral flexion is performed in extension and eased when performed in flexion. Similarly, when right lateral flexion is sustained (a movement that produced the right suprascapular pain) and flexion is added, the pain eases; when extension is added, the pain increases. When each of these movements is done in extension, the pain is increased, but when performed in flexion, it is eased. Thus the general technique of right lateral flexion is initially performed in flexion and then progressed to extension as the symptoms improve.

Similar principles can apply when using accessory movements. Considering the aforementioned example, unilateral posteroanterior pressure on the right C4-5 zygapophyseal joint may produce maximal symptoms when the cervical spine is placed in the position of right lateral flexion and right rotation. Unilateral pressure on the right of C4, pushing the inferior articulation of C4 caudad, may be performed with the head and neck in the neutral position, and this can be progressed to performing the same procedure with the head and neck in right lateral flexion and right rotation as the symptoms improve. The physical therapist would commence by performing the technique in the neutral position and then progress to the most painful combined position.

Irregular Movement Responses

The direction of movement chosen as treatment when there are irregular movement responses also may be the most painful movement performed in the least painful way. For example, if right lateral flexion produced right suprascapular pain that eases when done in extension and worsens when performed in flexion, then the chosen direction of treatment would be right lateral flexion in extension. However, when there is an irregular movement response, the response to treatment is less predictable. In other words, performing right lateral flexion in extension (the least painful position) may improve the most painful examination movement (lateral flexion in flexion), or the treatment technique may actually increase the pain experienced (e.g., there may be a random response to the technique).

When the disorder is characterized by severe pain or is very irritable, the least painful direction of movement should be used as a technique in the least painful combined position.

Techniques of Treatment

It is not possible in an introductory chapter such as this to describe the many positions that may be selected in treatment. A manual of technique would be required for that purpose.[11] However, five treatment techniques are described in this chapter. Most cervical physiological movements are examined in the upright position. As a consequence, the following first four techniques are performed in that position and are described for C4-5:

1. Right rotation in the neutral position (Figure 9-21). The therapist stands on the right side of the patient. The pad of the left middle finger is placed over the left

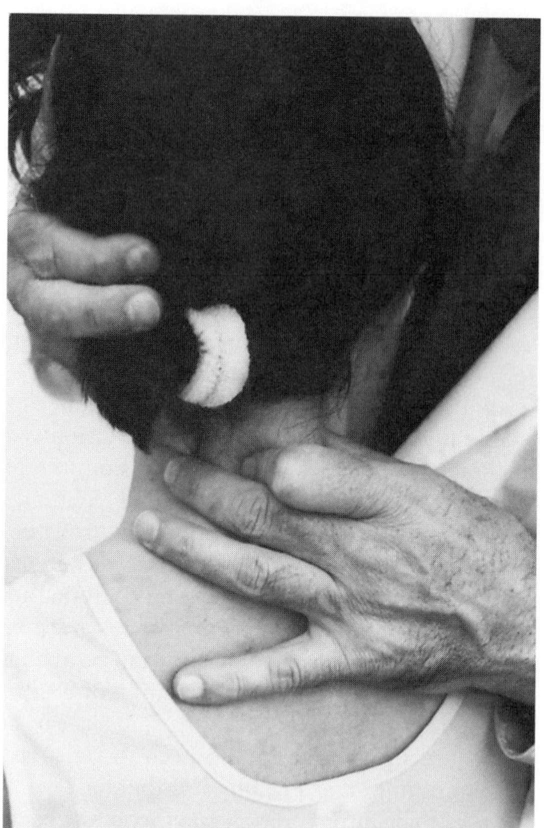

Figure 9-21
Right rotation in the neutral position.

superior articulation of C5. The pad of the left index finger is placed on the left side of the spinous process of C4, with the left thumb on the right superior articulation of C5. The right arm holds the patients head so that the right middle finger is placed on the left inferior articulation of C4. In this position, mobilization of C4 is performed by moving the right arm while stabilizing C5 with the left hand.

2. Right rotation in the flexion position (Figure 9-22). The same hand positions are adopted as described for right rotation in neutral, but the cervical spine is in flexion.
3. Right lateral flexion in the neutral position (Figure 9-23). The therapist's left hand is placed in the same position as described previously. The therapist's right little finger is placed over the left inferior articulation of C4, with the fingers of the right hand spread over the left side of the cervical spine. Right lateral flexion is done with the right hand laterally flexing at C4 while C5 is fixed by the left hand.
4. Right lateral flexion in the flexion position (Figure 9-24). The same hand positions are adopted as described for right lateral flexion in neutral, but the cervical spine is in flexion.
5. Right unilateral posteroanterior pressure in right rotation and flexion (Figure 9-25). The patient lies prone with neck flexed and rotated to the right. The therapist's thumbs are placed on the right C4-5 zygapophyseal joint, with the fingers placed lightly over either side of the cervical spine. The direction of the mobilization is cephalad.

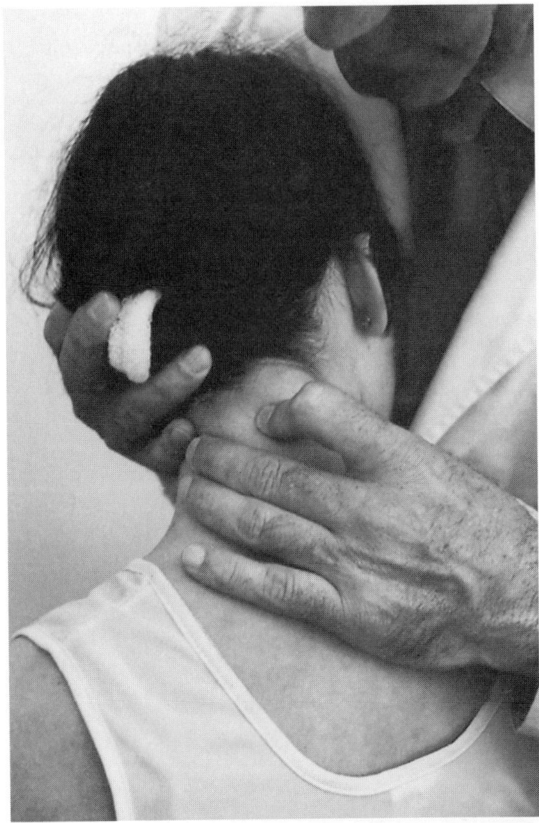

Figure 9-22
Right rotation in the flexion position.

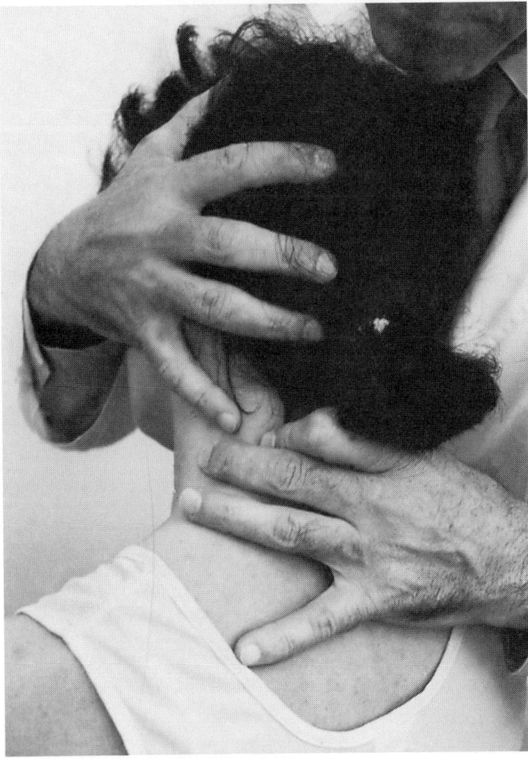

Figure 9-23
Right lateral flexion in the neutral position.

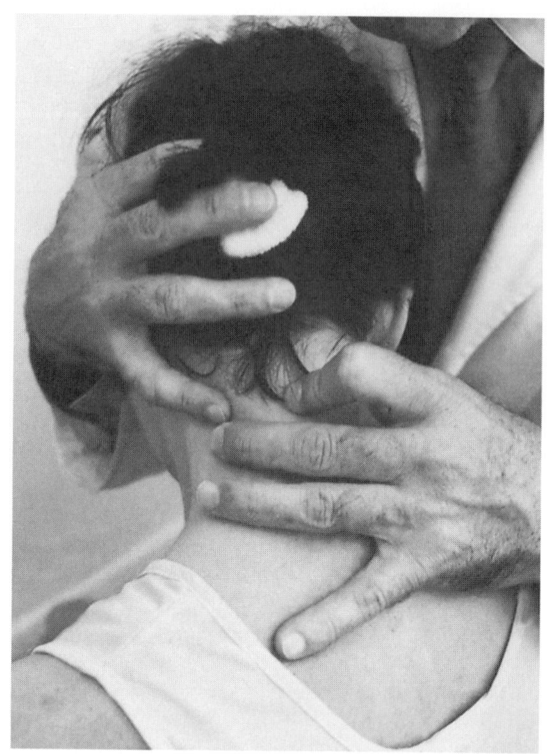

Figure 9-24
Right lateral flexion in the flexion position.

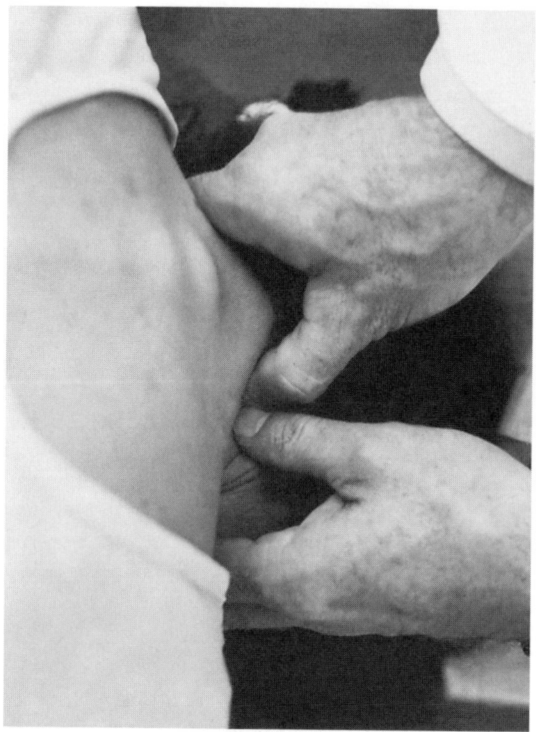

Figure 9-25
Right unilateral posteroanterior pressure in right rotation and flexion.

Predicting the Response to a Technique

The use of combined movements and movement responses can assist in predicting the result of treatment. With regular patterns of movement, the least painful movement on examination improves before the most painful. For example, if right lateral flexion in a neutral position produces the patient's right suprascapular pain and this pain is worsened when the movement is done in extension, then right lateral flexion in neutral will improve before right lateral flexion in extension.

It also may be expected that a treatment technique of right lateral flexion done in flexion, found on examination to be a painless position, will be unlikely to make the symptoms worse.

The response in the case of irregular movement responses is not as predictable, and the improvement in the symptoms may occur in an apparently random fashion. Most examinations of the cervical spine are carried out in the upright position; however, the treatment techniques commonly are performed with the patient prone or supine. Because of the altered weight distribution and position of canal structures when adopting the positions of supine, prone, or side-lying, there may be some alteration in the pain response when the movements are compared with those in the upright position. It is important therefore that, for a technique chosen because it produced particular symptoms in the upright position, the treatment position adopted be adjusted in such a way as to produce the same signs and symptoms.

LOWER CERVICAL SPINE (C6-T1)

Because of the change in shape from lordosis in the midcervical spine to kyphosis in the thoracic spine, the change in shape of the vertebral bodies, and the attachment of the first rib to the first thoracic vertebra, the lower cervical spine should be examined as a separate unit.

Examination by Combined Movements

The same principles of combining movements as for the middle cervical spine (C2-5) apply; however, the first rib limits the amount of movement available. The techniques of examination, although the same as for the middle cervical unit, must include palpation of the first rib. This should be performed with the lower cervical spine in combined movement positions. Figures 9-26 and 9-27 illustrate palpation techniques for the lower cervical spine.

Anterior Palpation of the Right Lower Cervical Spine with the Head and Neck in Flexion and Left Rotation (Figure 9-26). With the patient supine, the therapist places his or her left hand under the occiput and flexes and rotates the patient's head and neck to the left. The therapist's right thumb pad is placed over the right inferior articulation of C6 anteriorly. If pressure is directly caudally at this level, it will tend to decrease the effect of the right rotation between C6 and C7.

Anterior Palpation of the Right First Rib with the Head and Neck in Flexion and Left Rotation (Figure 9-27). The position of the patient and of the therapist's left hand is described for Figure 9-26. With this technique, however, the therapist's right thumb pad is placed anteriorly over the first rib, and mobilization is carried out. The lower cervical spine, including the first rib, is an area that causes a large percentage of symptoms distributed to the upper thoracic and upper limb areas. A combina-

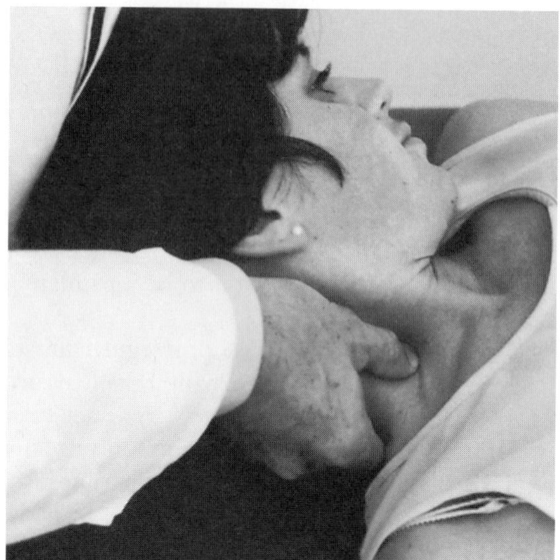

Figure 9-26
Anterior palpation of the right lower cervical spine in flexion and left rotation.

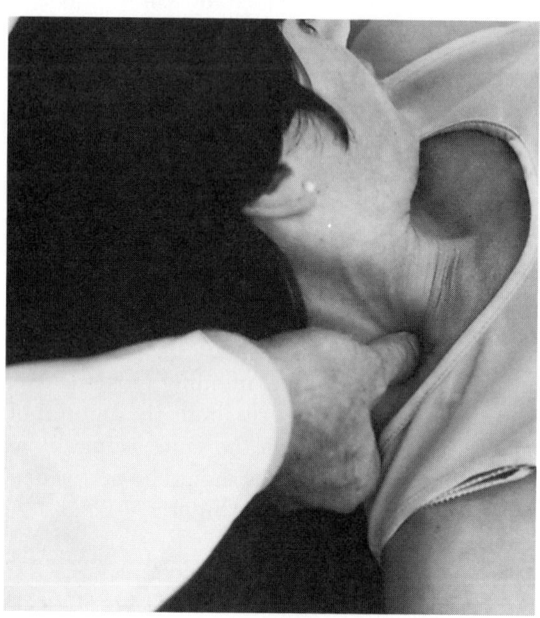

Figure 9-27
Anterior palpation of the right first rib with the neck in flexion and left rotation.

tion of anterior palpation in combined positions of the neck, as well as palpation of the first rib, is an important diagnostic procedure for pain distributed to the upper limbs. In carrying out these testing procedures, care must be taken so that the shoulder and the arm *remain in the neutral position.*

Treatment

The palpation procedures are carried out in the neutral position for the offending joint, and as the symptoms improve, the position is progressively changed to the most painful position.

SUMMARY

The importance of relating symptoms and signs to physiological movements in combined positions has been emphasized. Not only will combined movements highlight clinical findings, but they will also reveal movement responses that will assist in selection of treatment techniques and in predicting response to treatment.

ACKNOWLEDGMENT

The author would like to thank Mr. D. Watkins, photographer, School of Physiotherapy, Curtin University of Technology, Perth, Western Australia, for his assistance with the photographs.

References

1. Stoddard A: *Manual of osteopathic practice*, ed 1, London, 1969, Hutchinson.
2. Stoddard A: *Manual of osteopathic technique*, ed 1, London, 1962, Hutchinson.
3. Jackson R: Headaches associated with disorders of the cervical spine, *Headache* 6:175, 1967.
4. Braakman R, Penning L: *Injuries of the cervical spine*, Amsterdam, 1971, Excerpta Medica.
5. Mimura M, Moriya H, Watanabe T et al: Three-dimensional motion analysis of the cervical spine with special references to the axial rotation, *Spine* 14:1135-1139, 1989.
6. Worth DR, Selvik G: Movements of the craniovertebral joints. In Grieve GP, editor: *Modern manual therapy of the vertebral column*, Edinburgh, 1986, Churchill Livingstone.
7. Edwards BC: Combined movements of the lumbar spine: examination and clinical significance, *Aust J Physiother* 24:147, 1979.
8. Edwards BC: Combined movements in the cervical spine (C2-7): their value in examination and technique choice, *Aust J Physiother* 26:165, 1980.
9. Edwards BC: Combined movements in the lumbar spine: their use in examination and treatment. In Grieve GP, editor: *Modern manual therapy of the vertebral column*, Edinburgh, 1986, Churchill Livingstone.
10. Edwards BC: Examination of the high cervical spine (occiput-C2) using combined movements. In Grieve GP, editor: *Modern manual therapy of the vertebral column*, Edinburgh, 1986, Churchill Livingstone.
11. Edwards BC: Manual of combined movements, Oxford, England, 1999, Butterworth-Heinemann.

CHAPTER

10 Muscles and Motor Control in Cervicogenic Disorders

Vladimir Janda

It is no longer necessary to stress the importance of muscles in the pathogenesis of various pain syndromes of the musculoskeletal system. This is because of the now well-recognized fact, applied in clinical practice, that effective protection of the joints depends largely on the appropriate functioning of the muscle system. It has also been recognized that the dysfunctions of muscles and joints are so closely related that the two should be considered as a single inseparable functional unit and should be assessed, analyzed, and treated together. Although the causal relationship between muscles and joints in the pathogenesis of individual syndromes may still be a matter of discussion, practical clinical experience shows that the predominant influence of all (or almost all) techniques used in modern manual therapy is on muscles. Improvement of joint function depends to a large extent on the improvement in function of those muscles that have an anatomical or functional relationship to that joint. This is true even for those manipulative techniques using high-velocity thrust (with impulse), which were initially thought to influence the restriction of joint movement only. It is even truer for the soft mobilization techniques, muscle energy procedures, and postisometric relaxation or myofascial release techniques, to mention only those most frequently used. In this respect, the entire philosophy of how a particular therapeutic procedure works has to be reevaluated.

In conditions with acute pain, the increase in muscle tone plays the decisive role in pain production. In this respect, it has been suggested[1,2] that the increased muscle tone (muscle spasm) is probably the necessary link in the pathogenetic chain to perceive a joint dysfunction as a painful condition. Without the development of muscle spasm, the joint dysfunction usually remains painless. For this reason, muscle spasm should be given special attention in both the assessment and treatment of painful disorders of the cervical and thoracic spine. According to this view, use of the term *painful joint* when analyzing the function of many body structures within the range of musculoskeletal disorders may be simplistic and misleading, and it should perhaps be used as a clinical descriptor only.

Muscles play an extremely important role in the pathogenesis and management of various syndromes. It is therefore surprising that the analysis of muscle function has not been developed as precisely as has the examination of joints. Many therapists underestimate the importance of precise muscle analysis and are therefore likely to misinterpret clinical findings. For example, painful areas on the occiput are often considered to reflect periosteal pain or a painful posterior arch of the atlas,[3] despite the fact that they may well be occurring at the insertions of muscles in spasm.

Although the treatment of acute painful dysfunctions is less challenging, the treatment of chronic disorders—and particularly the prevention of recurrences of acute pain—are major challenges. It should be mentioned that from the socioeconomic aspect, chronic disorders of the spine are extremely costly. Although they represent only about 6% to 10% of all painful conditions of the musculoskeletal system, they consume about 80% of the costs.[4] The high incidence of neck pain amongst the general public demands that special attention be given to determining its origin, so that appropriate preventive and therapeutic measures may be taken.

ROLE OF MUSCLES AS A PATHOGENETIC FACTOR IN PAIN PRODUCTION

When considering the role of muscles in a specific syndrome, physical therapists must consider at least two factors: the presence of an acutely painful condition and the background against which this painful condition developed.

In acute pain, the role of a muscle as a pathogenetic factor can be explained in the following ways:

- Irritation from pain produces increased muscle tone, which leads to placing the involved spinal segment in a painless position.[5] In this case, the irritation and altered proprioceptive input from the joint are probably essential in producing muscle spasm, whereas a decrease in spasm leads to the relief of pain.
- An initial increase in muscle tone decreases mobility in the involved spinal segment (joint blockage) and causes pain. This is illustrated by the tension headache, which is triggered by increased muscle tone, such as in stress-induced situations (through increased activity of the limbic system) or as a defensive reaction associated with overactivation of virtually all of the neck muscles. Trigger points develop in predictable locations, with local and referred pain occurring in typical patterns.[6] The trigger points also represent areas of increased localized muscle tone.

A poor body alignment with a forward head posture and typical muscle imbalance is not only a predisposing but also a perpetuating factor in chronic disorders, episodic pain, and chronic discomfort and may lead to chronicity as well as to accidental decompensation and recurrent episodes of various acute pain syndromes. Considering the role of muscles in the development of neck pain, the function of muscles of the shoulder as well as the neck merits a review.

The cervical spine is the most intricate region of the spine, and so are the muscles of this region. All movements of the arm, whether fast or slow, resisted or unresisted, require activation of the shoulder or neck musculature or both—in particular the upper trapezius, levator scapulae, and deep intrinsic muscles. Muscle recruitment will be more pronounced if the patient carries heavy loads or has developed poor motor habits.

Muscles of the neck and shoulder region always function as a unit, and there is no movement in the upper extremity that would not be reflected in the neck musculature. However, in some activities, this coordination can only be hypothesized, because it is very difficult to measure the activation of the deep intrinsic muscles. Because the coactivity of the neck and shoulder musculature is reflected in the mechanics of the entire shoulder and neck complex, it is often difficult to estimate whether the shoulder or neck was the primary source of a particular dysfunction or pathology. A detailed evaluation usually reveals changes in both areas.

Muscles of the head, neck, and shoulder region can be divided into several groups as follows:

1. A superficial spinohumeral layer attaching the shoulder girdle to the spine
2. An intermediate spinocostal layer, which includes the serratus posterior superior and inferior, and deep layers, incorporating the true muscles of the back
3. The anterior neck muscles
4. The hyoid muscles
5. The facial muscles
6. The masticatory muscles

Muscles and Central Nervous System Regulation

Muscles should be considered as lying at a functional crossroads, being strongly influenced by stimuli coming from both the central nervous system (CNS) and the osteoarticular system.[7-9] In many ways the musculature should be understood as a sensitive, labile system that constantly reflects not only changes in the motor system, but changes in all parts of the body. This is so with respect to the neck muscles in particular.

Although this chapter is oriented toward clinical practice, a reference to relevant neurophysiological factors provides a basis for understanding the presentations and assessments of disorders of the cervical and thoracic spine. CNS mechanisms regulate the posture and position of the body in space, and this is reflected in adaptive reactions of the position of the head.[10,11] The latter are in turn reflected in the mechanics of the cervical joints and neck muscles in particular. These reactions must be taken into consideration because they can play a hidden or unrecognized role in understanding a specific syndrome. If the central regulation is impaired, the dysfunction of the musculoskeletal system becomes more apparent.

On the other hand, the compensatory reflex responses can be effectively used in treatment. For example, the compensatory eye movements may help to relax or inhibit or facilitate specific neck muscle groups. This effect is widely used as a supportive factor in mobilization techniques involving the upper part of the body, particularly in the postisometric relaxation and proprioceptive neuromuscular facilitation (PNF) techniques.[12] According to clinical experience, a more pronounced relaxation of the neck muscles can be achieved while sitting with crossed legs than sitting with the legs parallel. This observation can be applied effectively in physical therapy to achieve a better relaxation of the neck muscles before a specific treatment. It could also be used to help the patient to relax at work when a constrained position creates discomfort in the neck muscles. Furthermore, the brainstem reflexes commonly used in motor reeducation in cases of upper motor neuron lesions can be effectively used in improving upper body control. It has to be borne in mind that the neck muscles not only have a motion and stabilization function but are also strongly involved in the regulatory mechanism of posture. Indeed, this proprioceptive function of short, deep neck extensors is so strong that these muscles are often considered more as proprioceptive organs than as activators of movement.[13]

Neck muscles show a strong tendency to develop hypertonus and spasm, not only for the aforementioned reasons. It has been shown[14] that afferent fibers constitute up to 80% of neck muscles, in comparison to most other striated muscles, which contain approximately 50% of such fibers. This may explain a greater sensitivity of the neck musculature to any situation that alters the proprioceptive input from cervical structures. Joint-motion restriction is such a situation. The shoulder and neck muscle complex belongs to the part of the body that is strongly influenced by the functional status of the CNS, particularly of the limbic system. This is reflected primarily in an increase in tone in terms of muscle spasm and by a decreased ability to perform fine, economically coordinated movements.

The role of the limbic system in motor control and the quality of muscle tension has been a neglected area in physical therapy. The limbic system is a phylogenetically old part of the brain and in humans is entirely covered by the more recently evolved neocortex. It comprises a number of structures with numerous connections to the frontal motor cortex, hypothalamus, and brainstem. The limbic system was originally and imprecisely named the *rhinencephalon (olfactory brain)*.[10]

The limbic system regulates human emotions, and this control involves somatomotor, autonomic, and endocrine systems. It is closely associated with learning (including motor learning) and motor activation. It serves as a trigger to voluntary movements and regulates pain perception and motivation.[10,15] All of these functions can substantially influence a physiotherapeutic result. The greatest influence of the limbic system is on the shoulder and neck area, and it is therefore not surprising that any function of the limbic system will be more evident there than in another part of the body.

Because the limbic system is very sensitive to stress,[15] it is not difficult to understand that its dysfunction, which influences numerous functions of the human body, can be reflected in an industrialized society by a gradually increasing number of disorders marked by musculoskeletal pain. This is particularly so with respect to various cervicocranial syndromes. An improved function of the limbic system, with a consequent improvement in the general regulatory system of the body, can be mistakenly explained as a positive result of a local physiotherapeutic procedure. For example, in an unpublished study conducted by our group, a 4-week therapeutic stay in a spa facility, the main focus of which was treatment of chronic low back pain syndromes, produced the greatest improvement in cervicogenic syndromes, although they were not specifically treated. It might be hypothesized that the calming environment of the spa influenced the function of the limbic system, which contributed significantly to the general therapeutic effect. This observation should be a reminder that evaluation of a particular therapeutic procedure, particularly one involving the neck area, should be done under conditions of careful control.

Of particular importance to conditions affecting the shoulder and neck muscle complex are the defense reflexes and defense behavior, which are closely associated with the limbic and hypothalamic systems. These are expressions of anger and fear in humans. Besides the autonomic reactions, which are mainly associated with increased activity of the sympathetic system, there is a strong reaction in the head, neck, and shoulder muscles, with their increased activation resulting in the adoption of a typical posture intended to protect the head. The head is poked forward and retracted between the elevated shoulders. This position is exactly the same as occurs in the upper crossed syndrome (Figure 10-1). Both the defense reaction and the muscle imbalance can thus potentiate the overstress of predicted segments, resulting in typical syndromes.

Although under physiological conditions both the postural reflexes (tonic neck reflexes, deep tonic neck reflexes, righting reflexes) and the statokinetic reflexes are suppressed and inhibited (but not abolished), they influence the fine control of posture of the body and of the head in particular. This is associated especially with an increased activation of the neck and head extensors. Although these reflexes are difficult to measure under physiological conditions in humans, their influence has to be presumed and should be reflected in physical therapists' thinking.

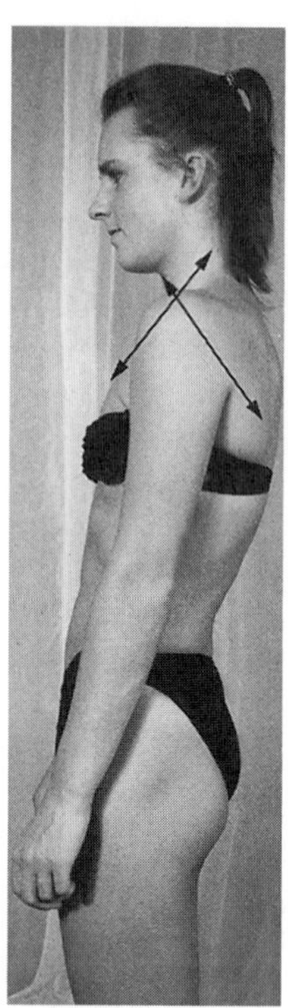

Figure 10-1
The upper crossed syndrome.

Other important functional relationships also affect the shoulder and neck muscle complex, although the associated activity may often be remote. For example, the neck muscles are included in one of the most important life-preserving movement patterns—the prehension pattern—and because of this, any movement of the upper extremity must be associated with at least some activation of the neck muscles. This activation is initiated by the reflex mechanism and continued by biomechanical reaction. Therefore, as previously stated, any movement of the upper extremity has an influence on head and neck position.

The position of the head and cervical spine—and therefore the activation of muscles in these areas—adapts to any alteration of position of the lower part of the body, particularly of the pelvis. Any scoliosis or scoliotic posture or asymmetrical position of the pelvis caused by dysfunction of the pelvis itself or as a response to, for example, a leg-length asymmetry will be reflected in the regulatory readjustment of the neck muscles to maintain equilibrium and an adequate position of the head. This regulatory control is primarily triggered reflexively, although it is potentiated by necessary biomechanical compensation.

The mutual influence of remote areas of the body on the neck muscles occurs, however, in even less obvious situations. An unpublished electromyographic (EMG) study conducted by our group, demonstrated that even an unresisted but not well-coordinated hip extension movement performed in a prone position is associated with an unwanted, increased activation of a majority of neck and shoulder muscles, resulting in a rotation and anterior tilt of the vertebrae of the lower cervical spine. Hyperextension of the hip joint is an essential part of the normal gait pattern. It can therefore be hypothesized that such a rotation and anterior tilt, which is no doubt the result of activation of the deep intrinsic neck muscles, will occur during each step of walking. This means that the lower cervical spine is exposed to repetitive, constrained additional and unwanted movements. This mechanism might help to explain the recurrence of neck syndromes or discomfort. It should be kept in mind that the muscular response in such reflex mechanisms usually occurs early and distinctly.

The muscles of the upper part of the body have been studied electromyographically to a much lesser extent than those of the lower body. There are several reasons for this. A partial, obvious explanation is the larger size and greater accessibility of muscles of the lower part of the body. Furthermore, the study of the upper body muscles requires more sophisticated EMG techniques; indeed, some muscles are accessible only under radiographic control.

The biomechanical function of the upper body muscles is also less well known, more controversial, and more complex than that of the lower body muscles. This is true not only for the primary function of muscles or muscle groups but also with respect to their synkinetic functions. For example, the explanation of the function of the accessory muscles of respiration has greatly changed[16,17]: the synkinetic movements of the head during chewing remain almost totally neglected; and the paradoxical function of the scaleni has not yet been analyzed. Particular attention should also be paid to the hyoid muscles. Although they may be a frequent source of headache[6] and other syndromes, they are not investigated as they should be. Neglecting them may lead to an incorrect diagnosis and disappointing results of therapy.

SIGNIFICANCE OF MUSCLE IMBALANCE AND ALTERED MOVEMENT PATTERNS

From the functional viewpoint, the following three basic dysfunctions should be considered in connection with disorders involving the muscles of the head and neck:

1. Muscle imbalance characterized by the development of impaired relationships between muscles prone to tightness and those prone to inhibition and weakness
2. Altered movement patterns, usually closely related to muscle imbalance
3. Trigger points within muscles as well as local and referred pain originating from these points

Muscle imbalance describes the situation in which some muscles become inhibited and therefore weak, whereas others become tight, losing their extensibility. Muscle tightness is generally a consequence of chronic overuse, and tight muscles therefore usually maintain their strength. However, in extreme or long-lasting tightness, a decrease in muscle strength occurs. This phenomenon has been described as "tightness weakness."[18] Stretching of tight muscles may lead to recovery of their strength. In addition, stretching of tight muscles results in improved activation of the antagonist (inhibited) muscles, probably mediated via Sherrington's law of reciprocal inhibition.

Muscle tightness (decreased flexibility or decreased extensibility, muscle stiffness, tautness) should not be confused with other types of increased muscle tone because each type is of different genesis and requires a different type of treatment. This confusion occurs particularly in relation to the scaleni because inhibition and commonly spasm and trigger points in these muscles are mistakenly diagnosed as tightness. In the proximal part of the body, the following muscles tend to develop tightness: pectoralis major and minor, upper trapezius, levator scapulae, and sternocleidomastoid. Although detailed analysis of the following muscles still remains to be undertaken, it is considered that the masseter, temporalis, digastric, and the small muscles connecting the occiput and cervical spine (the recti and obliques) also tend to become tight. Muscles that tend to develop weakness and inhibition are the lower stabilizers of the scapula (serratus anterior, rhomboids, middle and lower trapezius), deep neck flexors, suprahyoid, and mylohyoid.

The reaction of the longus colli, longus capitis, rectus capitis anterior, subscapularis, supraspinatus, infraspinatus, and teres major and minor remains unclear. It should be emphasized that knowledge of the function of the muscles of the neck region is inadequate and that many current concepts relating to them may well undergo change.

The tendency of some muscles to develop inhibition or tightness is not random but occurs as a systematic dysfunction associated with "muscle imbalance patterns."[7-9] The muscle imbalance does not remain limited to a certain part of the body but gradually involves the entire muscle system. Because the muscle imbalance usually precedes the appearance of a pain syndrome, a thorough evaluation can be of substantial help in introducing measures to prevent this.

In adults, a muscle imbalance is usually more evident in the lower part of the body and may precede the development of muscle imbalance in the upper part. The imbalance in the upper part of the body forms the "proximal or shoulder crossed syndrome." This is characterized by tightness and increased activation of the levator scapulae, upper trapezius, sternocleidomastoid, and pectoral muscles and by weakness of the lower stabilizers of the scapula and the deep neck flexors. Topographically, when the weakened and shortened muscles are connected, they form a cross (Figure 10-1). This pattern of muscle imbalance produces typical changes in posture and motion. In standing, elevation and protraction of the shoulders are evident, as are rotation and abduction of the scapulae, a variable degree of winging of the scapulae, and a forward head posture. This altered posture is likely to stress the cervicocranial and cervicothoracic junctions and the transitory segments at the level of C4 and C5. Furthermore, the stability of the glenohumeral joint is decreased because of the altered angle of the glenoid fossa. According to Basmajian,[19] almost no muscle activity is needed to keep the head of the humerus firmly in the glenoid fossa under normal conditions. In the proximal crossed syndrome, however, the biomechanical conditions change substantially. The plane of the glenoid fossa becomes more vertical because of the abduction, rotation, and winging of the scapula. Maintaining the humeral head in the glenoid fossa then provokes increased activity in the levator scapulae and trapezius. This occurs not only when the arm is used in vigorous movements but also with the arm hanging by the side of the body. Such increased activity tends to lead to spasm and tightness in these muscles, which in turn augment the improper position of the scapula; thus a vicious cycle develops. It may be hypothesized that abnormalities in proprioceptive stimulation result and lead to dystrophic changes in the shoulder joint.

Muscle imbalance in children, in contrast to that in adults, usually starts in the upper part of the body. Why this development in children contrasts with that in adults has not been satisfactorily explained. It is presumed that the main reason concerns the relatively large and heavy head of the child, which is supported by comparatively weak neck muscles and by the fact that the center of gravity of the child's head is located forward but is gradually shifted backward into a well-balanced position during growth. In accord with the more evident muscle imbalance in the upper part of the body in children is the clinical observation that various syndromes originating in the neck, such as acute wry neck or "school headache," are common in children, whereas syndromes related to other segments of the spine are rare.

The muscles involved in the layer (stratification) syndrome[20] in the proximal part of the body are the same as those involved in the proximal (shoulder and neck) crossed syndrome.

EVALUATION OF MUSCLE IMBALANCE AND ALTERED MOVEMENT PATTERNS IN THE UPPER BODY

The assessment of muscle imbalance and altered movement patterns is undertaken in three stages: evaluation during standing, examination of muscle tightness, and examination of movement patterns. A great part of the assessment is based on visual observation. However, deep palpation helps to evaluate muscle tone, whether increased or decreased, and helps in estimating the type of increase in muscle tone. Limbic dysfunction in the upper part of the body will include hypertonicity of mimetic, masticatory, and hyoid muscles, as well as of the whole shoulder and neck region, including the short neck extensors. The most obvious palpatory findings are in the area of the upper trapezius, levator scapulae, and deep short extensors of the neck. In this type of muscle hypertonicity, constant EMG activity at rest can generally be found.[21] At trigger points, increased tone and taut bands can be palpated, as described in detail by Travell and Simons.[6]

Analysis of Muscles in Standing

The analysis of the muscles of the lower part of the body in standing has been described elsewhere.[22] In this chapter, attention will be focused on analysis of the muscles in the upper part of the body, although the evaluations in the two regions cannot be separated. In addition, all other deviations of posture should be taken into consideration.

The patient is first observed from behind, noting particularly any changes in the interscapular space and in the position of the scapulae. Where there is weakness of the interscapular muscles (rhomboids, middle trapezius), the interscapular space will appear flattened (Figure 10-2). In the case of a pronounced weakness already associated with some atrophy, a hollowing instead of a flattening may appear. In addition, the distance between the thoracic spinous processes and the medial border of the scapula is increased because of the rotation of the scapula. Improper fixation of the inferior

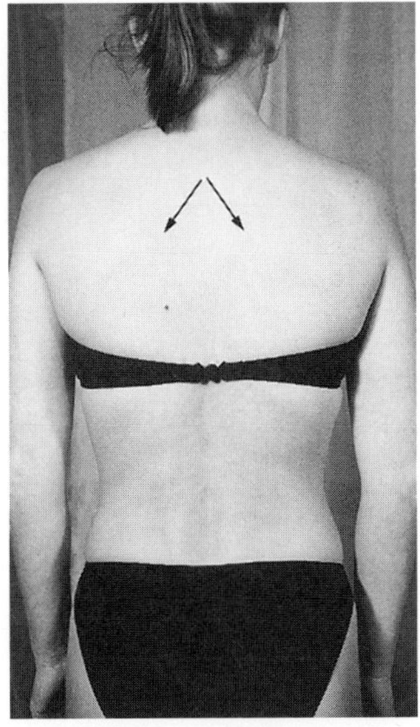

Figure 10-2
Flattening of the interscapular space as a sign of weakness of the rhomboids and middle trapezius muscles.

angle to the rib cage and a winging scapula indicate weakness of the serratus anterior muscle.

Tightness of the upper trapezius and levator scapulae muscles, which almost invariably accompanies this weakness, can be seen in the neck and shoulder line. Where there is tightness of the trapezius only, the contour will straighten. If the tightness of the levator scapulae predominates, the contour of the neckline will appear as a double wave in the area of insertion of the muscle on the scapula. This straightening of the neck and shoulder line is sometimes described as "gothic" shoulders because it is reminiscent of the form of a gothic church tower. In addition, there is an elevation of the shoulder girdle. Observation and palpation of the descending fibers of the trapezius along the cervical spine may reveal broadening and changed elasticity. Where there are tight pectoral muscles, there may be protraction of the shoulder girdle.

When observing the patient from the front, the physical therapist should observe the belly of the pectoralis major first. The tighter (or stronger) the muscle, the more prominent it will be. Typical imbalance will lead to rounded and protracted shoulders and slight medial rotation of the arms (Figure 10-3).

Much information can be obtained from observation of the anterior neck and throat. Normally, the sternocleidomastoid is just visible. Prominence of the insertion of the muscle, particularly of its clavicular insertion, is a sign of tightness. A groove along this muscle is an early sign of weakness of the deep neck flexors (Figure 10-4). The deep neck flexors tend to weaken and atrophy quickly, and this sign, among others, has therefore been proposed as a reliable way in which to estimate biological age.[23] Straightening of the throat line is usually a sign of increased tone of the digastric muscle. Palpation frequently reveals trigger points. Careful examination of this muscle is extremely important because pain referred from it is often misinterpreted.[6]

Head posture should also be observed. From the viewpoint of muscle analysis, a forward head posture is a result of weakness of the deep neck flexors and dominance or even tightness of the sternocleidomastoid. During observation of the forward head posture, it is important to note the degree of cervical lordosis and the extent of the thoracic kyphosis.

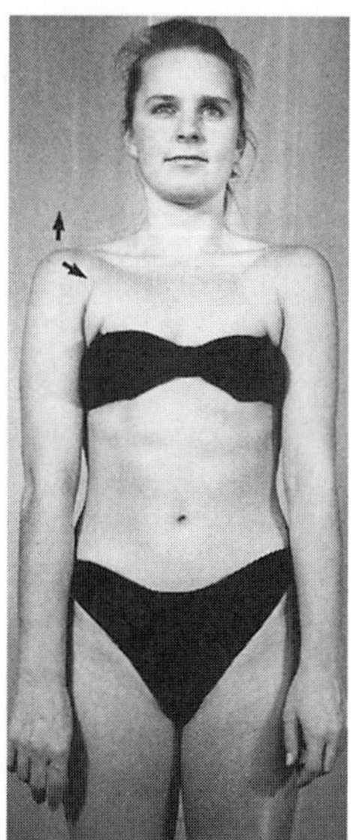

Figure 10-3
Protracted, elevated, and medially rotated shoulders as a sign of a combined tightness of the pectoralis major, upper trapezius, and latissimus dorsi muscles.

Testing of Muscle Tightness (Flexibility, Extensibility, Stiffness, Tautness)

Although it is highly important, flexibility of the muscles of the upper part of the body is often ignored in examination of the cervical and thoracic spine, and even worse, muscle tightness may be confused with increased activation of the particular muscle, with hypertonicity of various types,[21] and most frequently with trigger points. (Trigger points in muscles and myofascial pain in general are considered to be important components of pathological changes in muscles. Physical therapists should be familiar with the palpatory techniques used in their assessment.[5,6]) Although a combination of signs can be found simultaneously in a single muscle, an exact differential diagnosis is the basic presumption for successful and rational treatment.

Because tight muscles influence movement patterns and, as clinical experience reveals, contribute substantially to inhibition of their antagonists, the evaluation of muscle tightness should precede the evaluation of movement patterns and of weakness. It can, however, be combined with palpation and the evaluation of muscle tone.

In the upper part of the body, the upper trapezius, levator scapulae, and pectoralis major are the principal muscles of concern. Other muscles, even the sternocleidomastoid, are difficult to evaluate because their ranges of movement are limited by joints and ligaments.

The extensibility of upper trapezius and levator scapulae is best examined with the patient in the supine position. For testing of the upper trapezius, the patient's head is passively inclined to the contralateral side and flexed while the shoulder girdle is stabilized. From this position, the shoulder is moved distally (Figure 10-5). Normally, there is free movement with a soft motion barrier. However, when tightness is present, the range of movement is restricted, and the barrier is hard. Testing of the levator is done in a similar manner, except that in addition, the head is rotated to the contralateral (i.e., nontested) side (Figure 10-6). If the muscle is tight in addition to the movement restriction, a tender insertion of the levator can be palpated.

The pectoralis major is tested with the patient in the supine position with the arm moved passively into abduction. It is important that the trunk be stabilized before the arm is placed into abduction because a twist of the trunk might suggest a normal range of movement. The arm should reach the horizontal (Figure 10-7). To estimate the tightness of the clavicular portion, the arm is allowed to loosely hang down while the examiner moves the shoulder posteriorly (Figure 10-8). Normally, only a slight barrier is felt, but where there is tightness this barrier is hard.

Evaluation of the sternocleidomastoid is difficult and imprecise because this muscle spans too many motion segments. The short deep posterior neck muscles

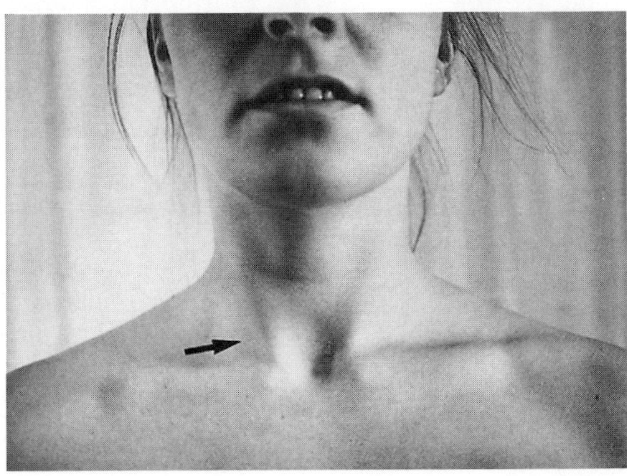

Figure 10-4
Deepening along the sternocleidomastoid muscle as a sign of weak or atrophied deep neck flexors.

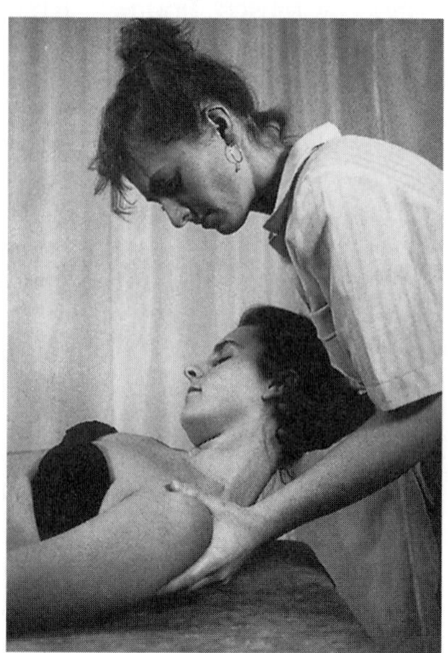

Figure 10-5
Evaluation of the tightness of the upper trapezius.

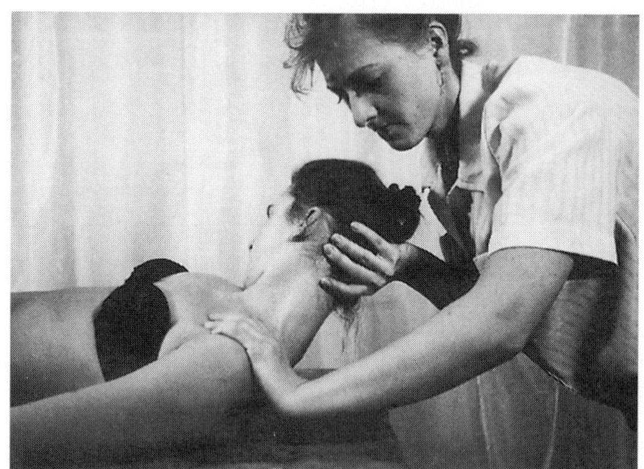

Figure 10-6
Evaluation of tightness of the levator scapulae.

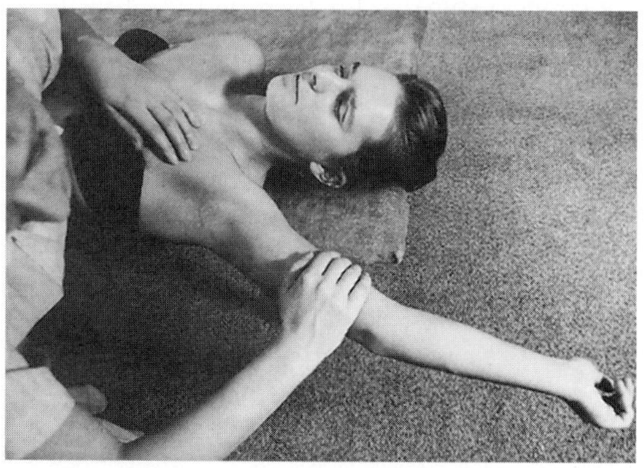

Figure 10-7
Evaluation of tightness of the sternal portion of the pectoralis major.

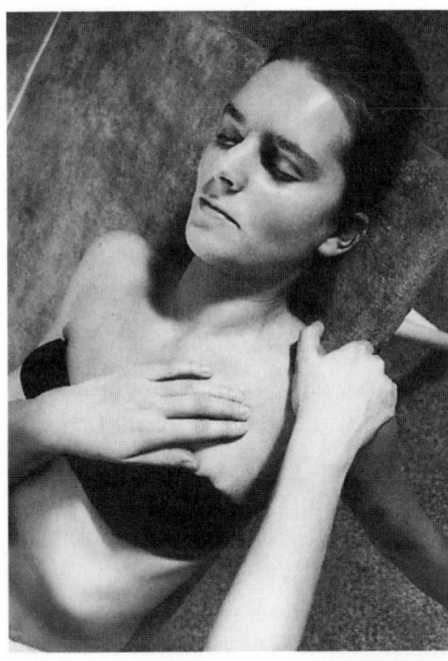

Figure 10-8
Evaluation of the tightness of the clavicular portion of the pectoralis major.

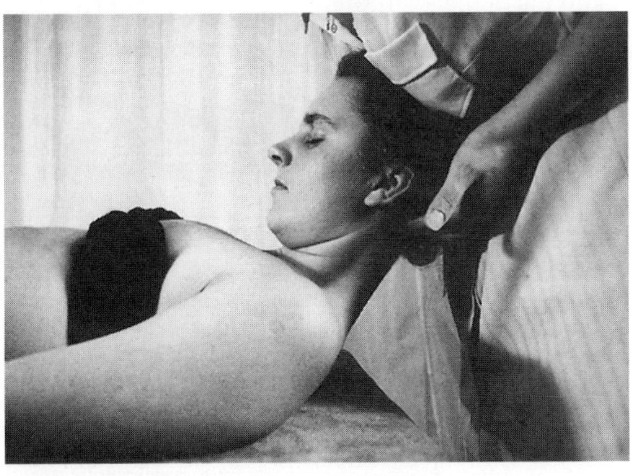

Figure 10-9
Evaluation of the deep short neck extensors.

(recti and obliques) can be palpated only while the upper cervical segments are passively flexed (Figure 10-9). Resistance felt on palpation of the proximal segments of the cervical spine is, however, not necessarily indicative of tight musculature.

More specific details of tests of muscle flexibility may be found in texts devoted to this subject.[24,25]

Examination of Movement Patterns and Weakened Muscles

Testing of individual muscles may help to estimate muscle weakness and differentiate weakness resulting from a lower motor neuron lesion from weakness caused by tightness, joint position (stretch), trigger points, or weakness of arthrogenic origin. The detailed description of all individual muscle tests is beyond the scope of this chapter; such information can be found in other sources.[24-29]

In musculoskeletal disorders, evaluation of the basic movement patterns of different regions of the body is of paramount importance. In the upper body, three movements are of particular value: the push up, head-forward bending, and abduction of the shoulder. An evaluation of movement patterns is usually more sensitive than testing of individual muscle groups because it reveals minute changes in the coordination and programming of movements. These changes may often be more important for the diagnosis and treatment of a spinal disorder than a simple estimation of individual muscle strength would be. In other words, the therapist is more concerned with the degree of activation of all of the muscles recruited during a particular movement than with any single muscle, regardless of whether a particular muscle is biomechanically capable of producing that movement.

Head flexion is tested in the supine position. The subject is asked to slowly raise the head in the habitual way. When the deep neck flexors are weak and the sternocleidomastoid strong, the jaw is seen to jut forward at the beginning of the movement, with hyperextension at the cervicocranial junction. An arclike flexion follows after approximately 10 degrees of head elevation from the plinth has been achieved. If the pattern is unclear, slight resistance of about 2 to 4 g (one or two fingers' pressure) against the forehead may be applied to make the hyperextension more evident. This test provides the therapist with information about the interplay between the deep neck flexors (which tend to become weak) and the sternocleidomastoids (which are usually strong and taut). If the test is performed by jutting the jaw forward, overstress of the cervicocranial junction is likely to exist (Figures 10-10 and 10-11).

Push-up from the prone position gives information about the quality of stabilization of the scapula. During push-up, and particularly in the first phase of lowering the body from maximum push-up, the scapula on the side on which stabilization is im-

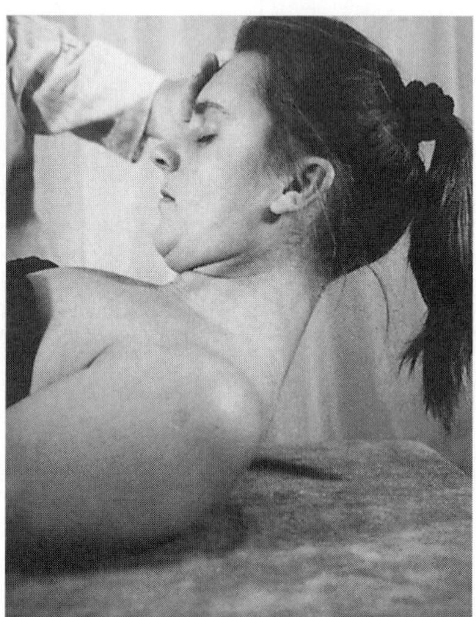

Figure 10-10
Head flexion pattern: evaluation of weak deep neck flexors.

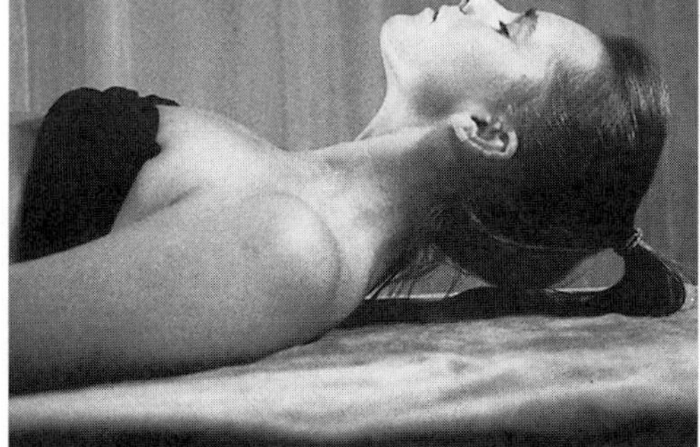

Figure 10-11
Head flexion pattern: head "pushed forward" position as a sign of the predominance of the sternocleidomastoid muscle.

paired glides over the thorax, shifting outward and upward or rotating, or both (Figure 10-12). If the serratus anterior does not function properly, winging of the scapula will result. The entire movement must be performed very slowly, or slight muscle weakness and incoordination may be missed. The pathological performance reveals that the movements of the upper extremity are somewhat impaired and that increased stabilization of the cervical spine is needed.

Shoulder abduction is tested in sitting with the elbow flexed. Elbow flexion controls undesired humeral rotation. The subject slowly abducts the shoulder (Figure 10-13). During this action, three components of the complex movement are evaluated: abduction at the glenohumeral joint, rotation of the scapula, and elevation of the whole shoulder girdle. Movement is stopped at the point at which shoulder girdle elevation commences. This usually occurs when 60 degrees of abduction at the glenohumeral joint has been achieved. The therapist should not be misled by some activation of the trapezii at the start of shoulder abduction. This activity is necessary to stabilize the cervical spine and prevent lateral flexion of the head.

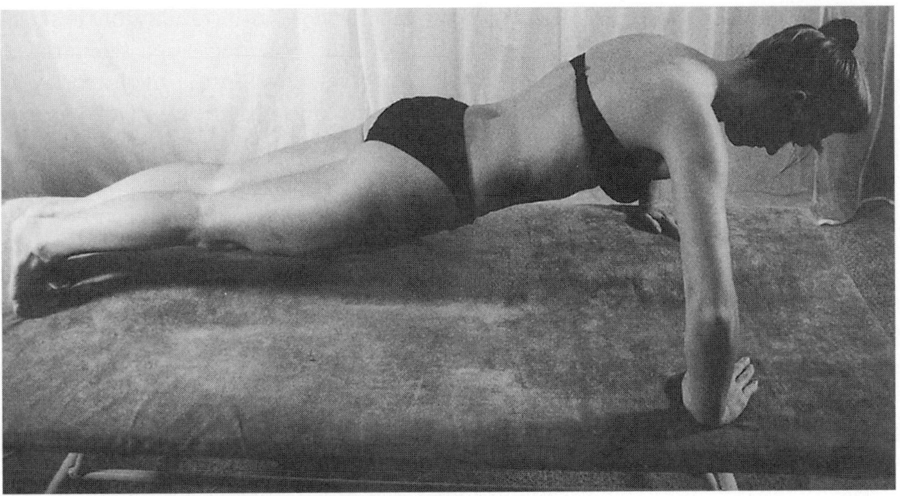

Figure 10-12
The push-up position for evaluation of weak lower stabilizers of the scapulae.

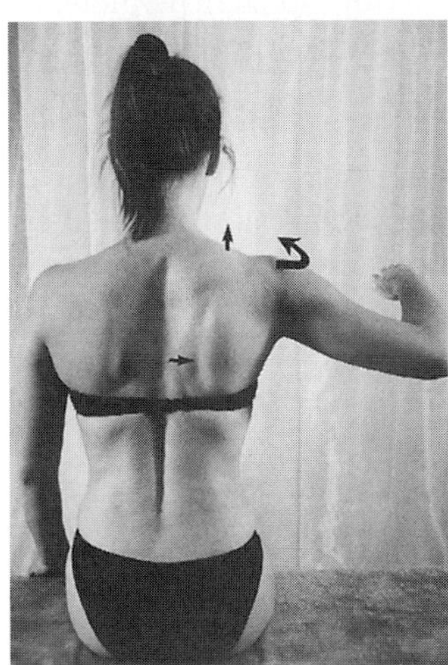

Figure 10-13
Evaluation of shoulder abduction pattern. Note that three components are evaluated: abduction at the glenohumeral joint, rotation of the scapula, and elevation of the whole shoulder girdle.

By itself, testing of the movement patterns provides only a basic clinical orientation to a patient's condition. To obtain comprehensive information, it is necessary to evaluate muscles and movements with multichannel EMG. However, this method is unrealistic in a busy practice because it is extremely time consuming as well as expensive.

HYPERMOBILITY

Muscles can be involved in many other afflictions. With regard to musculoskeletal syndromes, constitutional hypermobility should be considered.

Constitutional hypermobility is a vague, nonprogressive clinical syndrome, not strictly a disease. It is characterized by a general laxity of the connective tissue, ligaments, and muscles, although not to the same extent as in Ehlers-Danlos or Marfan syndromes. Its etiology is unknown, although a congenital insufficiency of mesenchymal tissue is postulated. Although it has not been confirmed that "hypermobile" subjects are more prone to musculoskeletal pain syndromes, an instability of these subjects' joints may be evident. The muscles in general show decreased strength and, when subjected to a strength-training program, never develop the hypertrophy and strength of "normal" subjects' muscles. The muscle tone is decreased when assessed by palpation, and there is an increased range of joint movement.

Constitutional hypermobility involves the entire body, although its different parts may not be affected to the same extent, and a slight unilateral asymmetry can be observed. It is more common in women than men and seems to involve the upper part of the body more commonly than the lower. In middle age, the hypermobility decreases in correspondence to the general decrease in range of movement that is seen with aging.

Muscle tightness may also develop in constitutional hypermobility, although this is not so obvious. In clinical practice, such tightness is mainly considered an expression of a compensatory mechanism for improving the stability of the joints. Therefore stretching should be performed carefully and gently and should be applied only to key muscles. Stretching is indicated only in a limited number of cases and should be done only after a thorough evaluation. Because the muscles in cases of constitutional hypermobility are generally weak, they may be easily overused, and trigger points may therefore develop easily in muscles and ligaments.

There is no effective treatment for the syndrome of constitutional hypermobility. However, reasonably prolonged strengthening and sensorimotor programs are usually helpful.

The identification of constitutional hypermobility requires a differential diagnosis because this clinical entity should not be confused with other possible sources of decreased muscle tone and increased range of motion. Among the most frequent errors in the diagnosis are confusion of constitutional hypermobility with the hypotonia in syndromes affecting the afferent nerve fibers, oligophrenia, and cerebellar and extrapyramidal insufficiency.

EVALUATION OF HYPERMOBILITY IN THE UPPER PART OF THE BODY

The assessment of hypermobility is in principle based on the estimation of muscle tone and range of movement of the joints. In clinical practice, orientation tests are usually sufficient for such as assessment. In the upper body, the most useful tests are head rotation, the high-arm cross, touching of the hands behind the neck, crossing of the arms behind the neck, extension of the elbows, and hyperextension of the thumb.[25]

Head rotation is tested in a sitting position, with the patient first actively turning the head. At the end of this active range-of-motion phase, an attempt is made to increase the range passively. The normal range is about 80 degrees to each side, and the ranges of active and passive movement are almost the same.

In the high-arm cross, the patient—while standing or sitting—puts the arm around the neck from the front to the opposite side. Normally the elbow almost reaches the median plane of the body, and the fingers reach the spinous processes of the cervical spine.

Touching of the hands behind the neck is tested with the patient standing or sitting. The patient tries to bring both hands together behind the back. Normally the tips of the fingers can touch without any increase in the thoracic lordosis.

Crossing of the arms behind the neck is again tested in either the sitting or standing positions. The patient puts the arms across the neck with the fingers extended in the direction of the shoulder blades. Normally the fingertips can reach the spines of the scapulae.

Extension of the elbows is better tested in the sitting than in the standing position. The elbows and lower arms are pressed together in maximal flexion of the elbows. The patient then tries to extend the elbows without separating them. Normally the elbows can be extended approximately 110 degrees.

In hyperextension of the thumb, the examiner performs a passive extension of the thumb and measures the degree of the achieved hyperextension. Normally it is up to 20 degrees in the interphalangeal joint and almost 0 degrees in the metacarpophalangeal joint.

IMPLICATIONS FOR TREATMENT

A number of points should be drawn together in concluding this chapter, and it must be emphasized that detailed controlled studies of various assessment and management techniques remain to be undertaken.

Muscle imbalance is an essential component of dysfunction syndromes of the musculoskeletal system. The overall treatment program for such syndromes includes techniques that depend on recognizing factors that perpetuate the dysfunction and methods directed toward its correction. This is true regardless of whether muscle imbalance is considered to cause joint dysfunction or to occur in parallel with it.

Because increased tone in a muscle that is in a functional relationship with a particular joint plays an important role in the production and perception of pain, it could be argued that the first goal of treatment should be to decrease this tone. The choice of a therapeutic technique for this may be less important than using the approach in which the clinician is most skilled. Physiologically there is probably not a substantial difference between the effects of "classical" gentle mobilization and techniques based on postfacilitation inhibition. Clinically, however, techniques based on postisometric relaxation (postfacilitation inhibition)[9,11,30] have been found to be most effective in treating musculoskeletal dysfunction. In conditions marked by acute pain, changes in muscle can be considered to be principally reflexive, and hard or vigorous stretching techniques are therefore not a treatment of choice. In chronic pain or in the painless period between acute attacks of pain, strong stretching is necessary.

Regardless of how effective they may be in decreasing muscle tone, the techniques selected for treatment must influence the basic impairment of CNS motor regulation and the concomitant muscle imbalance. In the long term, treatment of impaired muscle function has as its objective the restoration of muscle balance, with the achievement of optimal flexibility of muscles that are prone to tightness and improved strength in muscles prone to inhibition and weakness. This must be followed by the realization of a second objective—the establishment of sound and economic movement patterns for the patient. This approach is time consuming and demands advanced skill on the part of the therapist as well as good cooperation on the part of the patient. In addition it is tiring, because it requires the total concentration of both the therapist and patient. Moreover, because patients do not necessarily use "artificially" learned movement patterns in their everyday activities, the results of treatment are sometimes disappointing.

As a consequence, and based on some ideas of Freeman,[31,32] a program of "sensorimotor stimulation" has been developed.[33] Current knowledge stresses the important contribution of the cerebellum in the programming of primitive or simple movement patterns.[34] Consequently, a program of exercises has been developed to preferentially activate the spinovestibulocerebellar and subcortical pathways and regulatory circuits so as to increase proprioceptive flow from the peripheral parts of the musculoskeletal system. It is believed that this makes it possible to include an inhibited muscle more easily and effectively in important movement patterns such as gait.[35] Because this is achieved more on a reflex, automatic basis, the technique requires less voluntary control by the patient. It is less tiring and can be satisfactorily realized as a home program. It is beyond the scope of this chapter to do more than briefly mention this approach.

No therapeutic approach is sufficient unless body posture generally is improved. Whatever the cause of the patient's problem, special attention should be given to it. Overall, improvement of posture is time consuming, and because both the therapist and the patient are often satisfied by the immediate alleviation of symptoms, treatment is discontinued and posture correction not infrequently neglected. However, a strongly prophylactic approach promises good long-term results and the prevention of recurrences of acute episodes of dysfunction.

Despite the very encouraging long-term results of clinical treatment of muscle imbalance in patients with chronic pain syndromes, scientifically controlled studies of such treatment remain to be conducted. Enthusiastic but premature clinical claims may leave in their wake a tide of skepticism that may well prevent future progress in this important area.

ACKNOWLEDGMENT

I wish to thank Professor Margaret Bullock and Dr. Joanne Bullock-Saxton, Department of Physiotherapy, University of Queensland, Australia, for their willing assistance in preparing this chapter.

References

1. Maigne R: *Orthopaedic medicine*, Springfield, Ill, 1979, Charles C Thomas.
2. Bourdillon JF, Day EA, Bookhout MA: *Spinal manipulation*, Edinburgh, 1992, Butterworth Heinemann.
3. Lewit K: *Manipulative therapy in rehabilitation of the motor system*, Oxford, England, 1985, Butterworth-Heinemann.
4. Frymoyer JW, Gordon SL, editors: *New perspectives in low back pain*, Park Ridge, Ill, 1989, American Academy of Orthopaedic Surgeons.

5. Kraus H: *Diagnosis and treatment of muscle pain*, Chicago, 1988, Quintessence.
6. Travell JG, Simons GD: *Myofascial pain and dysfunction: the trigger point manual*, Baltimore, 1983, Williams & Wilkins.
7. Janda V: Introduction to functional pathology of the motor system. In Howell ML, Bullock MI, editors: *Physiotherapy in sports*, ed 3, Brisbane, Australia, 1982, University of Queensland.
8. Janda V: *Muscles, central nervous motor regulation, and back problems.* In Korr IM, editor: *The neurobiologic mechanisms in manipulative therapy*, New York, 1978, Plenum Press.
9. Janda V: *Evaluation of muscle imbalance.* In Liebenson C, editor: *Rehabilitation of the spine: a practitioner's manual*, Philadelphia, 1996, Williams & Wilkins.
10. Schmidt RF: *Fundamentals of neurophysiology*, New York, 1985, Springer.
11. Fisher AG, Murray EA, Burdy AC: *Sensory integration*, Philadelphia, 1991, FA Davis.
12. Voss DE, Ionta MK, Myers BJ: *Proprioceptive neuromuscular facilitation*, Philadelphia, 1985, Harper & Row.
13. Abrahams VC, Lynn B, Richmond FJR: Organization and sensory properties of small myelinated fibres in the dorsal cervical rami of the cat, *J Physiol (Lond)* 347:177, 1984.
14. Abrahams VC: The physiology of neck muscles: their role in head movement and maintenance of posture, *Can J Physiol Pharamacol* 55:332, 1977.
15. Guyton AC: *Basic human neurophysiology*, Philadelphia, 1981, Saunders.
16. Janda V: Some aspects of extracranial causes of facial pain, *J Prosthet Dent* 56:484, 1986.
17. Widmer CG: Evaluation of temporomandibular disorders. In Kraus SL, editor: *TMJ disorders*, New York, 1988, Churchill Livingstone.
18. Janda V: *Muscle strength in relation to muscle length, pain, and muscle imbalance.* In Harms-Rindahl K, editor: *Muscle strength*, New York, 1993, Churchill Livingstone.
19. Basmajian JV: *Muscles alive*, Baltimore, 1974, Williams & Wilkins.
20. Janda V: Die muskulären Hauptsyndrom bei vertebragenen Beschwerden. In Neumann HD, Wolff HD, editors: *Theoretische Fortschritte und Praktische Erfahrungen der Manuellen Medizin*, Konkordia, 1979, Bühl.
21. Janda V: Muscle spasm: a proposed procedure for differential diagnosis, *J Manual Med* 6:136, 1991.
22. Jull G, Janda V: Muscles and motor control in low back pain. In Twomey LT, Taylor JR, editors: *Physical therapy for the low back*, ed 2, New York, 1987, Churchill Livingstone.
23. Bourliere F: The assessment of biological age in man, WHO public health papers 37, Geneva, 1979, World Health Organization.
24. Kendall FP, McCreary EK; *Muscles, testing, and function*, ed 3, Baltimore, 1983, Williams & Wilkins.
25. Janda V: *Muscle function testing*, Oxford, England, 1983, Butterworth-Heinemann.
26. Daniels L, Worthingham C: *Muscle testing*, Philadelphia, 1986, WB Saunders.
27. Cole JH, Twomey LT: *Muscles in action: an approach to manual muscle testing*, Melbourne, 1988, Churchill Livingstone.
28. Clarkson HM, Gilewich GB: *Musculoskeletal assessment*, Baltimore, 1989, Williams & Wilkins.
29. Lâcote M, Chevelier AM, Miranda A et al: *Clinical evaluation of muscle function*, Edinburgh, 1987, Churchill Livingstone.
30. Mitchell FL, Moran PS, Pruzzo NA: *An evaluation and treatment manual of osteopathic muscle energy procedures*, East Lansing, Mich, 1979, Mitchell, Moran, and Pruzzo Associates.
31. Freeman MAR: Instability of the foot after injuries to the lateral ligament of the ankle, *J Bone Joint Surg* 47B:669, 1965.
32. Freeman MAR, Dean MRE, Hanham IWF: The etiology and prevention of function instability of the foot, *J Bone Joint Surg* 47B:678, 1965.
33. Janda V, Vávrová M: Sensory motor stimulation (video presented by J Bullock-Saxton, Body Control Videos, Box 730, Brisbane 4068, Australia).
34. Lehmkukl LD, Smith LK: *Brunnstrom's clinical kinesiology*, Philadelphia, 1987, FA Davis.
35. Bullock-Saxton JEW, Janda V, Bullock MI: Reflex activation of the gluteal muscles in walking, *Spine* 18:704, 1993.

CHAPTER 11

Upper Limb Neurodynamic Test: Clinical Use in a "Big Picture" Framework

David S. Butler

In the first edition of this text,[1] the *upper limb tension test (ULTT)* as it was then known, was presented in a mechanical and peripheralistic way that reflected the neurobiological knowledge and manual therapy approaches at the time. In the second edition,[2] the ULTT was presented under a framework of hypothesized pain mechanisms, with some direction to view the test responses in relation to proposed peripheral and central pain mechanisms. In this edition, a name change for the test is proposed, and the focus will be on the clinical use of the test considering current "big picture" evidence.

UPPER LIMB NEURODYNAMIC TEST

Instead of the commonly used term *upper limb tension test*, the term *upper limb neurodynamic test (ULNT)* is now proposed. The word tension is considered mechanistic and conceptually limiting. The term *neurodynamic*, as suggested by Shacklock,[3] allows consideration of movement-related neurophysiological changes and also the neuronal dynamics that surely occur in the central nervous system (CNS) during physical and mental activity.

The aim of the ULNT is to load parts of the upper limb nervous system and thus to test its physical health and associated mechanosensitivity. It is of course impossible to avoid load on other tissues, including other nerves, so at best the test allows a bias toward the median nerve and the middle and lower nerve roots. The symptomatic responses to the test[1] suggest that the median nerve may be responsible for symptoms. With different combinations of movements, it appears that other nerve trunks and parts of the plexus are tested.[4] Basic neurobiomechanics was discussed in earlier editions of this text and in Butler.[4,5] For recent work, see Kleinrensink et al,[6,7] Wright et al,[8] Zoech et al,[9] and Szabo et al,[10] among others.

Figure 11-1 presents the sequences of the standard ULNT probably used widely around the world. From original work by Elvey,[11] the test evolved to this particular sequence by trial and error, clinical observation, careful attention to anatomy, and available research findings. The components have been kept as simple as possible and

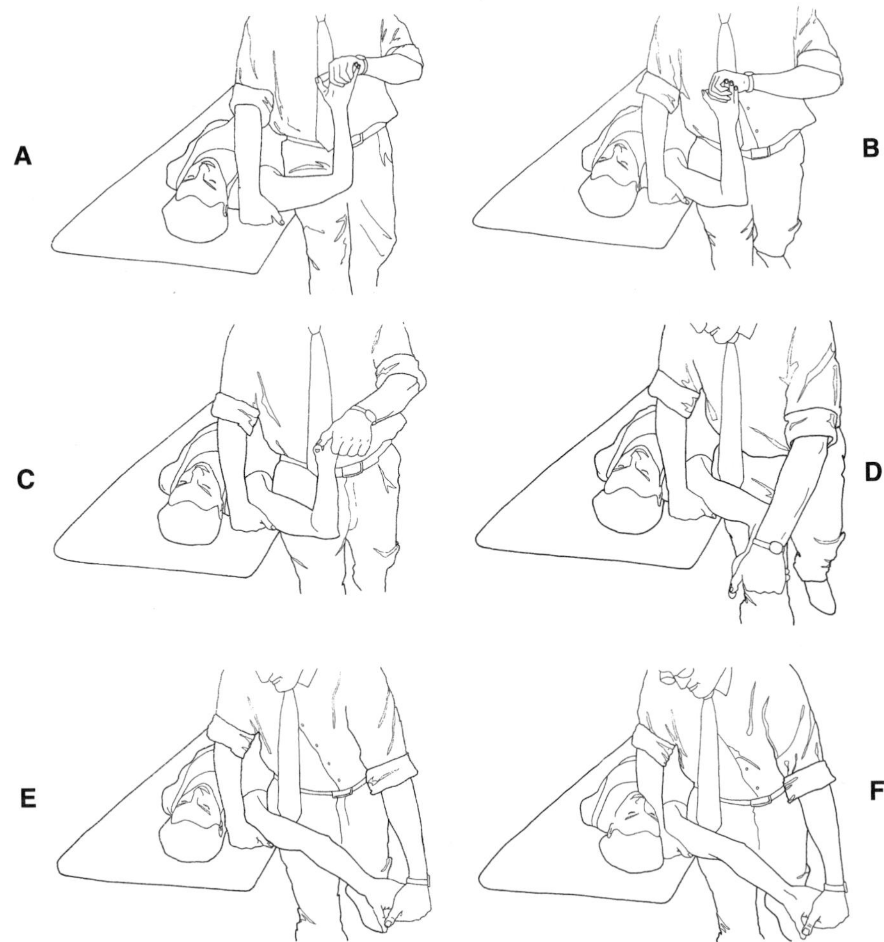

Figure 11-1
The upper limb neurodynamic test. **A,** Starting position. Note finger and thumb control, the fist on the bed prevents shoulder girdle elevation during abduction; the patient's arm rests on the clinician's thigh. **B,** Shoulder abduction. Take the arm to approximately 110 degrees or onset of symptoms. **C,** Forearm supination and wrist extension. **D,** Shoulder lateral rotation. **E,** Elbow extension. **F,** Neck lateral flexion. Lateral flexion away from test side usually increases symptoms, and lateral flexion toward test side decreases symptoms. Clinicians should be aware of symptoms evoked at each stage of the test.
(From Butler DS: *The sensitive nervous system,* Adelaide, Australia, 2000, Noigroup Publications.)

in the coronal plane to facilitate easy replication. (See Butler[4,5] for more specific details on handling skills.)

ULNT and Challenges for Manual Therapy Practice

Neurodynamic tests are frequently used in clinical practice[12] and have been introduced into many textbooks (e.g., Magee[13] and Brukner and Khan[14]). Their popularity may be increasing. This is at a time when there are unprecedented forces on manual therapy practice to adapt and modernize. In addition to restless patients and clinicians, pressures to adapt come from two main areas—from the growing emphasis on evidence-based practice and from neurobiological science. These two linked areas must provide the big-picture framework for the clinical and experimental use of neurodynamic tests such as the ULNT.

'BIG-PICTURE' EVIDENCE-BASED PRACTICE: WHAT WORKS?

The following is a very broad list of management features that have been shown to help patients with acute and chronic musculoskeletal pain.[15-19]

1. Educate the patient and relevant associates about the nature of the whole problem, including health status of the tissues, role of the nervous system, and results of investigative tests. Such information must make sense to the patient and be continually updated during management.
2. Provide prognostication and make realistic goals, which include clear recommendations about activities and progression, with the patient.
3. Promote self-care and self-motivation, which are closely related to the first two points.
4. Get the patient active and moving as early as possible and appropriate after injury, by any safe means possible. Use activities that the patient enjoys.
5. Decrease unnecessary fear related to movements, leisure, and work activities. This may mean challenging some beliefs and superstitions. It also requires that clinicians understand peripheral and central mechanisms of pain.
6. Help the patient identify and experience both success and a sense of mastery of the problem.
7. Perform a skilled physical evaluation that may well be more "low tech" and functional in more chronic pain states and more specific in acute and tissue-based problems. Results should be communicated immediately to the patient.
8. Make any treatment strategy as closely linked to evidence of the biological nature of the patient's problem as possible, in addition to the current syndromal, geographical, and temporal diagnostic constructs. In some pain states, specific techniques for specific population groups may help.
9. Use any measures possible to reduce pain, especially in the acute stage, and use patient-controlled analgesia when possible.
10. In chronic pain states, use multidisciplinary management if necessary.

A clinician operating under this broad framework could be said to be working under best evidence. To some extent, it may not matter what the therapy is or which school of thought is followed, as long as it fits in the aforementioned list. However, it is this big picture that allows a framework for reasoned use of specific techniques such as the ULNT.

Points 5, 7, and 8 suggest that the use of tests and the meaning of test responses may vary depending on the biological processes related to pain and whether the pain state is acute or chronic. Pain states are currently categorized by time (e.g., acute or chronic), causative forces (e.g., whiplash, repetition strain injury), or body part (e.g., lateral elbow pain). This labeling presents some difficulties because it does not predict outcome, give guidance to treatment, allow a search for risk factors, or identify subcategories that may be responsive to certain therapies. In particular, the terms *acute* and *chronic* are very polarized. For some years, there have been calls for bigger and better classification categories.[20-22] The suggestions by Woolf et al[22] mirror an underlying theme from the International Association for the Study of Pain and from the leading pain text[23] that pain can be categorized in terms of its mechanisms or processes—thus essentially, its biochemistry.

THE ULNT AND CURRENT UNDERSTANDING OF THE NERVOUS SYSTEM

A ULNT has traditionally been considered a test of the mechanosensitivity of the median nerve and associated roots. This view needs to be extended to consider not only upper limb anatomy but also the representation of the arm, in particular the median nerve and its innervated tissues in the CNS. Such a shift in thinking begins by recalling the well-known sensory homunculus[24] and considering that the ULNT, like all arm movements, is surely a test of the stability of the arm representation in the brain (Figure 11-2).

Brain functional concepts have changed rapidly in the last 10 years because of the new measurement tools of functional magnetic resonance imaging (fMRI), positron emission topography (PET), and magnetoencephalography. In particular, the distributed nature of neuronal activity after inputs and the enormous plasticity of the system are far greater than previously thought. Modern nervous system descriptive terms would include *associative*, *mutable*, *reactive*, *distributed*, and *representational*. The nervous system is associative in that the effects of any input will be determined by coexisting inputs. It is mutable, meaning that the system is extremely plastic, with receptive fields being dynamically maintained. It is reactive—that is, it has the potential to give value

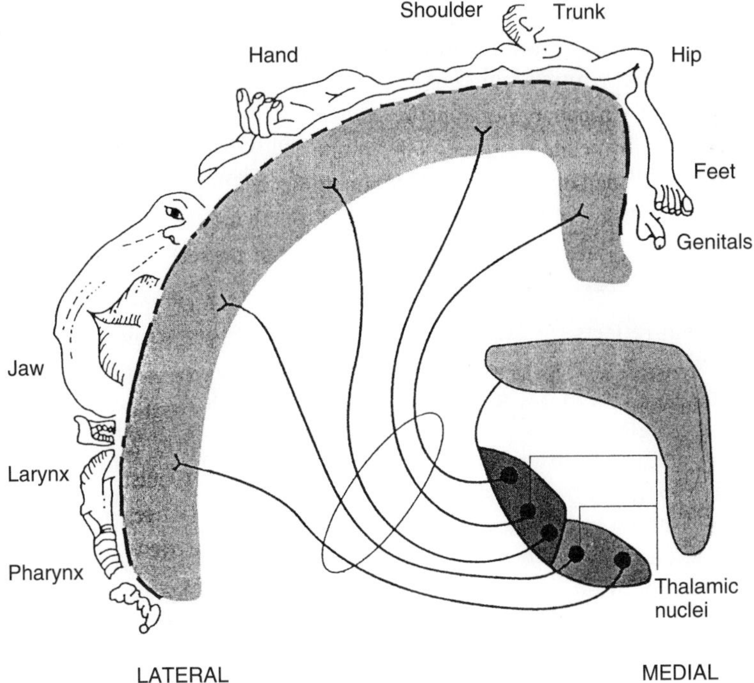

Figure 11-2
The primary somatosensory homunculus.
(Modified from Pritchard TC, Alloway KD: *Medical neuroscience*, Madison, Wis, 1999, Fence Creek.)

to all inputs and react via multiple systems, such as the endocrine and motor systems, or process input in terms of available response systems.[25] The system is distributed in that there is no one master pool of neurons for any one sensation or function. With noxious stimuli, brain areas such as the contralateral insular cortex, the cerebellar vermis, the thalamus, the contralateral anterior cingulate, and the premotor cortex, all areas that have roles other than pain perception,[26] will be active. Perhaps *representational* is the best descriptor. Through its transmitters, modulators, architectural hardware, and the aforementioned features, the system has the ability to represent the bodily parts and sensory, emotional, and cognitive aspects of injuries in ways that allow maximal survival and comfort in society. The ULNT may suddenly seem crude and far away, but it must somehow fit into this big picture. Notions of receptive fields can help.

Concept of Receptive Field

Since Sherrington's[27] time, a receptive field (RF) has been considered the region of sensory surface that must be stimulated to obtain a response in any given neuron or group of neurons. This definition is dated.[28] The simplest RF belongs to a peripheral sensory neuron, with the field being a tiny piece of skin. Because of convergence, second-order projection neurons in the spinal cord carry the receptive fields of a number of primary neurons, although the extent may depend on associated inhibitory or excitatory neurons. Third-order neurons will carry the RFs of second-order neurons, although with an exponential number of possible inhibitory and excitatory influences. Thus the receptive fields become larger, more complex, and more dynamic with each stage of information processing.

Neurons in the primary somatosensory cortex (S1) (Figure 11-2) have receptive fields, such as the sensory homunculus, that form maps of the body. The maps have fine delineations (i.e., individual fingers are mapped). At least 11 other homunculi have been discovered in S1. Some will respond to deep stimulation and others to skin stimulation,[29] and there are other homunculi elsewhere in the motor cortex, thalamus, and cerebellum. Movements are represented through changing homuncular arrangements in the brain.[30,31]

Receptive Fields Reflect the Stimulus History

A receptive field reflects the stimulus history and will change with trauma, practice, misuse, and disuse. This is particularly so in the cortex. This means, for example, that a finger representation in S1, instead of being a neatly delineated group of neurons with RFs for a single digit, may lose its fine definition and that neurons would expand RFs to include other digits or the whole hand. Researchers and clinicians have been aware of this process in the spinal cord for some years.[32] Experience-based reshaping of S1 has been shown in owl monkey studies by Byl and colleagues,[33-35] and degraded finger representations have been shown in patients with focal dystonia, particularly musicians and repetition strain-injury sufferers.[36,37] Evidence of plasticity at spinal, supraspinal, and cortical levels has also been shown in carpal tunnel syndrome,[38] a syndrome with symptoms likely to be reproduced by a test such as the ULNT.[39]

Phantom-limb pain, once consigned to a medical oddity basket, has now provided, with the new measurement tools, a remarkable new view of the brain and perhaps a fresh look at the ULNT. A common feature of phantom-limb pain is the development of trigger zones for the phantom or parts of the phantom. Ramachandran et al[40,41] described several patients with upper limb phantom pains that could be elicited by trigger zones on the ipsilateral face. The phantoms elicited were topographically precise. Amputation means that a portion of brain no longer has an anatomical input; however, the representation of the amputated part is sufficiently complex to be intact although somewhat unstable. It appears that neighboring neurons with intact RFs now "invade" the RFs of the amputated limb. In the somatosensory homunculus, the body is broken up; the hand is near the face; thus the hand area is easily invaded by the face area. The actual mechanism of takeover is unknown. There may be some sprouting of neurons, but with speed of takeover (i.e., minutes to hours), most authors use the term *unmasking of preexisting connections*.[42]

Links to the amount of cortical reorganization and the magnitude of phantom-limb pain have been shown.[43,44] The greater the pain, the greater the cortical reorganization. There is no cortical reorganization in amputees without a phantom or in subjects with congenital absence of an upper limb.[45] In addition, a recent study by Flor et al[46] points to somatosensory cortical degradation in chronic low back pain with high correlations between magnitude of reorganization and chronicity.

Although it provides a dramatic example, amputation is not necessary for representational changes. Sensory input, learning, and experience may also change the representations. For example, violinists, cellists, and guitarists have a greater cortical activation from fingertip stimulation[47] than nonmusicians. Braille users have an increase in finger representation in the sensory and motor cortices.[48,49] Surgical fusion of two digits in primates will result in a merging of their cortical zones in the sensory cortex.[50] In primates, reversibility of degraded representations can occur.[31,51] A number of recent reviews related to cortical plasticity exist.[52-57]

The ULNT and CNS Plasticity

Two proposals are made for clinicians to contemplate. First, during performance of a ULNT, there will be considerable activity in the brain, especially in cortical areas related to input from the upper limb. This activity will depend on handling skills, therapist-patient relationship, previous experiences of the patient, and meaning of the test, in addition to the particular anatomy and pathoanatomy of the upper limb. The ULNT could be considered a test of the patency of receptive fields in the brain as well as of tissues in the arm and neck.

Second, in patients for whom the ULNT is sensitive and relevant to the disorder, there will be changes in the relevant receptive fields in the spinal cord and brain, particularly when the pain state is chronic. This increases the likelihood that an input such as the ULNT will be maladaptively processed and highly depend on associative neural activity. In addition—and perhaps linked to variable pain responses—altered motor, autonomic, and endocrine systems may also come into play. Byl and Melnick[56] provide a nice example. In patients with focal dystonia, a stimulus such as vibration to an involved digit will result in a cocontraction of flexors and extensors, something not seen in asymptomatic individuals. With likely loss of delineated RFs, gross and maladaptive responses rather than specific output may occur. It is essentially a short circuit.

Simply, a ULNT may evoke symptoms as a result of excitation of neurons that are not normally excited. Sensory and motor responses may be enhanced, and brain centers for processing emotions, and fears and memories also may be activated. Some of the more variable and odd responses commonly evoked on an ULNT may begin to make more sense.

THE ULNT IN ASSESSMENT: KEY POINTS

Analysis of Sensitive ULNTs

The only information provided by a sensitive ULNT is that the person tested has a sensitive movement. This alone says nothing about anatomical sources of symptoms, nor does it impart any information about pathobiological mechanisms behind the symptoms, the role of psychological inputs, or the location of the pathologies along the nervous system. The responses may even be normal or from nonneural tissues, and other movements may be more sensitive. Perhaps a few evoked "pins and needles" or symptoms in a neural zone may point to a neural contribution, but further data are necessary to make clinical judgments on the test.

At the time of the physical evaluation, clinical data from a subjective evaluation should already be at hand, and external evidence, such as scans, should be used. Indeed, a reasoning clinician will expect certain findings on physical evaluation. Examples of support data could include area of symptoms (e.g., neural zone symptoms), behavior of symptoms, (e.g., after discharge, symptoms on activities that pinch or elongate nerves, psychological stress that increases pain), other physical findings (e.g., diminished reflex, stiffness in neighboring joints) and tests such as a nerve conduction test or patient self-assessment test. In-depth reasoning processes in orthopedic evaluation are discussed in Chapter 6 and elsewhere.[58]

Determining the Clinical Relevance of the Test

A ULNT is not pathognomic, nor should it ever be called a test for a syndrome, such as carpal tunnel. The tests will provide information about only one aspect of the big picture. Even the best-researched neurodynamic test, the straight leg raise (SLR) test, can only provide supporting evidence to a nerve root or discogenic problem.[59]

Asymptomatic individuals will all have varying sensitivity to the ULNT, as will patients. The following guidelines may help determine the relevance of a test.

Symptoms evoked on a ULNT can be inferred to be neurogenic if the test reproduces symptoms or associated symptoms, if structural differentiation (discussed in the next section) supports a neurogenic source and if there are differences left to right and to known normal responses. Further support for a neurogenic inference will come from other clinical data, such as history, area of symptoms, type of symptoms, and results from imaging tests.

However, this process of additive hypothesis support or rejection is just the first step to a clinical diagnosis. It is important to remember that the sensitivity could be from a combination of primary (tissue-based) or secondary (CNS-based) processes.

A test may appear positive, but is it clinically relevant? That is, is it a movement that would be worth addressing to reduce sensitivity, improve quality and range of motion, and assist restoration of function? Furthermore, if used as a reassessment tool, would a change in this movement be a worthwhile indicator of progression? Here is an area for fruitful research. However, for clinical use, the following guidelines to the determination of test relevance are suggested:

- If this movement is improved, will it help the patient function better? To make this judgment, physical therapists must have knowledge about current goals and activity levels and must perform physical examinations with skill. For example, minor limitations and hyperalgesia in a test that loads the radial nerve may well be relevant in a professional tennis player with lateral elbow pain. Similar minor findings in a patient with a widespread and long-standing pain state such as fibromyalgia may be less relevant.

- A clinical judgment on pain processes in operation may help. For example, history and symptom patterns may allow a clinical judgment that a maladaptive central sensitization process is in operation and that management may be better directed at altering threshold control of the CNS via education, fear reduction, and improvement movement quality as well as tissue health. More peripheral processes would suggest that the focus may shift, although not exclusively, to tissue function and health. Further discussion on integrating pain mechanisms into practice can be found elsewhere.[5,60-63]
- Relying on favorite hypotheses is a common clinical-reasoning error in manual therapy. Any innervated tissue is a potential source of symptoms and a contributor to peripheral and central pain mechanisms. Modern clinicians need clinical appreciation of all tissues and all processes related to pain. Because neurodynamics are somewhat new, clinicians must resist the urge to use the movements as the latest and trendy technique.

Concept of Structural Differentiation

During the ULNT, a forearm symptom made worse by neck lateral flexion away from the test side is also said to infer that symptoms are neurogenic.[4,64] Although this is an attractive and often exciting clinical finding for patients and clinicians, it does not mean much in terms of biological mechanisms. Such tests may preferentially load one tissue and assist in a clinical diagnosis but should not lead to an instant diagnosis of "neural tension" or "altered neurodynamics" and an immediate vision of a physically compromised nerve. A problem with structural differentiation occurs particularly in more chronic cases, wherein additional inputs may well be normal inputs—even A beta inputs—which, in the presence of a sensitized system, can be upregulated,[65] and the patient's CNS actively constructs a pain experience. Thus a ULNT may evoke a shoulder pain and the addition of wrist extension may increase the symptoms by adding further normal input to an already sensitized system. Care in interpretation and in attention to likely pain processes in operation is therefore needed.

Active and Passive Movements

In practice, it is suggested that the tests, including structural differentiation, be performed actively before being carried out passively. It may be that the observation of good range and movement quality in a particular movement would preclude passive performance of a test. When a passive evaluation follows, the patient will be better informed and allow better performance of the test. For the active performance of the ULNT, first ask the patient to look at the palm with the elbow flexed, then to extend the arm and abduct it to about shoulder height, and then to look away from the arm. Further protocols for active neurodynamic test evaluation are suggested in Butler.[5]

Pinch and Stretch

Neurodynamic tests tend to focus on elongation of the nervous system, perhaps at the expense of pinching forces. The neuroanatomical design is also such that the system can adapt to compressive forces and the "closing down" of tissues around the nerve. For example, spinal extension, lateral flexion, and rotation toward the test side close down intervertebral foramina and may pinch contained neural tissues. Whether the movement is reactive in the presence of neuropathy may depend on the dynamic roominess of the intervertebral foramen.[66] A similar concept applies to the median nerve at the wrist; there may be pinching forces on the median nerve during wrist flexion. This should serve as a reminder that when considering the physical health of nerves, physical therapists must give some thought to the neighboring structures of the nervous system in a static and a dynamic sense. Clinically, the ULNT may seem quite normal when there are signs and symptoms of nerve root irritation or compression. This may be caused by the nerve requiring a pinch stimulus rather than elongation. In addition, the plexus arrangements and intradural rootlet connections[67,68] are likely to prevent specific root testing. This finding is also supported by Kleinrensink's anatomical evaluation of the ULNT.[6]

USE OF THE ULNT IN PATIENT-MANAGEMENT STRATEGIES

Once a reasoned judgment is made that a test is reflective of part of the patient's problem and worthy of incorporating into management, there are a number of ways in which it can be used.

Using Concepts of Neurodynamics to Explain Aspects of Sensitivity and Tissue Health

Wrist pain worsened by laterally flexing the neck away from the test side demands an explanation from a patient. These symptoms can be simply explained in terms of transmission of load through a continuous sensitive structure and may well form part of a rationale for proposing that a more physically healthy neck would be advantageous to the wrist. When the sensitivity appears more centrally related, the finding can still be useful for explaining that a sensitive nervous system in operation is amplifying or magnifying symptoms. Explanation is treatment in its own right, and it forms a critical alliance with passive and active movement therapies. Easing various stressors such as fear and lack of diagnosis will have neurobiological consequences, such as altering body levels of noradrenaline and cortisol and easing demands on cell nuclear machinery to produce noradrenaline and glutamate receptors.

Knowledge of neurodynamics also relates to the art of listening and providing appropriate empathy. The quality of interaction is enhanced when a clinician can listen to a patient's story because it makes sense rather than the patient feeling they have to prove something is wrong.[69] Concepts of neurodynamics, especially when linked to knowledge of modern pain neurobiology, will assist in making sense out of some of the more bizarre symptoms of which patients complain.

Neurodynamics Tests and Passive Mobilization

In the current emphasis on self-care, the role of passive-movement therapies is being reevaluated. Passive movement in its various forms may assist in restoring tissue health, and the handling may result in the patient remembering an active treatment prescription more accurately. Good handling, a supportive treatment environment, and appropriate passive movement can be a collection of inputs into the CNS and can signal that performing a certain movement and perhaps experiencing a little pain without evoking a stress response is possible. Passive techniques, in addition to any tissue benefit, are also learning experiences for patients. It also should be remembered that when education is a critical aspect of management, the person who has skillfully touched and examined the painful areas may be the one whose advice is taken and complied with.

Some Suggestions Related to Passive Techniques. The following suggestions related to passive techniques are put forward:

- Passive techniques should form part of a management strategy that is likely to include active movements, education, fitness, work adjustments, and so on. They are unlikely to form treatments by themselves, and there is a limit to their use. When possible and relevant, alter CNS sensitivity first.
- Variations on the neurodynamic tests may be necessary. These may include variations to access other nerves, order of movement changes, or even fine movements to engage individual fingers. This is discussed elsewhere.[2,5]
- A passive movement prescription will depend on the healing state of tissues, the extent of damage, and likely operant pain mechanisms. Further details and discussion can be found elsewhere.[5,60,61] Likely candidates will have a well-reasoned and supported clinical diagnosis of specific physical dysfunction of the nervous system.
- Start movements away from a presumed site of pathology. This was probably taken to extremes in the past,[4,70] but it is useful. It should enhance safety and may allow less focus on the painful area. For example, in the patient with wrist trouble, movement of the elbow and shoulder girdle will glide and strain neural tissue at the wrist. In more sensitive states, movements from the nonpainful or less painful side, which are likely to have more processing and reflexive than mechanical effects, could be useful.
- When patients understand the rationale for mobilization, some movements can be coaxed into pain. Some old and stable peripheral neurogenic pain states may be treated by challenging tissue stiffness, although it is better to get the patients to progress actively and methodically when and if more vigorous movements are required. Many chronic pain patients will need to move with pain yet know that the pain does not necessarily signal a harmful experience.
- When the nervous system is physically unhealthy, neighboring structures are also likely to be unhealthy. For example, management of a patient with a carpal tunnel syndrome could involve (if assessed and deemed to be appropriate) active and passive mobilization of the carpal bones, massage of the skin across the tunnel, attention to a tight pectoralis minor muscle and the postures that have lead to it, some scapular stabilization work and attention to the cervical and thoracic spines, in addition to movements aimed at the physical health of the nervous system.

Role of the ULNT in Active Mobilization

Passive techniques may be converted into specific more functional and meaningful active exercises, and they can be used as part of a paced movement program. The tests could be used as a warm-up or a cool-down or as movements to "feed the representations" in the various homunculi. With integration of the movements, remember the big-picture evidence list at the beginning of the chapter and consider active movements for their likely beneficial inputs to both the physical health of neural and other tissues and for modification of the threshold controls of the CNS. If patients have learned to experience movement as painful, movement needs to be presented to the CNS in ways that are not painful.

Suggestions Related to Active Movements

Use of Meaningful Activities When Possible. *Activity* is a better word than *exercise*. The term *exercise* instantly evokes negativity in many people, particularly those in pain. Many activities mobilize various nerve tracts and presumably activate their CNS receptive fields, including adaptive or maladaptive links. Throwing objects, graduating from small balls, such as a table tennis ball, to a basketball and doing graded push-ups are activities that would mobilize the median nerve and activate its representations. It is possible to challenge the ulnar nerve by drying the back with a towel, adjusting collars, and encouraging grooming with the sensitive side. The radial and, indeed, all nerves and receptive fields are surely challenged during disco dancing, flamenco dancing, and movement activities such as tai chi. Memorably, Maitland[64] once said "technique is the brainchild of ingenuity." The brain is a hungry organ that always seeks to reward itself, and it will enjoy such an approach. Movements that are meaningful, familiar, goal-linked and prescribed by a trusted therapist are likely to be best accepted by the patient's CNS without maladaptive responses.

Use in Movement Breakdowns. Neurodynamic tests are sensitive in many pain states, more so than in control groups.[5] To fulfill the evidence-based demand of early active movements after injury, the physical therapist can break down the movements for use. Gentle progressive movement with the body placed in varying degrees of nervous system load can be performed. To exercise the neck in rotation in a patient with a sensitive neck and neural structures, for example, make sure the arms are folded and perhaps the shoulder girdle elevated. Subsequent neck exercises can be performed with the arms by the side or even in a neurally loaded position. This is the concept of the continuum of the nervous system. Along similar lines, the wrist could be moved in sensitive acute states with the rest of the limb in varying degrees of neural loading.

Use in Pacing. Physiotherapists are traditionally well versed in graded exercise prescription, ranging from cardiovascular to sports rehabilitation. Graded activity can also be used for chronic pain. Programs using operant conditioning were first described by Fordyce et al[71,72] and have good outcome data.[73] The essence is still the same as is used today.[74,75] A pacing prescription involves determining a level of realistic pain-free activities and following with a gradual increase in activity, guided by joint patient-clinician agreements. In patients with more chronic pain, written exercise timetables, guidance over time, and flare-up contingency plans are needed. The key point is that patients use time or number—and not pain level—as their guide to stopping and changing activity or posture.[76]

Tissue-beneficial effects may initially be minimal, but the CNS has a chance to retrain. Movements that have always been painful for patients (who may have learned this pain by association to other inputs) automatically will cause stress responses. Here is a chance to retrain. Many things can be paced, such as taking a collar off, going for a walk, ironing, participating in feared activities, performing a particular exercise, hearing noise, and even facing psychosocial forces. Activity could be paced in regard to pain, sweating, nausea, or any other symptoms. Neurodynamic tests or broken-down neurodynamic tests can also be activities that are paced or incorporated as meaningful movements. For discussions on the practicalities of pacing, see Harding[74] and Shorland.[75]

Use of "Slider and Tensioner" Movements and Order of Movement. Physical therapists can use the concept of sliders and tensioners to promote both variety of movement and large movements. A slider occurs when a person elevates the arm and then looks at the hand. If the individual were to do the same arm movement and look away it would be termed a (more aggressive) *tensioner.* Sliders allow larger ranges of motion, provide a means of distraction from the painful area, and should provide multitissue, nonpainful, and it is hoped, fear-reducing novel inputs into the CNS. Variations for all nerves are suggested elsewhere[5] but should not be difficult to make up. Tensioners may better challenge stiffness and more long-lasting physical dysfunction.

In addition, altering the order of movement and using "trick" movements are useful for establishing activity and perhaps providing a variety of input to the CNS. Performing the same movement in a different sequence provides fresh inputs. Arm elevation may be achieved differently by extending hand and elbow first instead of shoulder first. Removing gravity is the simplest trick. To elevate the shoulder, get the patient to lean over and swing the arm as in a pendulum. Use combinations of shoulder girdle movements and rotation. Turning the body while keeping the neck still is effectively rotating the neck. The brain might get some novel, nonpainful input from activities that were once painful and respond appreciatively with favorable and novel output. It makes sense from a CNS-plasticity viewpoint that additional inputs such as different movement environments, visual input from looking at the part exercised, and feeding the brain with big bilateral movements rather than with individual isolated movements alone should be beneficial.

Use in Postural and Ergonomic Advice

Neurodynamics has an important contribution to make to ergonomics. Detailed knowledge of dynamic neural relations with surrounding tissues in various movements must form a basis of ergonomic design.[5] It may be as simple as being aware of the potential risks for a patient in a wheelchair who is resting the arms on the wheelchair table at about the level of the cubital tunnel or for a typist who uses excessive wrist extension when typing.

Some advice could be offered in regard to sleeping positions. For example, patients with nonresolving cubital tunnel syndrome may beneficially alter their nocturnal elbow flexion patterns by sleeping with a small bean bag cushion in the cubital fossa.[77] In some acute states, it may be as simple as keeping the knees flexed to enhance sleeping.

FUTURE OF THE ULNT

The ULNT has not been accorded the experimental attention equivalent to its current clinical use. There is limited evidence-based work that demonstrates that the inclusion of specific upper limb neural mobilization will improve patient outcomes. However, there is plenty of big-picture evidence that suggests that patients can benefit if they can improve tissue and cardiovascular fitness as well as CNS representations via therapeutic activity input and changes in beliefs, superstitions, and environmental forces that hinder health. The ULNT currently should be approached modestly, as qualitative,[78] anatomical,[6] diagnostic,[39,79,80] and outcome[81,82] research continues to refine and define the test.

Uncorrupted clinical-reasoning science under the framework of big picture evidence, including the base science of neurobiology, must be the context for the continuing use of the test.

References

1. Kenneally M, Rubenach H, Elvey R: The upper limb tension test: the SLR of the arm. In Grant R, editor: *Physical therapy of the cervical and thoracic spine*, New York, 1988, Churchill Livingstone.
2. Butler DS: The upper limb tension test revisited. In Grant R, editor: *Physical therapy of the cervical and thoracic spine*, ed 2, New York, 1994, Churchill Livingstone.
3. Shacklock M: Neurodynamics, *Physiotherapy* 81:9, 1995.
4. Butler DS: *Mobilisation of the nervous system*, Melbourne, 1991, Churchill Livingstone.
5. Butler DS: *The sensitive nervous system*, Adelaide, Australia, 2000, Noigroup Publications.
6. Kleinrensink GJ, Stoeckart R, Mulder PGH et al: Upper limb tension tests as tools in the diagnosis of nerve and plexus lesions, *Clin Biomech* 15:9, 2000.
7. Kleinrensink GJ, Stoeckart R, Vleeming A et al: Mechanical tension in the median nerve: the effects of joint positions, *Clin Biomech* 10:240, 1995.
8. Wright TW, Glowczewski F, Wheeler D et al: Excursion and strain of the median nerve, *J Bone Joint Surg* 78A:1897, 1996.
9. Zoech G, Reihsner R, Beer R et al: Stress and strain in peripheral nerves, *Neuro-Orthopedics* 10:73, 1991.
10. Szabo RM, Bay BK, Sharkey NA et al: Median nerve displacement through the carpal canal, *J Hand Surg* 19A:901, 1994.
11. Elvey RL: Brachial plexus tension tests and the pathoanatomical origin of arm pain. In Idczak R, editor: *Aspects of manipulative therapy*, Melbourne, 1979, Manipulative Physiotherapists Association of Australia.
12. Foster NE, Thompson KA, Baxter DG et al: Management of non-specific low back pain by physiotherapists in Britain and Ireland, *Spine* 24:1332, 1999.
13. Magee D: *Orthopedic physical assessment*, ed 3, Philadelphia, 1997, WB Saunders.
14. Brukner P, Khan K: *Clinical sports medicine*, New York, 1993, McGraw-Hill.
15. Frank JD: *Persuasion and healing*, Baltimore, 1973, John Hopkins University Press.
16. Linton SJ: The socioeconomic impact of chronic back pain: is anyone benefiting? *Pain* 75:163, 1998.
17. Waddell G: *The back pain revolution*, Edinburgh, 1998, Churchill Livingstone.
18. Gerteis M, Edgman-Levitan S, Daley J, editors: *Understanding and promoting patient-centered care: through patients' eyes*, San Francisco, 1993, Jossey Bass.
19. Kendall NAS, Linton SJ, Main CJ: *Guide to assessing psychosocial yellow flags in acute low back pain: risk factors for long-term disability and work loss*, Wellington, New Zealand, 1997, Accident Rehabilitation & Compensation Insurance Corporation of New Zealand and the National Health Committee.
20. Deyo RA: Practice variations, treatment fads, rising disability: do we need a new clinical research paradigm? *Spine* 18:2153, 1993.
21. Cherkin DC: Primary care research on low back pain, *Spine* 23:1997, 1998.
22. Woolf CJ, Bennett GJ, Doherty M et al: Towards a mechanism-based classification of pain, *Pain* 77:227, 1998.
23. Wall PD, Melzack R, editors: *Textbook of pain*, ed 4, Edinburgh, 1999, Churchill Livingstone.
24. Penfield W, Boldrey E: Somatic, motor, and sensory representation in the cerebral cortex of man as studied by electrical stimulation, *Brain* 60:389, 1937.
25. Wall PD: Introduction to the fourth edition. In Wall PD, Melzack R, editors: *Textbook of pain*, Edinburgh, 1999, Churchill Livingstone.
26. Casey KL: Forebrain mechanisms of nociception and pain. Proceedings of the National Academy of Science, 96:7668, 1999.
27. Sherrington C: *The integrative action of the nervous system*, New Haven, Conn, 1906, Yale University Press.
28. Gilbert CD: Adult cortical dynamics, *Physiol Rev* 78:467, 1998.
29. McComas A: The world of touch: from evoked potentials to conscious perception, *Can J Neurol Sci* 26:7, 1999.
30. Nudo RJ, Jenkins WM, Merzenich MM et al: Neurophysiological correlates of hand preference in primary motor cortex of adult squirrel monkeys, *J Neurosci* 12:2918, 1992.

31. Nudo RJ, Milliken GW, Jenkins WM: Use-dependent alterations of movement representations of primary motor cortex of adult squirrel monkeys, *J Neurosci* 16:785, 1996.
32. Woolf CJ: The dorsal horn: state-dependent sensory processing and the generation of pain. In Wall PD, Melzack R, editors: *Textbook of pain*, Edinburgh, 1994, Churchill Livingstone.
33. Byl NN, Merzenich MM, Jenkins WM: A primate genesis model of focal dystonia and repetitive strain injury. I. Learning-induced differentiation of the representation of the hand in the primary somatosensory cortex in adult monkeys, *Neurology* 47:508, 1996.
34. Wang X, Merzenich MM, Sameshima K et al: Remodelling of hand representation in adult cortex determined by timing of tactile stimulation, *Nature* 378:71, 1995.
35. Topp KS, Byl NN: Movement dysfunction following repetitive hand opening and closing: anatomical analysis in owl monkeys, *Mov Disord* 14:295, 1999.
36. Byl N, Wilson F, Merzenich M et al: Sensory dysfunction associated with repetition strain injuries of tendinitis and focal hand dystonia: a comparative study, *J Orthop Sports Phys Ther* 23:234, 1996.
37. Bara-Jiminez W, Catalan MJ, Hallett M et al: Abnormal somatosensory homunculus in dystonia of the hand, *Ann Neurol* 44:828, 1998.
38. Tinazzi M, Zanette G, Volpato D et al: Neurophysiological evidence of neuroplasticity at multiple levels of the somatosensory system in patients with carpal tunnel syndrome, *Brain* 121:1784, 1998.
39. Coveney B, Trott P, Grimmer KA et al: The upper limb tension test in a group of subjects with a clinical presentation of carpal tunnel syndrome. Proceedings of the tenth biennial conference of the Manipulative Physiotherapists Association of Australia, Melbourne, 1997.
40. Ramachandran VS, Stewart M, Rogers-Ramachandran DC: Perceptual correlates of massive cortical reorganization, *Neuroreport* 3:583, 1992.
41. Ramachandran VS, Blakeslee S: *Phantoms in the brain*, New York, 1998, William Morrow.
42. Jacobs KM, Donoghue JP: Reshaping the cortical motor map by unmasking latent intracortical connections, *Science* 251:944, 1991.
43. Flor H, Elbert T, Knecht C et al: Phantom-limb pain as a perceptual correlate of cortical reorganization following arm amputation, *Nature* 375:482, 1995.
44. Birbaumer N, Lutzenberger W, Montoya P et al: Effects of regional anaesthesia on phantom-limb pain are mirrored in changes in cortical reorganization, *J Neurosci* 17:5503, 1997.
45. Flor H, Elbert T, Muhnickel W et al: Cortical reorganization and phantom phenomena in congenital and traumatic upper-extremity amputees, *Exp Brain Res* 119:205, 1998.
46. Flor H, Braun C, Elbert T et al: Extensive reorganization of primary somatosensory cortex in chronic back pain patients, *Neurosci Lett* 244:5, 1997.
47. Elbert TC, Pantev C, Wienbruch C et al: Increased cortical representation of the fingers of the left hand in string players, *Science* 270:305, 1995.
48. Pascual-Leone A, Cammaroya A, Wassermann EM et al: Modulation of motor cortical outputs to the reading hand of Braille readers, *Ann Neurol* 34:33, 1993.
49. Pascual-Leone A, Torres F: Plasticity of the sensorimotor cortex representation of the reading finger of Braille readers, *Brain* 116:39, 1993.
50. Allard T, Clark SA, Jenkins WM: Reorganization of somatosensory area 3b representations in adult owl monkeys after digital syndactyly, *J Neurophysiol* 66:1048, 1991.
51. Jenkins WM, Merzenich MM, Ochs MT et al: Functional reorganization of primary somatosensory cortex in adult owl monkeys after behaviorally controlled tactile stimulation, *J Neurophysiol* 63:82, 1990.
52. Kaas JH: The reorganization of sensory and motor maps after injury in adult mammals. In Gazzaniga MS, editor: *The new cognitive neurosciences*, Cambridge, Mass, 2000, MIT Press.
53. Ebner FF, Rema V, Sachdev R, et al: Activity-dependent plasticity in adult somatic sensory cortex, *Semin Neurosci* 9:47, 1997.
54. Nicolelis MAL: Dynamic and distributed somatosensory representations as the substrate for cortical and subcortical plasticity, *Semin Neurosci* 9:24, 1997.

55. Recanzone GH: Cerebral cortical plasticity. In Gazzaniga MS, editor: *The new cognitive neurosciences*, Cambridge, Mass, 2000, MIT Press.
56. Byl NN, Melnick M: The neural consequences of repetition: clinical implications of a learning hypothesis, *J Hand Ther* 10:160, 1997.
57. Johansson BB: Brain plasticity and stroke rehabilitation, *Stroke* 31:223, 2000.
58. Higgs J, Jones M, editors: *Clinical reasoning in the health professions*, ed 2, Oxford, England, 2000, Butterworth-Heinemann.
59. Supik LF, Broom MJ: Sciatic tension signs and lumbar disc herniation, *Spine* 19:1066, 1994.
60. Gifford L, Butler D: The integration of pain sciences into clinical practice, *J Hand Ther* 10:86, 1997.
61. Butler DS: Integrating pain awareness into physiotherapy: wise action for the future. In Gifford LS, editor: *Topical issues in pain*, Falmouth, United Kingdom, 1998, NOI Press.
62. Gifford LS, editor: *Topical issues in pain*, Falmouth, United Kingdom, 1998, NOI Press.
63. Butler DS, Shacklock MO, Slater H: Treatment of altered nervous system mechanics. In Boyling JD, Palastanga N, editors: *Grieve's modern manual therapy*, Edinburgh, 1994, Churchill Livingstone.
64. Maitland GD: *Vertebral manipulation*, ed 6, London, 1986, Butterworths.
65. Doubell TP, Mannion R, Woolf CJ: The dorsal horn: state dependent sensory processing, plasticity and the generation of pain. In Wall PD, Melzack R, editors: *Textbook of pain*, Edinburgh, 1999, Churchill Livingstone.
66. Penning L: Functional pathology of lumbar spinal stenosis, *Clin Biomech* 7:3, 1992.
67. Marzo JM, Simmons EH, Kallen F: Intradural connections between adjacent cervical spinal roots, *Spine* 12:964, 1987.
68. Tanaka N, Fujimoto Y, An HS et al: The anatomic relation among the nerve roots, intervertebral foramina, and the intervertebral discs of the cervical spine, *Spine* 25:286, 2000.
69. Hadler N: If you have to prove you are sick, you can't get well: the object lesson of fibromyalgia, *Spine* 21:2397, 1996.
70. Butler DS: Adverse mechanical tension in the nervous system: a model for assessment and treatment, *Aust J Physiother* 35:227, 1989.
71. Fordyce WE, Fowler R, Lehman J et al: Operant conditioning in the treatment of chronic pain, *Arch Phys Med Rehabil* 54:399, 1973.
72. Fordyce WE: Learning processes in pain. In Sternbach RA, editor: *Psychology of pain*, New York, 1987 Raven Press.
73. Lindstrom I, Ohlund C, Eek C: The effect of graded activity on patients with subacute low back pain: a randomized prospective clinical study with an operant-conditioning behavioral approach, *Phys Ther* 72:279, 1992.
74. Harding V: Application of the cognitive-behavioural approach. In Pitt-Brooke J, editor: *Rehabilitation of movement*, London, 1998, WB Saunders.
75. Shorland S: Management of chronic pain following whiplash injuries. In Gifford LS, editor: *Topical issues in pain*, Falmouth, United Kingdom, 1998, NOI Press.
76. Harding V, Williams A: Extending physiotherapy skills using a psychological approach: cognitive behavioral management of chronic pain, *Physiotherapy* 81:681, 1995.
77. Seror P: Treatment of ulnar nerve palsy at the elbow with a night splint, *J Bone Joint Surg* 75B:322, 1993.
78. Coppieters MW, Stappaerts KH, Staes FF: A qualitative assessment of shoulder girdle elevation during the upper limb tension test 1, *Manual Ther* 4:33, 1999.
79. Selvaratnam PJ, Matyas TA , Glasgow EF: Noninvasive discrimination of brachial plexus involvement in upper limb pain, *Spine* 19:26, 1994.
80. Greening J, Smart S, Leary R et al: Reduced movement of the median nerve in carpal tunnel during wrist flexion in patients with non-specific arm pain, *Lancet* 354:217, 1999.
81. Rozmaryn LM, Dovelle S, Rothman ER et al: Nerve and tendon gliding exercises and the conservative management of carpal tunnel syndrome, *J Hand Ther* 11:171, 1998.
82. Hall TM, Elvey RL: Nerve trunk pain: physical diagnosis and treatment, *Manual Ther* 4: 63, 1999.

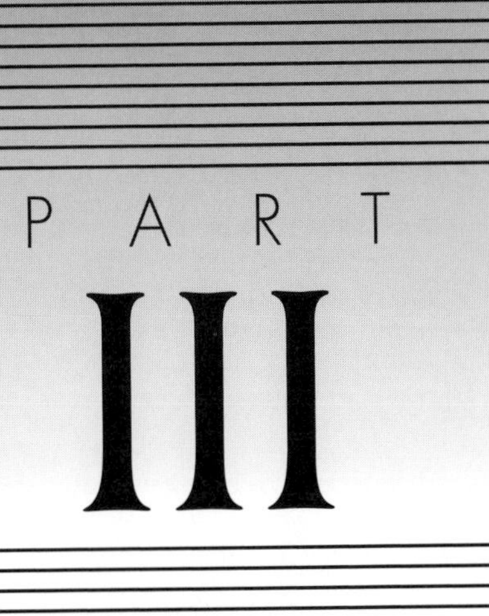

PART III

Clinical Management and Evidence-Based Practice

CHAPTER

12

Pain-Relieving Effects of Cervical Manual Therapy

Anthony Wright

The understanding of the effects and efficacy of manual therapy techniques applied to the cervical spine has improved significantly over the last decade. In the early 1990s there were only a few randomized controlled trials attesting to the efficacy of manual therapy techniques in the management of neck pain.[1-5] In the course of the last 10 years, we have seen more studies published. As a result it has been possible to conduct metaanalyses to pool the data from a number of randomized controlled trials and determine the efficacy of both mobilization and manipulation of the cervical spine.[6,7] The results of this process are encouraging, suggesting that manual therapy has a beneficial effect on neck pain within the first 4 weeks after treatment. Although there are still many questions to be addressed and the quality of evidence needs to be improved, the available data are beginning to suggest an affirmative answer to the question, "Does manual therapy work?"

It appears that manual therapy can exert a pain-relieving effect and contribute to improved function in patients with cervicogenic pain. The question of whether manual therapy is more efficacious than other treatments remains to be addressed, as does the question of cost effectiveness relative to other forms of treatment.

MODELS OF MANUAL THERAPY

If we accept that manual therapy has an effect in modulating pain, then the next important question becomes, "How does it work?" What is the mechanism by which manual therapy techniques produce pain relief? That question has been the focus of our research for much of the last decade. In the early 1990s models to explain the pain-relieving effects of manual therapy were still rudimentary and largely untested. It had been suggested that manual therapy activated the gate-control mechanism proposed by Melzack and Wall.[8,9] It also had been suggested that pain relief after manual therapy was related to a neural hysteresis effect.[10,11] In addition, the possibility that manual therapy techniques could trigger the release of endogenous opioids had been proposed.[12-14] Unfortunately, none of these theories had been subject to extensive investigation.

MULTIFACTORIAL MODEL OF MANIPULATION-INDUCED ANALGESIA

There was a clear need for a more comprehensive model of manual therapy-induced analgesia, and in the mid-1990s we proposed such a model (Figure 12-1).[15,16] This model drew on knowledge of the clinical characteristics of pain relief in patient populations, scientific information on endogenous analgesic systems, and the effect of movement in stimulating connective tissue repair. The essential features of the model were that pain relief from manual therapy treatments could not be ascribed to one specific mechanism. Rather, manipulation-induced analgesia was a multifaceted phenomenon. However, although it was thought that multiple effects may be important, it was suggested that they did not contribute equally in terms of either the magnitude of the effect or the time course of the effect. It was proposed that manual therapy techniques could relieve pain by the following means:

1. Stimulation of healing in peripheral joints
2. Modification of the chemical environment of peripheral nociceptors
3. Activation of segmental pain inhibitory mechanisms
4. Activation of descending pain control systems
5. Use of the positive psychological influences of the therapeutic interaction and the "laying on of hands"

The model was envisaged as being highly flexible. As well as there being variations in the time course of each of these effects, it was suggested that there might be variation in terms of the capacity of an individual to exhibit each of these responses. It also was suggested that by modifying the parameters of the manual therapy stimulus, therapists might be able to preferentially affect one or more of these mechanisms in a selective manner. For example, by applying a compressive stimulus as part of the treatment technique, it might be possible to have a more significant effect on stimulating connective tissue repair in injured joints.

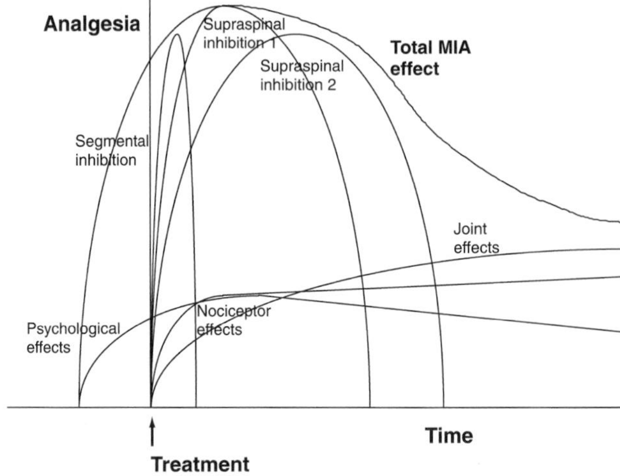

Figure 12-1
Schematic diagram of some possible components of the manipulation-induced analgesia effect. The diagram emphasizes the possibility that manipulation-induced analgesia is likely to be the result of a combination of effects and that the individual effects are likely to follow different time courses.

DESCENDING PAIN INHIBITORY SYSTEMS

In clinical practice, one cardinal feature of manual therapy techniques is that they induce a very rapid onset analgesic effect. Pain relief is apparent within minutes of applying a particular technique. This forms the basis of the reassessment process followed by most physical therapists. It was suggested that activation of descending pain inhibitory systems projecting from brain to spinal cord might be particularly important for mediating manipulation-induced analgesia in the period immediately after treatment application.[16] Because effects on peripheral repair processes might take some time to manifest and segmental inhibitory systems may be limited in their duration of effect, it was proposed that descending pain inhibitory systems influencing "the setting" of the spinal cord, might make a particularly strong contribution to manipulation-induced analgesia in the period immediately after treatment application.[16]

It is clear that there are several mechanistically distinct descending pain inhibitory systems.[17] In particular, studies of the periaqueductal gray (PAG) region of the midbrain have highlighted two distinct forms of analgesia.[18,19] The PAG region is an important integrating structure that plays a critical role in a variety of processes including vocalization, enhancement of pain perception, analgesia, sexual behavior, fear and anxiety, and cardiovascular control.[20,21] It has a characteristic columnar structure, with each of the columns exhibiting reciprocal connections with many areas of the forebrain and brainstem.[22,23] This connectivity provides the basis for the crucial integrating role that the PAG region plays in behavioral responses to life-threatening situations.[22-26]

The PAG region can be divided into functionally distinct dorsomedial, dorsolateral, lateral, and ventrolateral columns (Figure 12-2).[22,24-27] Stimulation of both the

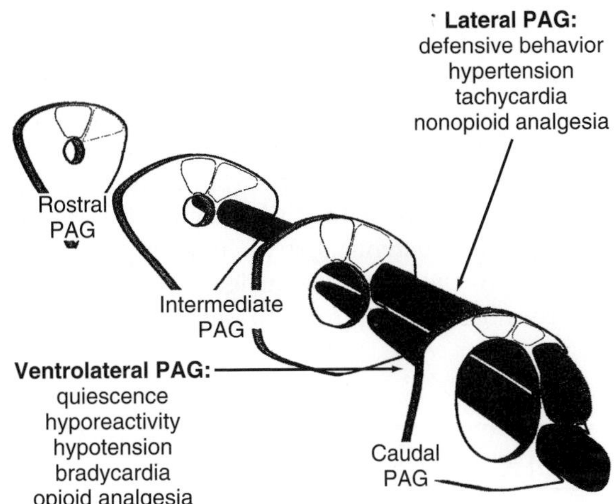

Figure 12-2

Columnar structure of the periaqueductal gray region showing the location of the lateral and ventrolateral columns.

(Modified from Bandler R, Shipley MT: *Trends Neurosci* 17[9]:379, 1994.)

lateral and ventrolateral columns using either electrical stimulation or iontophoretically applied excitatory amino acids produces analgesia in combination with changes in autonomic and motor function. However, the pattern of change in autonomic and motor function is distinctly different between these regions. Stimulation of the lateral column (also referred to as *dorsal PAG* in some nomenclatures) produces a sympathoexcitatory response and motor facilitation in addition to analgesia.[20,22,23] Blood flow is redirected from the viscera to the muscles in preparation for activity, and motor function is enhanced.[27-32] Stimulation of the ventrolateral column and the adjacent dorsal raphe nucleus has the opposing effect of inhibiting sympathetic nervous system function and reducing motor activity in addition to producing analgesia.[18,26,30,32,33] Blood flow is redirected from the limb musculature to the viscera, and rats exhibit a fixed posture with minimal movement (hyporeactive immobility).[26,30,32] This pattern of response is thought to be associated with the shock response that occurs after major trauma and blood loss and is considered to be a recuperative behavior.[34]

Although the analgesic effects produced by stimulating these regions are equipotent, the two forms of analgesia are mechanistically distinct. Stimulation of the ventrolateral column produces analgesia that is reversed by administering the morphine antagonist naloxone, exhibits tolerance with repeated stimulation and cross tolerance to stress-induced opioid-mediated analgesia.[35-38] This can be described as an opioid form of analgesia. Stimulation-produced analgesia from this region involves both ascending and descending efferent pathways.[28,39] Stimulation of the lateral column produces analgesia that is *not* reversed by the administration of naloxone and does *not* exhibit tolerance.[35,36,38] This is described as a nonopioid form of analgesia. Stimulation-produced analgesia from this region involves predominantly descending efferent pathways.[28,39]

It has been suggested that these response patterns subserve distinctly different behavioral situations. Stimulation of lateral PAG has been equated with a defensive pattern of behavior in which pain suppression is associated with motor activation.[24,29,40] Stimulation of ventrolateral PAG, on the other hand, is thought to equate to a situation in which the animal exhibits recuperative behaviors and reduces motor activity to facilitate tissue repair.[24,29,40] It is very clear from this body of research that in the natural situation, analgesia is never an isolated phenomenon. It is always associated with changes in other aspects of central nervous system (CNS) function that form part of a behaviorally important response pattern. This suggests that it may be possible to characterize naturally elicited forms of analgesia in terms of changes in other aspects of nervous system function, as well as the traditional pharmacological approach of classifying the analgesia as either opioid or nonopioid. Both of these approaches have been central to our research program over the last 10 years.

RESEARCH OBJECTIVES

Given this knowledge, our research over the last 10 years focused on three distinct objectives. They were as follows:

1. To determine whether it was possible to demonstrate an early onset analgesic effect after the administration of a cervical mobilization technique
2. To determine whether that analgesia was associated with concurrent changes in autonomic nervous system function and motor function and to characterize the pattern of that change

3. To determine whether the analgesia could be classified as either opioid or nonopioid using the classical pharmacological criteria for distinguishing these two forms of analgesia

MANIPULATION-INDUCED ANALGESIA

Characterizing early onset manipulation-induced analgesia as either opioid or nonopioid would help to demonstrate a physiological basis for the effects of manual therapy. Before the research reported in this chapter, there were only a few early studies investigating the effects of manipulation on pain perception.[41,42] They were not well described and lacked adequate controls. These studies suggested that manipulation of the cervical and thoracic spine could produce hypoalgesic effects as measured by changes in electrical pain thresholds and pressure pain thresholds.[41,42] They also suggested that these effects were demonstrable in both normal pain-free individuals[42] and individuals with painful cervical spine lesions.[41]

We used lateral epicondylalgia as a clinical model in which to determine the effect of mobilizing cervical spine segments on measures of hyperalgesia. Lateral epicondylalgia was selected as a clinical model for several reasons. First, we had previously conducted studies to characterize the pattern of hyperalgesia in this condition.[43,44] Second, several quantifiable and reliable measures were available to monitor hyperalgesia in this condition. These included measurement of pressure pain threshold,[43,44] measurement of the range of glenohumeral abduction in the radial nerve neural tissue provocation test,[44-46] and quantification of the grip force exerted before pain onset.[47,48] Impairments related to all of these measures had been demonstrated in patients with lateral epicondylalgia. In addition, we had evaluated thermal (heat and cold) pain thresholds in this population and had demonstrated that although there are no abnormalities in heat pain threshold, there is a subgroup of patients with lateral epicondylalgia who exhibit hyperalgesia to cold stimuli.[49]

This model also was selected because it had previously been demonstrated that manual therapy applied to the cervical spine had a beneficial influence on pain and function in the elbow region.[50] This meant that we could develop experiments in which the site of treatment would be separated from the site used to evaluate hyperalgesic responses. This was important to ensure that the effects of multiple testing of pain thresholds did not contaminate the effects of the treatment stimulus. It also provided an additional factor that contributed to blinding of the subjects and helped to ensure the double-blind nature of the studies. Use of this pain model in combination with the selected treatment technique also meant that we were investigating the effects of a technique that was unlikely to have any influence on local tissue pathology. The intention was not to negate the importance of local tissue effects in producing sustained pain relief but rather to create a contrived experimental situation in which the predominant effect was likely to be neurophysiologically based. An additional benefit of lateral epicondylalgia is that it has been used as a clinical pain model to evaluate a variety of physiological, pharmacological, and surgical treatments.[51]

Our more recent studies have used cervical zygapophyseal joint pain as a clinical model. This model is one of the most common clinical conditions for which manual therapy techniques are applied to the cervical spine. It therefore has the advantage of clinical relevance for testing the effects of manual therapy techniques applied to the cervical spine.

Table 12-1 Pattern of Response in Sympathetic Nervous System-Related Measures for Studies Evaluating the Posteroanterior Glide and Lateral Glide Techniques

Study	Technique	Skin Conductance	Skin Temperature
Petersen et al[71]	Anteroposterior glide	↑	↓
Vicenzino et al[72]	Lateral glide	↑	←→
Vicenzino et al[56]	Lateral glide	↑	↑
Chiu and Wright[69]	Anteroposterior glide	↑	←→
McGuiness et al[70]	Anteroposterior glide	NT	NT
Vicenzino et al[54]	Lateral glide	↑	↓
Vicenzino et al[73]	Lateral glide	NT	NT

↑, Increased value; ↓, decreased value; ←→, no change; *NT*, not tested.

In addition to studies using these patient populations, we also have investigated the effects of manual therapy techniques on normal, pain-free individuals using measures similar to those employed in our studies using clinical pain models.

All of our studies have compared treatment interventions to both active control and control conditions. In all cases the active control involved using the same hand contacts as were used for the treatment to control for the effect of manual contact and the "laying on of hands." The control condition involved no contact between the subject and the therapist. We ensured that researchers responsible for measurements were unaware of the experimental condition applied during any study session, and we used a variety of methods to try to ensure that subjects were unaware of the treatment component of the experiment.

The results of multiple studies clearly demonstrate that mobilization of the cervical spine induces an immediate-onset hypoalgesic or antihyperalgesic effect in patients with lateral epicondylalgia, patients with insidious onset, cervical zygapophyseal joint pain, and in pain-free, normal volunteers.[52-57] Our initial study of patients with lateral epicondylalgia represents the first double-blind, randomized controlled trial to clearly demonstrate an early onset hypoalgesic effect of a manual therapy treatment technique applied to the cervical spine and provides confirmation of the clinical observation that manual therapy techniques exert a very immediate influence on pain perception.[53] In addition, repeated applications of the manual therapy treatment over several days resulted in a cumulative increase in pressure pain thresholds. Table 12-1 provides a summary of the results of studies demonstrating a hypoalgesic effect of cervical manual therapy techniques.

Modality Specificity of the Hypoalgesic Effect

One interesting and very consistent observation in our research has been that the application of manual therapy treatment techniques produces a significant elevation of pressure pain threshold and other measures of mechanical hyperalgesia but that these treatments have absolutely no influence on thermal pain perception. This selective influence on mechanical as opposed to thermal pain perception now has been demonstrated in several studies.[15,52,54,56,57] This effect could be explained by the fact that patients with lateral epicondylalgia exhibit mechanical hyperalgesia and show no evidence of thermal (heat) hyperalgesia.[43,44,49] Therefore, if manual therapy were

Cutaneous Blood Flux	Respiratory Rate	Heart Rate	Systolic Pressure	Diastolic Pressure
NT	NT	NT	NT	NT
NT	NT	NT	NT	NT
NT	NT	NT	NT	NT
NT	NT	NT	NT	NT
NT	↑	↑	↑	↑
↑ elbow ↓ hand	NT	NT	NT	NT
NT	↑	↑	↑	↑

considered to have only an antihyperalgesic effect, it would be expected that this effect would be predominantly related to mechanical hyperalgesia in this population. Our studies on normal volunteers, however, clearly show that manual therapy techniques exhibit a hypoalgesic effect in individuals who do not exhibit hyperalgesia and that this hypoalgesic effect is selective for mechanical nociception.[15,56,58]

There is evidence from basic science research to suggest that processing and modulation of mechanical and thermal nociception involve distinctly different mechanisms.[59-62] It is therefore quite possible that a treatment might selectively influence one modality of nociception as opposed to the other. In particular, it appears that mechanical nociception is predominantly modulated by descending systems using noradrenaline as a neurotransmitter, whereas thermal nociception is predominantly modulated by descending systems that use serotonin (5-hydroxytryptamine) as a neurotransmitter.[60,62,63]

Somatotopic Organization of the Analgesic Effect

If manual therapy techniques produce a hypoalgesic effect, then it is of interest to determine how widespread that effect might be. Is it a generalized global effect, or is it relatively specific to the treated structures and segments? It appears that stimulation of the PAG elicits predominantly contralateral effects.[64] It is also of interest to note that the PAG exhibits a crude somatotopic organization, with rostral regions influencing discrete body sites and caudal regions influencing much larger body areas. There also is a dorsoventral somatotopic pattern, with dorsal sites eliciting analgesia of the ears and forepaws and more ventral sites eliciting analgesia of the hind paws and tail of the rat.[65]

We investigated the somatotopic organization of manipulation-induced analgesia in a controlled double-blind study using a unilateral anteroposterior mobilization as a treatment procedure in pain-free normal subjects. This study produced some interesting results in that mobilization of C5 on the right side produced significant mechanical hypoalgesia in the right upper limb. It also produced nonsignificant elevations of mechanical pain thresholds in the right lower limb and the right side of the head (Figure 12-3), but it showed absolutely no influence on mechanical pain thresholds on the left side of the body at any of the sites tested. This suggests that there is a crude somatotopic organization of the hypoalgesic effect produced by mobilization

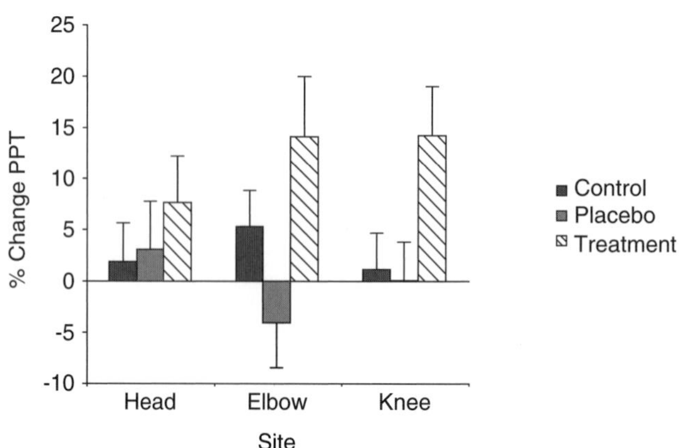

Figure 12-3
Percentage of change in pressure pain thresholds (PPT) at three sites (head, elbow, and knee) after a unilateral anteroposterior mobilization, an active control condition, or a no-contact control condition. Data are for the right side of the body only.

of spinal joint structures. This broad somatotopic organization parallels the rather generalized organization that is characteristic of the PAG.

To summarize, the combination of modality specificity and somatotopic organization of the hypoalgesic effect of manual therapy treatment techniques suggests that the pain relief produced by these interventions is not merely a generalized placebo effect. It would be anticipated that a generalized placebo response might influence all modalities of pain perception and that it might have a widespread influence on pain perception, particularly in normal individuals who had not been cued to expect a reduction in pain perception in any particular area. These findings suggest that there is a neurophysiological, as opposed to a psychological, basis to the observed effect.

INFLUENCE OF MANUAL THERAPY TECHNIQUES ON AUTONOMIC FUNCTION

Given the premise that manual therapy techniques exert at least part of their initial hypoalgesic effect by activating descending pain inhibitory systems from the frontal lobes, midbrain and brainstem and given that these systems are known to influence both autonomic and motor function, it becomes important to evaluate their influence on autonomic nervous system function. Early studies investigating the effect of manual therapy treatment techniques on autonomic nervous system function used a limited number of indirect measures and produced conflicting results.[66-68] A study by Harris and Wagnon,[66] for example, showed both increases and decreases in cutaneous temperature after spinal manipulation. These studies did not have adequate controls and did not use an adequate number of measures to provide some indication of the pattern of change in autonomic nervous system function.

We now have conducted multiple studies in patient populations (lateral epicondylalgia and insidius-onset cervicogenic pain) and normal pain-free individuals using a variety of measures that provide an indirect indication of autonomic, and particularly sympathetic, nervous system function.[52,54,69,73] The measures used included skin conductance, skin temperature, cutaneous blood flux, heart rate, respiratory rate, and systolic and diastolic blood pressure. We have evaluated the effects of the cervical lateral glide technique and the posteroanterior glide technique applied to the C5-6 motion segment in particular. A consistent pattern of response has emerged.

Posteroanterior Glide

In our initial study, we showed that a posteroanterior glide mobilization applied to the cervical spine in normal, pain-free subjects produced a significant and substantial increase in skin conductance (decrease in skin resistance) and a more modest decrease in skin temperature that was apparent only during the period of treatment application.[71] More recently we have shown that a posteroanterior glide applied to the same motion segment in patients with cervicogenic pain produces a similar increase in skin conductance and decrease in skin temperature measured on the palmar surface of the fingertips.[52] We also have shown that this treatment technique produces a significant elevation of respiratory rate, heart rate, and blood pressure during the period of treatment application.[72]

Lateral Glide

We completed a similar series of studies using the lateral glide treatment technique. Our initial study using this technique in pain-free subjects provided evidence of a large increase in skin conductance, although there was no significant change in skin temperature in the target limb.[72] Subsequent studies in patients with lateral epicondylalgia demonstrated an increase in skin conductance and showed significant reductions in skin temperature and cutaneous blood flux in the hand on the treated side.[54] More recently we have shown that the lateral glide technique produces significant increases in respiratory rate, heart rate, and blood pressure in normal pain-free subjects.[73]

We have interpreted this pattern of response as being indicative of increased sympathetic nervous system activity. Although there are variations among the studies (Table 12-2), the overall pattern of response is remarkably robust and consistent in both clinical populations and normal subjects.

Effect of Modifying Treatment Parameters

Two studies have clearly demonstrated that changing the parameters of the manual therapy stimulus can influence the sympathetic nervous system response. In an interesting study using the posteroanterior glide technique, Chiu and Wright[69] showed that by altering the frequency of joint oscillation in this technique, it was possible to significantly alter the skin conductance response produced by the treatment. Treatment at a rate of 2 Hz produced a significantly greater increase in skin conductance than treatment at a slower rate of 0.5 Hz, which was not significantly different from an active control condition that involved manual contact with the cervical spine without any movement of the motion segment.

Vicenzino et al[72] compared two experimental conditions in which the lateral glide technique was applied with the upper limb placed in two different positions. These positions approximated the radial nerve neural tissue provocation test and the original upper limb neural tissue provocation test. Both treatment procedures produced a greater increase in skin conductance than the active control or control conditions. It was apparent, however, that the technique applied with the arm in the radial nerve neural tissue provocation test position consistently produced a greater

Table 12-2 Pattern of Response in Pain-Related Measures for Studies Evaluating the Posteroanterior Glide and Lateral Glide Techniques

Study	Technique	Pressure Pain Threshold	Thermal Pain Threshold	Pain-Free Grip	Radial Nerve NTPT	Visual Analog Scale
Wright and Vicenzino[15]	Anteroposterior glide	↑	←→	NT	NT	NT
Vicenzino et al[56]	Lateral glide	↑	←→	NT	NT	NT
Vicenzino et al[53]	Lateral glide	↑	NT	↑	↑	←→ resting ↓ 24 hour
Vicenzino et al[54]	Lateral glide	↑	←→	↑	↑	
Vicenzino et al[55]	Lateral glide	↑	←→	↑	NT	NT
Sterling et al[52]	Anteroposterior glide	↑	←→	NT	NT	↓ resting ←→ end of range

NTPT, Neural tissue provation test; ↑, increased value; ↓, decreased value; ←→, no change; *NT,* not tested.

increase in skin conductance than the technique applied with the arm in the alternative position.[72]

These studies tend to suggest that the effect produced depends on specific parameters of the manual therapy treatment stimulus. The specificity of this response suggests that the changes observed are a specific physiological response to the treatment stimulus. Data from another study investigating a treatment technique applied to the thoracic spine suggest that the change in skin conductance is a very global response affecting both upper limbs, whereas the change in skin temperature is specific to the target limb.[74] Given that cutaneous sudomotor and vasomotor tone are controlled by different nuclei at the level of the medulla, it is feasible that one response might be much more widespread than the other.[75]

We also have investigated the effect of modifying the temporal characteristics of the manual therapy stimulus to determine how this influences the autonomic response. A study by Thornton[76] investigated the effect of repeating the posteroanterior glide treatment seven times. He showed that the change in skin conductance tends to peak during the first treatment application and that it diminishes with repeated applications, such that after five applications, there is no longer a significant increase in skin conductance evoked by the treatment stimulus.[76]

There is now a significant body of research that has investigated the effect of cervical mobilization techniques on indirect measures of sympathetic nervous system function. These studies provide convincing evidence that the following points do apply to manual therapy treatment techniques:

1. The techniques are an adequate stimulus for producing changes in autonomic nervous system function.
2. The degree of change is related to the parameters of the treatment stimulus.
3. There is a ceiling in terms of the degree of change that can be produced with repeated treatment applications.
4. The pattern of response is consistent and robust.
5. The pattern of change suggests increased sympathetic nervous system activity.

INFLUENCE OF MANUAL THERAPY TECHNIQUES ON MOTOR FUNCTION

Research investigating the influence of manual therapy treatment techniques on motor function is still at an early stage. However, we now have some preliminary evidence that manual therapy techniques can have a positive influence on motor function, particularly in clinical populations. The model that we have used investigates the effect of a posteroanterior glide technique on activation of the deep cervical flexor muscles using the staged craniocervical flexion test.[77] This test provides an indirect measure of deep cervical flexor function.

The procedure involves placing the subject in supine position with the cervical spine in a neutral position. A Stabilizer pressure biofeedback unit is placed under the cervical spine and inflated to 20 mm Hg. The subject is then asked to gently flex head on neck to increase the pressure in the biofeedback unit. In the staged test the subject is asked to progressively increase to target pressures of 22, 24, 26, 28, and 30 mm Hg.[77] Electromyography (EMG) signals are recorded from the superficial cervical flexors. The objective of the test is to produce controlled increases in pressure, associated with flattening the cervical lordosis, with minimal EMG activity in the superficial cervical flexor muscles. Performance on this test can be impaired in patients with cervicogenic headache.[78]

In a recent study we investigated the effect of a posteroanterior glide on performance of the staged craniocervical flexion test.[52] In comparison to active control and control conditions, subjects showed significantly lower levels of EMG activity in the superficial flexor muscles after the treatment intervention. Lower levels of normalized EMG activity are interpreted as indicating improved activation of the deep cervical flexor muscles. We interpreted this finding as providing preliminary evidence that manual therapy techniques may facilitate motor function.[52]

In a similar study on normal pain-free individuals, we were not able to demonstrate a consistent pattern of response, and so to date we have no evidence to suggest that manual therapy techniques have a positive influence on motor function in normals.[79] This leaves an open question as to whether improvements in motor function are simply an indirect effect of inhibiting pain perception or a primary effect of the treatment. Further research is required in normal pain-free individuals to determine whether manual therapy techniques can have a direct influence on motor function that is independent of the pain inhibitory effect.

Preliminary evidence gathered from the two studies[52,79] discussed here suggests that application of a manual therapy technique can enhance motor function in patients with cervicogenic pain, particularly in terms of control of the deep stabilizing muscles. More research is required to adequately investigate this effect and to determine whether facilitation of motor function is a distinct effect or simply a secondary consequence of pain inhibition.

INTERACTION AMONG PAIN, AUTONOMIC FUNCTION, AND MOTOR FUNCTION

If manual therapy techniques are an adequate stimulus to activate descending pain inhibitory systems projecting from the midbrain, then it would be expected that these techniques would produce concurrent changes in pain perception, autonomic function, and motor function. Although we have demonstrated changes in each of these domains in individual studies, it is important to evaluate multiple systems under the same study conditions to determine whether there is a relationship between changes occurring in each domain.

Pain and Autonomic Function

In a study using the cervical lateral glide technique applied to patients with lateral epicondylalgia, we investigated the relationship between changes in pain perception and changes in parameters related to sympathetic nervous system function.[54] The range of pain-related measures included pressure pain threshold, pain-free grip threshold, range of pain-free motion in the radial nerve neural tissue provocation test and thermal (heat) pain thresholds. The range of measures related to autonomic nervous system function included skin conductance, skin temperature, and cutaneous blood flux. Cutaneous temperature and blood flux were measured at both the elbow and the hand in the affected limb. We hypothesized a relationship between the hypoalgesic effect of the treatment and the sympathoexcitatory effect of the treatment rather than hypothesizing any relationship between specific measured variables. In this context, manual therapy-induced hypoalgesia and manual therapy-induced sympathoexcitation can be described as latent or immeasurable variables. Our experiment measured a number of related variables, but it did not specifically measure the latent variables (factors) of hypoalgesia and sympathoexcitation.

Fortunately, statistical techniques exist that allow us to use the measured variables to generate mathematical representations of the latent variables and then to test the relationship between those variables. We used confirmatory factor analysis[80,81] to model the data in terms of two latent variables, which we labelled *hypoalgesia* and *sympathoexcitation*, and we then tested the correlation between those variables. Two measures, thermal pain threshold and elbow skin temperature, were not included in the model. Neither of these measures exhibited any change related to the manual therapy treatment. The remaining measures were all included in the model (Figure 12-4).

The model provided an excellent representation of the data and met several important evaluation criteria. The independence model testing the hypothesis that all variables are not related was rejected, and the hypothesized model was strongly supported (nonsignificant χ^2 test and comparative fit index = 0.91). Use of the Lagrange multiplier and Wald tests[82] failed to identify additional parameters or produce a more parsimonious model by eliminating parameters. The correlation between each of the latent variables was r = 0.82 ($p < 0.05$).[54] This is a very strong correlation and sug-

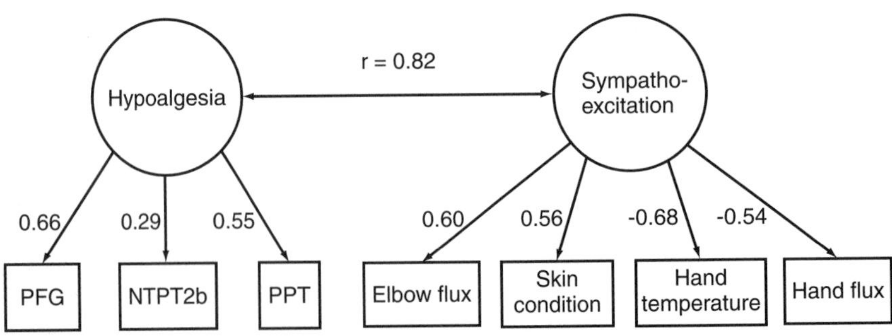

Figure 12-4
Confirmatory factor analysis model of the influence of the lateral glide technique on pain-related measures and measures related to sympathetic nervous system function.
(Modified from Vicenzino B et al: *J Manip Physiol Ther* 7(12):448, 1998.)

gests that those individuals who exhibited the most change in pain perception also were those who exhibited the most change in sympathetic nervous system function.

These findings suggest a coordinated change in both domains in response to the manual therapy treatment stimulus. This study therefore provides good evidence to suggest that the manual therapy stimulus is capable of activating brain regions rostral to the medulla that have the capacity to produce concurrent changes in nociceptive system function and autonomic nervous system function. The PAG is one such structure, although not the only potential point of control. However, given the specific pattern of change in terms of increased sympathetic nervous system activity, this might suggest a key role for the PAG in mediating this effect. This preliminary interpretation of the data requires further investigation using experimental approaches that can more specifically address the role of various brain structures in contributing to manipulation-induced analgesia. The nature of this future research is discussed later in this chapter.

PAIN, AUTONOMIC FUNCTION, AND MOTOR FUNCTION

In a study on patients with cervicogenic pain using the posteroanterior glide technique, we attempted to test the relationship between changes in pain perception, autonomic function, and motor function.[52] As reported previously, this study demonstrated improvements in pain-related measures and motor function as determined by the staged craniocervical flexion test. It also showed increased skin conductance and decreased skin temperature after treatment administration.[52] Attempts were made to model these data using confirmatory factor analysis. Unfortunately, it was not possible to successfully model the data and to test for relationships among the three latent variables. One specific reason for this was that the pattern of change in the EMG measures was distinctly different from the pattern of change in the other data sets.

In the EMG data, we noted that under the active control condition, EMG values actually increased relative to both the treatment condition and the control condition.[52] The other measures all exhibited a pattern of changes in which maximum change occurred in the treatment condition, less change occurred in the active control condition, and the least change occurred in the control condition. Because the pattern of the relationship among treatment, active control, and control measures was different among the three domains, this prevented us from successfully modelling the data. Although this study does demonstrate concurrent changes in each of the three domains, we must await the results of further studies before we can determine whether there is any statistical relationship among the changes occurring in the autonomic, motor, and nociceptive systems.

To summarize, one study has been published that clearly demonstrates a strong relationship between the pain-inhibitory effect of manual therapy and the sympathoexcitatory effect of the manual therapy stimulus.[54] This provides important evidence suggesting that a supraspinal control center may play a key role in mediating the pain-relieving effect of manual therapy treatment techniques. At this point we cannot be specific about the region of the brain responsible for controlling this response, although the pattern of change might suggest an important role for the PAG region. Further research is required to test this hypothesis. Another study attempted to test the relationships among pain inhibition, sympathoexcitation, and enhanced motor function.[52] Unfortunately, it was not possible to successfully model the data obtained from this study. Further investigations are therefore required to determine whether there is a relationship among the changes in each of the three domains induced by manual therapy treatment.

IS MOBILIZATION-INDUCED ANALGESIA AN OPIOID OR NONOPIOID FORM OF ANALGESIA?

One approach to characterizing endogenous forms of analgesia has been to determine whether they meet the pharmacological criteria to be classified as either an opioid or a nonopioid form of analgesia. Opioid analgesia has the following characteristics:

1. It is blocked or reversed after the administration of naloxone (morphine antagonist).
2. It exhibits tolerance after repeated administration of the analgesia-inducing stimulus.
3. It exhibits cross-tolerance with morphine.

Nonopioid forms of analgesia are by exclusion those forms of analgesia that do not exhibit the aforementioned three characteristics.[83] This is a rather arbitrary division, and in reality most forms of endogenous analgesia exhibit a varied response pattern that is difficult to classify into one category or the other. Nevertheless, this approach does help to provide a preliminary characterization of the analgesic effect and does help to guide subsequent research to determine the analgesic mechanism.

Naloxone is a drug used in clinical practice to reverse, or antagonize, some of the adverse effects of morphine administration, particularly respiratory inhibition. It has the ability to bind to opioid receptors in the nervous system, preventing morphine or endogenous opioids from acting on those receptors. In comparison to some newer drugs that are available for experimental studies, it does not have a high degree of specificity for any particular opioid receptor, although it does exhibit a preference for the mu receptor.

Analgesic tolerance can be defined as a decrease in a prescribed effect or a situation in which there is a need for a dose increase to maintain the effect after repeated administration.[84] It is a particular characteristic of morphine analgesia in experimental studies that if the same dose of drug is administered repeatedly over several days, the analgesic response will tend to diminish, such that after approximately 1 week there may be almost no analgesic effect of the drug. Tolerance can be tested by repeatedly administering an analgesia-inducing stimulus over several days and determining if the analgesic response tends to diminish.

Cross-tolerance means that when tolerance to morphine has been induced, there is concurrent tolerance to another analgesia-inducing stimulus. See Souvlis and Wright[84] for a more complete discussion of tolerance and its relevance to physiotherapy treatments.

NALOXONE REVERSIBILITY

Relatively few studies have attempted to characterize the analgesic effect of manual therapy treatments using this classification. An early study by Zusman et al[85] failed to demonstrate any reversal of analgesia induced in patients with cervicogenic pain using a variety of combined-movement manual therapy techniques. Although this study indicates that manipulation-induced analgesia may be a nonopioid form of analgesia, the authors did suggest some limitations of their study. In particular, they suggested that low-dose naloxone might be more effective in blocking and preventing analgesia from developing rather than actually reversing analgesia once it had become established. They therefore recommended administering naloxone before a manual therapy technique rather than after the technique.

We adopted this approach in a subsequent double-blind controlled study.[55] Three different experimental conditions were compared. In each case the lateral glide treatment technique was applied to the cervical spine in patients with lateral epicondylalgia. Pain-related measures similar to those listed previously were obtained before and after treatment. Before treatment, an injection of naloxone or saline or a control in which no injection was administered was carried out. The lateral glide treatment induced increases in the pain-free grip threshold and the pressure pain threshold indicative of a hypoalgesic effect.[55]

The data acquired showed no significant difference in the change in pressure pain thresholds or pain-free grip thresholds with each of the experimental conditions. There was a trend for the increase in pain-free grip threshold to be less with the naloxone condition, but this was not significant. This study therefore provides further evidence suggesting that the initial hypoalgesic effect of a manual therapy treatment is a nonopioid form of analgesia.

Tolerance

We also have investigated the development of tolerance after administration of the lateral glide treatment technique in patients with lateral epicondylalgia over six treatment sessions.[86] Once again, a hypoalgesic effect was apparent in terms of changes in pressure pain threshold and pain-free grip threshold but not thermal pain threshold. The main outcome measure used in this study was percentage of maximum possible effect (MPE). This measure often is used in experimental studies investigating tolerance, and it normally refers to the pain threshold expressed as a percentage of a maximum cut-off threshold used to ensure that the animal does not exhibit significant tissue damage. For example, in a study using the thermal tail flick test in the rat, a maximum response time of 10 seconds might be established. If the rat responds at 4 seconds and removes its tail from the heat source, then the MPE would be 40%. If the animal were analgesic and responded after 9 seconds, then the MPE would be 90%. The higher the percentage the greater the degree of analgesia. In the context of our lateral epicondylalgia clinical pain model, we determined the percent of MPE in the following manner. The change in pain thresholds from pretreatment to posttreatment was expressed as a percentage off the difference between baseline pain threshold in the affected limb and in the unaffected limb. Therefore if the pain threshold in the affected limb was increased to be equivalent to that of the unaffected limb, the response would be recorded as 100% MPE.

There were several interesting characteristics to the pattern of response to treatment over each of the six sessions. First there was evidence of a cumulative analgesic effect in that baseline pretreatment visual analogue pain scores decreased incrementally from day 1 to day 6. This is an interesting characteristic of the analgesic effect that is worthy of further investigation because it suggests that even if the effects of an individual treatment are relatively small, they are additive, and so a progressive normalization occurs over time. However, linear trend analysis showed no significant change in percentage of MPE for pressure pain threshold or pain-free grip threshold over the 6 days, suggesting that there was no analgesic tolerance with respect to these measures.[86] The average MPE was 4.87% for a pain-free grip threshold and 7.91% for a pressure pain threshold. Therefore although manipulation-induced analgesia does not appear to exhibit tolerance according to a technical definition, important changes do occur in the nature of the analgesic effect with repeated administrations over time.

Studies to determine the role of endogenous opioids in manipulation-induced analgesia are still at an early stage. The initial data suggest that the hypoalgesic effect of manual therapy treatment is a nonopioid form of analgesia. It appears to be nonnaloxone reversible,[55] and it does not exhibit tolerance.[86] There is a clear need for further research in this area. The studies to date have used relatively low doses of naloxone, comparable to the doses used to reverse adverse effects of morphine in clinical practice. Administering a higher dose of naloxone might result in some degree of reversal. It also is clear that although the manual therapy response does not exhibit tolerance in terms of any change in the percentage of MPE, there are cumulative changes in pain perception over repeated treatments. Further research is required to explore the patterns of response after multiple treatment applications. To date, no studies have been carried out to evaluate cross-tolerance with morphine, and only a limited number of studies have attempted to directly measure changes in the levels of endogenous opioids such as beta endorphin. A great deal of research is required before the involvement of endogenous opioids can be confirmed or refuted. However, the initial studies suggest a nonopioid form of analgesia.

FUTURE RESEARCH

Available evidence suggests that at least a component of the analgesic effect of manual therapy techniques may be caused by activation of a descending pain inhibitory system projecting from a structure located rostral to the medulla that has the capacity to concurrently modulate nociceptive, autonomic, and motor functions. We have speculated that this structure might be the lateral column of PAG because of the specific pattern of response that we have noted. However, none of the research that has been carried out to date provides conclusive evidence for the involvement of the PAG or any other structure in this effect. To implicate the PAG or any other brain structure in this effect, one must conduct studies that specifically demonstrate neuronal activity in that region or that show abolition of the effect as a result of pharmacological or anatomical lesioning of the structure. Detailed studies of this nature are best addressed in an animal model.

Developing an animal model of manipulation-induced analgesia is not a simple task. It involves developing a model of induced pain that mimics a musculoskeletal pain state and then modelling a particular manual therapy technique in a rat or other laboratory animal. Modelling the technique is difficult because of differences in relative size between humans and rats and because of differences in the anatomy of the spine and peripheral joints between the species. An additional factor is the need to establish a suitable outcome measure that provides a reliable evaluation of the hypoalgesic effect.

We have recently completed the first study to provide evidence of an antihyperalgesic effect of peripheral joint mobilization in the rat.[87] The pain model used was intraarticular injection of capsaicin, and the model manual therapy technique was a grade 3 extension of the knee joint with an anteroposterior glide of the tibia.[88] The hyperalgesic effect of capsaicin and the antihyperalgesic effect of the treatment were evaluated by testing mechanical pain thresholds on the plantar surface of the foot using von Frey filaments.[89] In this pain model, secondary mechanical hyperalgesia develops over the plantar surface of the foot within 2 hours after the capsaicin injection.[87] Five experimental conditions were compared. These were a no contact control condition, a manual contact control condition, and three treatment conditions in which the treatment technique was applied three times for three different durations (1, 3, and 5 minutes). Results showed that the treatment technique applied for a total of 9 minutes or 15 minutes produced a complete reversal of the hyperalgesia induced by capsaicin injection. This effect was apparent within 5 minutes and lasted for up to 45 minutes.

Further work is required to perfect this model; however, if a manipulation-induced analgesic effect can be modelled in the rat, then an array of studies can be carried out to determine the neurophysiological basis for this effect. Areas of neuronal activity in response to the manual therapy stimulus can be determined using an imaging technique such as functional magnetic resonance imaging. It also might be possible to record evoked activity from neurons in target structures. Pharmacological blockade of the induced effect can be attempted using antagonists for a variety of neurotransmitters, including endogenous opioids, noradrenaline, and serotonin. Drugs also can be administered to attempt to enhance particular components of the effect. Anatomical lesions can be performed to ablate key structures and determine the effect on the induced analgesia. Research over the next decade will use many of these experimental approaches to provide more detailed information about the neurophysiological basis of manipulation-induced analgesia.

DISCUSSION

Knowledge of the effects of manual therapy treatment techniques has improved considerably over the last decade. However, we still require a great deal more information before we can show categorically that joint mobilization activates a particular neurophysiological mechanism to modulate pain. Because of the pattern of pain modulation and other effects of joint mobilization that we have seen in a number of studies, we have suggested that the PAG may play an important role in this effect. A great deal more research is required to test this theory and to evaluate the role of many other structures that potentially might be involved.

One question that arises in relation to this is why should the CNS have acquired the ability to respond to particular joint movements by modulating pain perception. The answer may lie in reversing this question and asking what it is about manual therapy techniques that reflect stimuli that might induce analgesia in the natural situation. It has been postulated that activation of lateral PAG is particularly important for defensive situations.[19,40] The painting by Stubbs reproduced in Figure 12-5 shows a

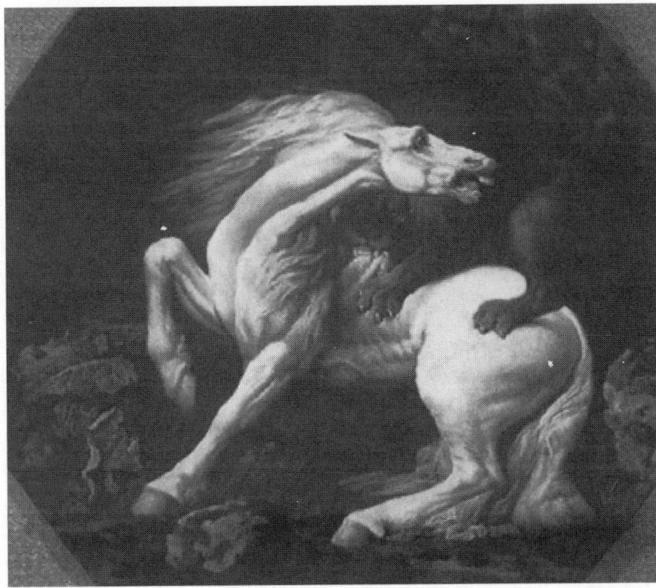

Figure 12-5
Horse attacked by a lion (George Stubbs, 1769). Note the arousal, the muscle activity, the extreme movements of head and neck and the penetration of the skin by teeth and claws.

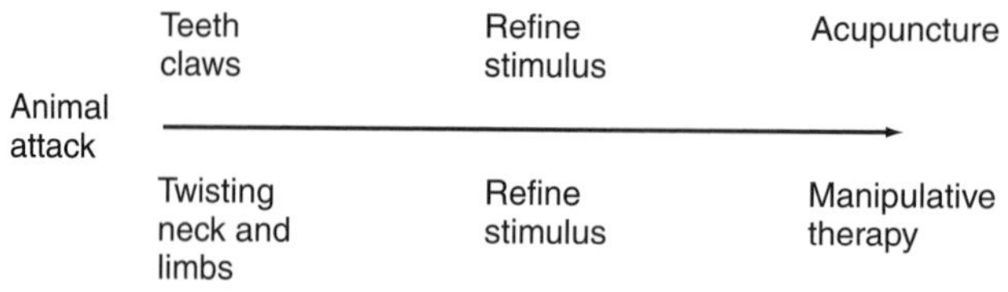

	Teeth claws	Refine stimulus	Acupuncture
Animal attack	→	→	→
	Twisting neck and limbs	Refine stimulus	Manipulative therapy

Figure 12-6
A conceptual mode of the transition from threatening stimuli to therapeutic interventions.

classic attack and defense situation. In this situation, the prey animal must exhibit a certain set of behaviors, including pain inhibition, if it is to have any prospect of survival. The painting clearly shows straining of muscles and extreme movements of joints that are likely to occur in these situations. It is easy to imagine the very rapid redirection of blood flow that the autonomic nervous system would have to accomplish to provide adequate oxygenation of the muscles. The physical stimuli triggering this response include penetration of the skin by the teeth and claws and marked rotation of the joints, particularly those of the cervical spine. If these stimuli were refined to arrive at the minimal stimulus that involves penetration of the skin and the minimal stimulus that involves rotation or translation of a specific spinal segment, then the resultant stimuli might be very similar to acupuncture and manual therapy (Figure 12-6). The concept is that these treatment approaches have evolved as a means of safely and relatively painlessly accessing a very potent pain-modulation system that has evolved over millions of years because of its survival benefit. Over the last few thousand years, humans have successfully developed therapeutic techniques that allow us to access the powerful pain-modulation systems that exist within the CNS.

CONCLUSION

It is likely that the pain-relieving effect of manual therapy techniques is a multifactorial phenomenon. Much work is still required to investigate all of the potential effects of manual therapy treatment techniques, especially the potential effects on tissue repair. A critical component of the initial pain relieving effect, particularly in the period immediately after treatment application, may be activation of endogenous pain modulation systems projecting from the brain to the spinal cord. It is now well established that when these systems are activated, analgesia is not produced as an isolated response but occurs in association with changes in both autonomic function and motor function that may be important for particular behavior patterns.

Research over the last decade has demonstrated consistent patterns of change in pain perception, autonomic function, and to a lesser extent, motor function after manual therapy treatment. The patterns of response that have been demonstrated provide indirect evidence of a potential role for the PAG in mediating this effect. Initial work now has been carried out to develop an animal model of manipulation-induced analgesia that may allow us to carry out much more detailed research over the next decade that will lead to a more specific elucidation of the neurophysiological basis of manipulation-induced analgesia. This work should bring us closer to providing an answer to the age-old question of how does manual therapy work.

References

1. Sloop PR, Smith DS, Goldenberg E, Dore C: Manipulation for chronic neck pain: a double-blind controlled study, *Spine* 7(6):532, 1982.
2. Mealy K, Brennan H, Fenelon GC: Early mobilization of acute whiplash injuries, *Br Med J (Clin Res Ed)* 292(6521):656, 1986.
3. Nordemar R, Thorner C: Treatment of acute cervical pain: a comparative group study, *Pain* 10(1):93, 1981.
4. McKinney LA, Dornan JO, Ryan M: The role of physiotherapy in the management of acute neck sprains following road-traffic accidents, *Arch Emerg Med* 6(1):27, 1989.
5. Brodin H: Cervical pain and mobilization, *Manual Med* 2:18, 1985.
6. Aker PD, Gross AR, Goldsmith CH, Peloso P: Conservative management of mechanical neck pain: systematic overview and meta-analysis, *Br Med J* 313(7068):1291, 1996.
7. Gross AR, Aker PD, Quartly C: Manual therapy in the treatment of neck pain, *Rheum Dis Clin North Am* 22(3):579, 1996.
8. Melzack R, Wall PD: Pain mechanisms: a new theory, *Science* 150(699):971, 1965.
9. Wyke BD: Articular neurology and manipulative therapy. In Glasgow EF, editor: *Aspects of manipulative therapy*, Edinburgh, 1985, Churchill Livingstone.
10. Zusman M: Spinal manipulative therapy: review of some proposed mechanisms and a new hypothesis, *Aust J Physiother* 32:89, 1986.
11. Zusman M: What does manipulation do? The need for basic research. In Boyling JD, Palastanga N, editors: *Grieve's modern manual therapy*, Edinburgh, 1994, Churchill Livingstone.
12. Vernon HT, Dhami MS, Howley TP, Annett R: Spinal manipulation and beta-endorphin: a controlled study of the effect of a spinal manipulation on plasma beta-endorphin levels in normal males, *J Manip Physiolog Ther* 9(2):115, 1986.
13. Sanders GE, Reinert O, Tepe R, Maloney P: Chiropractic adjustive manipulation on subjects with acute low back pain: visual analog pain scores and plasma beta-endorphin levels, *J Manip Physiolog Ther* 13(7):391, 1990.
14. Christian GF, Stanton GJ, Sissons D et al: Immunoreactive ACTH, beta-endorphin, and cortisol levels in plasma following spinal manipulative therapy, *Spine* 13(12):1411, 1988.
15. Wright A, Vicenzino B: Cervical mobilization techniques, sympathetic nervous system effects, and their relationship to analgesia. In Shacklock M, editor: *Moving in on pain*, Melbourne, 1995, Butterworth-Heinemann.
16. Wright A: Hypoalgesia post-manipulative therapy: a review of a potential neurophysiological mechanism, *Manual Ther* 1:11, 1995.
17. Cannon JT, Liebeskind JC: Analgesic effects of electrical brain stimulation and stress. In Akil H, Lewis JW, editors: *Neurotransmitters and pain control*, Basel, Switzerland, 1987, Karger.
18. Lovick TA: Interactions between descending pathways from the dorsal and ventrolateral periaqueductal gray matter in the rat. In Depaulis A, Bandlier R, editors: *The midbrain periaqueductal gray matter*, New York, 1991, Plenum Press.
19. Morgan MM: Differences in antinociception evoked from dorsal and ventral regions of the caudal periaqueductal gray matter. In Depaulis A, Bandler R, editors: *The midbrain periaqueductal gray matter*, New York, 1991, Plenum Press.
20. Behbehani MM: Functional characteristics of the midbrain periaqueductal gray, *Prog Neurobiol* 46(6):575, 1995.
21. Bernard JF, Bandler R: Parallel circuits for emotional coping behaviour: new pieces in the puzzle, *J Comp Neurol* 401(4):429, 1998.
22. Bandler R, Keay KA: Columnar organisation in the midbrain periaqueductal gray and the integration of emotional expression, *Prog Brain Res* 107:285, 1996.
23. Bandler R, Shipley MT: Columnar organisation in the midbrain periaqueductal gray: modules for emotional expression? *Trends Neurosci* 17(9):379, 1994.
24. Carrive P: The periaqueductal gray and defensive behavior: functional representation and neuronal organization, *Behav Brain Res* 58(1-2):27, 1993.
25. Lovick TA: Midbrain and medullary regulation of defensive cardiovascular functions, *Prog Brain Res* 107:301, 1996.

26. Morgan MM, Whitney PK, Gold MS: Immobility and flight associated with antinociception produced by activation of the ventral and lateral/dorsal regions of the rat periaqueductal gray, *Brain Res* 804(1):159, 1998.
27. Bandler R, Carrive P, Zhang SP: Integration of somatic and autonomic reactions within the midbrain periaqueductal grey: viscerotopic, somatotopic and functional organisation, *Prog Brain Res* 87:269, 1991.
28. Lovick TA: The periaqueductal gray-rostral medulla connection in the defence reaction: efferent pathways and descending control mechanisms, *Behav Brain Res* 58(1-2):19, 1993.
29. Lovick TA: Integrated activity of cardiovascular and pain regulatory systems: role in adaptive behavioural responses, *Prog Neurobiol* 40(5):631, 1993.
30. Carrive P, Bandler R: Control of extracranial and hind limb blood flow by the midbrain periaqueductal grey of the cat, *Exp Brain Res* 84(3):599, 1991.
31. Verberne AJ, Struyker Boudier HA: Midbrain central grey: regional haemodynamic control and excitatory amino acidergic mechanisms, *Brain Res* 550(1):86, 1991.
32. Zhang SP, Bandler R, Carrive P: Flight and immobility evoked by excitatory amino acid microinjection within distinct parts of the subtentorial midbrain periaqueductal gray of the cat, *Brain Res* 520(1-2):73, 1990.
33. Depaulis A, Keay KA, Bandler R: Quiescence and hyporeactivity evoked by activation of cell bodies in the ventrolateral midbrain periaqueductal gray of the rat, *Exp Brain Res* 99(1):75, 1994.
34. Henderson LA, Keay KA, Bandler R: The ventrolateral periaqueductal gray projects to caudal brainstem depressor regions: a functional-anatomical and physiological study, *Neuroscience* 82(1):201, 1998.
35. Cannon JT, Prieto GJ, Lee A, Liebeskind JC: Evidence for opioid and non-opioid forms of stimulation-produced analgesia in the rat, *Brain Res* 243(2):315, 1982.
36. Morgan MM, Liebeskind JC: Site specificity in the development of tolerance to stimulation-produced analgesia from the periaqueductal gray matter of the rat, *Brain Res* 425(2):356, 1987.
37. Terman GW, Penner ER, Liebeskind JC: Stimulation-produced and stress-induced analgesia: cross-tolerance between opioid forms, *Brain Res* 360(1-2):374, 1985.
38. Thorn BE, Applegate L, Johnson SW: Ability of periaqueductal gray subdivisions and adjacent loci to elicit analgesia and ability of naloxone to reverse analgesia, *Behav Neurosci* 103(6):1335, 1989.
39. Morgan MM, Sohn JH, Liebeskind JC: Stimulation of the periaqueductal gray matter inhibits nociception at the supraspinal as well as spinal level, *Brain Res* 502(1):61, 1989.
40. Bandler R, Depaulis A: Midbrain periaqueductal gray control of defensive behaviour in the cat and the rat. In Depaulis A, Bandler R, editors: *The midbrain periaqueductal gray matter*, New York, 1991, Plenum Press.
41. Vernon H, Aker P, Burns S et al: Pressure pain threshold evaluation of the effect of spinal manipulation in the treatment of chronic neck pain: a pilot study, *J Manip Physiolog Ther* 13:13, 1990.
42. Terret A, Vernon H: Manipulation and pain tolerance, *Am J Phys Med* 63(5):217, 1984.
43. Wright A, Thurnwald P, Smith J: An evaluation of mechanical and thermal hyperalgesia in patients with lateral epicondylalgia, *Pain Clin* 5(4):221, 1992.
44. Wright A, Thurnwald P, O'Callaghan J et al: Hyperalgesia in tennis elbow patients, *J Musculoskel Pain* 2(4):83, 1994.
45. Yaxley G, Jull G: A modified upper limb tension test: an investigation of responses in normal subjects, *Aust J Physiother* 37:143, 1991.
46. Yaxley GA, Jull GA: Adverse tension in the neural system: a preliminary study of tennis elbow, *Aust J Physiother* 39(1):15, 1993.
47. Burton A: Grip strength and forearm straps in tennis elbow, *Br J Sports Med* 19:37, 1985.
48. Stratford P, Levy D, Gowland C: Evaluative properties of measures used to assess patients with lateral epicondylitis at the elbow, *Physio Can* 45:160, 1993.
49. Smith J, O'Callaghan J, Vicenzino B et al: The influence of regional sympathetic blockade with guanethidine on hyperalgesia in patients with lateral epicondylalgia, *J Musculoskel Pain* 7(4):55, 1999.

50. Gunn C, Milbrandt W: Tennis elbow and the cervical spine, *CMAJ* 114:803, 1976.
51. Wright A: Lateral epicondylalgia. II. Therapeutic management, *Phys Ther Rev* 2:39, 1997.
52. Sterling M, Jull G, Wright A: Cervical mobilisation: concurrent effects on pain, sympathetic nervous system activity and motor activity, *Manual Ther* 6(2):72, 2002.
53. Vicenzino B, Collins D, Wright A: The initial effects of a cervical spine manipulative physiotherapy treatment on the pain and dysfunction of lateral epicondylalgia, *Pain* 68(1):69, 1996.
54. Vicenzino B, Collins D, Benson H, Wright A: An investigation of the interrelationship between manipulative therapy-induced hypoalgesia and sympathoexcitation, *J Manip Physiolog Ther* 21(7):448, 1998.
55. Vicenzino B, O'Callaghan J, Kermode F, Wright A: No influence of naloxone on the initial hypoalgesic effect of spinal manual therapy. In Devor M, Rowbotham MC, Wiesenfeld-Hallin Z, editors: Progress in pain research and management, vol 2, Seattle, 2000, IASP. Proceedings of the ninth World Congress on Pain, Vienna, Austria, 1999.
56. Vicenzino B, Gutschlag F, Collins D, Wright A: An investigation of the effects of spinal manual therapy on forequarter pressure and thermal pain thresholds and sympathetic nervous system activity in asymptomatic subjects: a preliminary report. In Shacklock M, editor: *Moving in on pain*, Melbourne, 1995, Butterworth-Heinemann.
57. Wright A, Vicenzino B: Cervical mobilisation techniques, sympathetic nervous system effects and their relationship to analgesia. In Shacklock M, editor: *Moving in on pain*, Melbourne, 1995, Butterworth-Heinemann.
58. Hennessey SM: The somatotopic organisation of analgesia following the application of a unilateral anteroposterior glide of the fifth cervical vertebra, honours thesis, Brisbane, 1997, University of Queensland (Australia).
59. Kuraishi Y, Kawamura M, Yamaguchi T et al: Intrathecal injections of galanin and its antiserum affect nociceptive response of rat to mechanical, but not thermal, stimuli, *Pain* 44:321, 1991.
60. Kuraishi Y, Harada Y, Aratani S et al: Separate involvement of the spinal noradrenergic and serotonergic systems in morphine analgesia: the differences in mechanical and thermal algesic tests, *Brain Res* 273:245, 1983.
61. Kuraishi Y, Hirota N, Satoh M, Takagi H: Antinociceptive effects of intrathecal opioids, noradrenaline and serotonin in rats: mechanical and thermal algesic tests, *Brain Res* 326(1):168, 1985.
62. Kuraishi Y, Satoh M, Takagi H: The descending noradrenergic system and analgesia. In Akil H, Lewis JW, editors: *Neurotransmitters and pain control*, Basel, Switzerland, 1987, Karger.
63. Fields HL, Baxbaum AI: Central nervous system mechanisms of pain modulation. In Wall P, Melzack R, editors: *Textbook of pain*, ed 2, London, 1943, Churchill Livingstone.
64. Soper WY: Effects of analgesic midbrain stimulation on reflex withdrawal and thermal escape in the rat, *J Comparat Physiolog Psych* 90(1):91, 1976.
65. Soper WY, Melzack R: Stimulation-produced analgesia: evidence for somatotopic organisation in the midbrain, *Brain Res* 251:301, 1982.
66. Harris W, Wagnon J: The effects of chiropractic adjustments on distal skin temperature, *J Manip Physiolog Ther* 10:57, 1987.
67. Ellestad S, Nagle R, Boesler D, Kilmore M: Electromyographic and skin resistance responses to osteopathic manipulative treatment for low-back pain, *J Am Osteopath Assoc* 88:991, 1988.
68. Yates RG, Lamping DL, Abram NL, Wright C: Effects of chiropractic treatment on blood pressure and anxiety: a randomized controlled trial, *J Manip Physiolog Ther* 11:484, 1988.
69. Chiu TW, Wright A: To compare the effects of different rates of application of a cervical mobilisation technique on sympathetic outflow to the upper limb in normal subjects, *Manual Ther* 1(4):198, 1996.
70. McGuiness J, Vicenzino B, Wright A: The influence of a cervical mobilization technique on respiratory and cardiovascular function, *Manual Ther* 2(4):216, 1997.

71. Petersen NP, Vicenzino GT, Wright A: The effects of a cervical mobilisation technique on sympathetic outflow to the upper limb in normal subjects, *Physio Theory Pract* 9:149, 1993.
72. Vicenzino B, Collins D, Wright A: Sudomotor changes induced by neural mobilisation techniques in asymptomatic subjects, *J Man Manip Therapy* 2(2):66, 1994.
73. Vicenzino B, Cartwright T, Collins D, Wright A: Cardiovascular and respiratory changes produced by the lateral glide mobilisation of the cervical spine, *Manual Ther* 3(2):67, 1998.
74. Slater H, Vicenzino B, Wright A: 'Sympathetic slump': the effects of a novel manual therapy technique on peripheral sympathetic nervous system function, *J Man Manip Ther* 2(4):156, 1994.
75. McAllen RM, May CN, Campos RR: The supply of vasomotor drive to individual classes of sympathetic neuron, *Clin Exp Hypertens* 19(5-6):607, 1997.
76. Thornton S: The effects of repeated applications of posteroanterior glides on the sympathetic nervous system in normal subjects, honours thesis, Brisbane, 1996, University of Queensland (Australia)
77. Jull GA: Management of cervical headache, *Manual Ther* 2:182, 1997.
78. Beeton K, Jull G: Effectiveness of manipulative physiotherapy in the management of cervicogenic headache: a single case study, *Physiotherapy* 80:417, 1994.
79. Luong P: The effect of a cervical mobilisation on the activity of the deep neck flexors, honours thesis, Brisbane, 1998, University of Queensland (Australia).
80. McDonald R: *Factor analysis and related methods*, Hillsdale, NJ, 1985, Lawrence Erlbaum Associates.
81. Bentler P: *EQS structured equation modeling*, ed 5, Encino, Calif, 1995, Multivariate Software.
82. Bentler P: *Lagrange multiplier and Wald tests for EQS and EQS/PC*, Los Angeles, 1986, BMDP Statistical Software.
83. Lewis JW, Sherman JE, Liebeskind JC: Opioid and non-opioid stress analgesia: assessment of tolerance and cross-tolerance, *J Neurosci* 1(4):358, 1981.
84. Souvlis T, Wright A: The tolerance effect: its relevance to analgesia produced by physiotherapy interventions, *Phys Ther Rev* 2:227, 1997.
85. Zusman M, Edwards BC, Donaghy A: Investigation of a proposed mechanism for the relief of spinal pain with passive joint movement, *J Man Med* 4:58, 1989.
86. Souvlis T, Kermode F, Williams E et al: Does the initial analgesic effect of spinal manual therapy exhibit tolerance? Proceedings of the ninth World Congress on Pain, Vienna, Austria, 1999.
87. Sluka KA, Wright A: Knee joint mobilisation reduces secondary mechanical hyperalgesia induced by capsaicin injection into the ankle joint, *Eur J Pain* 5(1):81, 2001.
88. Maitland GD: *Peripheral manipulation*, Oxford, England, 1991, Butterworth-Heinemann.
89. Sluka KA: Blockade of calcium channels can prevent the onset of secondary hyperalgesia and allodynia induced by intradermal injection of capsaicin in rats, *Pain* 71(2):157, 1997.

CHAPTER 13

Management of Cervicogenic Headache

Gwendolen A. Jull

It has long been known and accepted that cervical structures, particularly those innervated by the upper three cervical nerves, have the capacity to refer pain into the head,[1] and history has long recorded the occurrence of headache of a cervical origin.[2,3] It is now considered that headaches arising from musculoskeletal disorders of the cervical spine are not rare. In context, epidemiological data indicate a 1-month prevalence for cervicogenic headache of 2.5% in the general population[4] and for migraine, a 4% prevalence.[5] Tension headache is considered the most common form with a 1-month prevalence in up to 48% of the population.[5]

The anatomical substrate for cervicogenic headache and, indeed, other headache forms is the trigeminocervical nucleus.[6] Anatomically, any nociceptive activity arising from disease or disorders of upper cervical joint structures (Occ-3), muscles innervated by the upper three cervical nerves, or the nerves themselves can access the trigeminocervical nucleus and could be responsible for headache.[6] In 1983 Sjaastad et al[7] called for the recognition and classification of a syndrome that they named *cervicogenic headache*. A decade later the term was accepted by the International Association for the Study of Pain (IASP).[8] The term *cervicogenic* was used to recognize a potential spectrum of pain sources and pathologies in the upper cervical structures responsible for headache rather than to intimate that there was a discrete structure, pathology, or pathophysiological process responsible for headache.[9,10]

The pathogenetic mechanisms of cervicogenic headache are not well understood at this time.[11] It is postulated that pain stimuli from different anatomical structures of the cervical spine join up in a 'final common pathway' that underpins the relatively homogenous response pattern of cervicogenic headache.[12] These structures may become symptom sources through a variety of means.

Even though surgical intervention has allowed the identification of purportedly relevant pathology in a few cases,[13-15] a frustration that persists is the inability to make a pathologic diagnosis in the majority of cervicogenic headache patients. This situation is well known to practitioners dealing with neck and low back pain syndromes. It is thought that the most common causes of cervicogenic headache are degenerative joint disease or trauma that is either sudden (e.g., a motor vehicle accident) or gradual (e.g., that resulting from repetitive occupational or postural strain).[10,15,16]

It is evident in reading the literature that in clinical practice there are still some difficulties in determining the differential diagnosis of the common headache forms of cervicogenic, migraine without aura, and tension headache.[17,18] Because there can be some symptomatic overlap between these types of headaches, differential diagnosis becomes difficult in certain cases. However, the causes of the three headache forms are quite different.[19]

Physical therapies such as manipulative therapy and therapeutic exercise are suitable for the management of pain syndromes, in this case cervicogenic headache, that are caused by musculoskeletal disorders. However, if physical therapy management is to be efficacious, a first vital step is to accurately recognize the cervicogenic headache patient and not apply such treatments indiscriminately to a generic headache patient. Selecting the patient for whom physical therapy treatment is relevant is one of the primary factors that will influence efficacy of treatment. The second step in this era of evidence-based practice is to use management procedures that are relevant to the physical impairment associated with the pain state and for which ideally there is evidence of effectiveness. The third step is to critically review outcomes in the treatment process and ensure that appropriate measures are being used.

This chapter focuses on these factors. It does so recognizing that the clinical picture is not black and white but instead shaded. Musculoskeletal dysfunction has been reported in tension headache and migraine,[20,21] and some therefore infer causative associations.[22,23] The headache picture can be further confused by the presence of mixed headache forms that constitute combinations of cervicogenic, tension, and migraine headaches.[24-26] Nevertheless, a principal factor in diagnosis and management is knowing whether the musculoskeletal pain and dysfunction are the primary cause of headache or merely epiphenomena to the main cause of the headache. The treatment approach and the outcome expectations of the patient and clinician will vary accordingly.

DIFFERENTIAL DIAGNOSIS

Clinical criteria are still the mainstay for diagnosis of the primary headache forms of cervicogenic headache, migraine, and tension headache because knowledge of headache pathophysiology is incomplete, a result of which is the nonavailability of simple diagnostic laboratory and instrumental tests.[9,19,27] The International Headache Society (IHS)[28] has set diagnostic criteria for the different headache forms. Much of the research done to define the syndrome of cervicogenic headache and document the diagnostic criteria has been initiated and stimulated by Sjaastad and colleagues.[7,10,29] The diagnostic criteria used in classifying cervicogenic headache are presented in Box 13-1. For comparison, the criteria for migraine without aura and episodic tension headache are presented in Table 13-1.[28] In relation to cervicogenic headache, Sjaastad et al[10] considered that, particularly for the purposes of research, certain features needed to be present. These were precipitation of attack by neck movement, awkward postures of or pressure on the upper cervical area, a positive response to an anesthetic block of the C2 or greater occipital nerve (or joint block[30-32]), and unilaterality of headache without side shift. The absence of any of these features could compromise the strength of diagnosis.

Validity of the Criteria

Recently research has been undertaken to investigate the sensitivity and specificity of Sjaastad's criteria, although these studies have not included the response to anesthetic

Box 13-1

Diagnostic Criteria for Cervicogenic Headache

Major Symptoms and Signs

1. Unilateral, bilateral (unilaterality on both sides), no sideshift
2. Signs and symptoms of neck involvement
   a. Precipitation of attacks by:
      i. Neck movements, and/or sustained awkward postures
      ii. External pressure over the ipsilateral upper cervical or occipital region
   b. Ipsilateral neck pain
   c. Reduced ROM cervical spine
3. Confirmatory evidence by diagnostic anesthetic blocks (obligatory for scientific work)
4. Headache pain characteristics
   a. Moderate, nonthrobbing, nonlancinating pain, usually starting in the neck
   b. Episodes of varying duration
   c. Fluctuating, continuous pain
5. Other characteristics of some importance
   a. Only marginal effect or lack of effect of indomethacin
   b. Only marginal effect or lack of effect of ergotamine or sumatriptan
   c. Female sex
   d. Not infrequent occurrence of head or indirect neck trauma by history, usually of more than only medium severity

Other Features of Lesser Importance

6. Various attack-related phenomena, only occasionally present, and/or moderately expressed when present
   a. Nausea
   b. Phonophobia and photophobia
   c. Dizziness
   d. Ipsilateral blurred vision
   e. Difficulty swallowing
   f. Ipsilateral edema, mostly in the periocular area

Adapted from Sjaastad O, Fredriksen TA, Pfaffenrath V: *Headache* 38:442, 1998.

blocks as one of the criteria. This approach is more relevant to clinical practice, especially to physical therapy practice in which these diagnostic techniques are not used.

Vincent and Luna[33] used the cervicogenic headache criteria published by Sjaastad et al[29] in 1990 and those published by the IHS in 1988 for migraine and tension headache[28] to diagnose 33 cervicogenic headaches, 29 episodic tension headaches, and 65 migraines without aura. They then compared the frequency of patient responses for each criterion from their records to determine the accuracy with which the criteria could distinguish between the three headache forms. Using 18 individual cervicogenic headache criteria, cervicogenic headache could be differentiated from migraine with 100% sensitivity and specificity if at least seven of the criteria were present. Seven or

Table 13-1 The IHS Classification Criteria for Migraine Without Aura and Episodic Tension Headache[28]

Migraine Without Aura	Episodic Tension Headache
1. At least five headaches fulfilling criteria 2-4	1. At least 10 previous headaches fulfilling criteria 2-4
2. Headache attacks lasting 4-72 hours	2. Headache lasting from 30 minutes to 7 days
3. Headache has at least two of the following:	3. Headache has at least two of the following pain characteristics:
a. Unilateral	a. Pressing/tightening (nonpulsating) quality
b. Pulsating quality	b. Mild to moderate intensity (may inhibit, not prohibit activity)
c. Moderate to severe intensity (limits daily activity)	c. Bilateral location
d. Aggravated by walking stairs or routine physical activity	d. No aggravation by walking stairs or similar routine physical activity
4. During the headache at least one of the following:	4. During the headache both of the following:
a. Nausea and/or vomiting	a. No nausea or vomiting (anorexia may occur)
b. Photophobia and phonophobia	b. Photophobia and phonophobia are absent or one but not the other is present
5. Other causes of headache ruled out	5. Other headache forms ruled out

From International Headache Society Classification Committee: *Cephalalgia* 8:9, 1988.

more criteria were required to differentiate cervicogenic headache from tension headache with a sensitivity of 100% and a specificity of 86.2%. In reverse, using the 11 criteria for migraine without aura, migraine could be differentiated from cervicogenic headache with 100% sensitivity and 63.6% specificity if five or more migraine criteria were present. Using the 11 tension headache criteria, tension headache could be differentiated from cervicogenic headache with 100% sensitivity and 81.8% specificity if six or more criteria for tension headache were present. Vincent and Luna[33] concluded that the criteria were adequate to distinguish the three headache forms.

Bono et al,[34] in a similar study using the criteria set of Sjaastad et al,[29] estimated that between 70% and 80% of cervicogenic headache patients have five or more of the individual criterion. Within the two studies, the more distinguishing features of cervicogenic headache were unilateral, side-locked headache and headache associated with neck postures or movements, confirming the contention of Sjaastad et al.[10]

Van Suijlekom et al[18] recently conducted a very pertinent study in which they examined interobserver reliability for the diagnostic criteria for cervicogenic headache as published by Sjaastad et al[10] in 1998. The uniqueness of the study was that it was conducted prospectively in a clinical setting in the context of a patient examination. Six physicians examined subjects. They included two expert headache neurologists, two general neurologists, and two anesthesiologists, one of whom was an expert in pain management and the other an expert in head pain management. Each physician examined the 24 patients with headache.

The headache patients consisted of equal numbers of patients previously diagnosed (using Sjaastad's and IHS criteria) as suffering from cervicogenic headache, migraine, or tension headache. Subjects were examined using a semistructured interview.

The interview comprised a series of questions compiled from the criteria for the three headache types and included those criteria that would be required to make a diagnosis of each headache form. A physical examination was included that consisted of examination of cervical movements and palpation of the upper cervical and occipital region.

Agreement on headache diagnosis between pairs of examiners varied (kappa [κ] values 0.43 and 0.83) but indicated moderate to substantial agreement. The expert neurologists had the highest agreement for the diagnosis of the three headache forms. The lower values were observed between pairs of examiners in which there was a general physician. This, the authors considered, may have reflected a more strict employment of the criteria by the specialists. When the frequency of agreement for each of the three headache forms was calculated across examiners, it was discovered that agreement was highest, and virtually the same, for migraine and cervicogenic headache (77% and 76%, respectively).

Notably, tension headache presented the most difficulty in gaining observer agreement (48%). When agreement for the items from the interview were examined, κ values varied between 0.08 and 0.76. Those for the physical examination criteria were generally lower than those for symptomatic features and ranged from 0.16 to 0.59. Agreement for the presence of motion restriction was fair (all movements combined, $\kappa = 0.33$), and for the presence of pain on motion, it was moderate (all tests combined, $\kappa = 0.51$), but the agreement for palpation for tenderness in the upper cervical and occipital region ranged from only slight to fair ($\kappa = 0.16$ to 0.33). Van Suijlekom et al[18] recognized a potential weakness of their study in that the researchers had no standardized protocol for the physical examination and they offered no training to their physicians in standard physical examination procedures. Physical therapists, with their skills in physical examination, have the capacity to heighten the accuracy even further.

The results of these studies indicate that if the cervicogenic headache criteria are applied in the clinical examination of the headache patient, the practitioner can make an accurate differential diagnosis with reasonable certainty in most cases. What is absent from these criteria is a clear and comprehensive description of the physical impairment in the cervical musculoskeletal system, which would further differentiate cervicogenic headache from headache of other causes. This is an area where physical therapy research could make a substantial contribution.

Physical Criteria for Cervical Musculoskeletal Dysfunction in Cervicogenic Headache

The problem at this current time is that there is not as yet a comprehensive set of discrete physical criteria that definitively characterize the musculoskeletal dysfunction in cervicogenic headache in the clinical setting to aid in differential diagnosis from migraine and tension headache. This is readily observed in the descriptions and criteria nominated in Sjaastad et al's criteria,[10] as well as in those of the IHS[28] and IASP.[8] The physical criteria nominated are limited, and to a large extent, many are nonspecific (Table 13-2). This is reflected in several factors, including the potential spectrum of pain sources and pathologies in the upper cervical structures that relate to the entity of cervicogenic headache.[35] As a consequence, there are various physical reactions potentially possible in the cervical neuromusculoarticular system. It also reflects the comparative scarcity of research in the area of musculoskeletal impairment in cervicogenic headache.

Reflecting the lack of documented and reliable physical signs, there has been increasing research in medical circles regarding the use of diagnostic anesthetic blocks

Table 13-2 Current Criteria for Physical Dysfunction in Headache Classifications

International Headache Society*	International Association for the Study of Pain†	Sjaastad et al‡
Resistance to or limitation of passive neck movements	Reduced range of motion in the neck	Restriction of range of movement in the neck
Changes in neck muscle contour, texture or tone or response to active stretching or contraction	—	—
Abnormal tenderness in neck muscles	—	Pressure over the ipsilateral upper cervical or occipital region that reproduces headache

*International Headache Society Classification Committee: *Cephalalgia* 8:9, 1988.
†Merskey H, Bogduk N: *Classification of chronic pain,* ed 2, Seattle, 1994, IASP Press.
‡Sjaastad O, Fredrikson TA, Pfaffenrach V: *Headache* 38:442, 1998.

of the C2, C3, and greater occipital nerves and intraarticular blocks of the upper three cervical joints.[30,36-39] Relief of headache is generally regarded as a positive diagnostic response. It is now the opinion of some that the use of these nerve or joint blocks be included in the differential diagnosis of cervicogenic headache.[10,11,40] Nevertheless, their limitations have been debated. These limitations include (1) the sensitivity and specificity of especially single blocks, (2) the validity of interpretation of results, (3) the time taken for the procedure as well as associated cost when performed under x-ray control or placebo conditions, (4) the operator skill in the diagnostic method, and (5) widespread community applicability.[9,32,41-43]

Even taking a liberal view that diagnostic blocks are a current gold standard in diagnosis of cervicogenic headache, there are still other limitations in these diagnostic methods seen from the perspective of conservative examination and management. Pearce[43] pinpoints the problem, noting that relief of pain by an anesthetic nerve block does not necessarily imply that pain stems from the nerve, only that it is transmitted by that nerve. This may not be an issue when neurotomy or neurolysis is the method of treatment.[44-46] However, for the diagnosis and treatment of the cervicogenic headache patient using conservative physical therapies, it is necessary to be able to identify the nature of impairment in musculoskeletal structures, which then links the headache to musculoskeletal dysfunction.

It is pertinent to investigate studies that have examined the physical signs in the musculoskeletal system of cervicogenic headache sufferers to clarify or add to the IHS criteria. Not only is the detection of physical impairment in a reliable way important for diagnosis, but it is also important for determining the nature of the physical impairment, which will direct the type of physical therapy treatment to be used.

Postural Form. The IHS classification[28] nominates abnormal posture as one of the findings of radiographic examination in cervicogenic headache. Precise clarification of the nature of this abnormal sign was not provided. External observation of static postural form is a routine part of a physical therapist's assessment of patients with neck pain syndromes. Janda[47] (see also Chapter 10) has detailed an examination protocol for the observation of postural form that is inclusive of surface postural angles and, in line with the IHS description, changes in muscle contours, texture, and tone. No research has been found that has investigated observed muscle signs such as changes in contour, but there have been investigations into postural angles.

A more forward head posture is the postural anomaly that has commonly been associated with neck pain and cervicogenic headache. It is believed by clinicians that alterations in spinal alignment may lead to changes in muscle activity and altered loading on articular structures, which can be a factor causing or perpetuating neck pain and headache.[47] The angle of forward head posture is an external measure and is usually derived from a photograph. It is the angle formed between a line drawn from the tragus of the ear to the C7 spinous process and the line of the horizontal plane extending from C7.[48,49]

Grimmer[50] contends, quite correctly, that there is as yet no standard for defining poor head posture. Johnson[51] found no correlation between surface measures of head and neck posture and radiological measures of the anatomical alignment of the upper cervical vertebrae, even in those subjects who, from external assessment, would have been classified with an extreme forward head posture. Therefore the relationship between the measure and mechanical implications for soft tissues in the upper cervical region would seem tenuous in light of current knowledge.

Nevertheless, several studies have measured the postural position of the head to investigate any possible association between neck pain syndromes and a forward head posture, and results do lean toward an association. Watson and Trott[52] compared chronic cervicogenic headache subjects and age-matched controls and found that the cervicogenic headache subjects had a significantly more forward head posture. Griegel-Morris et al[53] also found that a forward head posture was associated with an increased incidence of neck pain and headache. However, the severity of postural abnormality did not correlate with severity and frequency of pain.

In contrast, Treleaven et al[54] failed to find a significant association between posture in a group suffering comparatively recent-onset, persistent headaches after head trauma in which other signs of cervical dysfunction were present. Haughie et al[55] measured the forward head position and compared the angles in two subject groups classified with relatively greater and lesser cervical pain syndromes. Interestingly, when posture was measured in subjects' natural sitting posture, simulating their work at a computer, the more symptomatic group had a significantly more forward head position. However, when measured in an erect sitting position, the difference in angles between the groups disappeared. The weight of evidence would suggest some relationship between an externally observed forward head position and pain. How sensitive the sign is for the presence of cervicogenic headache and the mechanical implications of such a position are yet to be elucidated.

Articular System. Painful cervical joint dysfunction is one of the primary features of cervicogenic headache.[10,15,37,39,56-60] This is accepted even though the precise pathology may not be clearly understood[61] and radiological evidence from plain and functional movement views is equivocal.[62-65] Relevant dysfunction should present within the upper three segments (Occ-C1, C1-2, C2-3) in accordance with their access to the trigeminocervical system. The upper cervical dysfunction may be accompanied by joint dysfunction in other regions of the cervical or thoracic spines.[37,64] In some cases, headache has been related to pathology in the lower cervical region.[66-68]

The physical impairment manifested by the joint dysfunction in a basic sense is an abnormality of motion, often accompanied by pain. Restrictions of general neck movement, reflecting reactions from painful abnormalities at the segmental level, are purported to characterize cervicogenic headache.[8,10,25,28] The challenge has been to reliably identify the presence of this articular dysfunction. The two conservative physical methods of examination are assessment of range of active cervical motion with the attendant pain response and manual examination to detect symptomatic cervical segments.

Active Range of Movement. Restricted range of movement is one of the diagnostic criteria for cervicogenic headache. Zwart[69] directly addressed this criterion by measuring quantitatively (Cybex, Lumex, Inc), cervical range of movement in cervicogenic, tension, and migraine headache sufferers and a control population. The results of this study can be viewed with some confidence because there were strict inclusion criteria for the study as per the headache classification criteria of the IHS for migraine and tension headaches and Sjaastad's criteria for cervicogenic headache (including response to anesthetic blocks). Furthermore, restricted cervical motion was not included as one of the criteria for cervicogenic headache to avoid a selection bias in the population.

Zwart[69] confirmed that motion was restricted in the cervicogenic headache group and was a characteristic of this group. There was significantly less range in flexion and extension and in rotation in the cervicogenic headache group when compared to the other three groups. Lateral bending did not demonstrate this difference (Table 13-3). What is notable in this study, in which accepted inclusion criteria were used, is the lack of difference in range of movement between the control, tension headache, and migraine groups despite the mean age and length of history of headache of subjects in these groups. This does not support a primary role of musculoskeletal dysfunction in these headache forms.

Segmental Joint Dysfunction. Manual examination is a clinical method of examination used by practitioners of manipulative therapy of all disciplines to determine the presence or absence of symptomatic spinal segmental joint dysfunction. Because diagnostic anesthetic joint blocks will be used only for a select group of patients, manual examination has the potential to have an important role in differential examination of the headache patient. It is a safe, noninvasive, and inexpensive method of examination and, as such, is suitable for use in clinical examination.

Manual examination has been used in a number of studies to detect the presence or absence of symptomatic upper cervical joint dysfunction to identify the cervicogenic headache subject or to identify cervical dysfunction in headache patients.[21,70-74]

Table 13-3 Population Characteristics and Measures of Cervical Motion

Diagnosis	Number of Subjects (M:F)	Mean Age (yr) (SD)	Mean Duration (yr)	Mean Rotation Degrees (SD)	Mean Flexion/Extension Degrees (SD)	Mean Lateral Flex Degrees (SD)
Cervicogenic	28 (7:21)	42.0 (8.8)	7.9	146 (23.4)	107 (17.6)	86 (12.9)
Migraine	28 (8:20)	39.5 (10.4)	13.4	174 (16.6)	133 (19.9)	91 (14.2)
Tension	34 (16:18)	38.0 (11.7)	10.4	168 (17.2)	127 (19.6)	91 (12.8)
Controls	51 (29:22)	42.8 (16.7)	—	170 (22.1)	129 (17.9)	94 (17.9)

Modified from Zwart JA: *Headache* 37:6, 1997.
SD, Standard deviation.

This method is still viewed with skepticism by some as being a very subjective exercise.[42] Indeed, there is no argument against calls for further investigation of its role as a diagnostic method in the examination of headache.[9]

Many of the controversial issues surrounding manual examination, and what it measures, can be side-stepped if a more robust question is asked; namely, can assessment by manual examination accurately detect and differentiate between symptomatic and dysfunctional spinal segments and asymptomatic segments? In this light, spinal manual examination can be regarded as a discrete pain provocative test. There have been several studies that have investigated the accuracy of manual examination in regard to detecting the presence or absence of painful cervical zygapophyseal joint dysfunction in which provoked tenderness was a criterion in the decision making. In one pivotal study, diagnoses determined by manual examination by a manipulative physical therapist was tested against diagnoses made by diagnostic anesthetic nerve or joint blocks in neck pain and headache patients.[75] Results indicated that manual examination performed by the examiner had a 100% sensitivity and specificity in identifying whether the patient's neck or neck and headache pain syndrome was related to a painful cervical zygapophyseal joint arthropathy.

In another controlled study, manual examination was used to identify whether painful zygapophyseal joint dysfunction was present in subjects with postconcussional headache for whom a cervical cause was postulated.[54,76] Examiner and subjects agreed to the presence and location of painful joints with an accuracy of 94%. In a further single blind study, Gijsberts et al[77] examined the intertherapist reliability between three pairs of manual therapists. Their task was to detect the presence or absence of painful joint dysfunction in a cohort of 105 headache subjects, 38 of whom were subsequently diagnosed as having cervicogenic headaches through a questionnaire (as per criteria of the IHS and Sjaastad). Intertherapist reliability was shown to be fair to good (Intraclass correlation coefficients [ICCs] 0.67 to 0.88). The provoked pain also accurately distinguished the cervicogenic headache group from the other types of headache. A further intertherapist study indicated excellent to complete agreement between pairs of physical therapists in regard to differentiating cervicogenic headache patients from nonheadache control subjects.[78]

In a related study, Schoensee et al[73] tested the intertherapist reliability for decisions made as a result of the examination of the upper three cervical segments in five cervicogenic headache subjects and revealed that reliability was good ($\kappa = 0.79$).

Thus evidence is accumulating that supports the potentially important role of manual examination in the differential diagnosis of headache. Upper cervical joint dysfunction is one of the primary impairments thought to be pathognomonic of cervicogenic headache. Further research is required to test the sensitivity and specificity of manual spinal joint examination in the differential diagnosis of different headache forms based on the detection of relevant joint dysfunction.

Muscle System. The IHS[28] diagnostic criteria for muscle dysfunction in cervicogenic headache are expressed in general terms (Table 13-2). It is appropriate to review studies that have investigated the muscle system and to seek any evidence of more specific impairments that may characterize cervicogenic headache.

Muscle Tenderness. The presence of tender points or trigger points in muscles has been investigated in cervicogenic headache, migraine, and tension headache, as well as in asymptomatic populations.[21,71,79-84] Bovim[79] compared muscle tenderness in the three headache forms. Pressure pain thresholds (PPTs) were measured at 10 points on the cranium, especially over the temporalis muscle and occipital and suboccipital region. In contrast to other studies,[83] Bovim[79] found that when PPTs from all sites were summed, the scores for the cervicogenic headache group were significantly lower than those for tension and migraine headache subjects and control subjects. This might indicate that specific tender points in muscles could be used in differential diagnosis. However, although the results were not uniform, the occipital part of the head on the symptomatic side did exhibit the lowest PPTs. This potential sign has not been documented in other studies of cervicogenic headache which Jaeger,[71] for example, reported findings more often in the temporalis muscle with only a 30% incidence in posterior cervical muscles.

Muscle tenderness and trigger points in muscles are likely to be present in cervicogenic headache subjects, but the sign has little specificity in relation to diagnosis. What is still debatable is whether this muscle tenderness represents a specific primary hyperalgesia[85] or, more likely, a secondary hyperalgesia perpetuated by either a peripheral cervical nociceptive source or a centrally sensitized state in the trigeminocervical system.[86] Indeed, the relative roles of central and peripheral mechanisms in the perception of pain and other associated symptoms in cervicogenic headache continues to be debated.[87,88]

Muscle Length. Research into the prevalence of muscle tightness in cervicogenic headache is sparse. This probably reflects the difficulty in gaining true quantitative measures representing the length of selected muscles in the cervicothoracic region. Two studies have used conventional clinical tests of muscle length to assess those muscles purported, clinically, to be prone to developing tightness—the upper trapezius, levator scapulae, scalene, and upper cervical extensor muscle groups.[47] Limitations of the subjective nature of the tests were recognized. Jull et al[89] compared responses in 15 subjects with cervicogenic headache with those of 15 asymptomatic age- and gender-matched control subjects, whereas Treleaven et al[54] examined 12 subjects with postconcussional headache with signs of cervical joint dysfunction and compared them with asymptomatic control subjects. The results of both studies revealed that muscle tightness could be present in the headache groups, but it was not exclusive to those groups.

Normal responses to stretch were reported in many of the muscles examined in both headache and control groups in each study. Abnormal findings were more prevalent in the headache groups, but in both studies, this failed to reach significance. The exception was the upper trapezius muscle in the study by Jull et al,[89] which might provide clinical support for the findings of heightened electrical activity (measured by electromyography [EMG]) in the upper trapezius muscle in cervicogenic headache sufferers found by Bansevicius and Sjaastad.[90]

It would seem that the presence of muscle tightness may be found in cervicogenic headache sufferers, but this impairment is not necessarily present in all patients. More research needs to be undertaken into the prevalence and relevance of abnormal response to stretch, although the initial results of these studies suggest that muscle length would not be a powerful discriminating feature for cervicogenic headache.

Muscle Contraction. Muscles will react in response to joint pain and dysfunction, and these responses are readily appreciated in the extremity joints, where they are often visible. Deficits in muscle performance have been identified in cervicogenic headache patients. Placzek et al[91] examined the strength of contraction in flexion and extension of 10 women with chronic headache. The authors made a presumption of cervical involvement in these chronic headache subjects, but no attempt was made to include subjects on the basis of any recognized criteria for cervicogenic headache. They did, however, detect restricted cervical motion in this group, suggesting at least a cervical component. Noting this deficit, results revealed that neck flexor and extensor strengths were significantly reduced in the headache group as compared to an asymptomatic control group.

The consideration of muscle strength is one feature of muscle function, but such measures may simplify the complex interactions required of the cervical muscle system in normal activities. With the number of muscles in the craniocervicoaxial region, as well as their intricate morphology, it is not surprising that the head-neck region is thought to be the most complex neuromechanical system in the body.[92]

The flexible cervical column must function to allow appropriate head movements in three dimensions in space, to maintain mechanical stability of the head-neck system at a given orientation, and to distribute load from the weight of the head, as well as from intrinsic and extrinsic loads of the upper limb function. To add to the complexity, the muscle system of the neck is intimately related to reflex systems concerned with stabilization of the head and the eyes, vestibular function, and proprioceptive systems that serve not only local needs but also the needs for postural orientation and stability of the whole body.[92-94] Therefore the cervical spine presents a multisegmental, multimuscle complex that is required to switch its control operations between intrinsic kinetic and mechanical demands and proprioceptive reflexes and vestibulocollic reflexes and still achieve an appropriate coordinated response.[94]

Muscle interactions are complex, and often a single muscle may perform multiple tasks.[95] Most of the research on the patterns of neck muscle behavior during orientating and stabilizing activities has been performed on animal models. Knowledge of how this integrated function is achieved in humans is limited in main part because of the ethical limitations of invasive procedures such as insertion of fine wires into multiple and deep muscles of the neck.[96] This has limited EMG experiments to superficial muscles in the main, and much remains uncertain. Nevertheless, such studies have shown that movement is produced and controlled by complex patterns of muscle action involving various muscle synergies.[93,96-101]

In recent times there has been interest in how the muscle system controls and supports the spine. In relation to spinal stabilization, a functional although interdependent division has been proposed between the superficial, more multisegmental muscles and the deeper muscle layers.[102-104] It is considered that control of spinal orientation is more reliant on the superficial multisegmental muscles, whereas the deep muscles have a greater role in control of the segmental relationships (i.e., segmental control).

Clinical research has been conducted in low back pain patients in whom specific deficits have been found in the muscle system, one of the primary impairments being in the deep muscles of the trunk and abdomen.[105,106] There is evidence that the deep muscles react to pain and injury with inhibition or altered patterns of recruitment and that their interaction with the more superficial muscles of their functional group may be altered.[105-107] The problems therefore appear to be related more to those of neuromuscular control within and between groups rather than only general strength of the whole group.

Although there is no question that all muscles contribute to head and neck stabilization and control, evidence is now emerging that an analogous situation may exist in the neck in deep and superficial muscle interactions in relation to spinal control and support (Figure 13-1). This model makes a division that may oversimplify some complex interactions between various neck muscles. Nevertheless, there is evidence to support the basic model.

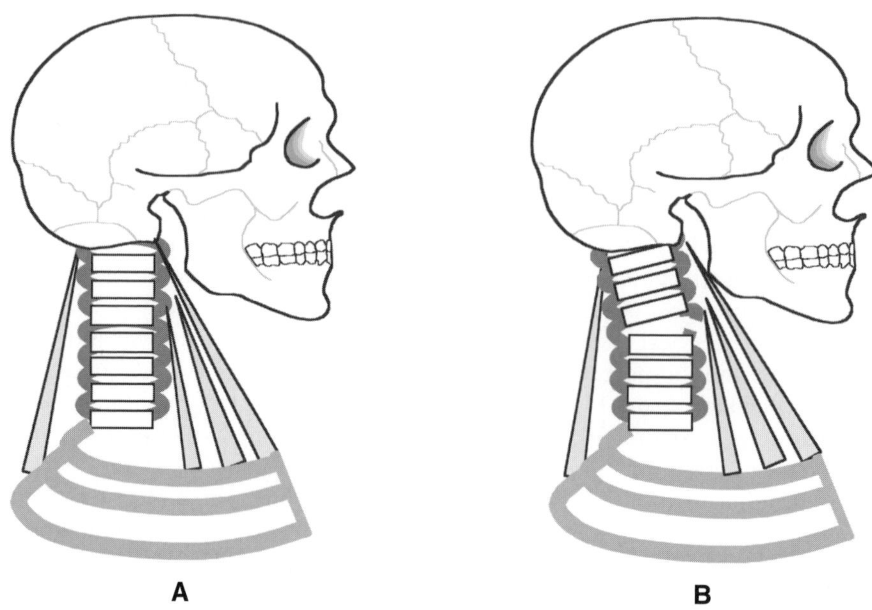

Figure 13-1
A, A schematic model that depicts the role of the deep muscles with their segmental attachments for segmental control and the role of the more superficial muscles that span the region for control of spinal orientation. **B,** The cervical segment may lose functional active support even in the presence of normally functioning superficial muscles.

There is growing recognition of the importance of the deep cervical flexor and extensor muscles in providing spinal segmental support and control.[92] Several authors have identified the particular role of the deep neck flexors, including longus capitus and longus colli, in this function of postural and segmental control.[108-110] These muscles also are important in the support of the spinal curve against bending moments caused by the contraction of the extensors and in the compression forces induced by the load of the head.[92,111]

There is evidence that these deep cervical flexors lose their endurance capacity in cervicogenic headache patients.[52,70,89] Concomitant with this is the evidence that there is muscle fiber transformation in the direction of type1 (tonic) fibers to type 2 (phasic) fibers in subjects with neck disorders irrespective of the nature of the pathology.[112,113] The transition occurs first in the neck flexors.[114] Problems also have been identified in the dorsal neck muscles. Hallgren et al[115] and McPartland et al[116] used magnetic resonance imaging to detect atrophy and fatty infiltration in the deep suboccipital extensors in patients with chronic neck pain. This distinguished the chronic neck pain patients from asymptomatic subjects.

The challenge has been to develop clinically applicable tests to detect this deep flexor and extensor muscle dysfunction. Progress has been made with the flexor muscles. A low-load craniocervical flexion test has been developed to assess a patient's ability to perform in a staged manner—a slow and controlled upper cervical flexion action (the anatomical action of longus capitus and colli)—and hold progressively inner range positions (Figure 13-2). This test has been used to examine subjects with

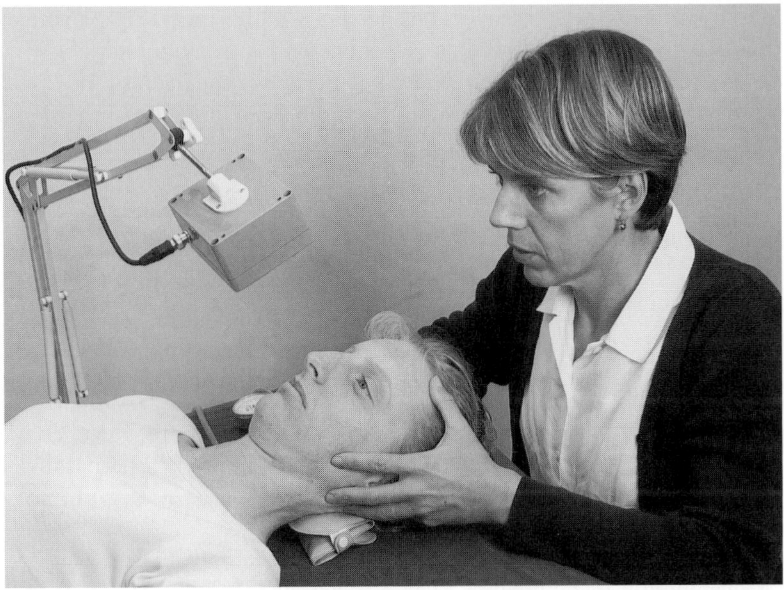

Figure 13-2
The craniocervical flexion test is conducted in the supine lying position. This action of the deep flexors is tested under low-load conditions to reflect the muscles' tonic function and to discourage unwanted recruitment of synergistic flexors that would be predicted in high-load tests. Because the target muscles are deep and cannot be palpated directly, an indirect method is used to gain some quantification of performance. An inflatable air-filled pressure sensor (Stabilizer, Chattanooga) is positioned suboccipitally behind the neck to monitor the subtle flattening of the cervical curve, which occurs with the action of longus colli. It is pre-inflated to 20 mm Hg, and in the test, patients are required to slowly perform craniocervical flexion to progressively target pressure increases of 2 mm Hg from 22 to 30 mm Hg. At each level, the ability to target the pressure and hold the position for at least 5 seconds is monitored and performance judged by the pressure level achieved with a slow and controlled action. Unwanted contributions from the superficial neck flexors that anatomically do not perform this action are measured with surface EMG or monitored clinically by palpation of onset of superficial muscle contraction. (See the Appendix for a detailed description.)

cervicogenic headache and subjects with persistent neck pain syndromes after a whiplash injury.[89,117] Both studies revealed significantly inferior performances in the symptomatic groups compared to asymptomatic control subjects.

The symptomatic subjects were less able to control the craniocervical flexion action and achieved pressure levels significantly lower than their asymptomatic counterparts. Furthermore, when EMG was included in the measurements, symptomatic subjects used their superficial flexors at significantly higher levels in attempts to achieve target pressures.[117] Thus the test appears to detect poorer motor control in the neck flexor synergy in symptomatic subjects, the increased coactivation of the superficial neck flexors being a likely compensation for reduced deep neck flexor function.

This research has identified a specific impairment in the muscle system linked to cervicogenic headache subjects and directs a specific approach in rehabilitation.

Research to investigate the sensitivity and specificity of this muscle impairment for the differential diagnosis of cervicogenic headache is currently underway.

Clinical tests have yet to be developed specifically for the deep suboccipital extensors. In light of the findings of atrophy in these muscles in neck pain patients,[115,116] there can be some reasoned expectation that there will be dysfunction in the cervicogenic headache patient.

In line with the joint and muscle dysfunction in cervical pain syndromes, there is growing evidence of kinesthetic deficits accompanying injury and degenerative disease.[116,118-120] The role of the cervical muscles, and particularly the deep upper cervical extensor muscles, as dynamic proprioceptors is well known. It is likely that there is a close relationship between the deep muscles' role in joint support and in neck kinesthesia. It has been shown that comparatively simple tests of cervical kinesthesia can sensitively detect deficits in reposition sense in neck pain patients that is not evident in asymptomatic control subjects.[118-120] Furthermore, Revel et al[121] were able to demonstrate that after training, improvement in kinesthesia paralleled a decrease in neck pain, indicating that the measure was related to symptomology and sensitive to change.

The other muscle dysfunction that has been linked clinically to cervical pain syndromes is dysfunction in the axioscapular muscles.[47,122] The importance of scapular stability and the correct transference of loads from upper limb function to the axial skeleton are well recognized, as is the need for appropriate scapular movement and control in relation to glenohumeral joint dysfunction.[123-126] In respect to the cervical spine, poor function in the scapular stability synergy can change load distribution to the axial skeleton. It is considered that poor postural function of muscles such as the serratus anterior and lower and middle fibers of the trapezius may be associated with altered scapular position. Compensatory increased activity in muscles, such as levator scapulae, which, with its suspension from the cervical region, may increase loads on cervical joints.[47,127] No research could be found that specifically addressed this occurrence in cervicogenic headache, but clinical experience would support the relative common finding of poor scapular control and poor tonic capacity of muscles such as the serratus anterior and the middle to lower portions of the trapezius in static and dynamic postural function.

Neural Structures. Direct physical compromise of neural structures can contribute to the pathogenesis of some cervicogenic headaches, and nerves may become physically painful. Greater occipital nerve and C2 root allodynia may be present in cervicogenic headache,[9,10] and Sjaastad et al[10] rate this sign with some significance. Nevertheless, the sensitivity of the sign and indeed the accuracy with which allodynic nerves can be differentiated from other myofascial and articular structures in the occipital, suboccipital region has been challenged.[6,43,128]

Cervicogenic headache is principally recognized as a *referred pain*,[6] but a neurogenic origin from physical compromise of the upper cervical nerve roots or the dorsal root ganglion and the greater occipital nerve has been recorded in a few case reports of cervicogenic headache subjects. Those identified surgically include (1) fibrosis of the greater occipital nerve in its course before its perforation through the tendinous lamina of the upper trapezius muscle, (2) spondylitic changes or scar tissues around the nerve root, and (3) compression of the C2 root by vascular structures.[13,14,129-132]

The dura mater of the upper cervical cord and the posterior cranial fossa receives innervation from branches of the upper three cervical nerves[6] and is capable of being one of the causes of cervicogenic headache. Pearce[133] contends that a feasible hypothesis for headache associated with spondylotic changes in the disc or zygapophyseal joints in the older age group could be nociceptive stimuli caused by irritation of the pain-sensitive dura in the upper cervical region. Recent years have seen a particular interest by physical therapists in this role of neural structures as a pain source in craniocervicobrachial syndromes when they are sensitized or their free movement is compromised by pathology or the pathological process.[134]

Case reports have been published claiming association of cervicogenic headache with pain-provocative mechanical tests of dural movement,[135] but the frequency of this occurrence and the accuracy of the claims have yet to be substantiated. Nevertheless, anatomical studies have demonstrated fibrous connections between the rectus capitus posterior minor and the cervical dura mater,[136] and continuity has been observed between the ligamentum nuchae and the posterior spinal dura at the first and second cervical levels.[137] Such connections indicate the mechanical interdependence of neural, ligamentous, and muscular structures in movements and postures of the upper cervical spine.

Cervical muscle reactivity has been demonstrated with noxious stimulation of cervical meningeal tissues.[138] Therefore it is feasible that the pathomechanics of the upper cervical region in cervicogenic headache could, in some cases, involve the upper cervical dura mater.

In the clinical setting, the movement of upper cervical flexion is used in attempts to identify such involvement.[139] Restriction of motion and pain provoked by this test movement could implicate the cervical dura or articular and muscular structures, which also are stressed by the test. Structural differentiation is attempted clinically with selective pretensioning of neural structures from a caudal source, either with the legs prepositioned in a straight leg raise or the arms in a position that tensions the brachial plexus.[134,140] The sensitivity of the clinical test and the prevalence of involvement of the cervical dura in cervicogenic headache are unknown.

Status of Diagnostic Criteria

Cervicogenic headache has been well characterized symptomatically, but the differential diagnosis could be enhanced further with the availability of more discrete indicators of the musculoskeletal impairment. Such indicators would assist clinicians to differentiate cervicogenic headache from other common headache forms of migraine and tension headache and also would facilitate reasonable estimates of cervical musculoskeletal contributions to mixed headache forms.

Box 13-2 tries to define more precisely the physical impairments that might characterize cervicogenic headache. It is based on the research to date but also contains impairments that could reasonably be expected to be present but are yet to be researched in the cervicogenic headache patient. Perhaps an equally important need for such criteria is in directing relevant and research-based physical therapy interventions. The quantification of these impairments are ideal outcomes for both clinical practice and research because it would test both the efficacy of the interventions on the physical impairments and the relationship between improvement in these impairments and improvement in the cervicogenic headache syndrome.

Box 13-2

Proposed Musculoskeletal Signs to Characterize Cervicogenic Headache

Major and Mandatory Signs

Reduced range of neck movement with or without associated neck pain

Joint pain and dysfunction in the upper cervical joints

Dysfunction in the neck flexor synergy, implicating the deep muscles

Dysfunction in the neck extensor synergy, implicating the deep suboccipital muscles

Dysfunction in the scapular muscle stabilizing synergy

Global strength deficits in neck musculature

Kinesthetic deficits

Other Clinical Signs That May Be Present

Forward head posture

Poor postural control

Tightness in selected axioscapular muscles

Muscle trigger or tender points

Mechanosensitivity of neural structures

TREATMENT OF CERVICOGENIC HEADACHE

The treatments documented for cervicogenic headache are manifold. In the conservative area, headache has been managed with pharmaceutical agents (simple analgesics and nonsteroidal antiinflammatory drugs [NSAIDs])[9,11,141,142] or with a variety of physical therapies, including manipulative therapy, traction, trigger point therapy, muscle stretching, cold packs, heat packs, and transcutaneous electrical stimulation.[70,74,143-146] Cognitive behavioral programs also have been trialed.[80] In addition, there are a variety of medical and surgical procedures being used in management, including anesthetic blocks to muscle trigger points, joints, and nerves; percutaneous radiofrequency neurotomies; radiofrequency therapy to the external surface of the occipital bone; and C2 ganglionectomy and surgical decompression or fusion.*

This array of treatments may reflect the spectrum of pathologies and physical reactions that might present in the cervicogenic headache syndrome. They may mirror the characterized progression of the disorder[8] for which, with time and disability level, more radical surgical interventions may be warranted for some patients.[11] The variety of treatments also may reflect the limited understanding that still exists about

*References 14, 44, 46, 57, 80, 142, 147, 148.

the pathophysiology and the nature of the physical dysfunction and impairments present in cervicogenic headache. The bias of the practitioner treating the cervicogenic headache sufferer also will likely have an influence. Whatever the reasons, and there are doubtless many, the situation reflects that the optimal treatment or treatment schema for cervicogenic headache is unknown at this time.

Sjaastad et al[11] recently reviewed the therapies for cervicogenic headache. They present the possible therapies in a hierarchical order. These begin with the most uncomplicated measures inclusive of physical therapy, NSAIDs or mild analgesics, the use of repeated (e.g., weekly) injections of local anesthetics, with or without corticosteroids, into the greater or lesser occipital nerves and progress to the more invasive procedures. Sjaastad et al[11] list approximately 20 different surgical techniques that have been used for the management of cervicogenic headache and suggest that these treatment alternatives are expanding.

Despite the burgeoning increase in surgical procedures, it is advocated that conservative therapies should be the treatment of choice for the vast majority of cervicogenic headache sufferers.[9] Nevertheless, there is a paucity of research investigating the effectiveness of conservative therapies for cervicogenic headache, even though formal criteria for the headache form were described by Sjaastad et al in 1989.[7] Table 13-4 presents summaries of the studies and reports found in the English literature since Sjaastad's classification that have specifically addressed the management of the cervicogenic headache syndrome by physical therapies. These included subjects on the basis of either the IHS description[28] or Sjaastad's criteria.[7,29] Two reports are included in the table that did not formally use these criteria, but their intention was clearly to treat dysfunction of the cervical spine as the primary cause of headache.[72,146] The type of treatment, dosages, and outcomes of each of the studies are detailed in the table. (There have been other studies of the efficacy of physical therapies for headache, but these addressed other headache forms such as migraine or tension headache, or the headache form was not specified.[22,23,149-153]) The studies in Table 13-4 provide some indication that physical therapies could have some effect on cervicogenic headache, but the quantity and quality of research preclude definitive conclusions, and follow-up periods, in the main, have been in the short term. There is an obvious need for more research in this area.

Manipulative therapy dominates as the conservative physical therapy investigated for the management of cervicogenic headache. Manipulative therapy will address the upper cervical joint pain and dysfunction that is a primary impairment in the syndrome. However, as suggested in Box 13-2, other impairments, particularly those in the muscle system, have been linked to cervicogenic headache. The management of cervicogenic headache needs to be broadened to include management of these other factors because there is no evidence or guarantee that there will be spontaneous recovery of the muscle dysfunction. Furthermore, any exercise program should be designed to address the impairments in the muscle system that have been identified in cervicogenic headache. A management program based on the identified impairments in the musculoskeletal system in cervicogenic headache is outlined in Box 13-3.

The program addresses the potential impairments in each system. It is inclusive of manipulative therapy as a treatment of the joint pain and dysfunction. There is initial evidence of the efficacy of this treatment approach. The goal of the exercise program is to reverse the proven impairments in the deep and supporting muscle system to enhance joint support and control. It is based on the principles of training for the restoration of active segmental stabilization.[154]

In contrast to conventional exercise interventions, this program focuses on using specific low-load exercises to target and retrain the activation and tonic endurance ca-

Text continued on p. 260

Table 13-4 Studies on the Treatment of Cervicogenic Headache by Physical Therapies

Authors	Criteria	Design	Number of Subjects	Interventions	Treatment Period	Outcome Measures	Results Population Means
Nilsson et al[145*]	IHS	RCT	53 (28)	Group 1: Manipulation (toggle recoil, upper cervical, diverse techniques, low cervical spine)	3 wks 2 Tx/wk	HA duration (hr/day)	Pre Tx – Post Tx Group 1 = 5.2 – 2.0 Group 2 = 4.0 – 2.4
			(25)	Group 2: Low-level laser to upper cervical region (sham)		HA intensity (VAS, 100-point scale)	Group 1 = 44 – 28 Group 2 = 41 – 36
				Deep frictions to low cervical and upper thoracic regions (including trigger points)		No. analgesics/day	Group 1 = 1.5 – 0.8 Group 2 = 1.0 – 0.7
Jensen et al[72]	Posttraumatic headache with cervical spine signs	RCT	19 (10)	Group 1: Manipulative therapy (manipulation, mobilization and muscle energy techniques)	4 wks 2 Tx total	HA intensity (mean % of baseline)	PreTx-PostTx-FU (4 wks) Group 1 = 100 – 43 – 84 Group 2 = 100 – 108 – 107
			(9)	Group 2: Cold packs		Presence of associated symptoms (mean % of baseline)	Group 1 = 100 – 52 – 90 Group 2 = 100 – 90 – 88 (approx)
						Analgesic use (mean % of baseline)	Group 1 = 100 – 36 – 100 Group 2 = 100 – 100 – 80
Schoensee et al[73]	IHS	Single case studies A-B-A	10	Passive mobilization Occ-3 (Maitland, Paris)	4-5 wks	HA frequency (days)	PreTx-PostTx 2.9 – 1.0
					2-3 Tx/wk	HA duration (hours)	5.4 – 3.4
					total 9 – 11	HA intensity (VAS, 10-point scale)	3.4 – 1.6

							PreTx-Tx-FU (6 wks)
Beeton and Jull[70]	IHS	Single case study A-B-A	1	Passive mobilization (Maitland)	6 wks	HA frequency (days)	5 − 6 − 1 (No. in 6 wks)
						HA intensity (VAS)	2.5 − 1.9 − 2.5
				Low-load exercise program for deep and postural muscles (Jull)	10 Tx total	*Physical assessments	
						Posture CV angle	51.5 − 53.6 − 51.8
						ROM (total LF)	91 − 104 − 117
						LC1-2 motion	mod − sl − sl hypo
						Muscle length scalenes	mod tight-sl-normal
						Deep neck flexor, 10-sec holds	3 − 10 − 10
						Headlift test endurance	21 − 55 − 105
						Scapular holding test	Improved
							PreTx-PostTx-4 wk FU
Martelletti et al[144]	Sjaastad et al[29]	Case series	36	Manipulative therapy (diverse techniques)	4 wks	Total pain index (HA freq,intens, dur)	6 − 1 − 1 (approx)
				Medication as required	3 Tx/wk	Drug intake index	3 −1 − 1 (approx)
							PreTx − Tx − Post Tx
Whittingham et al[74]	Unilateral HA with joint signs Occ-C1, C1-2	Case series	26	Toggle recoil technique C1	2 wks	HA duration (hr)†	110.1 − 54.4 − 25.0
					2 Tx/wk	HA intensity† (VAS 6-point scale)	55.5 − 33.4 − 22.8
	Sjaastad part criteria					HA frequency (days)†	18.7 − 11.4 − 7.1

IHS, International Headache Society, RCT, random controlled trial; *HA*, headache; *PreTx*, before treatment; *PostTx*, after treatment; *VAS*, Visual Analog Scale; *FU*, follow up; *ROM*, range of motion; *LF*, lateral flexion; *freq,intens,dur*, frequency, intensity, duration.

*Sample results only are included.

†Scores for each factor were summed for all subjects over 2-week periods.

Continued

Table 13-4 Studies on the Treatment of Cervicogenic Headache by Physical Therapies—cont'd

Authors	Criteria	Design	Number of Subjects	Interventions	Treatment Period	Outcome Measures	Results Population Means
Vernon[146]	Headache neck pain and dysfunction	Case reports	3	Manipulation	4-8 wks (includes FU period)	HA intensity (VAS 10-point scale)	*PreTx – FU* 10 – 0
					5-8	Medication use	Stopped all medication use PreTx-PostTx 2.25-6 yr FU
Jaeger[71]	Sjaastad et al[7] Active myofascial triggers, upper cervical joint signs	Case series	11	Passive mobilization (Maitland, Grieve) Postural awareness Spray and stretch exercises Moist heat Relaxation training Cognitive skills training	6 wks (?)	HA intensity (VAS 100 point scale)	54 – 8 (approx)* (effect maintained at FU)
						MPQ (4 subscales analyzed)	Sensory 16–4 (approx) Affective 3-0 (approx) (effect maintained)
						HA frequency per month (5 subjects)	6.8-1.4-2.25
Graff-Radford et al[80]	Chronic neck pain/ headache with active myofascial triggers, upper cervical joint signs	Case series	25	Passive mobilization (Maitland, Grieve) Postural awareness Spray and stretch exercises Moist heat Relaxation training Cognitive skills training	6 wks (?)	HA intensity (VAS 100 point scale)	*PreTx – PostTx-3,6,12 month FU* 52.5 – 3.8* (effect maintained through the 12 m FU)
						MPQ (four subscales analyzed)	Sensory 12-4 (approx) Affective 2-0 (approx) (effect maintained)
				Medication		Medication intake (index)	89.5% reduction (effect maintained)
Farina et al[143]	Sjaastad et al[7]	Case series	10	Transcutaneous nerve stimulation	10 days	HA index (not described)	*PreTx – PostTx* 2 subjects 40%-60% relief
					Daily	2-month mean	8 subjects > 60% relief

Box 13-3

A Management Program for Cervicogenic Headache

Articular Dysfunction

Manipulative therapy

Therapeutic exercise to restore muscle control of cervical segments

Muscle Dysfunction

Reeducation of neuromuscular control of the deep neck flexors and flexor synergy: training and assessment using the pressure biofeedback unit; aim to achieve holding capacity at 28 or 30 mm Hg without dominant activity in the superficial neck flexors as an outcome of training

Scapular control: retraining of the serratus anterior and lower trapezius, in relative isolation in the first instance, incorporating exercises into postural control and functional activities

Postural reeducation: correction through pelvic position to upright neutral position, plus control of scapular position

Cocontraction exercises: training in the correct sitting posture, use of rotation for cocontraction of neck flexors and extensors (note 10% to 20% MVC)

Muscle-lengthening exercises if necessary

Reeducation of movement patterns: cervical flexion pattern on return from extension, training in the prone position resting on elbows and progression to sitting

Kinesthetic retraining: exercises to retrain joint position sense

Neural System

Treatment of joint dysfunction first to assess effect on neural system

Gentle mobilization of neural system, Note that positions for deep neck flexor and scapular muscle retraining may have to be modified if neural system is sensitized

Ergonomics

Correction of work practices; work environment, most important component of management

Patient must practice postural correction and control preventatively in sedentary postures

Effective Home Program

Patient participation in treatment essential, taking responsibility for self-management

Outcome Measures

Critical evaluation of effectiveness of management; knowledge of effect in the long term essential; use of outcome tools for headache intensity, frequency, and duration and quantifiable measures of physical impairments

MVC, Maximum voluntary contraction.

pacity of the deep neck and shoulder girdle muscles in line with their functional requirements of support of the cervical joints. (See the Appendix at the end of this chapter for specific details of the neck flexor training.) It is a process of reeducation of muscle control to retrain the appropriate interaction between the superficial and deep muscle layers to facilitate their supporting role in both static and dynamic function. The involvement of the patient in the management program is emphasized, as is the need for suitable outcome measures. This treatment approach has recently been evaluated in a randomized controlled trial.[155] Results of the trial indicate the effectiveness of the program and, most important, gains from treatment were maintained over the 12-month follow-up period.

There is yet another issue to be considered in treatment. Although conservative treatment may be advocated as the treatment of choice for cervicogenic headache, it should be recognized that there are some pathologies associated with cervicogenic headache that, either by their nature or magnitude, may be beyond the realms of conservative care and may require surgical management. For example, there are documented case series of patients who had unremitting and severe neck pain and headache after cervical trauma and who were not responsive to conservative care but did respond to more radical radiofrequency neurotomy.[156] A further example could be those cervicogenic headaches resulting from compression of the C2 root by vascular structures.[14,129-131] How this small group of patients is recognized definitively is a matter of debate.[157,158] However, the challenge for clinicians and researchers is ultimately to have criteria that will identify the cervicogenic headache sufferer most likely to be responsive to conservative care.

CONCLUSION

Cervicogenic headache is being recognized increasingly as a distinct headache syndrome. Diagnostic criteria have been set and their sensitivity and specificity established. Use of these criteria, along with performance of a precise physical examination, will ensure correct selection of the headache patient most suitable for physical therapies rather than simply applying such therapies in a nondiscriminatory manner to any persons with headache. Knowledge of the precise nature of the physical impairment in the cervical spine linked to cervicogenic headache is increasing, and with this new knowledge comes the ability to apply the most relevant treatment methods. The evidence base for the effectiveness of conservative care needs further development, and part of this development must be the establishment of clear indications of the cervicogenic headache sufferers who are likely to be responsive to physical therapies. This will be achieved through careful documentation of outcomes, both in the clinical and the research arenas.

References

1. Feinstein B, Langton JNK, Jameson RM, Schiller F: Experiments on referred pain from deep somatic tissues, *J Bone Joint Surg* 36A:981, 1954.
2. Bartschi-Rochaix W: Headaches of cervical origin. In Vinben PJ, Bruyn GW, editors: *Handbook of clinical neurology*, vol 5, Amsterdam, 1968, North Holland Publishing.
3. Hunter CR, Mayfield FH: Role of the upper cervical roots in the production of pain in the head, *Am J Surg* 78:743, 1949.
4. Nilsson N: The prevalence of cervicogenic headache in a random population sample of 20- to 59-year-olds, *Spine* 20:1884, 1995.

5. Rasmussen BK, Jensen R, Schroll M, Olesen J: Epidemiology of headache in a general population: a prevalence study, *J Clin Epidemiol* 44:1147, 1991.
6. Bogduk N: Anatomy and physiology of headache, *Biomed Pharmacother* 49:435, 1995.
7. Sjaastad O, Saunte C, Hovdahl H et al: "Cervicogenic" headache: an hypothesis, *Cephalalgia* 3:249, 1983.
8. Merskey H, Bogduk N: *Classification of chronic pain*, ed 2, Seattle, 1994, IASP Press.
9. Pollmann W, Keidel M, Pfaffenrath V: Headache and the cervical spine: a critical review, *Cephalalgia* 17:801, 1997.
10. Sjaastad O, Fredriksen TA, Pfaffenrath V: Cervicogenic headache: diagnostic criteria, *Headache* 38:442, 1998.
11. Sjaastad O, Fredriksen TA, Stolt-Nielsen A et al: Cervicogenic headache: a clinical review with a special emphasis on therapy, *Funct Neurol* 12:305, 1997.
12. Pfaffenrath V: Cervical headache, *Cephalalgia* 15:334, 1995 (editorial).
13. Hildebrandt J, Jansen J: Vascular compression of the C2 and C3 roots: yet another cause of chronic intermittent hemicrania, *Cephalalgia* 4:167, 1984.
14. Pikus HJ, Philips JM: Outcome of surgical decompression of the second cervical root for cervicogenic headache, *Neurosurg* 39:63, 1996.
15. Trevor-Jones R: Osteoarthritis of the paravertebral joints of the second and third cervical vertebrae as a cause of occipital headache, *S Afr Med J* 38:392, 1964.
16. Bogduk N: Cervical causes of headache, *Cephalalgia* 9:172, 1989.
17. Niere K: Can subjective characteristics of benign headache predict manipulative physiotherapy treatment outcome? *Aust J Physiother* 44:87, 1998.
18. van Suijlekom HA, de Vet HC, van den Berg SG, Weber WE: Interobserver reliability of diagnostic criteria for cervicogenic headache, *Cephalalgia* 19:817, 1999.
19. Lance JW: *Mechanism and management of headache*, ed 5, Oxford, England, 1993, Butterworth-Heinemann.
20. Kidd RF, Nelson R: Musculoskeletal dysfunction of the neck in migraine and tension headache, *Headache* 33:566, 1993.
21. Vernon H, Steiman I, Hagino C: Cervicogenic dysfunction in muscle contraction headache and migraine: a descriptive study, *J Manip Physiol Ther* 15:418, 1992.
22. Boline PD, Kassak K, Bronfort G et al: Spinal manipulation vs amitriptyline for the treatment of chronic tension-type headaches: a randomized clinical trial, *J Manip Physiol Ther* 18:148, 1995.
23. Tuchin PJ, Pollard H: Does classic migraine respond to manual therapy: a case series, *Phys Ther Rev* 3:149, 1998.
24. Gawel MJ, Rothbart PJ: Occipital nerve block in the management of headache and cervical pain, *Cephalalgia* 12:9, 1992.
25. Pfaffenrath V, Kaube H: Diagnostics of cervicogenic headache, *Funct Neurol* 5:159, 1990.
26. Saper JR: The mixed headache syndrome: a new perspective, *Headache* 22:284, 1982.
27. D'Amico D, Leone M, Bussone G: Side-locked unilaterality and pain localization in long-lasting headaches: migraine, tension-type headache, and cervicogenic headache, *Headache* 34:526, 1994.
28. International Headache Society Classification Committee: Classification and diagnostic criteria for headache disorders, cranial neuralgias, and facial pain, *Cephalalgia* 8:9, 1988.
29. Sjaastad O, Fredriksen TA, Pfaffenrath V: Cervicogenic headache: diagnostic criteria, *Headache* 30:725, 1990.
30. Barnsley L, Bogduk N: Medial branch blocks are specific for the diagnosis of cervical zygapophyseal joint pain, *Reg Anesth* 18:343, 1993.
31. Bogduk N, Marsland A: On the concept of third occipital headache, *J Neurol Neurosurg Psych* 49:775, 1986.
32. Lord SM, Barnsley L, Bogduk N: The utility of comparative local anesthetic blocks versus placebo-controlled blocks for the diagnosis of cervical zygapophyseal joint pain, *Clin J Pain* 11:208, 1995.
33. Vincent MB, Luna RA: Cervicogenic headache: a comparison with migraine and tension-type headache, *Cephalalgia* 19:11, 1999.

34. Bono G, Anonaci F, Ghirmai S et al: The clinical profile of cervicogenic headache as it emerges from a study based on the early diagnostic criteria (Sjaastad et al, 1990), *Funct Neurol* 13:75, 1998.
35. Sjaastad O, Salvesen R, Jansen J, Fredriksen TA: Cervicogenic headache: a critical view on pathogenesis, *Funct Neurol* 13:71, 1998.
36. Barnsley L, Lord S, Bogduk N: Comparative local anaesthetic blocks in the diagnosis of cervical zygapophysial joint pain, *Pain* 55:99, 1993.
37. Bovim G, Berg R, Dale LG: Cervicogenic headache: anesthetic blockades of cervical nerves (C2-5) and facet joint (C2 to C3), *Pain* 49:315, 1992.
38. Dreyfuss P, Rogers J, Dreyer S, Fletcher D: Atlanto-occipital joint pain: a report of three cases and description of an intraarticular joint block technique, *Reg Anesth* 19:344, 1994.
39. Lord SM, Barnsley L, Wallis BJ, Bogduk N: Third occipital nerve headache: a prevalence study, *J Neurol Neurosurg Psych* 57:1187, 1994.
40. Rothbart P: Cervicogenic headache, *Headache* 33:249, 1996 (letter to the editor).
41. Barnsley L, Lord S, Wallis B, Bogduk N: False-positive rates of cervical zygapophysial joint blocks, *Clin J Pain* 9:124, 1993.
42. Edmeads J: Plenary session on headache cervicogenic headache, *Pain Res Manage* 1:119, 1996.
43. Pearce JMS: Cervicogenic headache: a personal view, *Cephalalgia* 15:463, 1995.
44. Bovim G, Fredriksen TA, Nielsen AS, Sjaastad O: Neurolysis of the greater occipital nerve in cervicogenic headache: a follow-up study, *Headache* 32:175, 1992.
45. Lord SM, Barnsley L, Bogduk N: Percutaneous radiofrequency neurotomy in the treatment of cervical zygapophysial joint pain: a caution, *Neurosurg* 36:732, 1995.
46. Sjaastad O, Stolt-Nielsen A, Blume H et al: Cervicogenic headache: long-term results of radiofrequency treatment of the planum nuchale, *Funct Neurol* 10:265, 1995.
47. Janda V: Muscles and motor control in cervicogenic disorders: assessment and management. In Grant R, editor: *Physical therapy of the cervical and thoracic spine*, ed 2, New York, 1994, Churchill Livingstone.
48. Raine S, Twomey L: Posture of the head, shoulders, and thoracic spine in comfortable erect standing, *Aust J Physiother* 40:25, 1994.
49. Refshauge K, Goodsell M, Lee M: Consistency of cervical and cervicothoracic posture in standing, *Aust J Physiother* 40:235, 1994.
50. Grimmer K: An investigation of poor cervical resting posture, *Aust J Physiother* 43:7, 1997.
51. Johnson GM: The correlation between surface measurement of head and neck posture and the anatomic position of the upper cervical vertebrae, *Spine* 23:921, 1998.
52. Watson DH, Trott PH: Cervical headache: an investigation of natural head posture and upper cervical flexor muscle performance, *Cephalalgia* 13:272, 1993.
53. Griegel-Morris P, Larson K, Mueller-Klaus K, Oatis CA: Incidence of common postural abnormalities in the cervical, shoulder, and thoracic regions and their association with pain in two age groups of healthy subjects, *Phys Ther* 72:425, 1992.
54. Treleaven J, Jull G, Atkinson L: Cervical musculoskeletal dysfunction in post-concussional headache, *Cephalalgia* 14:273, 1994.
55. Haughie LJ, Fiebert IM, Roach KE: Relationship of forward head posture and cervical backward bending to neck pain, *J Man Manip Ther* 3:91, 1995.
56. Bogduk N, Corrigan B, Kelly P et al: Cervical headache, *Med J Aust* 143:202, 1985.
57. Bogduk N, Marsland A: Third occipital headache, *Cephalalgia* 5(suppl 3):310, 1985.
58. Ehni G, Benner B: Occipital neuralgia and C1-C2 arthrosis, *New Engl J Med* 310:127, 1984.
59. Hartsock CL: Headache from arthritis of the cervical spine, *Med Clin N Am* p. 329, March 1940.
60. Jull GA: Headaches associated with the cervical spine: a clinical review. In Grieve GP, editor: *Modern manual therapy of the vertebral column*, Edinburgh, 1986, Churchill Livingstone.
61. Bogduk N: The anatomical basis for cervicogenic headache, *J Manip Physiol Ther* 15:67, 1992.

62. Fredriksen TA, Hovdal H, Sjaastad O: Cervicogenic headache: clinical manifestations, *Cephalalgia* 7:147, 1987.
63. Hinderaker J, Lord SM, Barnsley L, Bogduk N: Diagnostic value of C2-3 instantaneous axes of rotation in patients with headache of cervical origin, *Cephalagia* 15:391, 1995.
64. Jensen OK, Justesen T, Nielsen FF, Brixen K: Functional radiographic examination of the cervical spine in patients with post-traumatic headache, *Cephalalgia* 10:295, 1990.
65. Pfaffenrath V, Dandekar R, Mayer ET et al: Cervicogenic headache: results of computer-based measurements of cervical spine mobility in 15 patients, *Cephalalgia* 8:45, 1988.
66. Michler RP, Bovim G, Sjaastad O: Disorders in the lower cervical spine: a cause of unilateral headache? A case report, *Headache* 31:550, 1991.
67. Perez-Limonte L, Bonati A, Perry M et al: Lower cervical pathology as a recognizable cause of cervicogenic headaches, *Cephalalgia* 19:435, 1999 (abstract).
68. Persson GCL, Carlsson JY: Headache in patients with neck-shoulder-arm pain of cervical radicular origin, *Headache* 39:218, 1999.
69. Zwart JA: Neck mobility in different headache disorders, *Headache* 37:6, 1997.
70. Beeton K, Jull GA: The effectiveness of manipulative physiotherapy in the management of cervicogenic headache: a single case study, *Physiotherapy* 80:417, 1994.
71. Jaeger B: Are cervicogenic headaches due to myofascial pain and cervical spine dysfunction, *Cephalalgia* 9:157, 1989.
72. Jensen OK, Nielsen FF, Vosmar L: An open study comparing manual therapy with the use of cold packs in the treatment of post-traumatic headache, *Cephalalgia* 10:241, 1990.
73. Schoensee SK, Jensen G, Nicholson G et al: The effect of mobilization on cervical headaches, *J Orthop Sports Phys Ther* 21:184, 1995.
74. Whittingham W, Ellis WB, Molyneux TP: The effect of manipulation (toggle recoil technique) for headaches with upper cervical joint dysfunction: a pilot study, *J Manip Physiol Therapia* 17:369, 1994.
75. Jull G, Bogduk N, Marsland A: The accuracy of manual diagnosis for cervical zygapophysial joint pain syndromes, *Med J Aust* 148:233, 1988.
76. Jull GA, Treleaven J, Versace G: Manual examination of spinal joints: is pain provocation a major diagnostic cue for dysfunction? *Aust J Physiother* 40:159, 1994.
77. Gijsberts TJ, Duquet W, Stoekart R, Oostendorp R: Pain-provocation tests for C0-4 as a tool in the diagnosis of cervicogenic headache, *Cephalalgia* 19:436, 1999 (abstract).
78. Jull G, et al: Inter-examiner reliability to detect painful upper cervical joint dysfunction, *Aust J Physiother* 43:125, 1997.
79. Bovim G: Cervicogenic headache, migraine, and tension-type headache: pressure-pain threshold measurements, *Pain* 51:169, 1992.
80. Graff-Radford SB, Reeves JL, Jaeger B: Management of chronic head and neck pain: effectiveness of altering factors perpetuating myofascial pain, *Headache* 27:186, 1987.
81. Jensen R, Rasmussen BK, Pedersen B et al: Cephalic muscle tenderness and pressure pain threshold in a general population, *Pain* 48:197, 1992.
82. Jensen R, Rasmussen BK: Muscular disorders in tension-type headache, *Cephalalgia* 16:97, 1996.
83. Langermark M, Jensen K, Jensen TS, Olesen J: Pressure-pain thresholds and thermal nociceptive thresholds in chronic tension-type headache, *Pain* 38:203, 1989.
84. Marcus DA, Scharff L, Mercer S, Turk DC: Musculoskeletal abnormalities in chronic headache: a controlled comparison of headache diagnostic groups, *Headache* 39:21, 1999.
85. Davidoff RA: Trigger points and myofascial pain: toward understanding how they affect headaches, *Cephalalgia* 18:436, 1998.
86. Sheather-Reid RB, Cohen ML: Psychophysical evidence for a neuropathic component of chronic neck pain, *Pain* 75:341, 1988.
87. Becser N, Sand T, Pareja JA, Zwart JA: Thermal sensitivity in unilateral headaches, *Cephalalgia* 18:675, 1998.
88. Vingen JV, Stover LJ: Photophobia and phonophobia in tension-type and cervicogenic headache, *Cephalalgia* 18:313, 1998.

89. Jull G, Barrett C, Magee R, Ho P: Further characterisation of muscle dysfunction in cervical headache, *Cephalalgia* 19:179, 1999.
90. Bansevicius D, Sjaastad O: Cervicogenic headache: the influence of mental load on pain level and EMG of shoulder-neck and facial muscles, *Headache* 36:372, 1996.
91. Placzek JD, Pagett BT, Roubal PJ: The influence of the cervical spine on chronic headache in women: a pilot study, *J Man Manip Ther* 7:33, 1999.
92. Winters JM, Peles JD: Neck muscle activity and 3-D head kinematics during quasi-static and dynamic tracking movements. In Winters JM, Woo SLY, editors: *Multiple muscle systems: biomechanics and movement organization*, New York, 1990, Springer-Verlag.
93. Dutia MB: The muscles and joints of the neck: their specialisation and role in head movement, *Prog Neurobiol* 37:165, 1991.
94. Keshner EA: Controlling stability of a complex movement system, *Phys Ther* 70:844, 1990.
95. Kamibayashi LK, Richmond FJR: Morphometry of human neck muscles, *Spine* 23:1314, 1998.
96. Keshner EA, Campbell D, Katz RT, Peterson BW: Neck muscle activation patterns in humans during isometric head stabilization, *Exp Brain Res* 75:335, 1989.
97. Keshner EA, Cromwell RL, Peterson BW: Mechanisms controlling human head stabilisation. II. Head-neck characteristics during random rotations in the vertical plane, *J Neurophysiol* 73:2302, 1995.
98. Keshner EA, Peterson BW: Mechanisms controlling human head stabilisation. I. Head-neck dynamics during random rotations in the horizontal plane, *J Neurophysiol* 73:2293, 1995.
99. Lu WW, Bishop PJ: Electromyographic activity of the cervical musculature during dynamic lateral bending, *Spine* 21:2443, 1996.
100. Vasavada AN, Li S, Delp SL: Influence of muscle morphology and moment arms on moment-generating capacity of human neck muscles, *Spine* 23:412, 1998.
101. Winters JM, Peles JD, Osterbauer PJ et al: Three-dimensional head axis of rotation during tracking movements: a tool for assessing neck neuromechanical function, *Spine* 18:1178, 1993.
102. Bergmark A: Stability of the lumbar spine: a study in mechanical engineering, *Acta Orthop Scand* 230(suppl):20, 1989.
103. Crisco JJ, Panjabi MM: The intersegmental and multisegmental muscles of the spine: a biomechanical model comparing lateral stabilising potential, *Spine* 7:793, 1991.
104. Panjabi MM, Abumi K, Durabceau J, Oxland T: Spinal stability and intersegmental muscle forces: a biomechanical study, *Spine* 14:194, 1989.
105. Hides JA, Richardson CA, Jull GA: Multifidus recovery is not automatic following resolution of acute first episode low back pain, *Spine* 21:2763, 1996.
106. Hodges PW, Richardson CA: Inefficient stabilisation of the lumbar spine associated with low back pain: a motor control evaluation of transversus abdominis, *Spine* 21:2640, 1996.
107. O'Sullivan PB, Twomey L, Allison GT, Taylor J: Specific stabilizing exercises in the treatment of low back pain with a clinical and radiological diagnosis of lumbar segmental "instability," Tenth Biennial Conference Manipulative Physiotherapists Association of Australia, Melbourne, 1997, Australian Physiotherapy Association.
108. Conley MS, Meyer RA, Bloomberg JJ et al: Noninvasive analysis of human neck muscle function, *Spine* 20:2505, 1995.
109. Mayoux-Benhamou MA, Revel M, Vallee C et al: Longus colli has a postural function on cervical curvature, *Surg Radiol Anat* 16:367, 1994.
110. Vitti M, Fujiwara M, Basmajian JV, Iida M: The integrated roles of longus colli and sternocleidomastoid muscles: an electromyographic study, *Anat Rec* 177:471, 1973.
111. Panjabi MM, Cholewicki J, Nibu K et al: Critical load of the human cervical spine: an in vitro experimental study, *Clin Biomech* 13:11, 1998.
112. Ulrich V, Russell MB, Jensen R, Olesen J: A comparison of tension-type headache in migraineurs and in non-migraineurs: a population-based study, *Pain* 67:501, 1996.
113. Weber BR, Uhlig Y, Grob D et al: Duration of pain and muscular adaptations in patients with dysfunction of the cervical spine, *J Orthop Res* 11:805, 1993.

114. Uhlig Y, Weber BR, Grob D, Muntener M: Fiber composition and fiber transformations in neck muscles of patients with dysfunction of the cervical spine, *J Orthop Res* 13:240, 1995.
115. Hallgren RC, Greenman PE, Rechtien JJ: Atrophy of suboccipital muscles in patients with chronic pain: a pilot study, *J Am Osteopathic Assoc* 94:1032, 1994.
116. McPartland JM, Brodeur RR, Hallgren RC: Chronic neck pain, standing balance, and suboccipital muscle atrophy: a pilot study, *J Manip Physiol Ther* 20:24, 1997.
117. Jull GA: Deep cervical neck flexor dysfunction in whiplash, *J Musculoskeletal Pain* 8:143, 2000.
118. Heikkila HV, Astrom P-G: Cervicocephalic kinaesthetic sensibility in patients with whiplash injury, *Scand J Rehab Med* 28:133, 1996.
119. Loudon JK, Ruhl M, Field E: Ability to reproduce head position after whiplash injury, *Spine* 22:865, 1997.
120. Revel M, Andre-Deshays C, Minguet M: Cervicocephalic kinesthetic sensibility in patients with cervical pain, *Arch Phys Med Rehab* 72:288, 1991.
121. Revel M, Minguet M, Gergoy P et al: Changes in cervicocephalic kinesthesia after a proprioceptive rehabilitation program in patients with neck pain: a randomized controlled study, *Arch Phys Med Rehab* 75:895, 1994.
122. Mottram S: Dynamic stability of the scapula, *Man Ther* 2:123, 1997.
123. Johnson G, Bogduk N, Nowitzke A, House D: Anatomy and actions of the trapezius muscle, *Clin Biomech* 9:44, 1994.
124. Ludewig P, Cook TM, Nawoczenski DM: Three-dimensional scapular orientation and muscle activity at selected positions of humeral elevation, *J Orthop Sports Phys Ther* 24:57, 1996.
125. Lukasiewicz A, McClure P, Michener L et al: Comparison of 3-dimensional scapular position and orientation between subjects with and without shoulder impingement, *J Orthop Sports Phys Ther* 29:574, 1999.
126. McQuade KJ, Dawson JD, Smidt GL: Scapulothoracic muscle fatigue associated with alterations in scapulohumeral rhythm kinematics during maximum resistive shoulder elevation, *J Orthop Sports Phys Ther* 28:74, 1998.
127. Behrsin JF, Maguire K: Levator scapulae action during shoulder movement: a possible mechanism of shoulder pain of cervical origin, *Aust J Physiother* 32:101, 1986.
128. Leone M, D'Amico D, Grazzi L et al: Cervicogenic headache: a critical review of current diagnostic criteria, *Pain* 78:1, 1998.
129. Jansen J, Bardosi A, Hilderbrandt J, Lucke A: Cervicogenic, hemicranial attacks associated with vascular irritation or compression of the cervical nerve root C2: clinical manifestations and morphological findings, *Pain* 39:203, 1989.
130. Jansen J, Markakis E, Rama B, Hildebrandt J: Hemicranial attacks or permanent hemicrania: a sequel of upper cervical root compression, *Cephalalgia* 9:123, 1989.
131. Pikus HJ, Phillips JM: Characteristics of patients successfully treated for cervicogenic headache by surgical decompression of the second cervical root, *Headache* 35:621, 1995.
132. Sjaastad O, Fredriksen TA, Stolt-Nielsen A: Cervicogenic headache, C2 rhizopathy and occipital neuralgia: a connection? *Cephalalgia* 6:189, 1986.
133. Pearce JMS: The importance of cervicogenic headache in the over-fifties, *Headache Quart Curr Treat Res* 6:293, 1995.
134. Butler D: *Mobilisation of the nervous system*, Melbourne, 1991, Churchill Livingstone.
135. Rumore AJ: Slump examination and treatment in a patient suffering headache, *Aust J Physiother* 35:262, 1989.
136. Hack GD, Koritzer RT, Robinson WL et al: Anatomic relation between the rectus capitis posterior minor muscle and the dura mater, *Spine* 20:2484, 1995.
137. Mitchell BS, Humphries BK, O'Sullivan E: Attachments of ligamentum nuchae to cervical posterior dura and the lateral part of the occipital bone, *J Manip Physiol Ther* 21:145, 1998.
138. Hu JW, Vernon H, Tatourian I: Changes in neck electromyography associated with meningeal noxious stimulation, *J Manip Physiol Ther* 18:577, 1995.

139. Jull GA: Headaches of cervical origin. In Grant R, editor: *Physical therapy of the cervical and thoracic spine*, ed 2, New York, 1994, Churchill Livingstone.
140. Elvey RL: The investigation of arm pain: signs of adverse responses to physical examination of the brachial plexus and related neural tissues. In Boyling J, Palasanga N, editors: *Grieve's modern manual therapy of the vertebral column*, ed 2, Edinburgh, 1994, Churchill Livingstone.
141. Bogduk N: Neck pain: assessment and management in general practice, *Mod Med Aust* vol 102, 1995.
142. van Suijlekom HA, van Kleef M, Barendse GA: Radiofrequency cervical zygapophyseal joint neurotomy for cervicogenic headache: a prospective study of 15 patients, *Funct Neurol* 13:297, 1998.
143. Farina S, Granella F, Malferrari G, Manzoni GC: Headache and cervical spine disorders: classification and treatment with transcutaneous electrical nerve stimulation, *Headache* 26:431, 1986.
144. Martelletti P, LaTour D, Giacovazzo M: Spectrum of pathophysiological disorders in cervicogenic headache and its therapeutic indications, *J Neuromusc System* 3:182, 1995.
145. Nilsson N, Christensen HW, Hartvigsen J: The effect of spinal manipulation in the treatment of cervicogenic headache, *J Manip Physiol Ther* 20:326, 1997.
146. Vernon H: Spinal manipulation and headaches of cervical origin: a review of literature and presentation of cases, *J Man Med* 6:73, 1991.
147. Jansen J, Vadokas V, Vogelsang JP: Cervical peridural anaesthesia: an essential aid for the indication of surgical treatment of cervicogenic headache triggered by degenerative diseases of the cervical spine, *Funct Neurol* 13:79, 1998.
148. Vincent M: Greater occipital nerve blockades in cervicogenic headache, *Funct Neurol* 13:78, 1998.
149. Bove G, Nilsson N: Spinal manipulation in the treatment of episodic tension-type headache, *J Am Med Assoc* 280:1576, 1998.
150. Hammill JM, Cook TM, Rosecrance JC: Effectiveness of a physical therapy regimen in the treatment of tension-type headache, *Headache* 36:149, 1995.
151. Hoyt WH, Shaffer F, Bard DA: Osteopathic manipulation in the treatment of muscle-contraction headache, *J Am Osteopathic Assoc* 78:322, 1979.
152. Parker GB, Tupling H, Pryor DS: A controlled trial of cervical manipulation for migraine, *Aust New Zeal J Med* 8:589, 1978.
153. Rundcrantz B, Johnson B, Moritz U, Roxendal G: Cervico-brachial disorders in dentists: a comparison between two kinds of physiotherapeutic intervention, *Scand J Rehab Med* 23:11, 1991.
154. Richardson CA, Jull GA, Hodges PW, Hides JA: *Therapeutic exercise for spinal segmental stabilization in low back pain: scientific basis and clinical approach*, Edinburgh, 1999, Churchill Livingstone.
155. Jull G, Trott P, Potter H et al: A randomised control trial of physiotherapy management of cervicogenic headache, *Spine* 2002 (accepted for publication).
156. McDonald GJ, Lord SM, Bogduk N: Long-term follow-up of patients treated with cervical radiofrequency neurotomy for chronic neck pain, *Neurosurg* 45:61, 1999.
157. Horwitz NH: Letter to the editor, *Neurosurg* 39:70, 1996.
158. Long DM: Letter to the editor, *Neurosurg* 39:70, 1996.

Appendix

TESTING AND RETRAINING THE DEEP CERVICAL FLEXORS

CLINICAL POINTERS

Testing and training the craniocervical flexion action to target the deep neck flexors may, from a superficial perspective, appear to be a simple procedure both to the clinician and patient. However, to the contrary, testing and helping the patient train the action requires skill by the clinician in teaching and assessing the pattern of motor control used by the patient. The following section presents a protocol in some detail and highlights some of the common substitution strategies that patients use to mask deficiencies in the neck flexor synergy.

TESTING THE CONTROL OF CRANIOCERVICAL FLEXION TO TARGET THE DEEP NECK FLEXORS

1. Patient position
   a. The test is conducted in a crook lying position with the craniocervical and cervical spine positioned in a midrange neutral position. For the neutral neck position, check for a horizontal face line and a horizontal line bisecting the neck longitudinally.
   b. Maintain the position, when required, with the appropriate thickness of folded towel layers placed under the head. Ensure that the edge of the towel is aligned with the base of the occiput and the upper cervical region is free.
2. Preparation of the pressure biofeedback unit (PBU)
   a. Concertina the blue airbag of the PBU and clip together. The clip attachments are on the outside layers with the section without the clip attachments in the middle.
   b. Position the folded bag under the neck so that it abuts against the occiput. Do not let it slide down to the lower cervical area.
   c. Inflate the bag to a baseline of 20 mm Hg. Do not inflate the bag before insertion behind the neck. For more rapid air distribution in the bag, it is helpful to gently squeeze the sides of the bag. Repeat the inflation and the gentle squeezing until the pressure is stabilized.
3. Patient instruction
   a. Turn the pressure dial of the PBU away from the patient.
   b. Explain that the test is one of precision and control; it is not a strength test, but one to test whether the patient can use the deep neck muscles and hold a contraction.
   c. Liken the test movement to gently nodding the head as if saying "yes." Let the patient practice the movement in the first instance. Encourage the patient to move gently and slowly. Some patients, who find this movement difficult, may need to simply practice a larger amplitude, craniocervical flexion and extension in the first instance, to learn the movement.
   d. Turn the pressure dial to the patient. Check that the baseline is 20 mm Hg. Reinflate if necessary to stabilize baseline. This should be the last time the pressure has to be adjusted.
   e. Instruct the patient to place the tongue on the roof of the mouth, lips together but teeth just separated. This will discourage substitution with the platysma or hyoid muscles.

   f. Instruct the patient to gently nod to target 22 mm Hg, that is, just one mark on the pressure dial. See whether the position can be held steadily. If successful at that pressure, relax and repeat at each target pressure separately. Progressively target 24 mm Hg, 26 mm Hg to a maximum of 30 mm Hg. Pressures higher than 30 mm Hg are not relevant.
   g. The pressure that the patient can hold steady with minimal superficial muscle activity is the one on which endurance capacity can be assessed (i.e., 10 repetitions of 10-second holds).
4. Assessment during testing
   a. Gentle mobilization of the trachea from side to side should be possible if the hyoid musculature is relaxed before the test. Jaw musculature also should be relaxed.
   b. The physical therapist monitors the anterior superficial neck muscles to determine that they are not overactive. This can be done with palpation in the first instance.
   c. Ensure that the patient is performing a pure nod. There is *no* head retraction and *no* head lifting.
   d. Ensure that the movement is slow and controlled. Performing the movement quickly or with phasic, jerky movements indicates a deficit in performance.
5. Correct performance
   a. The patient can perform the test to target at least 26 mm Hg in a slow controlled manner. This is a minimum requirement for a satisfactory performance, based on data from asymptomatic populations; 28 and 30 mm Hg are the ideal targets and should be the targets to be achieved in a rehabilitation process.
   b. The patient can hold a steady contraction for the 10-times, 10-second holding test.
   c. The patient should perceive it as an easy action (i.e., the patient cannot feel the contraction).
6. Poor performance
   a. Incorrect action—the patient is not able to easily perform an isolated nod of the upper cervical spine. The patient is unable to perform the movement or uses substitute movements such as retraction or head lift.
   b. The patient tends to retract the neck. This is a common substitution strategy. Observe that the patient is actually flexing the upper cervical spine by rolling the occiput on the bed.
   c. The movement is performed too quickly, often overshooting the target.
   d. The pressure change is achieved using superficial muscle activity. Phasic, erratic movements occur as the patient attempts to hold the target pressure. The needle on the pressure gauge trembles.
   e. The patient is activating the jaw and hyoid musculature to perform the craniocervical flexion action. By stabilizing the jaw, the patient is able to use the hyoid musculature to perform the upper cervical nod. Palpate the jaw musculature and mobility of the trachea to detect this substitution strategy.
   f. The pressure is unable to be maintained steadily and drops off the target, indicating fatigue.
   g. The patient feels that a strenuous exercise is being performed.

Specific Problems That May Impact on Testing and Training the Deep Neck Flexors

1. Neural system mechanosensitivity: Craniocervical flexion will move the neural tissue in the upper cervical region. If the neural tissue is mechanosensitive, the deep cervical flexor testing and training may be provocative, particularly of headache. If

neural tissue mechanosensitivity of the upper cervical spine is present, attempt testing and training in positions that will reduce tension on the neural system (e.g., a crook lying position with slight shoulder elevation and arms folded across the chest). If necessary, delay training of the deep neck flexors or attempt to find other positions of ease for the neural system. For severe problems, gentle static rotations or simple eye movements looking down may be all that can be tolerated in the first instance while treatment addressing the neural system is undertaken.

2. Incorrect pattern: The patient is unable to perform the simple craniocervical flexion action. To remedy this, it may be necessary in the first instance to perform an assisted active craniocervical flexion and extension concentrating on the roll of the head through a large range of flexion and extension to improve the overall pattern. The patient may merely need to practice the movement for a few days before progressing to the formal test and training. In this instance, the PBU is not recommended initially because it may only reinforce poor patterns in attempts to change pressure.
3. Overactive scalenes and sternocleidomastoid muscles: Some patients have particularly overactive anterior superficial muscles even at rest. It is necessary for the patient to learn to relax these in the first instance. This may be achieved by practicing relaxed diaphragmatic breathing. Use of EMG biofeedback to assist relaxation at rest also can be of benefit, progressing to use during the nodding action. Generally the PBU is not recommended at this stage until the patient has learned to relax these muscles. Feedback from two sources may become too confusing.
4. Overactive hyoids and jaw muscles: Emphasizing the relaxed jaw position is important. Use of the position of tongue on the roof of the mouth, lips together, and teeth apart or placing tongue between the teeth is helpful. The patient also can be taught to palpate the hyoid to ensure it remains mobile and to palpate the jaw musculature. EMG biofeedback may be useful to assist relaxation. Treat any concurrent temporomandibular joint problems as necessary.
5. Tightness of the upper cervical extensors: Tightness of upper cervical extensors or marked upper cervical joint restriction will make performance of the upper cervical flexion action more difficult. Treatment of these factors should occur concurrently. Persistent restriction will make higher levels of pressure difficult to achieve, but training can still be done at the lower pressure levels.

Retraining Motor Control of the Deep Cervical Flexors

1. Treatment: physical therapist's role
   a. Explain the importance of the deep supporting muscles and the way that the muscle system is the natural mechanism to protect and control joints. Explain the concept of exercising for deep segmental muscle control and support and the way it differs from conventional strength training. Explain the importance for specific facilitation and precise rehabilitation.
   b. Explain the concept that muscle control is for pain control and for prevention of pain and recurrence. Ensure the explanation is convincing to assist patient compliance with exercise.
   c. Demonstrate the muscle deficit to the patient quantitatively using the PBU in the test procedure. Explain what is considered an adequate performance.
   d. Explain the nature of the retraining. Exercises should be pain free, low load, precise, and specific. This may take concentration and time, and adequate practice is required.
   e. Help the patient plan times to undertake the specific craniocervical flexion training at home (e.g., first thing in the morning before getting out of bed and

again for a few minutes when in bed at night). Plan times and cues for other exercises during the working day. Let the patient see that it is easy to be compliant without disruption of often busy days.

f. Monitor the patient's performance, correcting and giving adequate feedback.

g. Progress the craniocervical flexion training program appropriately; do not progress too rapidly. Quality and accuracy of performance should not be sacrificed just to achieve a higher pressure level.

h. Specific low-load training of tonic endurance capacity of the deep neck flexors, cocontraction exercises of the neck flexors and extensors, scapular muscle retraining, and reeducation of posture and movement control are all necessary components of retraining. One aspect cannot be performed in isolation or used to substitute for another.

2. Treatment: patient's role
   a. Patient compliance is essential, and exercises need to be practiced in a specific, controlled, and accurate manner.
   b. The patient must understand that the formal exercises for the deep neck flexors need to be performed in the supine position, the starting neutral head position must be replicated, and exercises should be pain free and practiced at the correct level. The patient must understand and recognize fatigue and know that practice using an inappropriate substitution pattern is counterproductive.
   c. Formal training needs to be undertaken at least twice per day. Other components of the exercise program can be undertaken within daily activities.
   d. Patients should monitor their own performance of the craniocervical flexion action. Self-palpation to detect overactive superficial muscles and use of the PBU on loan at home may be necessary. Patients can position the arms on pillows across the chest to allow the PBU dial to be easily read without excessive use of arm musculature.
   e. Consistent exercise daily over at least a 6-week period may be necessary for reeducation. Regular self-checking of performance and continuation of a maintenance program at home 2 or 3 times a week, guard against recurrence.
3. General principles for retraining the activation of deep neck flexors
   a. Train the specific deep neck flexor muscle activation capacity initially, emphasizing precision and control. Training needs to be performed in supine lying with the patient positioned as per the test using feedback from the PBU. The clinician must ensure that the muscles are functioning correctly before there is any assurance that these muscles will be recruited in more functional weight-bearing exercise. No phasic, erratic movements should occur. Emphasize slow and controlled movement. Precision and control are the keys to successful training.
   b. Commence training at the pressure level that the patient can achieve and hold steadily with a good pattern, without substitution strategies. Progress the time that this pressure level can be held to 5 to 10 seconds. Training with feedback from the PBU unit is generally deemed essential. Patients tested after training without feedback have poorer results.
   c. EMG biofeedback also may be used to encourage relaxation in the superficial neck flexors. Self-palpation often is sufficient, especially if the patient has trouble coping with two feedback sources (i.e., pressure and EMG).
   d. Retraining kinesthesia. One method of retraining joint position sense can be incorporated with deep neck flexor training. The patient can practice targeting different pressures first with visual feedback and then without feedback with the eyes closed. Accuracy can be self-checked by the patient.

e. Emphasize patient compliance, and augment this with objective retesting with the PBU. Compliance is usually not a problem when patients gain control of pain with the exercise.
f. Feedback is essential for retraining the deep neck flexors and the neck flexor synergy, and it is preferable in many cases for patients to train with the PBU at home both for improving the activation capacity and for holding ability of the deep neck flexors. The visual feedback from the PBU needs to be gradually withdrawn once the patient is controlling and holding the action well so that he or she can successfully self-manage with the correct action in the long term. In preparation for this, the patient should practice to various levels of pressure with feedback, concentrating on the feeling of the muscle contraction, and then repeat the task with the eyes closed. Success can be confirmed by rechecking the PBU dial. Once the patient can perform the exercises accurately, the visual feedback can be withdrawn.

4. Training tonic endurance
   a. It is necessary to train the holding capacity of the craniocervical flexion action. Commence by holding the pressure level that has been achieved for 5 seconds. Stop at fatigue, because working into fatigue often will encourage unwanted activity in superficial muscles.
   b. Progression is made through increasing the number of repetitions and the time the position is held. Increase repetitions to 10; progress time to 10 seconds. Eventually increase the number of repetitions for each pressure level successfully achieved.
5. Reeducation of posture
   a. From the first treatment session, the deep neck flexor muscle training with scapular muscle training should be incorporated into postural reeducation in the upright posture. The facilitation and reeducation strategies for the scapular muscles must be conducted with precision equal to that of deep neck flexors.
   b. Correction of pelvic posture in the sitting to the upright neutral position with restoration of the normal low lumbar lordosis usually facilitates correct thoracic and cervical postures. If necessary, a subtle sternal lift rather than a shoulders-back action can be used to optimize thoracic posture. The arms and shoulders should remain relaxed with appropriate lower level contraction of the serratus anterior and the lower trapezius to correct scapular position. A subtle "occipital lift" or flexion may be necessary if craniocervical posture has not automatically assumed a neutral position.
   c. Postural retraining should be repeated numerous times throughout the day. Help the patient recognize cues to practice (e.g., when answering the telephone, at traffic lights, on public transport, during advertisements on TV, when drinking a cup of coffee).
6. Cocontraction: Further progression of the program includes cocontraction exercises of the neck flexors and extensors using low-resistance isometric rotation. These can be performed with patient self-resistance either in the supine or a correct upright sitting posture. Emphasize slow-onset and slow-release resistance-holding contractions.
7. Movement patterning
   a. Ensure the patient uses the deep neck flexors correctly in neck flexion-extension patterning. A correct pattern of movement from extension to neutral and neutral to flexion (leading with upper cervical flexion) may be practiced in a prone-on-elbows position with control of scapular position, as well as in a correct sitting position.

b. Ensure a neutral cervical spine posture can be maintained with performance of a slow, small-range rotation movement. This may be performed in a supine, a prone-on-elbows, or a correct upright posture.

Research is indicating that the deep neck flexor function does not return automatically without specific training. Research also is indicating that relief of joint pain with manual therapy techniques does not impact to any degree on the deep neck flexor activation capacity (Jull, unpublished data). The program outlined previously is conducted in concert with specific retraining of the scapular musculature in a comprehensive active stabilization program. If occupation or recreational activities require upper limb strength or postures in which the head is flexed or inclined forward for long periods, a higher level of control will need to be achieved. The program should be progressed to incorporate higher load stabilization and strengthening exercises once control by the deep muscle system of the cervical and scapular regions has been achieved.

ACKNOWLEDGMENT

To other members of the Whiplash Research Unit in the Department of Physiotherapy at The University of Queensland: M. Sterling, J. Treleaven, S. Edwards, and P. Dall'Alba for their assistance in the development of the exercise protocols.

CHAPTER 14

Management of Selected Cervical Syndromes

Patricia H. Trott

This chapter builds on the previous chapters of this book, particularly those relating to pain mechanisms and clinical reasoning. Physical therapists are required to evaluate and manage patients with cervical disorders of varying complexity. These range from those with clear anatomical patterns to those that seem bizarre in their presentation. The former are typical of input-dominant pain mechanisms, be they peripherally evoked or of a peripheral neurogenic nature. The latter are typical of a central neural processing problem.

The case histories presented in this chapter are examples of nociceptive and peripheral neurogenic pain mechanisms. The symptoms behave mechanically and originate in local tissues in the area of the symptoms. The patients have a reasonable understanding of and respond appropriately to their problems, and there are no cases in which maladaptive feelings or behaviors contribute significantly to the problems. Contributing factors, associated with the development and maintenance of the patient's symptoms, are limited to biomechanical examples and exclude those of a psychosocial nature.

Discussion is restricted to the presentation of basic concepts underlying the recognition of certain clinical patterns and to the selection of passive movement techniques for treating cervical syndromes. This is followed by the presentation of selected cervical conditions often seen by physical therapists; in the overall management of these cervical conditions, manual therapy (passive mobilization and manipulation) has a major role.

ISOLATION OF CERTAIN CERVICAL SYNDROMES

Patients who have a history of *symptoms occurring spontaneously*, or symptoms occurring after some trivial incident, have symptoms, signs, and histories that are easily recognized. These conditions have clear neuroanatomical patterns that are evoked by input-dominant pain mechanisms. They follow a predictable course, and their response to manipulative therapy also is predictable. Knowledge of the structures that can cause pain, the response to posture and movement, and the expected signs to be found on physical examination also assist the therapist in recognizing those conditions marked by a spontaneous onset of symptoms. This contrasts with patients who have a *history of injury*, such as a direct blow to the head, a fall, or surgery. In those cases the symptoms and signs vary, depending on which tissues are injured and the force of the injury; in such case the response to treatment is less predictable.

The suggestion that all patients fit neatly into specific categories is invalid; indeed, as stated before, patients often have symptoms and signs of more complex nociceptive patterns. As discussed in depth in Chapter 6, the organization of knowledge into schemata, such as clinical patterns or syndromes, facilitates the recall of that knowledge for use with each patient encounter. The separate presentation of some of these conditions in this chapter can help inexperienced therapists more easily recognize the components of two or more coexisting conditions and direct their treatment appropriately.

SELECTION OF PASSIVE MOVEMENT TECHNIQUES

The principles of selecting a technique for the diagnosis and treatment of conditions affecting the cervical spine are similar to those outlined for the lumbar spine[1] but are presented again with specific examples of disorders of the cervical spine.

DIAGNOSIS

Determining the specific diagnosis of a disorder of the cervical spine can be difficult because the etiology of such disorders often is multifactorial. For example, mechanical, inflammatory, and viral causes may coexist. Also, a pathological process can produce differing patterns of symptoms and signs. For example, a patient with a diagnosis of cervical spondylosis may experience severe low cervical and medial scapular pain that restricts cervical movement in all directions or may experience no pain but marked restriction of extension, rotation, and lateral flexion to one side. Pain patterns can range from more easily recognized peripherally evoked nociception (input mechanisms) to complex patterns arising from altered central neural processing mechanisms or an output pain mechanism such as an autonomic disorder (see Chapter 6).

For these reasons, the selection of physical treatment modalities for a disorder of the cervical spine is based on the patient's symptoms and signs and on the history of the disorder rather than on a diagnostic title. Particular attention is paid to the patterns of pain response that can occur during test movements because these are important in the selection of passive movement techniques. These considerations are discussed in more detail in the following sections.

PAIN-SENSITIVE STRUCTURES AND THEIR PAIN PATTERNS

See Chapter 4 for a discussion of available research on cervical pain mechanisms.

RANGE AND PAIN RESPONSE TO MOVEMENT

Test movements of the cervical intervertebral joints and neuromeningeal tissues produce the common patterns described in the following sections.

Stretching or Compressing Pain. Unilateral neck pain may be reproduced by either stretching (e.g., lateral flexion to the contralateral side) or by compressing the faulty tissues (e.g., lateral flexion toward the painful side).

End-of-Range or Through-Range Pain. Pain may be reproduced at the limit of a particular movement (i.e., when the soft tissue restraints are stretched) or during the performance of a movement, increasing near the limit of the movement. (This is common in joints in which there is a constant ache.)

Local and Referred Pain. In patients who have referred pain, the response to test movements influences the selection of passive movement techniques. For example, a patient in whom test movements immediately cause distal symptoms requires treatment with very gentle movement that does not provoke the distal symptoms. Test movements that cause latent referred pain or cause the referred pain to linger also indicate caution in treatment. In cases in which a test movement must be sustained at the end of a range of movement before the referred symptoms are provoked, sustaining the treatment technique also will be necessary.

History

The history of a disorder includes information about its onset and progression. Conditions that have a spontaneous (nontraumatic) onset have a characteristically progressive history; a degenerating disc or postural ligamentous pain, for example, have a typical pattern of progression. Knowing the history that is typical for these conditions helps the therapist recognize the current *stage of the disorder* and match it with the symptoms and signs to form a syndrome. Typical histories are included at the end of this chapter.

A detailed history also gives information about the stability of the disorder. This guides the extent and strength of the techniques used in identifying and treating it and may contraindicate certain techniques. This is particularly important in cases of radicular pain with worsening neurological signs, in which injudicious treatment may further compromise the affected nerve root. The progression of the disorder allows prediction of the *outcome of treatment*, the number of treatment sessions needed, and the long-term *prognosis*.

The following case history illustrates these aspects of history taking. A 40-year-old truck driver has a 10-year history of recurrent episodes of neck stiffness and left-sided low cervical pain. These symptoms occur for no apparent reason and last for 1 to 2 days. In the previous 2 years the pain has spread to his left shoulder, and on each occasion the pain has required treatment (heat and exercise). One week ago, after driving a long distance, the patient experienced his worst episode yet of severe neck pain, which spread further into his left arm; he also experienced paresthesia in his left thumb and index finger. His symptoms are not responding to heat and exercise, but he has been able to continue his work driving and lifting merchandise.

This history is typical of worsening zygapophyseal joint arthropathy, and the patient now has symptoms of C6 nerve root irritation. His cervical disorder is relatively stable in that he can continue his work without worsening of his symptoms. More specific treatment will be required and can be performed quite firmly without risk of exacerbating his symptoms. One would expect to make him symptom free but would also anticipate further episodes of his condition to occur because of its progressive nature.

SYMPTOMS

The area and the manner in which a patient's symptoms vary in relation to posture and movement assist in the recognition of their source and, if they match the response to physical examination, can assist in the selection of passive movement techniques. A movement or combination of movements that simulates a position or movement described by the patient as one that causes pain can be used as the treatment technique. The following case history illustrates this.

A woman complains of left-sided midcervical pain each time she twists to reach for her car seatbelt. In that position, her neck is extended, laterally flexed, and rotated to the left. Examination confirms that this combined position reproduces her pain, and testing of intervertebral movement reveals hypomobility of the left C3-4 zygapophyseal joint. An effective treatment would consist of placing the patient's neck in this combined position and passively stretching one or more of its components (localizing the movement to the C3-4 joint by use of local thumb pressures).

Two other important aspects of the patient's symptoms are the *severity of the pain* and the *irritability of the disorder. Severity* relates to the examiner's interpretation of the severity of the pain based on the patient's description and the functional limitations caused by the pain. The irritability or "touchiness" of a disorder is explained in Chapter 7. In relation to treatment, the most significant factor in irritability is the length of time the pain takes to subside after provocation. If, in the example given, the patient experiences a momentary pain each time she reaches for her seatbelt, her condition is nonirritable, and the treatment suggested is appropriate. However, if she is left with a residual ache for an hour after reaching once for her seatbelt, her condition is irritable, and the initial treatment technique should be performed with the patient's neck in a position of comfort and should not provoke pain.

SIGNS

Signs refer to physical examination findings and are discussed in Chapter 7. It is important to reach a mechanical diagnosis of neuromusculoskeletal tissue dysfunction through isolation of the structures at fault, based on knowing the distribution of pain and the response to physical tests. Knowledge of the movements that increase and decrease the pain response is a major determinant of the method to be used for applying passive movement in treatment.

SELECTION BASED ON THE EFFECTS OF THE TECHNIQUE

Passive movement as a treatment technique can be broadly divided into its use as *mobilization* (passive oscillatory movements) or *manipulation* (small-amplitude thrust and stretch performed at speed at the limit of a range of movement). Mobilization is the method of choice for most cervical conditions because it can be used as a treatment for pain or for restoring movement in a hypomobile joint. It can be adapted to suit the severity of the pain, the irritability of the condition, and the stability of the disorder. Also, gentle mobilization may be safely applied in conditions in which a manipulation is contraindicated (e.g., vertebrobasilar insufficiency [VBI]). Manipulation is the treatment of choice when an intervertebral joint is locked. When the aim is to regain mobility of an irritable joint, a single manipulation may be less aggravating than repeated stretching by mobilization.

Position of the Intervertebral Joint and Direction of the Movement Technique

Treatment by passive movement involves careful positioning of the affected intervertebral segment and selection of the most effective direction of movement. These steps are based on knowledge of spinal biomechanics and the desired pain response.

A manipulation is applied in the direction of limitation to stretch the tissues in that particular direction. For example, using biomechanical principles, the cervical spine is positioned (in lateral flexion and contralateral rotation) to isolate movement to the desired intervertebral segment, and a thrust is applied in the appropriate direction. When passive *mobilization* is used, both the position of the intervertebral joint and the direction of movement are varied according to the desired effect of the technique. Some examples follow.

Avoiding Discomfort or Pain. In cases in which pain is severe or a condition is irritable, the provocation of symptoms should be avoided. The cervical spine is positioned so that the painful intervertebral segment is pain free; the movement technique that is used also must be pain free.

Causing or Avoiding Referred Pain. Provocation of referred pain is safe when that pain is chronic, nonirritable, and not originating from a nerve root. To alter the condition, provocation of the symptoms in treatment may be necessary by positioning, by application of the treatment technique that is selected, or by both. However, if the pain is of nerve root origin (i.e., it is worse distally, and neurological changes are present), and particularly if the examination of movements reproduces distal pain, treatment techniques that provoke the distal pain should not be used.

Opening One Side of the Intervertebral Space. Techniques that open one side of the intervertebral space (i.e., widen the disc space and the foraminal canal) should be chosen in cases of nerve root irritation and compression and in cases of a worsening unilateral disc or zygapophyseal joint disorder.

Stretching Contracted Tissues. Joints that are both painful and hypomobile can respond differently to passive mobilization. The pain response during the performance of a technique, and its effect over a 24-hour period, will guide the therapist in determining the direction in which to move the joint and how firmly to stretch the contracted tissues. A favorable response to gentle oscillatory stretching occurs when there is a decrease in the pain experienced during the technique, thus allowing the movement to be performed more strongly. A worsening of the pain response indicates that this direction of movement is aggravating the condition.

Moving Intervertebral Joints or the Intervertebral and Foraminal Canal Structures. If, during the physical examination, movements of both the intervertebral joints and neural structures in the foraminal canals reproduce the patient's arm pain, treatment should be directed to the intervertebral joints in the first instance. The effect on the intervertebral joint signs and neural signs is noted, and if the neural signs do not improve, movement of the neural tissues should be added.

Performance of the Movement Technique

Selection of a treatment technique relates not only to the direction of movement but also to the manner in which it is applied.

The *amplitude* of a movement can be varied from barely perceptible to full use of the available range. The rhythm can be varied from smooth and evenly applied to staccato. Similarly, the speed and *position in range* in which the movement is performed can be altered.

A passive movement technique must be modified according to its desired effect, and this is based on the symptoms experienced by the patient during the technique, the quality of the movement, the presence of spasm, and the end-feel. A complete discussion of these details is beyond the scope of this chapter, but the two ends of the symptom spectrum are presented as follows: from a constant ache with pain experienced through the range of movement to stiffness with mild discomfort felt only at the end of the range of certain movements. A full description of the symptom spectrum may be found in Maitland.[2]

Constant Aching with Pain Through Range. The cervical spine must be placed in a position of maximal comfort (usually one of slight flexion and midposition for the other movements). The treatment technique is of small amplitude, performed slowly and smoothly (so that there is no discomfort or increase in the degree of aching). The movement technique may be a physiological or an accessory movement and should result in an immediate reduction in the degree of aching. In those patients in whom there is no immediate effect, the effect should be noted over a 24-hour period.

Stiffness with Mild Discomfort Felt Only at the End of Range of Certain Movements. The cervical spine is carefully positioned at or near the limit of the hypomobile directions of movement (i.e., in the position that best reproduced the symptoms of stiffness and discomfort). The treatment should put maximal stretch on the hypomobile intervertebral segment. The technique should be firmly applied, of small amplitude, and sustained. If the level of discomfort increases with the firm stretching, large-amplitude movements can be interspersed every 40 to 60 seconds.

CERVICAL SYNDROMES

In this section, some of the common clinical presentations with a history of spontaneous (nontraumatic) onset are discussed using typical case histories. The clinical reasoning related to management of these conditions by manipulative physical therapy is emphasized. It is beyond the scope of this chapter to describe patient self-management in detail, but it must be stressed that this aspect of treatment is integral to the management of all patients. Cervical vertigo and cervical headache are not included because these conditions are discussed in Chapters 8 and 13.

Zygapophyseal Joint Arthralgia

The zygapophyseal joints are a common source of pain in the cervical spine, particularly in the upper cervical spine, where they can cause local neck pain and pain referred to the head (see Chapter 4). Joints between C3 and C7 can refer pain to the supraspinous fossa and into the arm.[3] The area of pain strongly suggests the intervertebral source of the pain, but this must be confirmed by specific palpation for soft tissue changes (thickening of the tissues in the interlaminar space and around the zygapophyseal joint) and altered intervertebral movement (most often hypomobility). Seldom does pain arise from one joint alone; more commonly it arises from two or three adjacent joints. Joints may become symptomatic bilaterally or only on one side.

Osteoarthrotic changes (joint space narrowing, sclerosis, and osteophytosis) may or may not be evident on plain radiography, but Rees[4] found these changes to be common features in his tomographic studies of 2000 patients with cervical headache. In the elderly, low cervical (C4 to C7) spondylitic changes are more common than osteoarthrotic changes of the zygapophyseal joints, but the two kinds of changes often coexist. Specific examination will help to determine if symptoms are arising from the disc and/or the zygapophyseal joints.

Case Study 1

A 55-year-old housewife had a 3-year history of right-sided neck pain of gradual onset. When severe, the pain spread to the supraspinous fossa and upper lateral arm. The patient could not recall any specific incident having caused the onset of her pain, but it had been worse ever since she had hit her head 10 days earlier. Radiographs showed moderate spondylosis at C5-6 and mild bilateral osteoarthrosis of the C4-5 and C5-6 zygapophyseal joints.

Symptoms. The patient's mornings were symptom free, but by the end of each afternoon her neck ached, and the ache was worsened by activities involving cervical extension.

Physical Signs. Cervical flexion and left rotation (70 degrees) were slightly restricted but painless on passive overpressure. Extension was limited to half the normal range by right neck pain, and rotation to the right (40 degrees) reproduced pain in the right neck and supraspinous fossa. Intervertebral movement tests revealed hypomobility at the C3 to C6 zygapophyseal joints, which was more marked on the right. The pains in the cervical and supraspinous fossa were reproduced by right unilateral posteroanterior (PA) gliding (C3 to C6), whereas PA gliding on the left side revealed painless hypomobility.

Interpretation. The patient is a middle-aged woman with a stiff, degenerative, low cervical spine. The condition has been made worse by jarring of her neck. The area of pain and the patient's physical signs strongly suggest a zygapophyseal joint disorder. It would be appropriate to treat this with passive movement because both the symptoms and signs have a mechanical presentation. There are no contraindications to this, but at the first application it would be prudent to mobilize the joints short of producing discomfort. The presence for 3 years of symptoms in hypomobile degenerative joints suggests that a number of treatments (e.g., 5 to 10) may be required to progress both the firmness of stretching and the precision of application to the point of pain-free mobility. Examination for shortening of the cervical musculature must be included, and if any muscle groups are tight, then lengthening by relaxation techniques or stretching would be included. A home exercise program will be required to reduce the frequency of recurrence of the patient's symptoms.

Treatment

Day 1 (Treatment 1). With the patient prone and her neck supported comfortably in slight flexion, large-amplitude unilateral PA oscillatory pressures were applied over the right C3 to C6 zygapophyseal joints (Figure 14-1). The

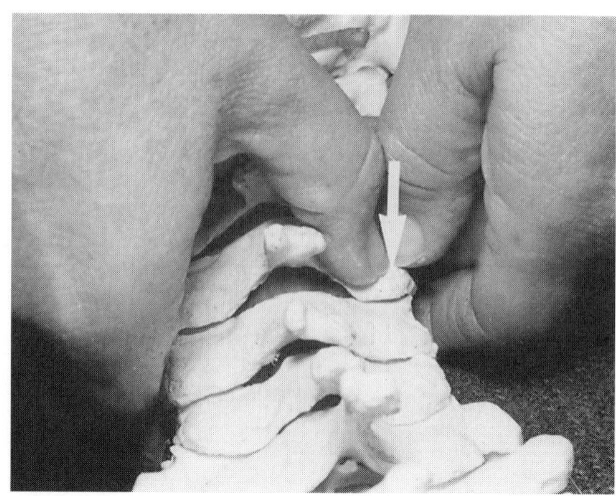

Figure 14-1
Unilateral posteroanterior (PA) gliding of the facets of the right C2-3 zygapophyseal joint.

oscillations were slow and rhythmic, with care being taken not to cause any discomfort during the technique. Reexamination showed an improvement of 10 degrees in the range of both cervical extension and right rotation. The patient was asked to perform mobility exercises twice daily after heating her neck under a warm shower. She was instructed to extend and to rotate her neck to each side, taking the movements to the onset of slight discomfort only.

Day 3 (Treatment 2). The patient reported that she had more mobility of her neck and less aching in the late afternoons. Physical examination showed that she had maintained the increased range gained at her first treatment. Unilateral PA pressures were applied further into range so that they stretched the hypomobile right C3 to C6 zygapophyseal joints, causing some discomfort. Two applications of this technique improved the range of right rotation to 60 degrees, but extension remained unaltered. The patient was asked to continue with her mobilizing exercises.

Day 5 (Treatment 3). The patient reported that her condition was improved. She had a mild ache on the right side of her neck at the end of the day but no referred pain to the supraspinous fossa or arm. Cervical extension remained at three fourths of the normal range, and right rotation remained at 60 degrees. Firmly applied unilateral pressures to the right C3 to C6 zygapophyseal joints restored a full pain-free range of right rotation, but extension of the patient's neck remained unchanged. (*Full range* refers to the full range for a patient's age and somatotype.)

Interpretation. Intervertebral movement tests demonstrated long-standing hypomobility of the C3 to C6 zygapophyseal joints bilaterally, but treatment had so far been directed unilaterally. Right rotation improved because it had been restricted predominantly at the symptomatic right zygapophyseal joints, which after treatment had improved mobility. However, extension involves movement of the zygapophyseal joints symmetrically and might have been restricted by the stiffness on the patient's left side. Therefore, in that case, treatment bilaterally would have been necessary to increase the patient's mobility, even though her symptoms were experienced unilaterally.

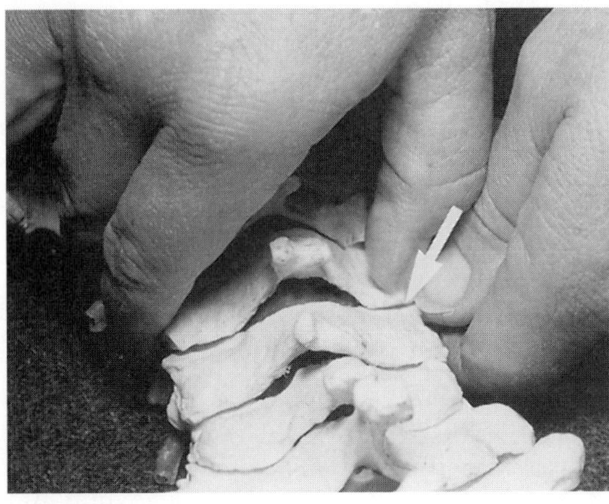

Figure 14-2
Medially directed unilateral PA gliding of the facets of the C2-3 zygapophyseal joint.

Day 5 (Treatment 3) Continued. Firm, sustained central and unilateral PA pressures (applied to each side) effected a marked increase in the range of low cervical extension and of both rotations (now 80 degrees).

The patient was asked to progress her exercises so that they applied a stretch into extension and both rotations. The degree of stretching was governed by the pain response, in which only discomfort (not pain) was to be experienced.

Day 7 (Treatment 4). The patient was delighted with her progress. She had experienced only two episodes of right-sided neck aching, this after cleaning windows. Her cervical extension and right rotation were full range, causing slight right low cervical discomfort. By directing the right unilateral PA pressure medially (a technique that glides the facets under some compression) on C4 and C5 (Figure 14-2), sharp local pain was elicited. This technique was used as a treatment. Three repetitions of oscillations lasting 30 seconds each were firmly applied to stretch the right zygapophyseal joints. Sharp pain was experienced on each occasion, but there was no aching afterward. Following this, extension and right rotation were painless on passive overpressure. Mobilizing exercises were reduced to once daily to maintain mobility of the patient's neck. The patient was shown how to use her hand to apply a firm stretch, and lateral flexion to each side was added.

Also, now that her symptoms were improving, tests for the length of the sternomastoid, upper trapezius, scalenes, and levator scapulae muscles were performed.[5] These muscles were not found to be tight, indicating that loss of cervical mobility was the result of joint hypomobility.

Day 12 (Treatment 5). The patient was asymptomatic and felt that her neck mobility was the best it had been for years. Slight discomfort was provoked by placing her neck in the combined position of extension and right rotation. With her neck in this combined position, firm unilateral PA pressures over the right C5-6 zygapophyseal joint caused sharp pain. Four repetitions of this technique for 30 seconds each, restored full range extension and right rotation with no discomfort on passive overpressure.

Treatment was discontinued, with an explanation to the patient that recurrences of her neck pain and stiffness were likely but would be less frequent if she maintained her cervical mobility with once-daily mobilizing exercises.

Acute Locking of Zygapophyseal Joint (Wry Neck)

Acute locking can occur at any intervertebral level but is most common at C2-3.[6] When locking occurs above this intervertebral level, there is usually a history of trauma, whereas locking in the low cervical levels is usually secondary to a disc disorder. Classically, locking follows an unguarded movement of the neck, with instant pain over the articular pillar and an antalgic posture of lateral flexion to the opposite side and slight flexion, which the patient is unable to correct. Locking is more common in children and young adults. In many the joint pain settles within 24 hours without requiring treatment (because the joint was merely sprained or because it unlocked spontaneously), but other patients will require a localized manipulation to unlock the joint. Some authors[6,7] postulate that the locking is the result of impaction of synovial villi or meniscoids between the facets of the zygapophyseal joint (see also Chapter 1). In older subjects the locking may result from the mechanical catching of roughened arthritic articular surfaces.[8] In both cases the innervated synovium and capsule would be stretched.[9]

Case Study 2

A 26-year-old man had a history of sharp left-sided neck pain of sudden onset when he turned his head rapidly to the right to catch a ball that morning. He found that he was unable to hold his head erect because of this sharp pain. He had no past history of cervical symptoms.

Symptoms. When the patient held his head flexed laterally to the right and in slight flexion, he had no pain—only a dull ache along the left side of his neck. On attempting to hold his head erect he experienced sharp, deep pain localized over the left C2-3 zygapophyseal joint. There were no symptoms of VBI.

Physical Signs. The patient's head was held in right lateral flexion and slight flexion. Attempts to correct this position actively or passively caused sharp pain over the left C2-3 zygapophyseal joint. With the patient's head in slight lateral flexion to the right, flexion and right rotation were full range and painless, upper cervical extension was slightly limited, and left rotation was 40 degrees, with both of these movements causing sharp left-sided cervical pain.

With the patient in the supine (nonweightbearing) position, it was possible to place his head in the midline position. With the head and neck in the neutral position, sharp pain was elicited on full upper cervical extension and at 50 degrees of left rotation. Testing of left lateral flexion at each intervertebral level confirmed a mechanical block to the movement at C2-3 with pain and spasm, whereas the movement was full range at the adjacent levels.

Treatment

Day 1 (Treatment 1). With the patient supine and his neck in a neutral position for the upper cervical spine, gentle manual traction was applied as a slow oscillation sustained for 30 seconds and then released. This was repeated 4 times, causing no discomfort. Because there was no improvement in the range of motion of his head, a relaxation technique was used in an attempt to reduce the spasm and so allow the joint to unlock spontaneously. The patient's head was rotated 45 degrees to the left, short of any discomfort, and a technique of reciprocal relaxation for the right cervical rotators was applied. Passive intervertebral lateral flexion to the left at C2-3 remained unchanged.

Interpretation. Because the patient's zygapophyseal joint would not unlock easily, it was necessary to "gap" the facets using a manipulation localized to the C2-3 intervertebral level. This is one condition in which it is not possible to fully perform the premanipulative screening tests for VBI[10] or for instability of the upper cervical spine.[11] In this particular case, there was no history of symptoms suggestive of VBI or of trauma or disease that might weaken ligamentous tissue. By careful positioning of the spine, the "thrust" technique should place minimal stretch on the segments above C2. Informed consent for the use of manipulation must be obtained from the patient.

Day 1 (Treatment1) Continued. A transverse thrust manipulation was applied to open the left C2-3 zygapophyseal joint. A description of the method of this technique can be found in Maitland.[2] Before the manipulation, the end position of the technique was sustained for 10 seconds to ensure that there would be no provocation of vertigo or nystagmus and was then released to note whether any latent symptoms occurred. The manipulation was performed after this.

After the manipulation, there was a full passive range of left lateral flexion at the left C2-3 zygapophyseal joint, but on assuming the sitting position, the patient again adopted a wry neck position. Active left lateral flexion was full but still painful. After the application of large-amplitude unilateral PA oscillatory pressures and ultrasound to the left C2-3 zygapophyseal joint, only slight discomfort was experienced on active left lateral flexion.

A soft collar was applied to protect the joint from jolting in the patient's car. The patient was advised to rest, with his head comfortably supported on one pillow, for the remainder of the day.

Day 2 (Treatment 2). The patient reported that because his neck ached on the way home, he had taken analgesics and rested. He had subsequently experienced one or two twinges of pain when turning in bed. On the morning of his second treatment his neck had felt "normal." In sitting, full left lateral flexion was painful over the left C2-3 joint. Passive left lateral flexion at this joint was painful when subjected to nonweightbearing testing but was of full range. Treatment consisted of three repetitions of large-amplitude unilateral PA pressures, each applied for 60 seconds over the left C2-3 zygapophyseal joint, after which left lateral flexion, performed in the sitting position, was pain free to passive overpressure. On the following day the patient telephoned to cancel his appointment because he had regained full pain-free mobility of his neck.

Recurrent Locking of Cervical Zygapophyseal Joints

Some individuals experience recurrent cervical zygapophyseal joint locking. Many are women who exhibit generalized joint hypermobility. The recurrence rate of this condition can be lessened by teaching these individuals exercises to improve both the strength and coordination of their cervical muscles, especially the deep muscles that span one to three segmental levels.

Discogenic Pain

The low cervical spine is a common site of spondylosis. From in vitro studies,[12] (see also Chapter 1) it has been noted that horizontal fissuring of the disc from the uncovertebral region begins in the first decade of life and is quite extensive by 20 to 30 years of age. In many cases, this degenerative process remains asymptomatic, but in others, symptoms develop either spontaneously or after postures involving sustained extension or flexion. Cases of spondylosis of traumatic origin are excluded from this discussion.

The clinical picture varies considerably. Hypomobility of the low cervical spine is common to all cases. This may progress to the stage at which loss of mobility interferes with daily activities; thus, for example, loss of extension and rotation make it difficult to turn the head to drive the car in reverse. Often stiffness of the cervicothoracic region causes the development of a kyphotic (dowager's hump) deformity. In other cases, aching and pain may develop. The stiff low cervical joints may be the source of pain, which often is described as a burning pain across the base of the neck, or the mobile midcervical joints may become symptomatic, the typical complaint being a central, deep midcervical pain. Pain also may be experienced in the medial scapular area.[13]

It is unusual for patients with spondylosis to complain of nerve root symptoms or to develop neurological signs. This contrasts with discogenic disorders of the lumbar spine, which often progress to the prolapse of nuclear material, causing nerve root symptoms and signs. In cervical discs the small nucleus pulposus is gradually lost via the posterior and lateral fissures and at the same time, undergoes metaplastic change from a soft gel into fibrocartilage. Any nuclear material remaining in young adults is more likely to herniate posteriorly into the spinal canal than laterally through the uncovertebral joints (see Chapter 1).

Case Study 3

A 60-year-old housewife had central low cervical pain of gradual onset over the preceding 3 weeks. She associated this with long hours of sustained neck flexion while sewing. Discogenic pain is likely to arise from mechanical stress (e.g., sustained flexion and anterior shear forces) on the annulus, the outer fibers of which are innervated.[14,15] The patient's symptoms began as stiffness on straightening her neck and some short-lived stiffness in the mornings. Movements of her neck would readily ease this. Her symptoms were worsening in that for the previous week she had been able to sew only for increasingly short periods before her symptoms appeared. Three days before visiting the physical therapist, she awoke with a very stiff neck and experienced left medial scapular pain each time she flexed her neck. She was unable to recall any neck symptoms in the past, but for 2 or 3 years had awakened with neck stiffness that she considered to have been "normal as one gets older." Radiographs of the cervical and thoracic spine showed mild narrowing of the C4-5 and C5-6 disc spaces.

Symptoms. The patient was unable to flex her neck because of sharp pain experienced medial to the spine of her left scapula. This pain would ease immediately on returning her neck to the upright position. This pain interfered with many of her daily activities, and by noon of each day, a constant, deep central ache (C5 to C7) had developed. Lying supine with her head on a thick pillow eased her pain after half an hour, but the ache would soon return once she was again upright and attempting household activities. In the mornings her neck was stiff and ached for half an hour.

Signs. The patient had a pronounced forward head posture (Figure 14-3, *A*), attempted correction of which by passive posterior gliding (Figure 14-3, *B*) reproduced both the low cervical and sharp left medial scapular pain. The following movements also reproduced both areas of symptoms: flexion (half range), extension (one-fourth range), and left rotation (45 degrees). The patient was instructed to perform these active movements only until the onset of discomfort.

On palpation, the spinous process of C4 was depressed, whereas that of C5 was prominent. The deep interspinous soft tissues between C4-5 and C5-6 were thickened, and this thickening was most pronounced on the left between C4 and C5. The C4 vertebra was very mobile to central PA pressures, whereas C5 was by contrast markedly hypomobile. Deep pain was elicited at both levels. The C4 to C7 zygapophyseal joints were of normal mobility and only mildly painful with unilateral PA pressure and testing of segmental physiological movements. Tests for the upper and midthoracic spine demonstrated painless hypomobility.

Because of the irritability of the patient's condition, muscle length and strength tests were deferred until the condition was no longer irritable.

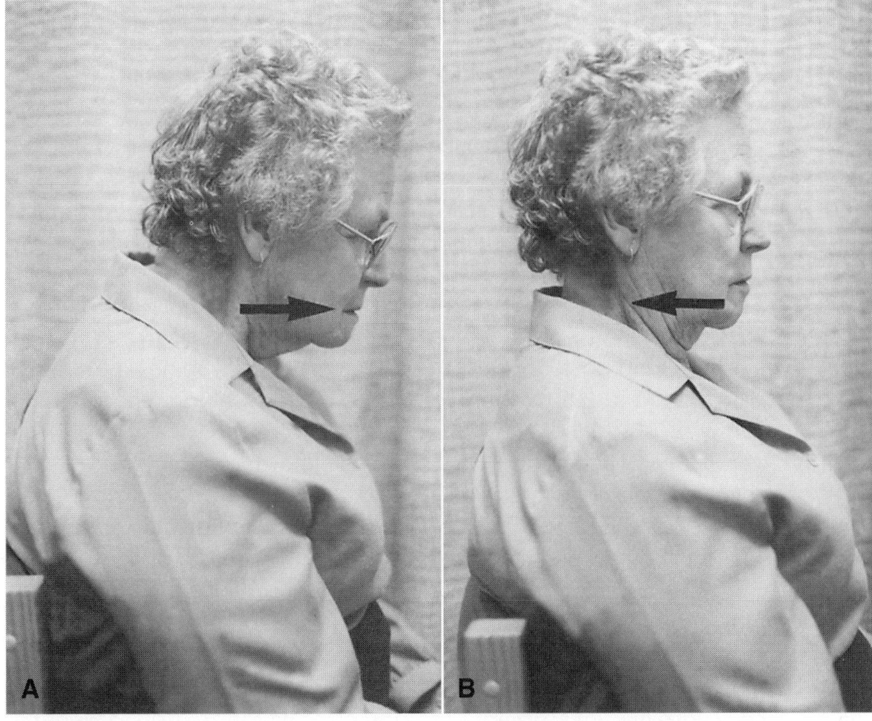

Figure 14-3
A, Lateral view of forward head posture. **B,** Correction of forward head posture by posterior gliding.

Interpretation. Discogenic disorders often commence insidiously, in this case with morning stiffness. A forward head posture coupled with long periods of sustained flexion puts an anterior shearing force on the low cervical discs, and in time, symptoms may develop. The area of pain, pattern of movement restriction, and palpation findings in this case were typical of a discogenic disorder. The lack of unilateral neck pain and normal mobility of the zygapophyseal joints for the patient's age and somatotype failed to implicate these joints as the source of her pain. Her disorder was worsening and irritable.

Although the symptomatic joints in a case such as this should settle in 1 or 2 weeks with treatment, the long-term relief of symptoms requires attention to correcting both the muscle imbalance and the forward head posture.

Treatment

Day 1 (Treatment 1). After the examination the patient experienced a constant deep central ache in the low cervical area. Because this was relieved by gentle manual traction, traction was chosen as the treatment technique. Traction was applied with the patient supine and with her head and neck supported comfortably on two pillows so that the head-on-neck position was neutral between flexion and extension, and the neck-on-thorax position was in approximately 35 degrees of flexion, which was the neutral position for the C4-5 intervertebral joint. Four pounds of traction was chosen because with that strength, movement could be palpated in the soft tissues in the interspinous space between C4 and C5 and because this effected a reduction in the patient's neck ache. Traction was applied for 7 minutes, and because of the irritability of the patient's disorder, her movement signs were not reassessed afterward.

The patient was given a soft collar as a temporary measure to support her neck and to prevent painful flexion. She was asked to wear the collar while upright but not when resting in bed.

Day 2 (Treatment 2). When seen the next day, the patient reported that her neck was more comfortable and that she had slept well. Cervical movements were unaltered. Traction was repeated at 4 lb for 15 minutes, after which all of the patient's cervical movements improved in range before medial scapular pain was produced. She was asked to continue wearing the collar.

Day 3 (Treatment 3). The patient had experienced no left medial scapular pain, and her neck felt less stiff on the morning of her third day of treatment. Flexion, extension, and posterior gliding of her low cervical spine were now at three-fourths range, and left rotation was at 70 degrees before sharp medial scapular pain was produced. Movement further into range was possible with central PA pressures over C4 and C5 before eliciting deep pain.

For treatment, central PA pressures (Figure 14-4) were applied slowly and rhythmically to C4 and C5 for 60 seconds, keeping short of producing any discomfort. This resulted in a definite improvement in the range of all movements. Because a second application of this technique caused a deep ache to develop, the technique was stopped and traction was applied using the same dosage as on the previous day. Reassessment showed a full range of all movement except for posterior gliding, which remained at three-fourths range and still produced sharp medial scapular pain. The patient was advised to wear her collar only if her neck or medial scapular pain returned, and she was taught correction of her forward head posture, taking the movement only to the onset of discomfort.

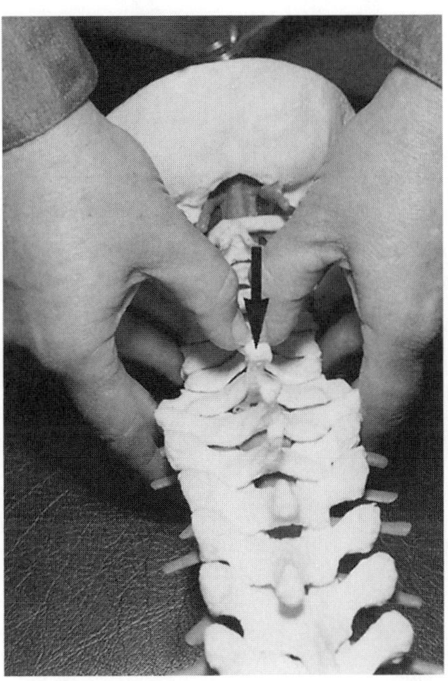

Figure 14-4
Central PA oscillatory pressures on spinous process of the C5 vertebra.

Day 4 (Treatment 4). The patient had been symptom free until late afternoon, when her central low cervical ache developed. This improvement was helped by the collar. Stiffness was now present for 5 minutes only in the mornings and was eased by a warm shower. Flexion and left rotation were full and painless to passive overpressure, extension was almost full range but caused pain centrally over C7, and the extreme range of posterior glide still caused slight left medial scapular pain. If PA pressures to C5 were directed toward the right (Figure 14-5), deep, sharp pain was elicited. Treatment consisted of three repetitions of central PA pressures applied for 30 seconds to C5, including some directed toward the right. This technique was performed as small oscillations at the end of the range of movement so as to obtain greater mobility. The treatment caused local pain that settled as soon as the stretching stopped. After each application, extension and posterior gliding improved, becoming full and painless to overpressure.

Interpretation. With a long-standing forward head posture, there is often an associated poking chin with adaptive shortening of the suboccipital muscles and weakness of the short flexor muscle group. Now that the discogenic disorder is no longer irritable, the neck muscles should be examined for tightness and weakness.

Day 4 (Treatment 4) Continued. With this particular patient, the craniocervical extensors were not tight, but the patient was unable to contract the deep craniocervical flexors without also activating the superficial cervical flexors. Specific retraining of the deep flexors consisted of teaching the patient how to position her head and neck in a neutral position in supine, using towels under

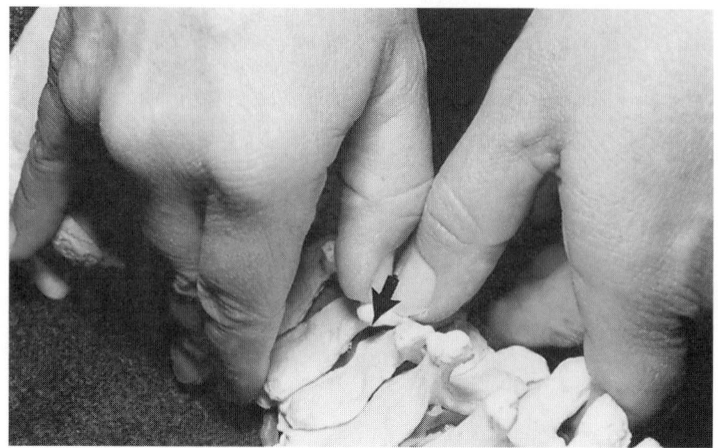

Figure 14-5
Central PA oscillatory pressures directed toward the right.

the occiput. Assisted active head-on-neck flexion (nodding) and extension was practiced in this neutral position, and the patient was shown how to palpate for unwanted activity in the superficial flexors.

The cuff of a pressure biofeedback unit (Chattanooga) was placed behind the neck and the cuff inflated to 20 mm Hg. At this pressure the patient was aware of the cuff against the skin of her neck. She was shown the pressure dial and asked to increase the pressure to 22 mm Hg by slowly and gently nodding her head. The patient was able to hold this pressure for 5 seconds and to perform five nods. The muscles tired after five repetitions, and attempts at a stronger contraction caused the superficial flexors to contract.

A biofeedback unit and written instructions were given to the patient for twice-daily exercises at home. Starting with five contractions at 22 mm Hg with a hold of 5 seconds, the patient was asked to gradually increase the number to 10 contractions, and once this was achieved, the holding time was to be incrementally increased to 10 seconds. Emphasis was placed on slow, steady, and gentle "nods" as shown on the dial of the biofeedback unit.

Day 12 (Treatment 5). The patient reported only two occasions when her neck had ached. Each occasion had followed sewing for 1 hour, and she had been able to stop the aching by repeated posterior gliding of her low cervical spine. On examination, her cervical movements were full and painless to passive overpressure, with the exception of sustained overpressure to posterior gliding, which caused a deep ache over C7. PA pressures to C5, when directed to the right, were stiffer than when directed to the left. Proficiency at the deep neck flexor exercises was checked using the biofeedback unit. The patient could easily perform 10 contractions at 22 mm Hg each with a hold of 10 seconds, and with no overflow into the superficial muscle groups.

Treatment consisted of four repetitions of PA pressure applied to C5 centrally and directed to the right. The oscillatory pressures were applied firmly and sustained for 60 seconds to stretch the restricted range of C5 on its adjacent vertebrae. At the end of the third and fourth applications, a deep ache developed but was eased by larger-amplitude PA pressures. After the mobilization, sustained overpressure to posterior gliding was pain free. Firm PA and lateral pressures from both sides were applied to the spinous processes of C7 to T5 vertebrae to mobilize the hypomobile kyphotic posture of the upper thoracic spine. Improved mobility in this area was likely to decrease the mechanical stress on the low cervical spine during daily activities. Because the short flexor muscle control had improved, the exercises were progressed to 24 mm Hg of pressure on the cuff. The patient was able to perform 10 contractions with a 5-second hold. She was asked to gradually build up to 10 contractions with a 10-second hold and, once this was achieved, to progress to 26 mm Hg of pressure.

Advice was given to the patient regarding self-management of her cervical disc problem. This included regular posture correction and instruction to break up long periods of sustained cervical flexion by regularly performing full-range low cervical extension and posterior gliding and to avoid lifting or pushing when she was tired or unwell (i.e., at times when the muscular protection of her neck is less efficient).

Day 33 (Treatment 6). When seen 3 weeks after her fifth treatment, the patient was symptom and sign free except for some residual hypomobility and soreness with PA pressures on C5. Her short flexor muscles were performing well (10 repetitions at 26 mm Hg for a 10-second hold). The patient was shown how to combine the "nodding action" with scapular depression and adduction. Home exercises consisted of this combined control of nodding (28 mm Hg) with scapular stabilization. After 3 weeks, the frequency was to be reduced to once daily.

The C5 vertebra was firmly mobilized, as was the upper thoracic spine. The persistence of continuing hypomobility of C5 was explained to the patient, and the need for regular posture correction and exercise was emphasized.

Discogenic Wry Neck

The exact pathoanatomical mechanism for the production of medial scapular pain and the associated antalgic posture of contralateral lateral flexion and flexion has not been reported, although the innervation of the outer annulus of the cervical discs has been described[14,15] and Cloward[13] demonstrated that pain can be referred from the cervical discs to the medial scapular area.

A wry neck position, or torticollis, secondary to a discogenic condition differs in the following respects from that secondary to a locked cervical zygapophyseal joint:

1. There is no history of a quick or unguarded movement resulting in a sudden onset of pain and locking; often the patient awakens with the pain, having been pain free the night before.
2. The distribution of the symptoms differs from the case of a locked cervical zygapophyseal joint; most commonly, sharp pain is experienced medial to one scapula with certain cervical movements and postures, but there is no pain in the neck. However, having to hold the wry position against gravity may result in some generalized aching in the cervical musculature.
3. The physical signs also are different. There is often a marked kyphotic deformity, and in the nonweightbearing position, a greater range of pain-free

movement is possible. In particular, ipsilateral lateral flexion is not mechanically locked but is limited by sharp referred pain (no local pain). Testing of passive accessory intervertebral movements demonstrates painful hypomobility with the application of central PA pressures, whereas unilateral PA oscillatory mobilization of the zygapophyseal joints is full range and painless.

Differentiation of the two distinct types of wry neck is important because the appropriate treatment for each differs. For a locked zygapophyseal joint, unlocking the joint (often by a manipulation) is essential, whereas manipulation is likely to irritate the discogenic type of wry neck.

Cervical Radicular Pain

A previously injured nerve root can give rise to pain if it is subjected to mechanical stimuli. The low cervical and upper thoracic nerve roots may be subject to injury because of the angulated course of the rootlets. Within the dura the rootlets run downward, but on piercing it they turn abruptly upward at an angle of between 30 and 45 degrees[16] to reach their relevant foramen. The angulation of these rootlets is increased during cervical extension,[6] and hence they are prone to injury during hyperextension injuries and if the neck is held in sustained extension (as in painting a ceiling).

The onset of nerve root involvement may be insidious or may follow unrecognized stress or trauma, such as sleeping in an awkward position, unusually prolonged cervical extension or flexion, or traction on an arm. Nerve root symptoms are unusual in young subjects unless there is a history of trauma, in which case the likely causes are posterolateral disc protrusion or zygapophyseal joint effusion.[17] In older individuals with established degenerative changes (regardless of whether they are symptomatic), the nerve root may be compromised as a result of foraminal encroachment by osteophyte formation at the margins of the facets of the zygapophyseal joint or disc-vertebral body margin. Nerve root compression also may be the result of fibrotic thickening of the dural sleeve.[18]

Case Study 4

Six months ago, a 50-year-old farmer experienced right-sided low cervical pain and stiffness after shoveling earth for 4 hours. The pain settled after a few days, but the patient subsequently noticed that any physical activity was followed by neck stiffness the next morning.

Four days ago the patient painted a ceiling. He woke the next morning with severe right shoulder and arm pain. During the day this pain worsened and spread into his forearm. He felt that his condition was worsening in that his fingers felt numb. Routine radiographs showed advanced spondylitic changes at C5-6 and C6-7 but no osteophytic encroachment of the neural foramina.

Symptoms. The patient complained of constant, severe pain that was worse in the right forearm and from which he was unable to find relief except by medication, which gave some short-term relief. Numbness of the right index and middle fingers also was present.

Physical Signs. The patient's head and neck were held rigidly in slight flexion, and he cradled his right arm with his left and supported it across his chest. Only two cervical movements were examined because of the severity of his pain and the irritability of the condition. Both extension (5 degrees) and right rotation (30 degrees) increased the patient's forearm pain. A neurological examination revealed that his right triceps power was only of half strength, his right triceps reflex was absent, and there was numbness of the pads of his right index and middle fingers. The first component of the upper limb tension test (ULTT) (shoulder girdle depression) increased the intensity of his forearm pain. Passive intervertebral movement tests and scanning tests for other sources of arm symptoms were not performed.

Interpretation. The early history of this case is typical of a chronic condition (there is insufficient information to incriminate a disc or a zygapophyseal joint disorder as the cause). Then, after sustained cervical extension, symptoms developed in the arm. The presence of neurological changes supports a diagnosis of right C7 nerve root compression.

Traction is the treatment of choice for severe nerve root pain of acute onset. It may take several days before the symptoms improve, although a slow, steady improvement in the physical signs is expected.

Treatment

Day 1 (Treatment 1). Traction was given with the patient supine. Positioning for maximal comfort is essential. Two pillows were required to place the low cervical spine in sufficient flexion, and another pillow was placed under the patient's right arm (to prevent the weight of the arm from retracting or depressing the shoulder girdle).

Seven pounds of traction was needed for the therapist to palpate movement occurring in the deep soft tissues at C6-7. The patient was asked to assess the intensity of his arm symptoms, after which the 7 lb of traction was applied and the intensity of the patient's symptoms was reassessed. Because the pain then worsened, the strength of the traction was halved and sustained for 10 minutes. Throughout the procedure, the patient's arm symptoms remained unchanged. After the traction was stopped, the patient continued to rest for half an hour, after which the traction was reapplied for another 10 minutes at the same strength. At the completion of another rest period, the patient reported that the intensity of his forearm pain had decreased. His physical signs were not reassessed. The patient was advised to rest in bed as much as possible, in a position of maximal comfort.

Days 2 and 3 (Treatments 2 and 3). The patient reported no symptomatic relief, and his cervical and neural signs were unchanged. Cervical traction was repeated, with two applications of 15 minutes at the second treatment and 20 minutes at the third treatment, interspersed with a rest period of 30 minutes. Neural conduction was unaltered, although the patient reported improvement in his forearm pain and finger sensation.

Day 4 (Treatment 4). The patient reported that he could sometimes completely ease his forearm pain by tucking his right thumb in his belt. Examination revealed that in this position his shoulder girdle was elevated, a position that reduces tension on the C7 nerve root. With the patient's right thumb tucked into his belt, his cervical extension and right rotation could be taken an extra 15 degrees before producing forearm pain. His nerve conduction signs were unchanged.

Interpretation. The signs in this case show that there is painful restriction of the normal distal movement of the C7 nerve root and that this also is limiting the range of cervical extension and right rotation. Rather than continue cervical traction, a more rapid symptomatic improvement is likely to occur from mobilization of the articular tissue (C6-7 intervertebral level and the first rib where the neural tissue passes between the clavicle and first rib) or the neural tissue, using a component of the ULTT. In view of the patient's previously worsening neurological status, it was decided to treat the articular component of his condition.

Day 4 (Treatment 4) Continued. With the patient lying prone, passive accessory movements isolated the maximal hypomobility and local discomfort to the right C6-7 zygapophyseal joint. This was then mobilized, using a combination of small- and large-amplitude movements and taking care not to refer symptoms to the arm. After this, the patient was able to hang his right arm by his side for 2 minutes before experiencing forearm pain. His cervical extension and rotation each improved by 15 degrees. A second application of passive mobilization was thought unwise, owing to the patient's unstable neurological status, but cervical traction, as for Treatment 3, was given. On completion of the traction there was definite improvement in the patient's triceps strength and reflex and in sensation in his finger pads.

Day 6 (Treatment 5). The patient was delighted with his progress. He experienced only occasional and less intense right forearm pain, and his finger sensation was normal. His triceps was five sixths of normal strength, and his triceps reflex was slightly depressed. It was necessary to combine low cervical extension with right rotation to reproduce his neurogenic forearm pain. Shoulder girdle depression was pain free, but the addition of 40 degrees of passive abduction brought on sharp forearm pain.

Interpretation. With such improvement in neural conduction, it is safe to more firmly mobilize the low cervical spine. Because neural tension signs more effectively reproduce the forearm pain, it may be necessary to add careful neural mobilization.

Day 6 (Treatment 5) continued. After three applications of firm passive mobilization of the C6-7 and adjacent levels, the patient's forearm pain could not be reproduced even by sustaining the combined position of extension and right rotation. After the first application of mobilization, the patient's neural mobility increased slightly (right shoulder abduction to 50 degrees), after which there was no further change. Before the treatment technique was changed to neural mobilization, the patient's neurological conduction was assessed and found to be unchanged. With the right shoulder girdle depressed, large-amplitude abduction, up to the onset of forearm pain, was performed. Only slight resistance to this movement was encountered. The technique was repeated, after which forearm pain was elicited at 65 degrees abduction.

Day 13 (Treatment 6). The patient was asymptomatic and had full recovery of C7 nerve root conduction. With the shoulder girdle depressed, abduction to 90 degrees was pain free, but the addition of 30 degrees of glenohumeral lateral rotation caused sharp forearm pain. On the left side, by comparison, the addition of lateral rotation and elbow extension components of the ULTT could be taken to full range and were painless. To lessen the likelihood of recurrence of the patient's symptoms, it was decided to stretch the right arm into lateral rotation (three firm stretches). The patient was asked to return in a fortnight because his neural tissue still lacked full mobility.

Day 27 (Treatment 7). The patient remained asymptomatic. Cervical and neural conduction signs were checked and found to be normal. The ULTT revealed a painless limitation of elbow extension of 20 degrees. Three firm stretches of elbow extension restored a full range of motion, and treatment was discontinued.

SUMMARY

This chapter highlights the application of manual therapy (passive mobilization and manipulation) in some cervical syndromes. Manual therapy is an effective and safe method of treatment if it is based on careful, thorough examination and regular assessment. In practice, it is essential that manual therapy be integrated with management of inadequate muscle protection and poor posture.

References

1. Trott PH, Grant ER: Manipulative physical therapy in the management of selected low lumbar syndromes. In Twomey LT, Taylor J, editors: *Physical therapy of the low back*, ed 3, New York, 2000, Churchill Livingstone.
2. Maitland GD: *Vertebral manipulation*, ed 5, London, 1986, Butterworths.
3. Aprill C, Dwyer A, Bogduk N: Cervical zygapophyseal joint pain patterns. II. A clinical evaluation, *Spine* 15:458, 1990.
4. Rees S: Relaxation therapy in migraine and chronic tension headaches, *Med J Aust* 2(2):70, 1975.
5. Kendall FP, McCreary EK, Provance PG: *Muscle testing and function: with posture and pain*, ed 4, Baltimore, 1993, Williams & Wilkins.
6. Grieve GP: *Common vertebral joint problems*, ed 2, Edinburgh, 1988, Churchill Livingstone.
7. Bourdillon JF: *Spinal manipulation*, ed 4, London, 1987, Heinemann, Appleton & Lange.
8. Stoddard A: *Manual of osteopathic practice*, ed 2, London, 1983, Hutchinson.
9. Giles LG, Taylor JR: Human zygapophyseal joint capsule and synovial fold innervation, *Br J Rheumatol* 26:93, 1987.
10. Australian Physiotherapy Association: Protocol for pre-manipulative testing of the cervical spine, *Aust J Physiother* 34:97, 1988.
11. Aspinall W: Clinical testing for the craniovertebral hypermobility syndrome, *J Orthop Sports Phys Ther* 12:47, 1990.
12. Taylor JR, Twomey LT: Acute injuries to cervical joints: an autopsy study of neck sprain, *Spine* 18:1115, 1993.
13. Cloward RB: Cervical discography: a contribution to the aetiology and mechanism of neck, shoulder, and arm pain, *Ann Surg* 150:1052, 1959.
14. Bogduk N, Windsor M, Inglis A: The innervation of the cervical intervertebral discs, *Spine* 13:2, 1989.
15. Mendel T, Wink CS, Zimney ML: Neural elements in human cervical intervertebral discs, *Spine* 17:132, 1992.

16. Nathan H, Feuerstein M: Angulated course of spinal nerve roots, *J Neurosurg* 32:349, 1970.
17. Simeone FA, Rothman RH: Cervical disc disease. In Rothman RH, Simeone FA, editors: *The spine*, vol I, Philadelphia, 1975, WB Saunders.
18. Frykolm R: Cervical root compression resulting from disc degeneration and root sleeve fibrosis, *Acta Chir Scand* Suppl:160, 1951.

CHAPTER 15

Sympathetic Nervous System and Pain: a Reappraisal

Helen Slater

In the second edition of *Physical Therapy of the Cervical and Thoracic Spine*, many authors[1-4] commented on the lack of fundamental anatomical, experimental, and clinical data in relation to the thoracic spine. Many manual therapy strategies that have been developed to manage idiopathic thoracic pain have been or are putative.[2] With the advent of evidence-based medicine, there is an increasing push in physical therapy to critically examine the effectiveness of currently accepted practices. This movement has been long overdue. As Jones[5] comments, physical therapy is vulnerable to misdirection with much of its current practice based on a combination of scientific and quasiempirical approaches.

This is not to suggest that clinical observations and related practices are to be disregarded as we await scientific corroboration but merely to balance scientific knowledge with clinical observations and implement research that explores the relationships between what we see, what it means, and how we can positively influence patient outcomes.[6] Such an approach offers critical yet creative clinical strategies. Not only should these practices be examined for effectiveness, but we also must develop a better understanding of the ways in which manual therapy treatments provide pain relief and help to restore normal neuromusculoskeletal function and improve quality of life.

This chapter is a synopsis of the current knowledge and thinking in relation to the role of the sympathetic nervous system (SNS) in musculoskeletal pain states relevant to the upper quarter (cervical and thoracic spines and the upper limbs). Recent findings on the ways in which specific manual therapy techniques influence manipulation-induced analgesia (MIA) will be discussed. Readers are presented with an overview of a biopsychosocial paradigm for management of complex regional pain syndromes (CRPSs), with specific emphasis on the role of physical therapy. It should be noted that at the time of writing this chapter, the International Association for the Study of Pain (IASP) had recently held a closed workshop on the issue of the classification of CRPSs, their proposed mechanisms, and implications for their management. The consensus statement from this workshop has yet to be released (see the list of

Websites at the end of chapter). Further detail is provided by other authors[7-9] (see also Chapter 4).

SYMPATHETIC NERVOUS SYSTEM: WHAT'S NEW?

Sympathetic (and central autonomic) regulation is coordinated through neuronal cell pools located in the brainstem (medulla oblongata, pons and midbrain), diencephalon, and telencephalon. The central autonomic network (CAN) has both direct and indirect reciprocal connections with the SNS and parasympathetic nervous systems from the spinal cord and cranial outflows.[7] It is thought that this reciprocal arrangement serves as a feedback mechanism to regulate sympathetic, parasympathetic, and neuroendocrine functions (Figure 15-1). There are also well-developed interconnections between the CAN and autonomic integrative centers, including the prefrontal and insular cortex, amygdala, hypothalamus, ventrolateral medulla, nucleus tractus solitarii (NTS), parabrachial nucleus, and periaqueductal gray (PAG) matter. Of particular note are the reciprocal connections between the NTS and the amygdala and between the amygdala and the limbic structures. This is an important area because the amygdala is involved in behavioral, neuroendocrine, and other autonomic functions related to injury and illness. Fear-related behaviors and sensory input from other brain nuclei are interpreted in the amygdala as either stressful or not.

Immune interactions with neurons in this and other brain regions activate cortisol-mediated restraint of the immune response and also induce behaviors that assist in recovery from illness and injury.[10] Cytokines from the body's immune system can signal the NTS and associated brain centers to induce behaviors linked with the stress response, such as fear-avoidance, anxiety, and other illness behaviors that are characteristic of the healing process.

The areas devoted to controlling sympathetic outflow include the following:

- Paraventricular hypothalamic nucleus
- A5 noradrenergic cell group
- Caudal raphe area
- Rostral ventrolateral medulla and the ventromedial medulla

From these nuclei fibers, descending projections terminate in the intermediolateral cell column of the lateral horn of the spinal thoracolumbar cord.

In summary, regulation of sympathetic (autonomic) function is mediated by reflex modulation of sympathetic and parasympathetic tone at the end-organ and by neurohumoral mechanisms. For example, a stressful situation may induce rapid reflex alterations that enhance the chances of survival; these include changes in heart rate, blood pressure, pupil size, and gastrointestinal function. Simultaneously, the neurohumoral system increases the level of cortisol in response to the perceived stress. This highly integrated and coordinated process not only involves physiological shifts in function but also manifests with changes in behavior.

SPINAL AND PERIPHERAL SYMPATHETIC NERVOUS SYSTEMS

The SNS regulates the function of all innervated tissues and organs throughout the body with a few exceptions, such as skeletal muscle fibers.[11] It forms the major efferent component of the peripheral nervous system.

The SNS has a special significance in the context of the mind-body interaction in health and disease. Mobilizing the human body during stress, the SNS also innervates immune organs such as the thymus, spleen, and lymph nodes and assists in the regu-

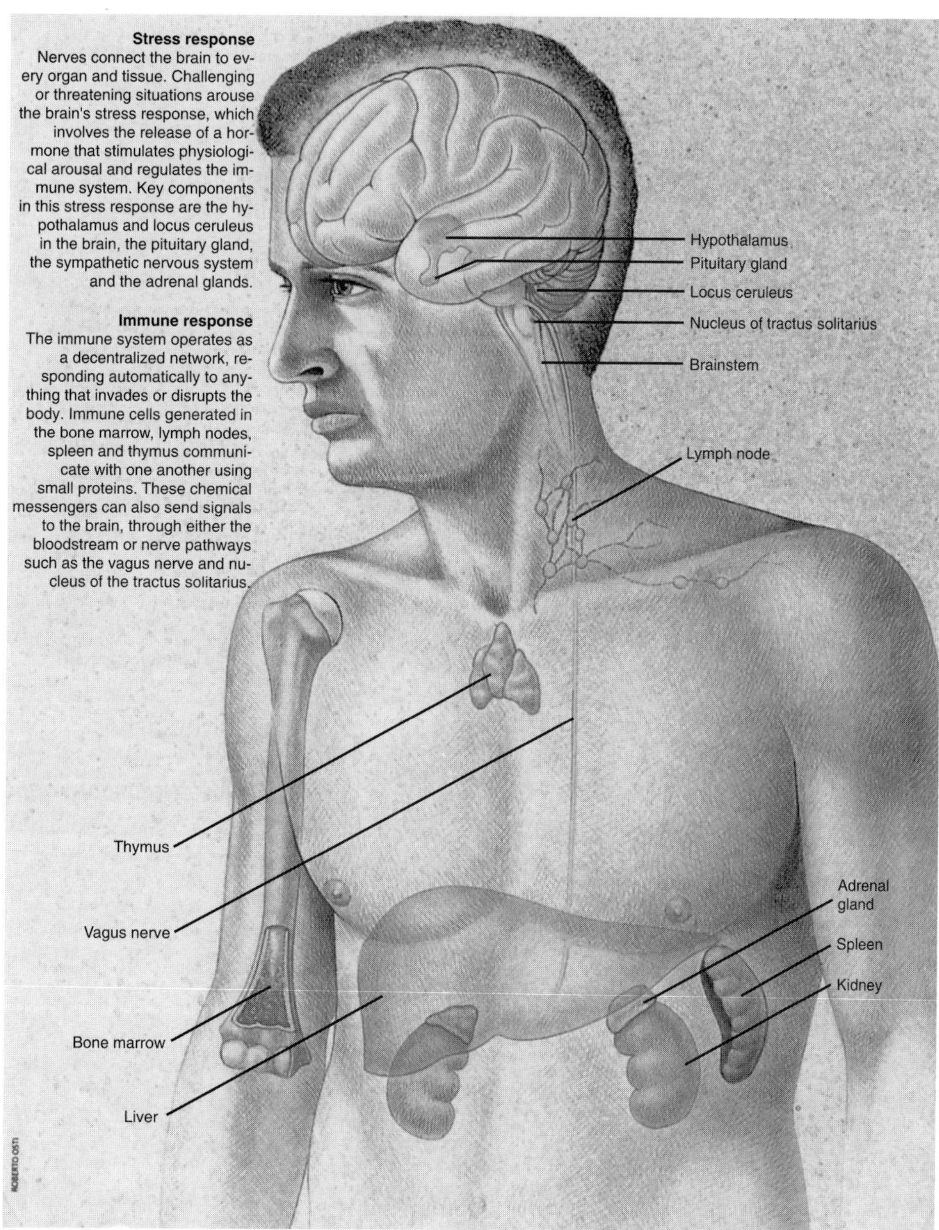

Stress response
Nerves connect the brain to every organ and tissue. Challenging or threatening situations arouse the brain's stress response, which involves the release of a hormone that stimulates physiological arousal and regulates the immune system. Key components in this stress response are the hypothalamus and locus ceruleus in the brain, the pituitary gland, the sympathetic nervous system and the adrenal glands.
Immune response
The immune system operates as a decentralized network, responding automatically to anything that invades or disrupts the body. Immune cells generated in the bone marrow, lymph nodes, spleen and thymus communicate with one another using small proteins. These chemical messengers can also send signals to the brain, through either the bloodstream or nerve pathways such as the vagus nerve and nucleus of the tractus solitarius.
Hypothalamus
Pituitary gland
Locus ceruleus
Nucleus of tractus solitarius
Brainstem
Lymph node
Thymus
Vagus nerve
Adrenal gland
Spleen
Kidney
Bone marrow
Liver
ROBERTO OSTI

Figure 15-1
Integration of sympathetic functions and neuroendocrine and immune systems.
(From Sternberg EM, Gold PW: *Sci Am* 7:9, 1997.)

lation of inflammatory responses throughout the body. Interactions between the SNS and the sensory apparatus in response to pain are also considered integral parts of the injury and tissue-repair process. They are especially relevant in the discussion on the role of the SNS in ongoing pain states.

Key Features of the Spinal and Peripheral Sympathetic Nervous System. Cell bodies located in the intermediomedial and interomediolateral columns of spinal cord segments T1 to L2 give rise to the thoracolumbar outflow, otherwise known as the *sympathetic outflow* (Figure 15-2).

The main features of the spinal and peripheral SNS are summarized next. When relevant, the clinical significance of the key features is discussed after each point.

1. Neurons arising from the cell bodies in the thoracolumbar region form the preganglionic efferent innervation to postsynaptic sympathetic neurons that are housed in the paravertebral ganglia, the prevertebral ganglia, or the previsceral ganglia.
2. Paravertebral ganglia are contained bilaterally in 22 pairs of ganglia, known as the *sympathetic trunk* or *chain*. There is some suggestion in the literature that the paravertebral ganglia and sympathetic trunks may hold particular interest to physical therapists working in the neuromusculoskeletal area.[1,9,12]

   Mechanical compromise of the sympathetic trunk has been hypothesized[1] as a potential contributor to alterations in physiology (via axonal transport mechanisms) of the sympathetic efferents. Many clinicians will have witnessed the profound changes that can occur in skin color, skin temperature, sweating, and reported pain in response to manual treatments directed at the thoracic spine. Readers will have noted the well-documented and apparently effective treatment strategies for T4 syndrome and chest pain masquerading as angina pectoris.[13,14] The mechanisms involved in such responses must be mediated via peripheral, spinal, and central autonomic interactions and interactions with the somatic and endocrine systems.

   Sympathetic ganglia are surrounded by a dense connective tissue capsule that is continuous with the epineurium of the preganglionic and postganglionic nerve trunks. The capsule is well innervated and therefore potentially reactive. Distortion and disruption of the ganglia has been linked with vertebrogenic autonomic syndromes.[15] Nathan[16] also documented the incidence of osteophytes of the spine compressing the sympathetic trunk and splanchnic nerves in the thorax. Appen-

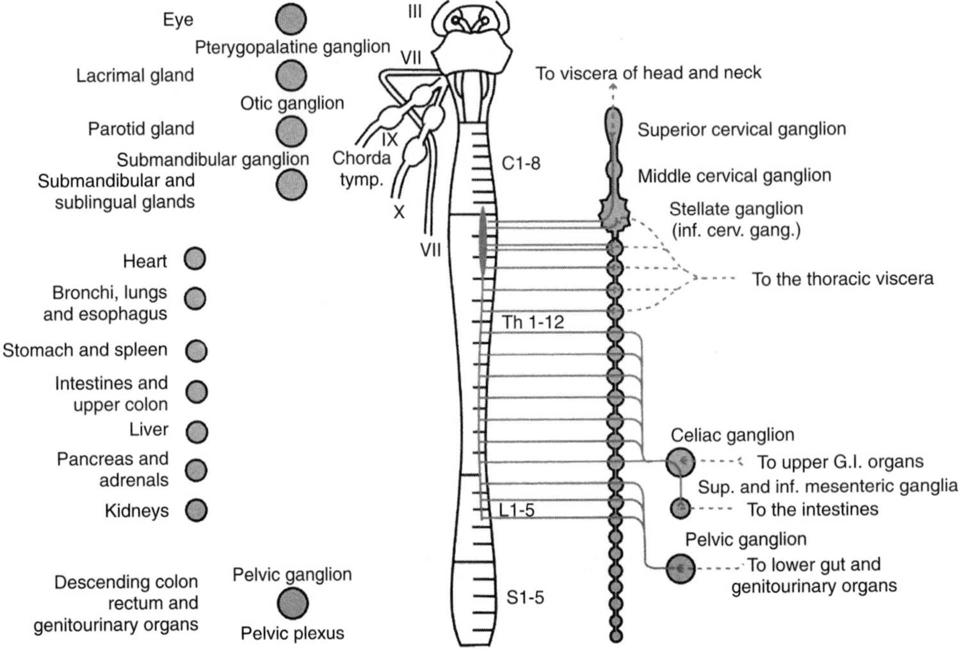

Figure 15-2
The spinal and peripheral sympathetic division of the autonomic nervous system.

zeller[17] has reported patches of excessive sweating confined to the shoulder, arm, or chest of patients with severe scoliosis. The pathophysiology of these epiphenomena remained unclear; however, Appenzeller[17] suggested spinal cord injury or injury to preganglionic neurons.

Further consideration must be given to the effects of chronic distortion of neural tissue from the work of Mackinnon and Dellon,[18] who have researched and documented the pathophysiology of double crush, reverse crush, and multiple crush syndromes. The concept of *crush* refers to compromise of the nervous system at one site that predisposes the system to serial impingement farther along the nervous system continuum. This means that patients with osteoarthritic changes in the cervical spine are more likely to develop a carpal tunnel syndrome than those without such changes (Figure 15-3). Patients with bilateral carpal tunnel syndrome have a 50% chance of developing ulnar nerve compromise at the wrist. The crush typically occurs at "vulnerable" sites,[19] such as tunnels (carpal tunnel, Guyon's canal, cubital tunnel) or areas where peripheral nerves divide (such as the radial nerve at the elbow) or emerge through unremitting fascia such as the thoracolumbar fascia.

The pathophysiology of these syndromes has been shown to relate primarily to changes in axonal transport. In peripheral nerve, axons are long relative to the size of their cell bodies. The transport of substances within the axoplasm of axons requires specialized mechanisms to allow for neurotransmitters, cytoskeletal elements, neurotrophic factors, and other chemicals to be carried the length of the axon. (These mechanisms are well-documented elsewhere.[20]) Axonal transport occurs in a bidirectional way, so there is a constant dialogue between the associated target tissues, the central processes of the axon (dorsal horn for a primary afferent neuron), and other neurons synapsing with the affected neuron.

With pressures below those recorded in patients with minor carpal tunnel syndrome, axonal transport can slow or stop.[19] Depending on the duration and magnitude of compression in these cases, the target tissues (e.g., extensor muscles in the forearm) may become painful, or there may be trophic changes in overlying skin or nails of the digits, possibly signs of neurogenic inflammation (a patch of swelling localized to a peripheral nerve innervation field) or a slower-than-expected rate of recovery from injury. Sensitization of the dorsal horn may also occur as the transport of chemicals to and from the nerve cell body is altered. Physical therapy assessment and management must not only focus on the state of the

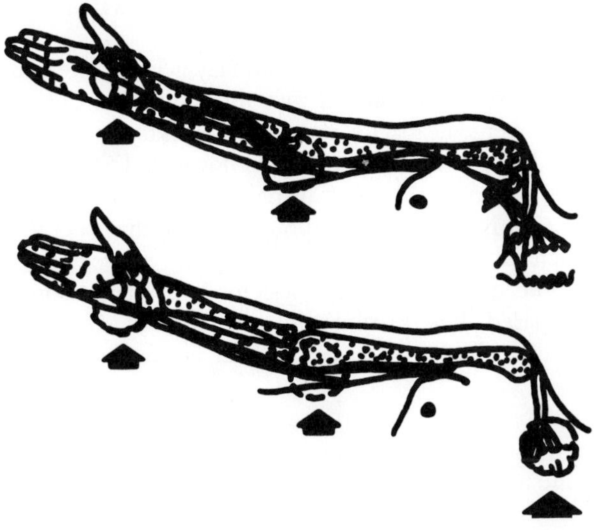

Figure 15-3
Serial impingement of the ulnar nerve at the cubital tunnel and Guyon's tunnel subsequent to compromise at the related intervertebral foramen in the cervical spine.

target tissues but also address the related peripheral nerve mechanical and physiological integrity.[1,19]

3. Postganglionic neurons contained in the paravertebral ganglia innervate target organs in somatic tissues, such as skeletal muscle, nerves, skin, and blood vessels. Pathophysiology of the sympathetic postganglionic neurons has the potential to affect a number of target tissues and possibly to influence the rate and extent of tissue repair after injury.
4. Prevertebral ganglia are midline structures positioned anterior to the vertebral column and aorta, whereas previsceral ganglia are small collections of sympathetic ganglia located close to target tissues.
5. Preganglionic sympathetic neurons are relatively short, are finely myelinated, and travel to the sympathetic trunk via the ventral nerve root and white rami communicantes. They may travel through several ganglia before synapsing on 4 to 20 postganglionic neurons. Each spinal level may synapse with multiple peripheral ganglia that supply multiple targets. This translates as a given spinal segment potentially influencing up to 100,000 postganglionic neurons.[21] This design feature serves as a potent reminder of the intrinsic ability of the SNS to exert widespread effects, albeit differentiated, on a number of target tissues.
6. Postganglionic fibers travel quite long distances before reaching their target organs. For example, in the upper limb, fibers must pass from the stellate ganglia through the brachial plexus to reach cutaneous and vascular structures in the hand.

   The nature of this design means that sympathetic postganglionic neurons are particularly susceptible to metabolic disorders (diabetes) and mechanical compromise such as double crush.[18] Horner's syndrome is an example of interruption of either the preganglionic fibers before reaching the superior cervical ganglion, or the compromise may occur in the exiting postganglionic fiber. The clinical manifestation of this is a drooping eyelid (ptosis), slight elevation of the lower lid, pupil constriction (miosis), the appearance of a sunken eye (enophthalmos), a loss of sweating (anhydrosis), and flushing of the skin. Lung disorders such as bronchiectasis , tumors, and tuberculosis have also been found to be associated with ipsilateral facial flushing resulting from mechanical irritation of the sympathetic trunk[17] (Figure 15-4).
7. The sympathetic pathways that originate in various cord segments may not be distributed to the same part of the body as the same segmental spinal nerves. The sympathetic neurons to the head and neck, for example, arise from T1-4; those to the upper limb from T1-9; to the thorax, T3-6; to the abdomen, T7-11; and the lower limb, T12-L2.

   In pain and injury states therefore, physical examination may need to extend to areas that are not routinely recognized as associated with the symptoms. For example, in patients suffering cervicogenic headache, it may be necessary to examine not just the upper cervical spine but also the thoracic spine down to T6, possibly lower. Many clinicians will have observed the relief of headache certain patients experience when the thoracic spine is mobilized. Although the mechanisms that explain the symptomatic and objective improvement are not well researched, the interaction between the autonomic and somatic input systems (possibly via somatovisceral reflexes) must be considered. The neurophysiological basis of MIA—and specifically the role of the SNS in analgesia—is discussed later in the chapter and further in Chapter 12.

   Readers are reminded that the relative importance of postural, movement, muscle, and motor control factors, which are critical parts of a comprehensive neuromusculoskeletal assessment and management of cervicogenic headache, must not be overlooked[22] (see Chapter 13).

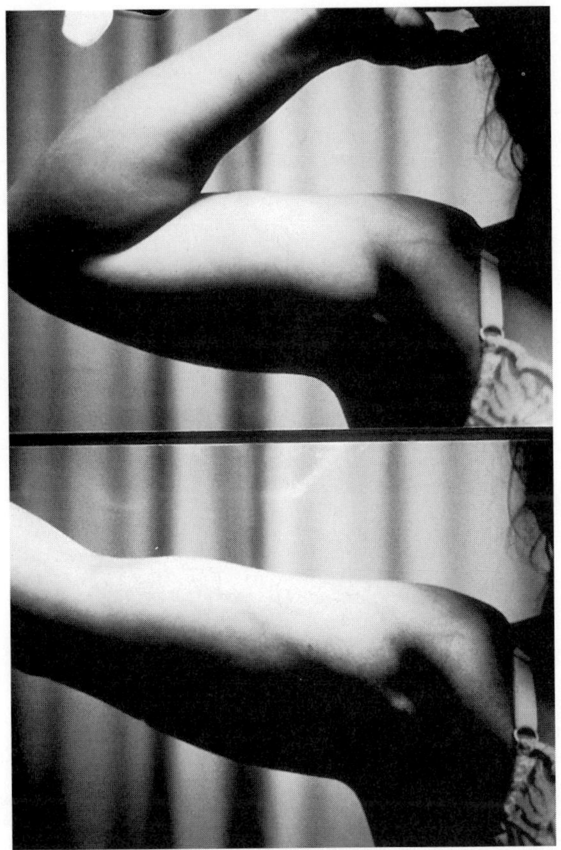

Figure 15-4
A clinical example of pathodynamics in the musculocutaneous nerve. Note the difference in prominence of the nerve with elbow extension compared with elbow flexion. This patient reported persistent pain and abnormal sweating of the right axilla subsequent to a right-sided thoracotomy. The pain and sweating could be altered by loading and unloading the neural tissues in the right arm and by mobilizing the thoracic spine.

8. Specific reflex pathways that are dedicated to the neuronal regulation of autonomic target organs exist in the spinal cord.[11] These reflex patterns are termed *functional fingerprints*. Essentially they are a physiological expression of the CAN organization. This is good design for a system that has such a diversity of effector organs, with both specific and wide-ranging effector responses. A number of functionally "dedicated" lines exist, each functional set of preganglionic neurons synapsing with a specific set of postganglionic neurons to effect a specific response at the target organ.

   Such sympathetic spinal functional units consist of sympathetic preganglionic neurons, interneurons, and the connections with afferent inflow from the periphery (e.g., muscle, fascia, and viscera) and receive descending input from the brainstem and hypothalamus (Figure 15-5). This organization is consistent with the spinal cord having a specific role in the responses of target organs to noxious, tissue-damaging events and the supraspinal structures having a more generalized effect. Links between the SNS and the immune system provide support for the likelihood of functional classes of neurons that innervate and regulate inflammatory responses throughout the body.[10]

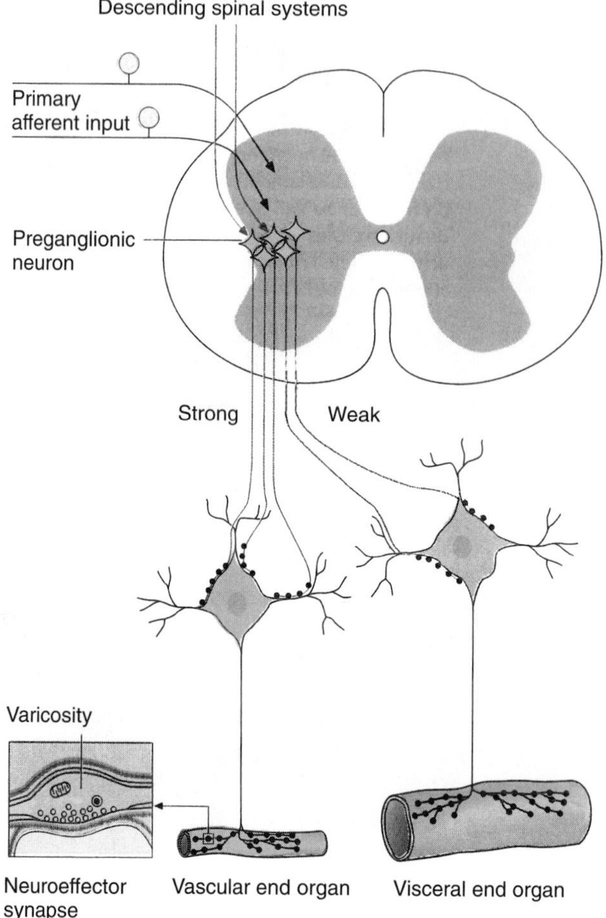

Figure 15-5
Organization of the sympathetic nervous system in functional units. Distinct functional pathways exist from the central nervous system to effector organs. Note the preganglionic neurons in the intermediate zone of the spinal cord. These neurons integrate signals from higher centers and segmentally from primary afferent fibers.

(From Slater H: In Van Den Berg F, editor: *Angewandte physiologie 2 organsysteme verstehen und beeinflussen,* Stuttgart, Germany, 2000, Thieme Verlag. Modified from Janig W, McLachlan EM: *J Autonomic Nervous Sys* 4:13, 1992.)

SYMPATHETIC NERVOUS SYSTEM IN INJURY AND ILLNESS

BRAIN STRESS RESPONSE—DEFENSE REACTION

The brain stress response is initiated in potentially threatening situations, stimulating physiological arousal via chemical messengers and acting to regulate the immune system. Hormones produced in immune cells "talk back" to centers in the brain, such as the NTS. This makes good sense; it means that the brain stress response is biologically beneficial in that it promotes physiological and behavioral changes that favor survival or recovery from injury or illness. A continuum whereby the brain stress re-

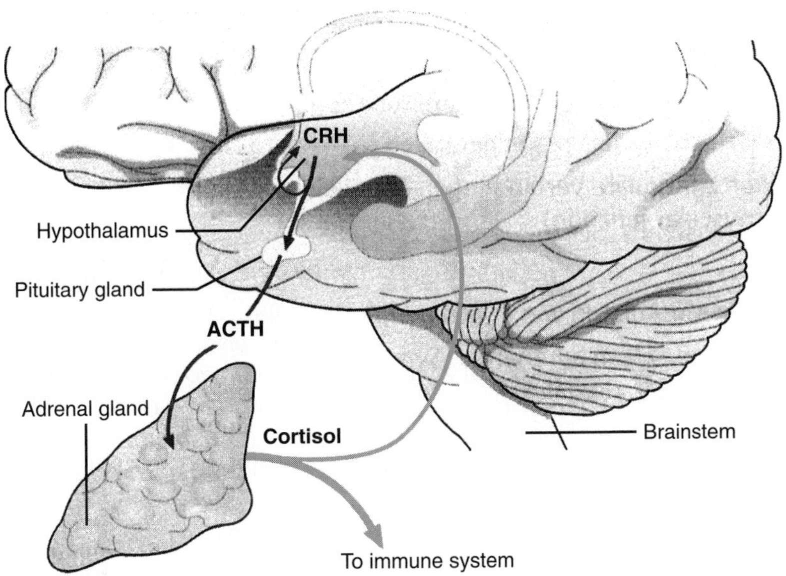

Figure 15-6
The hypothalamic-pituitary-adrenocortical (HPA) axis is a key element of the brain stress response. Corticotropin-releasing hormone (CRH) stimulates the pituitary gland to release adrenocorticotropin hormone (ACTH) into the bloodstream *(black arrows)*. This in turn stimulates the release of cortisol from the adrenal glands; the cortisol then feeds back to modulate the stress response *(gray arrows)*.
(From Slater H: In Van Den Berg F, editor: *Angewandte physiologie 2 organsysteme verstehen und beeinflussen*, Stuttgart, Germany, 2000, Thieme Verlag. Modified from Sternberg EM, Gold PW: *Sci Am* 7:11, 1997.)

sponse can be specific or more generalized—whatever is biologically appropriate—exists.

The key areas involved in the brain stress response include the hypothalamus and locus ceruleus in the brain, the pituitary gland, the SNS, and the adrenal glands (Figure 15-6). There is now a substantial body of research showing that under chronic (pathophysiological) conditions, the brain stress response may become misregulated, resulting in disorders of arousal, thoughts, and feelings. For clinicians dealing with patients suffering chronic pain, this is a common pattern of presentation. Recognizing the interactions between the brain and the neuroendocrine and immune systems should have implications for physical therapy management of patients recovering from or coping with disease and illness. For example, the likelihood of rapid recovery from a whiplash injury in a patient with a preexisting clinical depression may well be reduced. Tissue repair processes in patients with insulin-dependent diabetes are also likely to be delayed.

Brain Stress Response: Nociception and Analgesia

Integral to the brain stress response is the control of nociception and endogenous analgesia. A number of areas within the brain are dedicated to the control of pain. One of the centers of particular importance for endogenous pain control is the PAG region. In a highly coordinated fashion and in response to stressors, connections from the PAG to the intermediolateral horn of the spinal cord facilitate autonomic changes; connections from the PAG to the dorsal horn mediate analgesia and influence motor activity to the anterior horn. Patients rarely exhibit responses that do not involve alterations in all these dimensions (i.e., pain, motor function, and autonomic phenomena).

Various philosophies of manual therapy direct the focus of assessment and management strategies of patients with musculoskeletal and neurological disorders predominantly to one of the sensory, motor, or autonomic systems. Inherent in these approaches is a possible error of reasoning that does not adequately recognize the interplay between the sensory, autonomic, and motor systems. Physical therapists are well positioned in terms of knowledge and skills to apply an integrated examination and treatment and rehabilitation program that maximizes the interplay between all systems. Alert clinicians must recognize the potential of altered sensory input to drive pain states and abnormal motor patterns and conversely to alter motor patterns to favorably impact on sensory dimensions of pain.

Within the PAG are the following two discrete regions that mediate different forms of analgesia:

1. The dorsal system (dPAG): dorsolateral and dorsomedial and lateral subdivisions
2. The ventral system (vPAG): dorsal raphe nucleus and the ventrolateral subdivision

Analgesia from the dPAG is described as being nonopioid and is associated with an immediate defense response in relation to stressful situations. The associated physiological responses are consistent with sympathoexcitation and activation of alpha motoneurons at the spinal cord level.[23] Behavioral correlates support a defensive strategy by the central nervous system that favors survival and avoidance of threats. As the stress reduces and resolves, the form of analgesia shifts from nonopioid- to opioid-based analgesia via the vPAG. This is associated with sympathoinhibition and depression of motor activity. These physiological changes favor recuperative behaviors such as decreased cardiovascular output, respiratory demands, and reduced mobility.[24]

Mobilization Techniques, Sympathetic Nervous System Effects, and Analgesia

What evidence exists that spinal mobilization can result in hypoalgesia or analgesia in healthy subjects and in patients?

Recent research[12,25-32] (see also Chapter 12) has begun to explore the neurophysiological basis of MIA in relation to specific manipulative physical therapy techniques. It is thought that the initial hypoalgesic effect of MIA demonstrated in normal subjects may be mediated by descending pathways from the dPAG via nuclei in the ventrolateral medulla to the spinal cord. From these investigations, it appears that specific manipulative physical therapy techniques exert an initial sympathoexcitatory effect (within 15 seconds) that is most significant during the treatment procedure (Figure 15-7). The sympathoexcitatory effects have been shown to be technique specific and more effective than placebos. Results[28,30] have also supported a hypothesis that some manipulative physical therapy techniques produce a relative hypoalgesia to mechanical nociceptive stimulation. A strong correlation between activation of the peripheral SNS and analgesia was also demonstrated in patients with lateral epicondylalgia.[30]

Collectively the data generated from these studies suggest that the initial sympathoexcitatory effects of specific manipulative therapy techniques are associated with mobilization of the descending pain-control systems—in particular, with the noradrenergic system. The associated hypoalgesic or analgesic effect associated with this sympathoexcitation is likely to be mediated via the descending noradrenergic pathways and therefore be classified as nonopioid.[32] Associated changes in SNS parameters (i.e., blood pressure, heart rate, respiratory rate, skin conductance, and skin temperature) and functional measures beyond those attributable to placebo are consistent

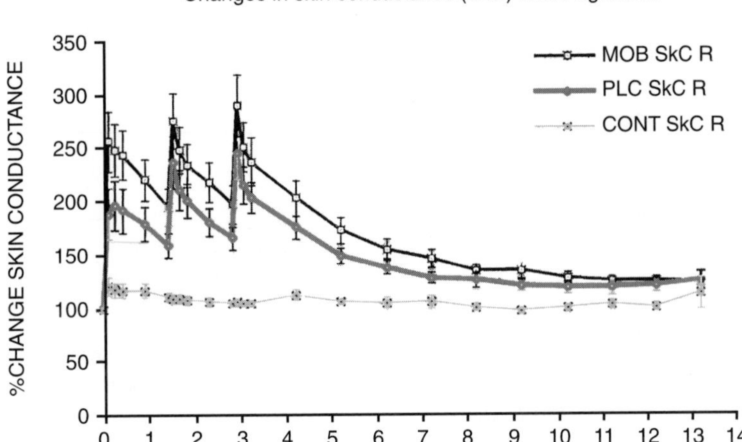

Figure 15-7
Changes in skin conductance in the right upper arm in response to the sympathetic slump. MOB, treatment group; PLC, placebo group; CONT, control group.
(From Slater H, Vicenzino B, Wright A: *J Manual Manip Ther* 2[4]:156, 1994.)

with a coordinated sensory-autonomic and motor response to the treatment condition. More research is needed to examine these effects in various patient populations as an attempt to support an evidence-based approach to physical therapy treatments.

Sympathetic Nervous System, Immune Responses, and Illness

It is clear that the mind can influence both susceptibility to and recovery from infections, inflammatory and autoimmune diseases, and associated mood disorders. This fact has long been observed in medicine, only to be trivialized in more recent times with the advent of more extensive and expensive pharmacopeia and technology diffusion.

This 'mind-disease influence' implies a network that links the immune and nervous systems. Such a network does exist. Chemicals produced by the immune system signal the brain, and in response, the brain replies with chemical signals that restrain the immune system (Figure 15-8). Behavioral responses to stress are influenced by these same chemicals.[10] Dysfunction of this communication network results in exacerbation of the diseases and disorders that the immune and nervous systems are designed to prevent and control.

The brain-stress response and the immune system function reciprocally to maintain homeostasis. The immune system does this by recognizing and destroying bacteria, viruses, other pathogens, and foreign bodies and by facilitating the tissue regeneration and repair processes.

The immune response is driven by the following two integrated functions:

1. A cellular response regulated by cytokines
2. A neurohumoral response mediated by antibodies

Cytokines are biological molecules that cells use to communicate. They are small proteins that target specific cell types, inhibiting or stimulating a response.[10] By this means, chemical messengers can signal the brain via the circulation or nerve pathways such as the vagus nerve and the NTS. During inflammation and other disease pro-

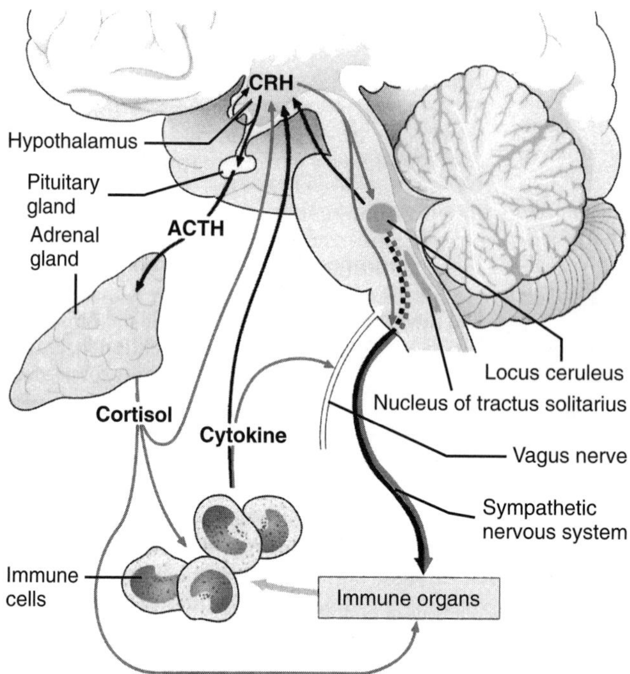

Figure 15-8
Interaction between the brain and immune systems. The brain and immune system have a reciprocal relationship. They can inhibit *(gray arrows)* or excite *(black arrows)* each other. Corticotropin-releasing factor stimulates the hypothalamic-pituitary-adrenocortical (HPA) axis; the release of cortisol "tunes down" the immune response. Corticotropin-releasing factor also stimulates the sympathetic nervous system, which in turn innervates immune organs and regulates inflammatory processes in the body. Disturbances in this loop may lead to greater susceptibility to autoimmune and inflammatory diseases and mood disorders. (From Slater H: In Van Den Berg F, editor: *Angewandte physiologie 2 Organsysteme verstehen und beeinflussen,* Stuttgart, Germany, 2000, Thieme Verlag. Adapted from Sternberg EM, Gold PW: *Sci Am* 7:9, 1997.)

cesses, the blood-brain barrier has increased permeability, enabling certain cytokines to travel across the barrier. This results in physiological and behavioral responses that are appropriate to illness and favor recovery.

Cytokines play a staggering number of roles in many neurobiological processes in the central and peripheral nervous systems, including the modulation of pain, mediation of inflammatory and noninflammatory processes, stimulation of hypothalamic hormone release, the initiation of neovascularization, an increase in cold-sensitive neuron activity (a feature of CRPSs), a decrease in appetite, and the promotion of sleep. Systemic illnesses, such as those caused by viruses, that have characteristics of lethargy, myalgia, arthralgia, headache, and hypotension are thought to be due to the actions of circulating cytokines on SNS neurons throughout the body.[34,35]

Sympathetic innervation of the thymus, lymphoid tissue, spleen, T cells, B cells, and monocytes allows sympathetic modulation of the immune response. In stressful situations, sympathetic function is increased, and this should be associated with an inhibition of immune function. This is supported by the effects on the immune response of chemical and surgical sympathectomy.

Brain and immune interactions are not only relevant in the context of illness and disease. In athletes, it is widely acknowledged that overtraining or chronic fatigue can affect the capacity of the immune system to resist infection or facilitate tissue repair. Excessive efforts during recovery from injury in athletes may provoke a chronic inflammatory response, with the possibility of incomplete repair or delayed recovery.[35,36] Conversely, moderate physical exercise seems to "boost" the immune system.[37] This knowledge needs to be incorporated into the clinical-reasoning process and should direct strategies to make management specific to each patient's needs and capabilities.

Sympathetic Contribution to Neurogenic Inflammation and Tissue Repair

With both tissue and nerve injury, not only does the immune system participate in the process of inflammation and repair, but the nervous system does too. *Neurogenic inflammation* refers to the neurally mediated part of the normal adaptive inflammatory response to tissue injury. It promotes rapid increases in tissue substrates, activates cells for local defense (e.g., mast cells), and facilitates the transport of water to isolate and dilute foreign bodies.

Of particular interest is the role of the primary afferents and sympathetic postganglionic neurons in releasing neuropeptides and neurotransmitters from their terminals. These substances can act as inflammatory mediators, influencing the inflammatory response by initiating processes such as plasma extravasation. Substance P is the most well-recognized proinflammatory mediator released by the primary afferent, and its effects can be augmented by substances released from sympathetic postganglionic neurons. In addition to this function, substances such as prostaglandins, purines, neuropeptide Y, and norepinephrine from the sympathetic efferents can enhance or inhibit plasma extravasation and interact with other nonneural factors to influence inflammation.[38] Ultimately this interaction assists in modulating the degree of tissue injury as opposed to tissue repair.

Sympathetic efferent and primary afferent contributions to inflammation may also help make sense of the development of rheumatoid arthritis after cerebrovascular accidents but with only minimal signs of the disease on the affected side. One of the aims of management of such patients must be to assist with stress-management strategies as an integral part of managing the disease and any associated impairment or disability.[6]

The relationship between inflammation and tissue repair is such that increased plasma extravasation results in reduced tissue injury. This suggests that the plasma extravasation operates partly as a tissue-protective process during the inflammatory response.[39] Clearly the observation that chemical and surgical sympathetectomy actually decreases plasma extravasation and tissue injury suggests that other neurobiological interactions between the sympathetic postganglionic neurotransmitters and nonneural components facilitate some of the degradative elements of inflammation. The role of nonsteroidal antiinflammatory drugs in inflammatory states has been questioned[40] because they reduce plasma extravasation and may aggravate tissue injury or delay tissue repair.

EFFERENT SYMPATHETIC NERVOUS SYSTEM AND PAIN

Although the pathophysiology continues to be hotly debated, the fact that the SNS is associated with pain is well recognized. Janig[11] stated that the SNS can be associated with pain in two ways. The first relates to the generalized and specific localized reactions in response to noxious, tissue-damaging inputs. These responses have been discussed previously as part of the brain stress response. The interaction between the neuroendocrine and immune system and the SNS should be considered as part of the body's response to pain. Similarly, nociceptive and central nervous system processing changes associated with pain must also be considered in terms of somatomotor programs.

The key elements of the generalized response can be seen as components of different patterns of defense and recuperation behaviors. In a biologically meaningful situation, defense and flight behaviors are associated with activation of the dPAG, initiated from the body surface and mediated via endogenous nonopioid analgesia. The transition to endogenous opioid analgesia occurs via the vPAG and is associated with recuperative, quiescent behaviors. These preprogrammed basic biological behaviors allow us to deal with pain or prepare for impending pain that is related to both dangerous situations and potentially tissue-damaging events.[11]

The second way in which the SNS is associated with pain is after tissue damage in the extremities. This may occur in association with or in the absence of any frank nerve lesion, the clinical sequelae of which may be diffuse burning pain and hyperalgesia in the involved extremity (features of CRPSs). Sympathetic epiphenomena may also be present and include alterations in blood flow and temperature, sweating, and trophic changes in skin, subcutaneous tissues, fascia, and bone. Changes in motor patterns may be expressed as physiological tremor and dystonias. Surgical and sympathetic blockade may alleviate the pain and dysesthesias although there is no consistent evidence that phentolamine or guanethidine intravenous blockade is effective, even when repeated.[41] The SNS may also be causally linked with pain of visceral organs (e.g., irritable bowel syndrome and angina pectoris) and hyperalgesia associated with inflammatory processes.[11]

Definitions and Diagnosis of Complex Regional Pain Syndromes

There is a consensus that it is the contribution of the SNS to pain *after traumatic injury to the extremities* that has created much confusion and controversy. However, much of what has been previously documented and described in pain states in relation to the causative role of the SNS in generating and maintaining pain is being challenged. Long-held beliefs that an increase in sympathetic drive is a basis for pain are no longer tenable. Consequently, both reflex sympathetic dystrophy and causalgia have been redefined using the descriptive terms of *complex regional pain syndrome (CRPS) type 1* and *type 2*, respectively.[42,43] These definitions are shown in Box 15-1.

This redefinition is an attempt to shift towards a clearer understanding of the etiology of complex regional pain syndromes without implicating either specific pain mechanisms or suggesting any associated aberration of sympathetic function. Ultimately it is hoped that the reevaluation of the links between the efferent SNS and pain will provide a more rational approach to the clinical diagnosis and management of patients with complex regional pain syndromes. This classification is open to revision contingent upon future basic and clinical research. However, questions have already been raised as to the external validity of these criteria—that is, the ability of the International Association of the Study of Pain criteria to discriminate between CRPS patients and non-CRPS neuropathic pain (e.g., postherpetic neuralgia, diabetic neuropathy). A recent study[44] found that these criteria and decision rules—such as signs or symptoms of edema, color, or sweating changes—discriminated significantly between groups. However, although sensitivity was high (0.98), specificity was poor (0.36), and a positive diagnosis of CRPS was likely to be correct in only 44% of cases.

Box 15-1

Definitions and Diagnostic Criteria for Complex Regional Pain Syndromes Types I and II

CRPS is a term describing a variety of painful conditions following injury which appears regionally, having a distal predominance of abnormal findings, exceeding in both magnitude and duration the expected clinical course of the inciting event, often resulting in significant impairment of motor function and showing progression over time.

CRPS I (Formerly "Reflex Sympathetic Dystrophy")

1. Type I is a syndrome that develops after an initiating noxious event
2. Spontaneous pain or allodynia/hyperalgesia occurs, not limited to the territory of a single peripheral nerve, and is disproportionate to the inciting event
3. There is or has been evidence of edema, skin blood flow abnormality, or abnormal sudomotor activity in the region of the pain since the inciting event
4. This diagnosis is excluded by the existence of conditions that would otherwise account for the degree of pain and dysfunction

CRPS II (Formerly "Causalgia")

1. Type II develops after a nerve injury. Spontaneous pain, allodynia or hyperalgesia occurs, is not necessarily limited to the territory of the injured nerve
2. There is or has been evidence of edema, skin blood flow abnormality, or abnormal sudomotor activity in the region of the pain since the inciting event.
3. This diagnosis is excluded by the existence of conditions that would otherwise account for the degree of pain and dysfunction

Adapted from Stanton-Hicks M, Baron R, Boas R et al: *Clin J Pain* 14:155, 1998.

A decision rule that required at least two sign categories and four symptom categories to be positive optimized diagnostic effectiveness. This meant that an accurate diagnosis was likely in up to 84% of cases, and a diagnosis of non-CRPS neuropathic pain likely to be accurate in 88% of cases.

Subsequent to the findings of this study, modified research criteria have been suggested. However, until sufficient research criteria are available, the recommendation is to continue to work with the current diagnostic criteria. Revisions of CRPS criteria will ultimately contribute to improved clinical diagnosis. A web site has been listed at the end of the chapter and readers can keep informed of ongoing changes in this area.

Pathophysiology of Complex Regional Pain Syndromes

The pathophysiology of CRPS remains unclear. No longer is the inference that the SNS is *causally* involved in the generation of pain. Readers are referred to Janig[11] for a comprehensive overview of pathophysiology. The IASP Special Interest Group for Sympathetic Nervous System also provides regular bulletins to update such knowledge as it becomes available. Table 15-1 summarizes hypotheses on the pathophysiology of CRPSs.

Clinical Diagnosis of Complex Regional Pain Syndromes

The diagnostic criteria listed in Table 15-1 can be used as an integral part of subjective inquiry strategies in patients when it is considered relevant. Research has yet to reveal the predictors of developing CRPS after trauma and the criteria to differentiate between patients with a posttraumatic response that subsides within expected tissue-

Table 15-1 Hypotheses on the Pathophysiology of Complex Regional Pain Syndromes

Hypothesis	Pathophysiological Mechanisms
1. Sensitization of nociceptive (and possibly other small diameter) fibers by initial trauma	Damaged primary afferents generate ongoing activity, reduced threshold to mechanical, chemical and thermal and stimulation Generation of ectopic impulses from damaged primary afferents Altered processing of nociceptive and non-nociceptive information at spinal cord level Alteration of descending pain control from supraspinal systems Nociceptive afferents spontaneously active in deep soma Low-rate continuous input ? activates sensitized dorsal horn neurons
2. Coupling between sympathetic post-ganglionic and afferent neurons	Noradrenergic postganglionic neurons coupled to primary afferent neurons (nociceptive and non-nociceptive), resulting in abnormal afferent impulse traffic Coupling may occur via upregulation of alpha-adrenoceptors in primary afferent neurons, novel appearance of adrenoceptor mRNA; via dorsal root ganglion to afferent neurons; indirectly via the microvascular bed or non-neural cells close at afferent receptors; via postganglionic noradrenergic sensitizing primary afferent neurons following inflammation Ephaptic coupling between sympathetic and afferent fibers
3. Activity in sympathetic neurons	Alteration of sympathetic discharge pattern in response to sensitization of primary afferents and dorsal horn neurons
4. Sympathetic target organs	Following nerve lesions, possible hyperreactivity of blood vessels to circulating catecholamines; changed pattern of blood vessel regulation: alteration of pre/post capillary control by afferent neurons
5. Somatomotor system	Sensitization of spinal neurons may result in an altered discharge pattern in alpha and gamma motoneurons leading to reduction in active range of movement, muscle strength and physiological tremor
6. Tissue changes	Generation of swelling and trophic changes related to indirect effects of abnormal blood flow through affected area on afferent unmyelinated neurons

Adapted from Janig W: In Janig W, Stanton-Hicks M, editors: *Reflex sympathetic dystrophy: a reappraisal*, Seattle, 1996, IASP Press.

healing timeframes and patients who suffer from CRPS. In the early stages the differentiation can be difficult, and because the specificity of clinical examination can be poor,[44,45] improved diagnostic criteria are essential.

Physical Examination Strategies. Given these caveats, some of the recommended tests that should assist in supporting or negating a clinical diagnosis of CRPS include the following:

Sensory Tests

- Evaluation of impairment of sensation (light touch and pinprick), not only on the affected and unaffected extremities but also recommended on the entire body surface, as the incidence of hemisensory impairment has been documented as 33%.[46] In the same study, sensory abnormalities in patients with left-sided CRPS were more commonly demonstrated (77%) than in patients with right-sided CRPS (18%). Mechanical allodynia and mechanical hyperalgesia also were observed in a higher percentage of patients with hemisensory deficit or impairment in the upper quadrant (92%) than in patients with a sensory deficit isolated to the affected limb (17%).
- Note that sensory abnormalities may be evident as hypoesthesias, hyperesthesias, or dysesthesias.
- Temperature testing using a metal or plastic device. Normal subjects perceive the metal side as being cooler than the plastic side, although there is no major temperature difference. Further tests of tolerance and perception of hot (38° C) and cold (22° C) can be performed using the standard test tubes.
- Stereognosis. Identification of familiar objects, such as keys and coins, can be assessed.
- Two-point discrimination.
- Graphesthesia. Recognition of different numbers traced bilaterally on the backs of the hands, arms, trunk, and dorsum of the feet.
- Vibratory sense 256 cps (knuckles of both hands as well as both ankles). The vibration scale can be set at the tip of the acromion. With the measurement being recorded as n/8:0/8 vibration is not perceived: 8/8 vibration is perceived up to the final swing.[46]

Motor Tests

- Measurements can be made of active ranges of motion and muscle strength or using a handheld manometer, if appropriate.
- Observation of any contractures.
- Evidence of any resting or physiological tremors.
- Evidence of dystonic postures.
- Routine reflex testing may not reveal any differences; however, in some patients an alteration of reflexes will be demonstrated. The incidence of motor impairment is reported to be higher in patients with generalized sensory changes in comparison with patients who have spatially restricted sensory alterations.[46]
- Note that the motor changes can spread proximally and may involve the ipsilateral side of the body.
- There appears to be a higher frequency of motor impairment in patients with generalized sensory deficits.

Target Tissue Examination

- Observation of trophic changes in skin, hair, and nails should be sought, although in the early stages of examination these changes may not be evident.
- Examine for any signs of persistent neurogenic inflammation.

Palpation. Routine palpation may reveal temperature differences and tissue sensitivity (mechanical allodynia and mechanical hyperalgesia). The focus should be localized not only to the symptomatic region but also to the spinal regions appropriate to that area. This may reflect changes in somatotopic organization in response to the injury at the spinal cord level. Responses may occur in a pattern that is suggestive of reorganization at supraspinal levels rather than at spinal cord levels. Here it is routine to see areas anatomically separate from the area of injury; for example, stroking the face may elicit arm pain.[47]

Neurodynamic Tests. The upper limb neurodynamic tests—the straight leg raise test, the slump test, and the sympathetic slump bias—may also be useful indicators of peripheral and central nervous system sensitization (see Chapter 11). Although the specificity and sensitivity of these tests has not been established, they are useful in forming a working hypothesis as part of the clinical picture in a clinical context. The change in the CRPS paradigm means that interpretation of any physical test should be considered within this context. A sympathetic slump test that reproduces hand pain may indicate sensitivity of the peripheral SNS in response to a sensitized dorsal horn or sensitized target tissues. It does not implicate the sympathetic trunk as the *cause* of the pain. It does not indicate that the source of symptoms is the sympathetic trunk.

In patients with costovertebral osteoarthritis, the effect of distortion of the sympathetic trunks on axonal transport mechanisms and associated target tissue sensitivity may be considered a factor that contributes to the patient's presentation.[9] The physiological effects of the sympathetic slump on the peripheral SNS have been investigated in normal subjects and in a patient population.[12,48]

Nerve palpation may also be a useful test of peripheral nerve sensitivity in patients with a peripheral neuropathy (e.g., patients with diabetes). It is possible to feel changes such as thickening, swelling, neuromas, neurofibromas, or alterations in sensitivity to palpation in peripheral nerves. Readers are referred to Butler[19] for details of peripheral nerve palpation techniques and interpretation of findings.

Physical Therapy Management of Complex Regional Pain Syndromes

The gold standard for management of CRPS is recognized as a multidisciplinary approach that minimizes the role of sympathetic blockade.[49] Figure 15-9 illustrates the current IASP algorithm for CRPS. Notice the central role of physical therapy in the management of patients with these disorders.

At first glance the IASP algorithm appeals in the approach it takes with CRPS patients. The intersection of pain control, psychotherapies, and physical therapy should offer an optimal environment for the patient's physical and psychological rehabilitation. However, it should be emphasized that a clear set of clinical predictors and indicators for diagnosing CRPS does not yet exist. It should also be stressed that patients often have clinical patterns that suggest multiple problems, not only CRPS. Rehabilitation must take a balanced approach to the presentation and seek an access that offers pain control while allowing reeducation of motor programs, optimizing function, and enhancing quality of life.

The clinical-reasoning framework will offer clinicians a way in which they can make management situation specific rather than recipe driven. The IASP algorithm should not be seen as a recipe for management. The context of the injury and rehabilitation will significantly influence management. A simplified explanation of proposed mechanisms for CRPS is important. Drawing diagrams to illustrate possible sites of pathophysiology may be useful for the patient. Gaining the patient's confi-

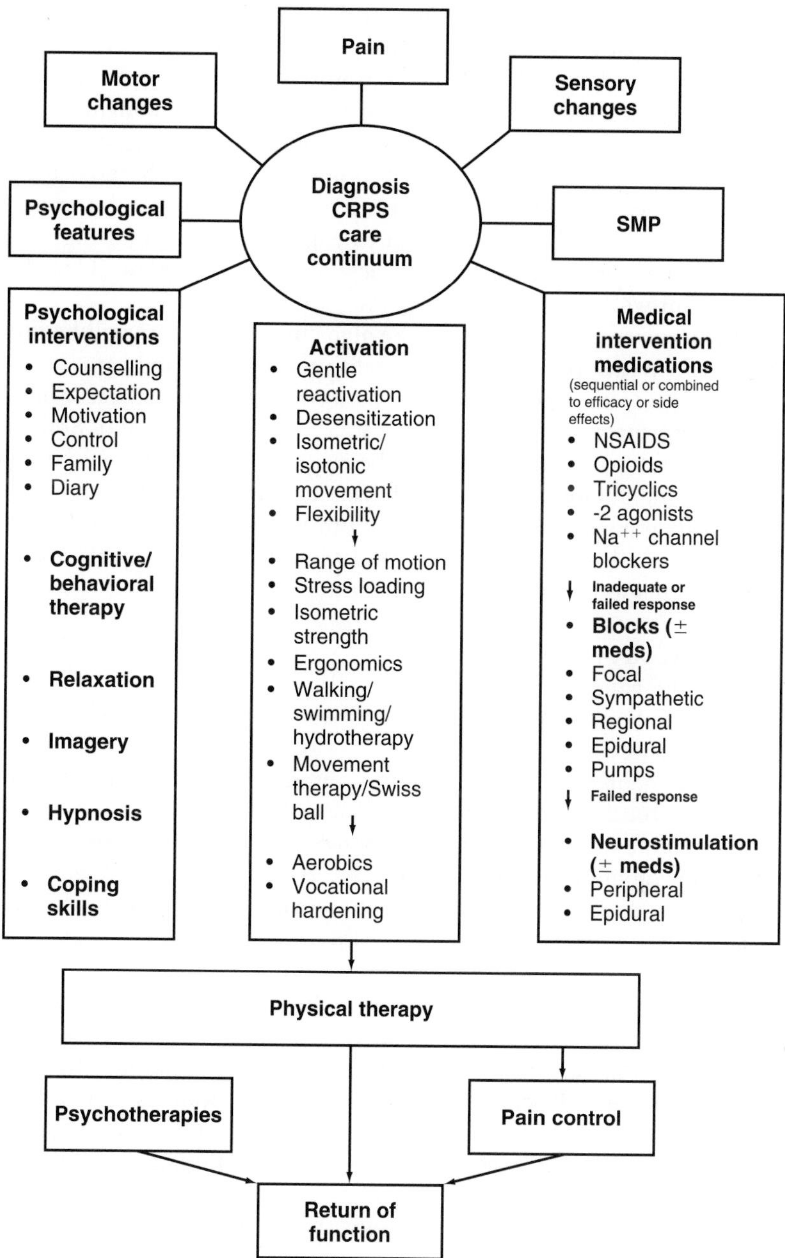

Figure 15-9
International Association for the Study of Pain (IASP) algorithm for complex regional pain syndromes.
(Adapted from Stanton-Hicks M, Baron R, Boas R et al: *Clin J Pain* 14:155, 1998.)

dence will assist in minimizing anxiety in response to examination and management strategies.

Guidelines for Management of CRPS. The following guidelines are based on the IASP algorithm, with modifications drawn from clinicians' experiences and knowledge. It is recommended that therapists use these guidelines in a clinical-reasoning framework as described in Chapter 6. Setting short- and long-term goals with input from the patient—and when appropriate, from other disciplines—is to be encouraged. If indicated, appropriate medication should help to control pain during the rehabilitation process. In particular, control of mechanical allodynia through the use of oral adrenergic agents, analgesics, topical alpha2 agonists, or regional anesthetic blocks, should facilitate the approach to physical therapy. Some pain clinic facilities may recommend minimal or no pharmacological pain control. For example, a patient with chronic pain who participates in a cognitive behavioral program may be required to undergo detoxification before beginning the program. This should be taken into account when setting patient goals.

The time to move from one step of the algorithm to the next will be influenced by factors specific to each patient (e.g., irritability, mechanisms and nature of any concurrent pathology, coping mechanisms, and pain control). Generally, it would be reasonable to expect progressing between steps in a 2- to 4-week period. Some form of cognitive-behavioral management will also be required. This may be especially so in the case of CRPS in children, when the behavioral management is thought to be very critical in providing coping mechanisms for both the child and parents. In a private practice setting, it is advisable for physical therapists to initiate set goals with input or collaboration from appropriate psychotherapies.

Gentle Reactivation and Desensitization

- Explain what the patient can do safely.
- Educate patients about limiting the nervous system stimulants, including caffeinated drinks and cigarettes.
- Educate the patient (e.g., with diagrams, literature, discussion of other case examples).
- Emphasize the role of the brain stress response in terms of recovery (e.g., positive state of mind promoting tissue healing).
- Encourage a breathing pattern that is diaphragmatic rather than accessory muscle focused
- Suggest relaxation tapes when appropriate.
- Contrast baths within thermal pain thresholds (cold, 8° to 10° C, and warm, 40° to 45° C). Duration varies depending on patient tolerance. Start with cold for 30 seconds to 2 minutes, interspersed with warm bath for 3 to 5 minutes. Increase exposure to cold as tolerated. Cycles should average 20 to 30 minutes. These are easy for the patient to do at home.
- Encourage patient to "play" with materials that have different textures (e.g., pasta, clay, and sand).
- Encourage gentle self-massage within limits of mechanical allodynia/hyperalgesia.

Isometric Movement and Flexibility. Avoiding aggressive range-of-movement activities should help to minimize proprioceptive input to an already sensitized dorsal horn. Transcutaneous electrical nerve stimulation may be tried as a pain control measure during exercise. Hydrotherapy may be useful in the early stage of management when weightbearing may be too provocative. The water temperature will need to be considered when choosing this option (preferably 28° C or higher). Exercise bicycles with mobile handles and pedals may also be helpful for both upper and lower limb rehabilitation. Again, focus on what is achievable and enjoyable for the patient. This progress may involve exercises that are specific for each patient; for example, children may enjoy using Swiss balls to increase load on joints and improve balance and truncal control. The Pilates method of floor and reformer table exercises may offer another method of progressing the program, especially for those who have poor dynamic muscle control as a contributing factor to their presentation.

Guidelines: Progression of Management Paradigm

- Revisit the explanation of the pathophysiology of the disorder and the importance of the brain stress response to recovery.
- Progress the sensory program, increase time and decrease temperature, and explore more sensory options (e.g., graphesthesia).
- Begin with nonweightbearing activity that loads the affected area.
- Progress to loadbearing as tolerated; intersperse with nonweightbearing as described.
- Aim to increase cardiovascular fitness as a strategy to improve blood flow to the extremities, to assist in controlling edema, and to improve general postural tone and psychological well-being.
- Encourage use of yoga, tai chi, or other forms of slow, gentle, active range-of-movement activities, which can be performed safely at home.

Ergonomics and Vocational Retraining. As patients progress through the algorithm, the appropriate time for addressing ergonomic and vocational retraining will need to be decided. This should be a cooperative effort between the patient and all the involved medical and allied disciplines. The role of the psychotherapies may be particularly relevant in addressing anxiety about return to work, the risk of reinjury, the ability to cope with the demands of work, and possibly a different job and different environment, all of which contribute to stress. When possible, the ergonomic site should be assessed and modified as required. For children, it may be valuable to do an on-site school visit to assess any specific requirements to allow for regular play and schooling.

Readers are recommended to follow any specific work- or home-related management approach for each patient on an individual level, recruiting input from occupational physical therapists as required.

Guidelines: Progression of Management Paradigm

- Progression of the sensory program as described
- Continuous increases in cardiovascular fitness
- Incorporation of other forms of exercise as appropriate (e.g., swimming, aqua aerobics, Feldenkrais training)
- Work-site, home-site, or school visit
- Suggestion for ergonomic adjustments

Passive Mobilization in Patients with CRPS. Although passive mobilization does not specifically form part of IASP CRPS algorithm, it may be considered as an option in therapy if appropriate. It appears both from the current research and from clinical experience that in some cases the use of manual mobilization techniques may be helpful. Their use should not be overemphasized and should be omitted if thought to be a contributing factor.

The use of the clinical-reasoning framework may suggest in certain cases that this strategy will offer a favorable outcome. For example, after a Colles' fracture in the wrist, a patient develops a CRPS type I. In combination with the strategies that have already been discussed, mobilization of a stiff or painful inferior radioulnar joint may decrease a constant nociceptive input from this site. The grade of movement would be guided by the severity and irritability of the disorder[13] and would rely on the mechanical allodynia being well controlled. Similarly, mobilization of the contained neural tissue via an upper limb neurodynamic test (and its variations) may be indicated at some stage of the treatment process. Care must be taken with mobilizing sensitized neural tissue because the potential for aggravation of the symptoms is substantial. In this example, the therapist may choose to use the contralateral arm to gently decrease or increase movement and "load" on median nerve in the injured wrist.

Performed at the appropriate time and in a clinically reasoned framework, this may improve axonal transport to the wrist structures and improve blood flow, helping to desensitize the target tissues around the wrist. These changes may ultimately assist in "damping down" peripheral and central sensitization. Neurodynamic tests can also be performed actively, incorporated into a hydrotherapy or tai chi program.

COMPLEX REGIONAL PAIN SYNDROMES IN CHILDREN AND ADOLESCENTS

CRPSs occur not just in adults; both children and adolescents are also affected. As Stanton-Hicks[49] points out, CRPS in children should be viewed as a separate entity from the adult disease.

The epidemiological profile for this group shows that female patients are predominantly affected more often than male patients; the suggested ratio is 4:1.[50] Lower limbs are more likely to be affected than upper limbs; the ratio is 5.3:1. The average age of onset is 12.5 years, yet children as young as 3 years old have been reported to have developed CRPS II after intraneural injection of antibiotics into the sciatic nerve. The history of the inciting event may be trauma (fracture, injection, and injury), although there may be no apparent predisposing factor. There is little support for a preemptive psychopathology. This is not to underestimate the influence of external stressors such as academic pressures and family stressors. These are recognized as amplifying both the severity of the symptoms and the family's reaction to the child's problem.[50]

The focus of rehabilitation of children and adolescents with CRPS is physical therapy. Children rarely require interventional treatment. Management should be as enjoyable and relevant for the child and adolescent as possible. Very young children can be encouraged to play with a variety of toys and different textures to facilitate the normalization of sensibilities. Young children may find the use of a skateboard an effective and fun way of mobilizing without having to load the lower limb in the early stages of rehabilitation. Swiss balls are a useful and fun tool for progressing weightbearing for both the upper and the lower limbs (Figure 15-10). Similarly,

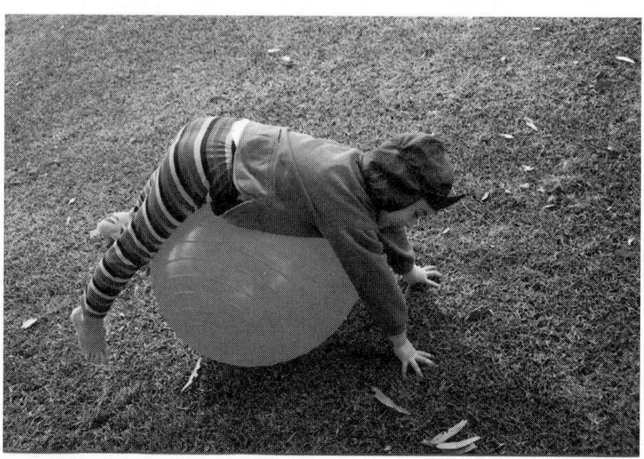

Figure 15-10
The use of Swiss balls can be a fun and effective way to facilitate rehabilitation of sensorimotor function in both children and adults after a complex regional pain syndrome.

hydrotherapy can be used as an alternate or adjunctive management. This means that other family members can be involved, and the child can move into an environment of well-being as opposed to rehabilitating in a medical setting.

CONCLUDING COMMENTS

Although the preceding text focused specifically on the SNS, it is emphasized that the separation from peripheral and central nervous systems and the endocrine and immune systems is purely artificial. The intimate relationship between the SNS and the neuroendocrine and immune systems emphasizes the potential for mind states to influence illness and wellness. Changing the way patients feel—changing their understanding of a problem and their ability to positively influence a problem—can beneficially change not only their behavior but also the physiology of their autonomic, neuroendocrine, and immune systems.[6,9]

For all patients, regardless of the pathology and dominant pain mechanisms, optimal rehabilitation must incorporate approaches that reflect the interaction of all systems. Ongoing collaboration through basic and clinical research is necessary to better understand the complex interactions between the therapist and the patient. Indeed, this will reveal more about the ways in which physical therapy works and how we can then maximize management approaches in consultation with the patient.

References

1. Butler DS, Slater H: Neural injury in the thoracic spine: a conceptual basis for manual therapy. In Grant R, editor: *Physical therapy of the cervical and thoracic spine*, ed 2, New York, 1994, Churchill Livingstone.
2. Bogduk N, Valencia F: Innervation and pain patterns of the thoracic spine. In Grant R, editor: *Physical therapy of the cervical and thoracic spine*, ed 2, New York, 1994, Churchill Livingstone.
3. Grant R: Manual therapy: science, art and placebo. In Grant R, editor: *Physical therapy of the cervical and thoracic spine*, ed 2, New York, 1994, Churchill Livingstone.
4. Lee D: In Grant R, editor: *Physical therapy of the cervical and thoracic spine*, ed 2, New York, 1994, Churchill Livingstone.
5. Jones MA: Clinical reasoning and pain. In Shacklock MO, editor: *Moving in on pain*, Melbourne, 1995, Butterworth-Heinemann.
6. Gifford LS: Pain physiology. In van Den Berg F, editor: *Angewandte physiologie 2 organsysteme verstehen und beeinflussen*, Stuttgart, Germany, 2000, Thieme Verlag.
7. Barron KD, Chokroverty S: Anatomy of the autonomic nervous system: brain and brainstem. In Low PA, editor: *Clinical autonomic disorders*, Boston, 1993, Little, Brown.
8. Mosqueda-Garcia R: Central autonomic regulation. In Robertson D, Low PA, Polinsky RJ, editors: *Primer on the autonomic nervous system*, San Diego, 1996, Academic Press.
9. Slater H: Physiology of the autonomic nervous system. In Van Den Berg F, editor: *Angewandte physiologie 2 organsysteme verstehen und beeinflussen*, Stuttgart, Germany, 2000, Thieme Verlag.
10. Sternberg EM, Gold PW: The mind-body interaction in disease: mysteries of the mind, *Sci Am* 7(special issue), 1997.
11. Janig W: The puzzle of "reflex sympathetic dystrophy": mechanisms, hypotheses, open questions. In Janig W, Stanton-Hicks M, editors: *Reflex sympathetic dystrophy: a reappraisal*, Seattle, 1996, IASP Press.

12. Slater H, Vicenzino B, Wright A: Sympathetic slump: the effects of a novel manual therapy technique on peripheral sympathetic nervous system function, *J Manual Manip Ther* 2(4):156, 1994.
13. Maitland GDM: *Vertebral manipulation*, ed 5, London, 1986, Butterworths.
14. Grieve GP: The autonomic nervous system in vertebral pain syndromes. In Boyling JD, Palastanga N, editors: *Modern manual therapy: the vertebral column*, ed 2, Edinburgh, 1994, Churchill Livingstone.
15. Giles LGF: Paraspinal autonomic ganglion distortion due to osteophytosis: a cause of vertebrogenic autonomic syndromes, *J Manip Physiol Ther* 15:551, 1992.
16. Nathan H: Osteophytes of the spine compressing sympathetic trunk and splanchnic nerves in the thorax, *Spine* 12:527, 1986.
17. Appenzeller O: *The autonomic nervous system: an introduction to basic clinical concepts*, Amsterdam, 1990, Elsevier.
18. Mackinnon SE, Dellon AL: Double and multiple "crush" syndromes, *Hand Clin* 8:369, 1992.
19. Butler D: *Mobilisation of the nervous system*, Melbourne, 1991, Churchill Livingstone.
20. Lundborg G: *Nerve injury and repair*, Edinburgh, 1988, Churchill Livingstone.
21. Hamill RW: Peripheral autonomic nervous system. In Robertson D, Low PA, Polinsky RJ, editors: *Primer on the autonomic nervous system*, San Diego, 1996, Academic Press.
22. Jull GA: Headaches of cervical origin. In Grant R: *Physical therapy of the cervical and thoracic spine*, ed 2, New York, 1994, Churchill Livingstone.
23. Lovick TA: Interactions between descending pathways from the dorsal and ventrolateral periaqueductal gray matter in the rat. In Depaulis A, Bandlier R, editors: *The midbrain periaqueductal gray matter*, New York, 1991, Plenum Press.
24. Fanselow MS: The midbrain periaqueductal gray as a coordinator of action in response to fear and anxiety. In Depaulis A, Bandlier R, editors: *The midbrain periaqueductal gray matter*, New York, 1991, Plenum Press.
25. Petersen NP, Vicenzino GT, Wright A: The effects of a cervical mobilisation technique on sympathetic outflow to the upper limb in normal subjects, *Physiother Theory Pract* 9:149, 1993.
26. Vicenzino B, Collins D, Wright A: Sudomotor changes induced by neural mobilisation techniques in asymptomatic subjects, *J Manual Manip Ther* 2:66, 1994.
27. Yelland SR, Wright A: The effects of spinal manipulative therapy on the sympathetic nervous system of subjects with upper limb pain. Proceedings of the fourteenth international congress of the Australian Physiotherapy Association, Bali, Indonesia, 1994.
28. Vicenzino B, Gutschlag F, Collins D, Wright A: An investigation of the effects of spinal manual therapy on forequarter pressure and thermal pain thresholds and sympathetic nervous system activity in asymptomatic subjects: a preliminary report. In Shacklock MO, editor: *Moving in on pain*, Melbourne, 1995, Butterworth-Heinemann.
29. Chui TTW, Wright A: Comparing the effects of two cervical mobilization techniques on sympathetic outflow to the upper limb in normal subjects, *Hong Kong Physiother J* 16:13, 1998.
30. Vicenzino B, Collins DM, Benson HAE, Wright A: The interrelationship between manipulation-induced hypoalgesia and sympathoexcitation, *J Manip Physiol Ther* 7:448, 1998.
31. Vincenzino B, Cartwright T, Collins DM, Wright A: An investigation of stress and pain perception during manual therapy in asymptomatic subjects, *Eur Pain J* 3:13, 1999.
32. Wright A, Vincenzino B: Cervical mobilization techniques, sympathetic nervous system effects and their relationship to analgesia. In Shacklock MO, editor: *Moving in on pain*. Melbourne, 1995, Butterworth-Heinemann.
33. Arnason BGW: The sympathetic nervous system and the immune response. In Low PA, editor: *Clinical autonomic disorders*, Boston, 1993, Little, Brown.
34. Beck KD, Valverde J, Alexi T et al: Mesencephalic dopaminergic neurons protected by GDNF from axotomy-induced degeneration in the adult brain, *Nature* 373(6512):339, 1995.

35. Harrelson GL: Physiological factors of rehabilitation. In Andrews JR, Harrelson GL, editors: *Physical rehabilitation of the injured athlete*, Philadelphia, 1992, WB Saunders.
36. Pyne D: Recovery and the immune system. *Sports Coach Aust Coach Mag* 17(3):13, 1994.
37. Verde TJ, Thomas RW, Moore PN et al: Immune response and increased training of the elite athlete, *J Appl Physiol* 73(4):1494, 1992.
38. Heller PH, Green PG, Tanner KD et al: Peripheral neural contribution to inflammation. In Fields HL, Liebeskind J, editors: *Progress in pain research*, vol 1, Seattle, 1994, IASP Press.
39. Coderre T, Chan AK, Helms C et al: Increasing sympathetic nerve-terminal—dependent plasma extravasation correlates with decreased arthritic joint injury in rats, *Neuroscience* 40:185, 1991.
40. Heller PH, Gear R, Levine JD: Short-term pain control: long-term consequences? *Am Pain Soc Bull* 2:12, 1992.
41. Kingery WS: A critical review of controlled trials for peripheral neuropathic pain and complex regional pain syndromes, *Pain* 73:123, 1997.
42. Janig W, Blumberg H, Boas RA, Campbell JA: The reflex sympathetic pain syndrome: consensus statement and general recommendations for diagnosis and research. In Bond MR, Charlton JE, Woolf CJ, editors: Proceedings of the sixteenth World Congress on Pain, Pain Research, and Clinical Research, vol 4, Amsterdam, 1991, Elsevier.
43. Merskey H, Bogduk N, editors: *Classification of chronic pain: descriptors of chronic pain syndromes and definition of terms*, ed 2, Seattle, 1994, IASP Press.
44. Bruehl S, Harden NR, Galer BS et al: External validation of IASP criteria for complex regional pain syndrome and proposed research diagnostic criteria, *Pain* 81:147, 1999.
45. Field J, Atkins RM: Algodystrophy is an early complication of Colles' fracture: what are the implications? *J Hand Surg* 22B:178, 1997.
46. Rommel O, Gehling M, Dertwinkel R et al: Hemisensory testing in patients with complex regional pain syndromes, *Pain* 80:95, 1999.
47. Schultz G, Melzack R: A case of referred pain evoked by remote light touch after partial nerve injury, *Pain* 81:199, 1999.
48. Slater H, Wright A: An investigation of the physiological effects of the sympathetic slump on peripheral sympathetic nervous system function in patients with frozen shoulders. In Shacklock MO, editor: *Moving in on pain*, Melbourne, 1995, Butterworth Heinemann.
49. Stanton-Hicks M: Management of patients with complex regional pain syndromes: a publication on pain and the sympathetic nervous system, Seattle, 1998, IASP Press.
50. Wilder RT: Reflex sympathetic dystrophy in children and adolescents: differences from adults. In Janig W, Stanton-Hicks M, editors: *Reflex sympathetic dystrophy: a reappraisal—progress in pain research management*, vol 6, Seattle, 1996, IASP Press.

Websites

http://noigroup.com
http://www.pain.com
http://www.ampainsoc.org/links
http://www.rsdhope.org/
http://www.halcyon.com/iasp/

CHAPTER

16 Manual Therapy for the Thorax

Diane Lee

What is manual therapy? In the broadest terms, it means "treatment that involves the use of the hands." What manual therapists do with their hands—and the reasons for their selection of a technique—varies widely according to what the therapist perceives the problem to be. This perception comes from educational and clinical experiences.

With respect to movement disorders of the thorax, manual techniques can be used to identify and treat the articular, myofascial, and neural systems. This chapter will focus on how these techniques can be used in conjunction with the biomechanical model outlined in Chapter 3 to assess and treat the articular system. Although the variability and flexibility of motion patterning within the thorax should be acknowledged, this biomechanical model is still useful for the selection of manual therapy techniques. Ultimately, the goal is to restore effortless motion with adequate control and strength necessary to meet whatever load is being imposed on the thorax. When used in conjunction with education and exercise, manual therapy following this biomechanical model can be effective in facilitating recovery.

EXAMINATION OF SEGMENTAL MOTION WITHIN THE THORAX

When an abnormal pattern of motion is noticed during active movement testing of the thorax, an examination of segmental motion is required to isolate the level of dysfunction. This examination includes active physiological mobility tests, passive physiological mobility tests, passive accessory mobility tests, and passive stability tests. The findings from these tests determine which manual therapy techniques will be used to treat the movement disorder.

Active Physiological Mobility Tests

Active physiological mobility tests examine the movements of the bones both in space and relative to one another (osteokinematic analysis). The motion of two adjacent thoracic vertebrae and the two ribs that attach to these vertebrae is analyzed.

The ability of the thoracic vertebrae to rotate in the sagittal plane is examined as follows. The transverse processes of two adjacent vertebrae are palpated with the index finger and thumb of both hands (Figure 16-1). The patient is instructed to forward- or backward-bend the trunk, and the symmetry of motion is noted. Both index fingers should travel superiorly an equal distance. Asymmetry is not indicative of any particular dysfunction; it merely implies that a less than optimal pattern of motion is occurring.

The relative osteokinematic motion between a thoracic vertebra and the rib is examined as follows. The transverse process is palpated with the thumb of one hand. The rib is palpated just lateral to the tubercle and medial to the angle with the thumb of the other hand (Figure 16-2). The index finger of this hand rests along the shaft of the rib. The patient is instructed to forward- or backward-bend the trunk, and the relative motion between the transverse process and the rib is noted. To interpret the findings from this test, the relative flexibility between the thoracic spinal column and the rib cage needs to be considered. There are three motion patterns that are considered normal, and understanding the biomechanical model is essential when interpreting the test results.

At the end of the forward-bending motion, the rib anteriorly rotates farther than the spine flexes in the mobile thorax. Thus the tubercle of the rib is felt to travel further superiorly than the transverse process at the end of the range. In the stiff thorax, the spine flexes farther than the rib anteriorly rotates; therefore the transverse process travels farther superiorly than the tubercle of the rib. When the relative mobility between the thoracic vertebra and the rib is the same, no motion occurs between the vertebra and the rib during forward bending. To determine the patient's normal

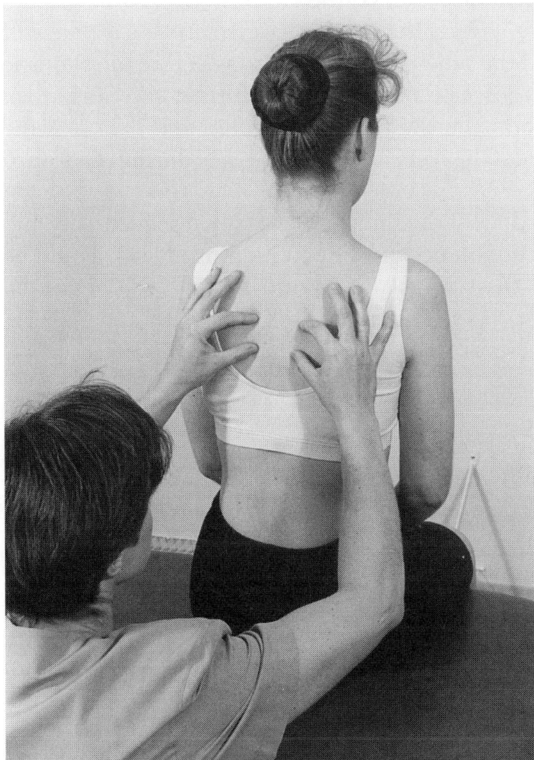

Figure 16-1
Examination of active physiological mobility at T5-6.
From Lee D: *Manual therapy for the thorax,* Delta, British Columbia, Canada, 1994, DOPC.)

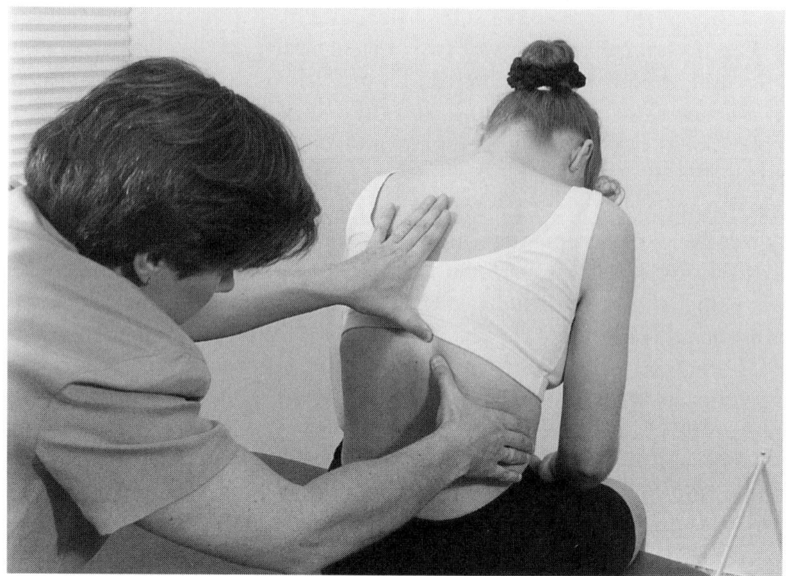

Figure 16-2
Examination of active physiological mobility of the right ninth rib and T9.
(From Lee D: *Manual therapy for the thorax,* Delta, British Columbia, Canada, 1994, DOPC.)

movement pattern, the physical therapist must evaluate levels above, below, and contralateral to the tested segment.

During backward bending of the mobile thorax, the rib posteriorly rotates, and the tubercle of the rib travels further inferiorly than the transverse process. In the stiff thorax, the rib posteriorly rotates, and the tubercle of the rib stops before full thoracic extension is achieved such that the transverse process travels further inferiorly than the rib. When the relative mobility between the thoracic vertebra and the rib is the same, no motion is palpated between the vertebra and the rib during backward bending.

When forward and backward bending of the thorax is performed sequentially, full osteokinematic and arthrokinematic motion occurs. The motion produced should be symmetric.[1,2] Therefore any disorder that affects motion of the joints or bones of the thorax will be evident during this test. If asymmetry of motion—or an apparent restriction of motion—is felt, further tests are required to determine the cause.

Passive Physiological Mobility Tests

Segmental passive physiological mobility tests provide information on movement resistance throughout the range as well as at the end. This information is essential not only for choosing a particular treatment technique but also for grading it appropriately to avoid aggravating any symptoms.

With the patient sitting and the arms crossed to the opposite shoulders, the clinician palpates the segment to be examined in the intertransverse space bilaterally with one hand. The other hand or arm supports the thorax and imparts the testing motion. The trunk is passively flexed, extended, laterally flexed, and rotated, and the motion resistance, or ease, is compared to levels above and below.

Passive Accessory Mobility Tests

The passive accessory mobility tests examine the ability of the joint surfaces to glide relative to one another (arthrokinematic analysis). In the thorax, the zygapophyseal joints and the costotransverse joints are examined.

Restricted movement during these tests does not necessarily incriminate the articular structures because excessive compression across the joint from hypertonic or tight muscles can limit the ability of the joint to glide.[3] The *quality* of the motion resistance gives the examiner more information regarding the etiology of the restriction. A stiff joint with a reduced neutral zone[4] of motion secondary to fibrosis of the articular capsule yields a consistently hard resistance through the entire range of motion. An overly compressed joint secondary to muscular hypertonicity also has a reduced neutral zone of motion; however, the size of this zone varies depending on the speed with which the joint surfaces are moved. Further range is gained if the motion is applied slowly. In addition, the end feel of motion is more elastic than when the neutral zone is reduced as a result of fibrosis. A joint fixation also has a reduced neutral zone; in fact, there is very little palpable movement, and the end feel is very blocked. In this situation, there is an obvious asymmetry in the position of the segment, and speed does not vary the amount of movement palpable.

Tests of Segmental Mobility. The following test is used to examine the ability of the right zygapophyseal joint at T4-5 to glide superoanteriorly (motion required for forward sagittal rotation). The inferior aspect of the left transverse process of T5 is palpated with the left thumb while the right thumb palpates the inferior aspect of the right transverse process of T4. The left thumb fixes T5, and a superoanterior glide is applied to T4 with the right thumb (Figure 16-3). The motion resistance or ease is compared to levels above and below.

The inferoposterior glide of the right T4-5 zygapophyseal joint is tested as follows. The inferior aspect of the right transverse process of T5 is palpated with the left thumb. The right thumb palpates the superior aspect of the right transverse process of T4. The left thumb fixes T5, and an inferior glide is applied to T4 with the right thumb. The motion resistance or ease is compared to levels above and below.

An inferior glide of the right costotransverse joint is required during full inspiration, left lateral bending, and right rotation of the thorax.[5,6] The following test is used to determine the ability of the right fifth rib to glide inferiorly relative to the transverse process of T5. With the patient prone and the thoracic spine in neutral, the inferior aspect of the right transverse process of T5 is palpated with the left thumb. The right thumb palpates the superior aspect of the right fifth rib just lateral to the tubercle. The left thumb fixes T5, and an inferior glide (allowing the conjunct posterior roll to occur) is applied to the fifth rib with the right thumb. The motion resistance or ease is compared to levels above and below.

A superior glide of the right costotransverse joint is required during full expiration, right lateral bending, and left rotation of the thorax. With the patient prone and the thoracic spine in neutral, the superior aspect of the transverse process of T5 is palpated with the right thumb. The left thumb palpates the inferior aspect of the right fifth rib just lateral to the tubercle. The right thumb fixes T5, and a superior glide (allowing the conjunct anterior roll to occur) is applied to the fifth rib with the left thumb.

Between T7 and T10, the orientation of the costotransverse joint changes such that the direction of the glide for inspiration is anterolateroinferior. The position of the right hand is modified to facilitate this change in joint direction so that the index

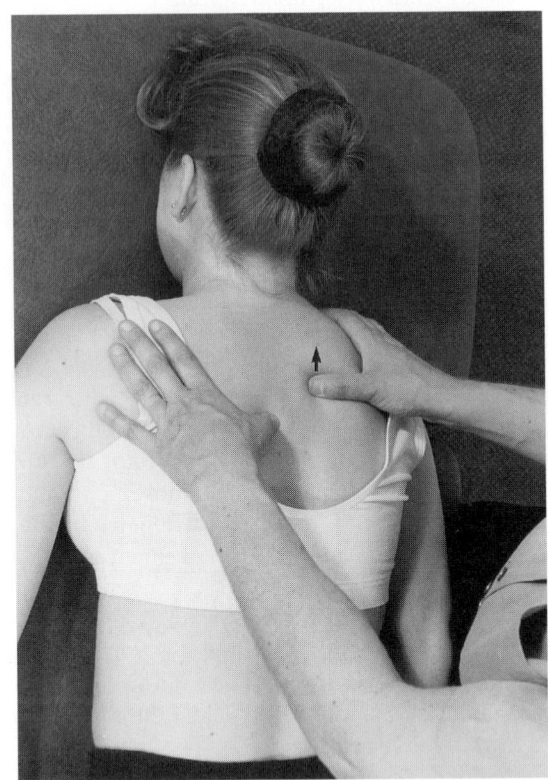

Figure 16-3
Examination of superoanterior glide at T4-5 on the right.
(From Lee D: *Manual therapy for the thorax*, Delta, British Columbia, Canada, 1994, DOPC.)

finger of the right hand lies along the shaft of the rib and assists in gliding the rib in an anterolateroinferior direction (Figure 16-4). For expiration, the direction of the glide is posteromediosuperior. Without changing the hand position, this glide is tested by fixing the transverse process with one thumb and gliding the rib in a posteromediosuperior direction.

Mediolateral translation in the transverse plane occurs during rotation of the thorax. This motion involves all of the bones and joints of the thoracic segment, and although the amplitude of the motion is very small,[1,2] it is essential for rotation to occur. The following test examines the ability of T5 and the right and left sixth ribs to glide to the right relative to T6 (anteromedial translation of the left sixth rib, posterolateral translation of the right sixth rib). The patient sits with the arms crossed to opposite shoulders. With the right hand or arm, the thorax is palpated above the sixth segmental ring. With the left hand, the transverse processes of T6 are fixed. With the right hand/arm the T5 vertebra and the ribs are translated *purely* to the right in the transverse plane (Figure 16-5). The motion resistance/ease is compared to levels above and below.

Stability Tests. Intertester studies for manual techniques that compare *quantity* of motion have consistently shown poor reliability in the spine and the pelvic girdle.[7-10] Intertester studies for manual techniques comparing *resistance* to motion (stiffness) have been more encouraging.[11] In an experimental model aimed to reproduce the linear elastic phase of the force-displacement curve of a posteroanterior pressure technique, four physical therapy students were able to demonstrate reliability. When the experiment was conducted in vivo on the lumbar spine, the

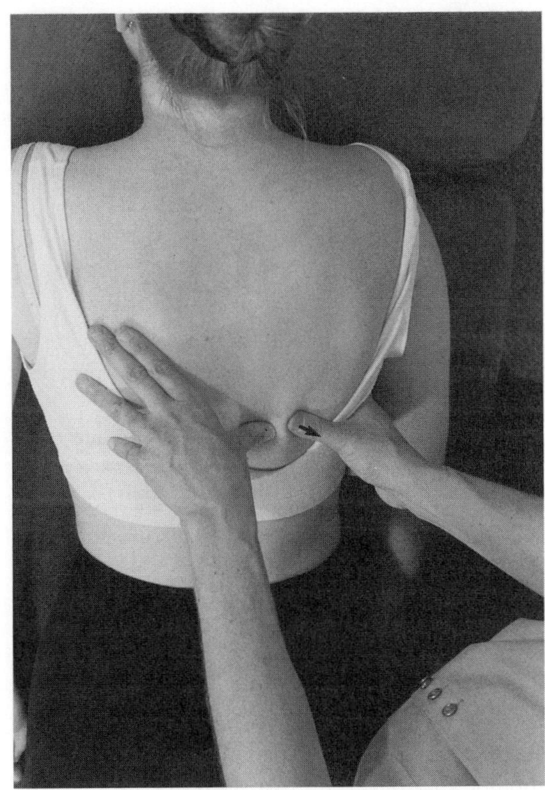

Figure 16-4
Examination of anterolateroinferior glide of the right ninth costotransverse joint.
(From Lee D: *Manual therapy for the thorax,* Delta, British Columbia, Canada, 1994, DOPC.)

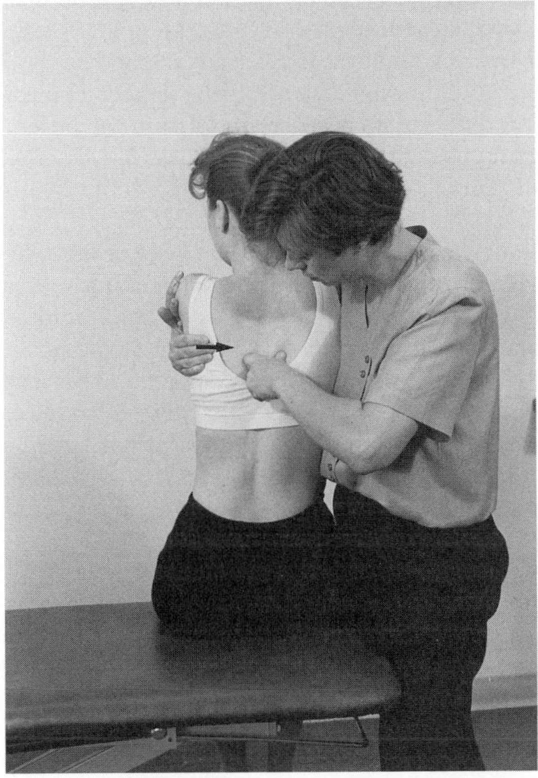

Figure 16-5
Examination of right mediolateral translation mobility between T5 and the sixth ribs and T6.
(From Lee D: *Manual therapy for the thorax,* Delta, British Columbia, Canada, 1994, DOPC.)

results were not as good because they had to interpret sensations from both the toe-phase (neutral zone) and the linear elastic phase (end feel) of the force displacement curve.

Stiff joints impart a high resistance to motion in both the toe-phase (smaller neutral zone) and the linear phase of the force displacement curve (harder end feel). Loose joints move more easily and provide less resistance when the same force is applied (larger neutral zone and a softer end feel). This does not mean that the loose joint is unstable; further analysis is required to make this diagnosis.

The passive stability tests examine the ability of the entire segment to resist anteroposterior, posteroanterior, rotational, and mediolateral shear forces in the transverse plane. The total quantity of motion is less significant than the amount of resistance felt in the toe-phase of the force displacement curve. This is where traumatic, degenerative and postural changes in neutral zone motion are felt.[3,4]

Dynamic stability (efficacy of the force closure mechanism[12-14]) is evaluated by reassessing the ability of the segment to resist linear translation in the transverse plane while the patient activates muscles that are supposed to stabilize the joint. When the force closure mechanism is intact, the transarticular compression prevents all linear translation.

Tests of Segmental Spinal Stability. The ability of the thorax to resist posterior translation is tested as follows. The patient is sitting with the arms crossed to the opposite shoulders. The thorax is stabilized with one hand or arm under or over (depending on the level) the patient's crossed arms, and the contralateral scapula is grasped. The transverse processes of the inferior vertebra are fixed with the dorsal hand. Passive stability is tested by applying an anteroposterior force to the superior vertebra through the thorax while fixing the inferior vertebra (Figure 16-6). Particular attention is given to the toe-phase of the force displacement curve, and the resistance to motion is compared to the levels above and below.

The force closure mechanism for dynamic stability of the segment can be tested in the same position by resisting elevation of the crossed arms. If the segmental musculature is able to control shear forces at the joint, no posterior translation will be felt. Instability is diagnosed if there is excessive posterior translation with less resistance to a consistently applied force (compared to levels above and below) and if activation of the segmental musculature does not prevent the posterior translation.

Stability for anteroposterior translation is tested with the patient lying prone. The transverse processes of the superior vertebra are palpated with one hand. The other hand fixes the transverse processes of the inferior vertebra, and a posteroanterior force is applied through the superior vertebra. Particular attention is given to the toe-phase of the force displacement curve, and the resistance to motion is compared to the levels above and below. Rotational stability is tested by applying a unilateral posteroanterior force to one transverse process of the superior vertebra while fixing the contralateral transverse process of the inferior vertebra.

Tests of Segmental Costal Stability. Posteroanterior stability of the costotransverse joint is tested with the patient prone. One hand fixes the contralateral transverse process of the thoracic vertebra while the other applies a posteroanterior force to the rib.

When the sternocostal or costochondral joints are unstable, the injuring force usually causes a separation of the joint. When this occurs, a gap or a step can be palpated at the joint line. The positional findings of the rib relative to the costal cartilage,

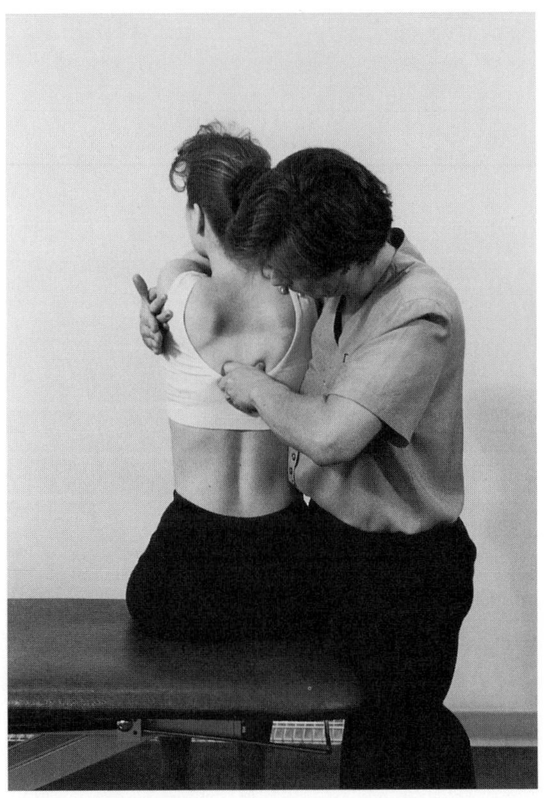

Figure 16-6
Examination of segmental posterior translation stability.
(From Lee D: *Manual therapy for the thorax,* Delta, British Columbia, Canada, 1994, DOPC.)

or the costal cartilage relative to the sternum, are noted before stability testing of the joint. When the sternocostal or costochondral joint is unstable, an anteroposterior force is often painful, and less resistance is felt in the toe-phase of the force displacement curve.

Test of Mediolateral Translation Stability: Spinal and Costal. Mediolateral translation in the transverse plane occurs during rotation of the thorax. For this motion to occur the ribs must be allowed to translate relative to the transverse process of the thoracic vertebra of the same number. When the ribs are compressed into the vertebral body there should be very little, if any, mediolateral translation between two thoracic vertebrae. The resistance is felt immediately, and the end feel is quite firm. For testing of the right mediolateral translation stability at T5-6, the patient sits with the arms crossed to the opposite shoulders. With the right hand or arm, the thorax is palpated so that the fifth finger of the right hand lies along the fifth rib. With the left hand, T6 and the sixth ribs are fixed bilaterally by compressing the ribs centrally towards their costovertebral joints (Figure 16-7). The T5 vertebra is translated through the thorax *purely* in the transverse plane. Particular attention is given to the toe-phase of the force displacement curve, and the resistance to motion is compared to the levels above and below. An unstable segment will still translate when the ribs are compressed and the resistance in the toe-phase of the force displacement curve is not altered by compressing the ribs medially. This is a key feature in rotational instability of the midthorax.[15]

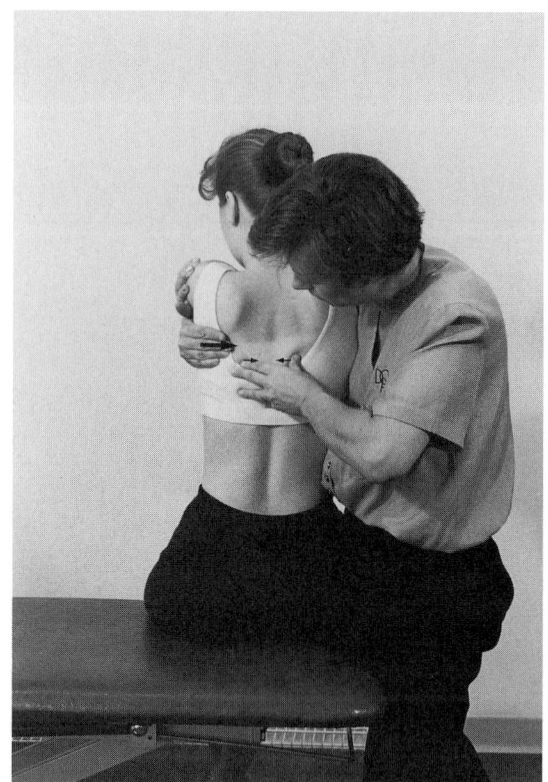

Figure 16-7
Examination of right mediolateral translation stability between T5 and the sixth ribs; and T6.
(From Lee D: *Manual therapy for the thorax*, Delta, British Columbia, Canada, 1994, DOPC.)

MANUAL THERAPY TREATMENT TECHNIQUES FOR THE MIDTHORAX

This section will review how manual therapy can be used in conjunction with the biomechanical model to restore motion when a segmental restriction is found in the midthorax. These techniques have a powerful effect on the afferent input from the segmental structures and should not be regarded as just articular in nature. In fact, it is impossible to touch the skin and not directly influence the nervous system and thus the myofascial system. Thus to assume that a specific mobilization aimed at restoring an arthrokinematic glide is affecting only the joint is very erroneous. The goal of the technique is to reduce the compressive force across the joint that is limiting its ability to move. The compression may be coming from the following:

- Fibrosis of the capsule
- Hypertonic muscles that increase transarticular compression
- Neural irritability or facilitation
- Altered emotional states

The technique selection in this model is based on the findings from the objective segmental motion examination. The grading of the technique depends on the irritability of the tissues and the presence or absence of pain, resistance, and spasm, otherwise known as the joint picture.[16] A stiff joint resulting from capsular fibrosis is mobilized with a sustained grade 4 passive technique. A joint that is compressed secondary to hypertonic transarticular muscles is mobilized with an active mobilization technique (muscle energy[17]) or a grade 3 oscillatory passive mobilization. A joint

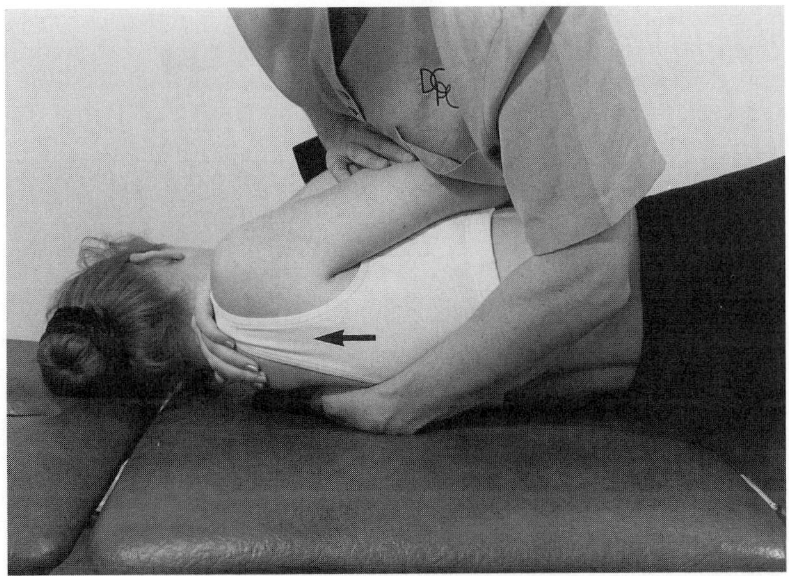

Figure 16-8
Mobilization for segmental bilateral superior glide of the zygapophyseal joints.
(From Lee D: *Manual therapy for the thorax,* Delta, British Columbia, Canada, 1994, DOPC.)

that is fixated (unstable and compressed) is mobilized with a grade 5 high velocity, low-amplitude thrust technique. An example that describes how each of these techniques can be used in the thorax will be given. Further examples of how manual therapy is used with this biomechanical model can be found elsewhere.[6,15,18]

BILATERAL RESTRICTION OF SEGMENTAL FLEXION: SPINAL COMPONENT

Longitudinal traction produces a superior glide of the zygapophyseal joint bilaterally. This is the arthrokinematic motion necessary to restore segmental flexion between two thoracic vertebrae. For the technique to be specific and segmental, it is best done with the patient in lying.

To begin, the patient is side-lying, with the arms crossed to the opposite shoulders. The therapist stands facing the patient with his or her feet in a forward stance position. The back leg or foot is the one closest to the table. The inferior vertebra of the segment to be mobilized is fixed by palpating the transverse process bilaterally with the tubercle of the scaphoid bone and the flexed proximal interphalangeals (PIP) joint of the long finger. The other arm lies across the patient's crossed arms to control the thorax. Segmental localization is achieved by flexing the joint to the motion barrier with the arm controlling the thorax. This localization is maintained as the patient is rolled supine *only until contact is made between the table and the therapist's dorsal hand.* From this position, a third vector,[19] which focuses the technique and reduces the amount of force necessary to achieve mobilization, is introduced. This vector is compression and is applied by the squeezing the thorax with the dorsal forearm. The ventral arm controls the segmental flexion, the dorsal hand fixes the inferior vertebra, and the dorsal forearm applies the third vector of compression. From this position, longitudinal traction is applied through the thorax to produce a superior glide of the zygapophyseal joint bilaterally (Figure 16-8). This motion is produced when the therapist shifts the body weight from the back leg to the front. The arms and hands focus the technique; the mobilization comes from the lower extremities. For this force to pass through the therapist's legs, pelvis, low back, and thorax to the arms, it is essential that the therapist understands the mechanism of core stabilization[20] and is able to activate the appropriate motor program to effectively and safely transfer forces through his or her own body.[20,21]

This passive technique can be graded from 2 to 5 with this approach. When the joint is compressed by hypertonic muscles, an active technique can effectively restore motion. When the motion barrier has been localized, the patient is instructed to gently elevate the crossed arms. The motion is resisted by the therapist, and the isometric contraction is held for up to 5 seconds, followed by a period of complete relaxation. The joint is then passively taken to the new motion barrier. The technique is repeated three times. Reevaluation will confirm whether the technique has been effective.

Unilateral Restriction of Segmental Flexion: Left T5-6

A unilateral restriction of flexion will produce a segmental rotoscoliosis as well as a compensatory multisegmental curve above and below the restricted level. Active forward bending of the trunk will reveal this asymmetry. A unilateral restriction of flexion on the left at T5-6 will produce a left rotation and left side-flexion position of T5 at the limit of forward bending. The right transverse process of T5 will travel further superiorly than the left. The left transverse process of T5 will be more dorsal than the right. Right rotation and right lateral bending of the trunk will be restricted and produce a kink in the midthoracic curve during these motions. The superior arthrokinematic glide of the left zygapophyseal joint at T5-6 will be restricted when either the joint is affected or the transarticular compressive force from the muscle system is excessive.

To begin, the patient is right side-lying, and the arms are crossed to the opposite shoulders. The therapist stands facing the patient with the feet in a forward stance position. The back leg or foot is the one closest to the table. The segment to be mobilized is localized by palpating the left transverse process of T6 with the tubercle of the scaphoid and the right transverse process of T5 with the flexed PIP of the long finger. The other arm lies across the patient's crossed arms to control the thorax. Segmental localization is achieved by right side-flexing the joint to the motion barrier with the arm controlling the thorax. This localization is maintained as the patient is rolled supine *only until contact is made between the table and the therapist's dorsal hand.* From this position, a third vector,[19] which focuses the technique and reduces the amount of force necessary to achieve mobilization, is introduced. This vector is compression and is applied by the squeezing the thorax with the dorsal forearm. The ventral arm controls the segmental side-flexion; the dorsal hand focuses the forces segmentally, and the dorsal forearm applies the third vector of compression. From this position, a right side-flexion force is applied through the thorax to produce a superior glide of the left zygapophyseal joint (Figure 16-9). This motion is produced when the therapist shifts the body weight from the back leg to the front. The arms and hands focus the technique; the mobilization comes from the lower extremities.

This passive technique can be graded from 2 to 5 with this approach. When the joint is compressed by hypertonic muscles, an active technique can effectively restore motion. When the motion barrier has been localized, the patient is instructed to gently elevate the crossed arms. The motion is resisted by the therapist, and the isometric contraction is held for up to 5 seconds, followed by a period of complete relaxation. The joint is then passively taken to the new motion barrier. The technique is repeated three times. Reevaluation will confirm whether the technique has been effective.

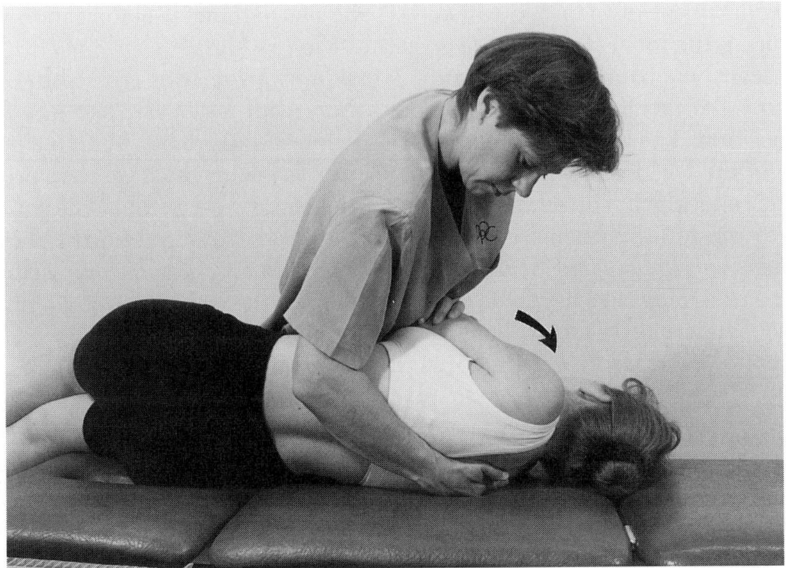

Figure 16-9
Mobilization for segmental unilateral superior glide for a left zygapophyseal joint.
(From Lee D: *Manual therapy for the thorax,* Delta, British Columbia, Canada, 1994, DOPC.)

Unilateral Restriction of Posterior Rotation: Right Fifth Rib

This restriction affects the motion of the rib necessary for full inspiration, left lateral bending, and right rotation of the thorax. When excessive myofascial compressive forces limit the arthrokinematic glide at the costotransverse joint, an active mobilization technique is useful for restoring motion. To begin, the patient sits with the arms crossed to opposite shoulders. The therapist stands at the patient's left side. With an open pinch grip of the thumb and index finger of the dorsal hand, the right fifth rib is palpated. The ventral arm or hand controls the thorax. The motion barrier is localized by left side-flexing and right-rotating the thorax. This combination of movements requires posterior rotation of the right fifth rib. From this position, the patient is instructed to hold still while the therapist applies resistance to the right rotation of the trunk. The isometric contraction is held for up to 5 seconds, after which the patient is instructed to completely relax. The new motion barrier of left side-flexion and right rotation is localized, and the mobilization repeated three times. Reevaluation will confirm whether the technique has been effective.

Fixated Right Fifth Costotransverse Joint

This situation is always the result of trauma. The injuring force causes the rib to move beyond its physiological motion barrier. At this time, the articular passive restraints are stretched, and a massive afferent input into the CNS causes an efferent motor response and excessive muscle activation. This results in the joint becoming compressed in a "malaligned" position. In the new model of altered neutral zone function[3] this dysfunction is classified as an unstable or compressed joint. A grade 5 high-velocity, low-amplitude thrust technique is the technique of choice. A grade 5 distraction of the costotransverse joint will release the myofascial compression, and the costotransverse ligament (ligament of the neck) will correct the malalignment. Stabilization therapy for restoring the force closure mechanism must follow.[15]

To begin, the patient is lying on the left side with the arms crossed to opposite shoulders. The therapist stands facing the patient with his or her feet in a forward stance position. The back leg or foot is the one closest to the table. With the proximal phalanx of the left thumb, the rib is palpated just lateral to the transverse process of the vertebra to which it attaches. The other arm supports the patient's thorax. Localization to the fifth costotransverse joint is achieved by rolling the patient over the dorsal hand *only until contact is made between the table and the dorsal hand.* Further axial rotation of the thorax against the fixed rib will distract the costotransverse joint. A low amplitude, high velocity thrust applied through the thorax in axial rotation will release the fixation. Very little force is required in this technique.

Left Lateral Translation and Right Rotation Fixation: Sixth Segment

This fixation (unstable or compressed joint) involves a complete thoracic segment, including two adjacent thoracic vertebrae, the intervertebral disc, the two ribs and their associated anterior and posterior joints, and the sternum. It occurs when excessive rotation is applied to the unrestrained thorax or when rotation of the thorax is forced against a fixed rib cage (e.g., seatbelt injury). According to the biomechanical model (see Chapter 3), at the limit of right rotation the superior vertebra has translated to the left, the left rib has translated posterolaterally, and the right rib has translated anteromedially. Further right rotation results in a right side-flexion tilt of the superior vertebra. As the passive restraints to this motion are stretched, excessive muscle activation occurs and compresses the segment, thus maintaining the abnormal position.[6,15] In the new model of altered neutral zone function[3] this dysfunction is classified as an unstable or compressed joint. A grade 5 high-velocity, low-amplitude thrust technique is the technique of choice. A grade 5 distraction combined with right translation of the sixth thoracic segment is required to release the myofascial compression.

To begin, the patient is in left side-lying with the arms crossed to the opposite shoulders. The therapist stands facing the patient with the feet in a forward stance position. The back leg or foot is the one closest to the table. T6 is fixed by palpating the transverse process bilaterally with the tubercle of the scaphoid bone and the flexed PIP joint of the long finger. Care is taken to ensure that the sixth ribs will be free to move relative to the transverse processes of T6. The other arm lies across the patient's crossed arms to control the thorax. Segmental localization is achieved by flexing the joint to the T5-6 level with the arm controlling the thorax. This localization is maintained as the patient is rolled supine *only until contact is made between the table and the dorsal hand.* From this position, a third vector[19] of compression is introduced by squeezing the thorax with the dorsal forearm. The ventral arm controls the segmental flexion, the dorsal hand fixes the inferior vertebra, and the dorsal forearm applies the third vector of compression. From this position, strong longitudinal traction is applied to the segment, followed by a high-velocity, low-amplitude thrust into right lateral translation (Figure 16-10). The longitudinal traction comes from a shift in body weight from the back to the front leg while the right lateral translation force comes from the entire trunk and upper body of the therapist. The arms and hands focus the technique; the manipulation comes from the body's core and the lower extremities. For this force to pass through the therapist and be effectively focused at T5-6, it is essential that the therapist know how to stabilize and transfer forces through his or her own body.[20,21]

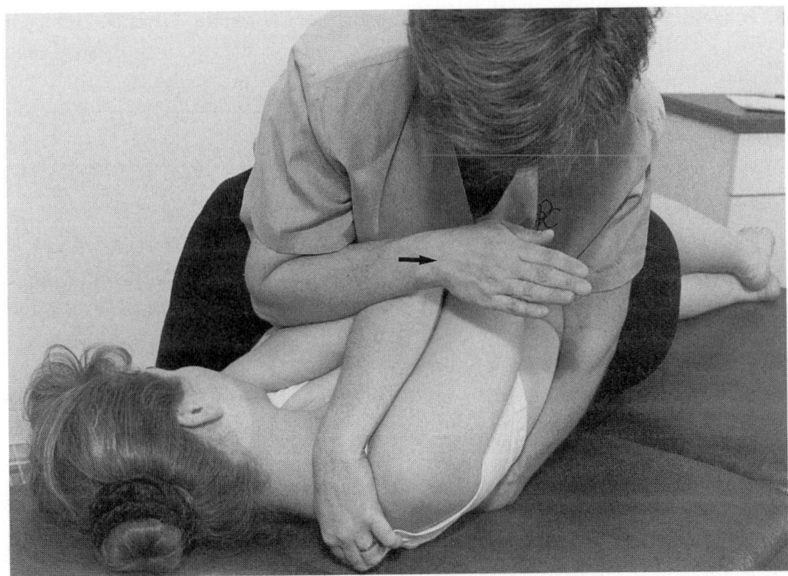

Figure 16-10
Manipulation for a left lateral translation fixation.
(From Lee D: *Manual therapy for the thorax,* Delta, British Columbia, Canada, 1994, DOPC.)

After release of the myofascial compression, the stability tests for mediolateral translation will reveal the underlying segmental instability of the ring. Stabilization and rehabilitation of the force closure mechanism is then required.[15]

CONCLUSION

Science is not about truth but about creating effective models.[22] The biomechanical model is useful for understanding segmental motion dysfunction in the thorax. However, models that consider only anatomy and biomechanics will always fall short of the clinical experience. Some people do not fit the model, and that means the model is too limited. In fact, a new model that incorporates anatomy, biomechanics, sensorimotor programming, emotions, awareness, and the impact of all of these on motion is being developed.[23] In this new model, manual therapy remains a powerful tool for effecting function because there will always be something very therapeutic about touch.

References

1. Panjabi MM, Brand RA, White AA: Mechanical properties of the human thoracic spine, *J Bone Joint Surg* 58A:642, 1976.
2. Willems JM, Jull GA, Ng JKF: An in vivo study of the primary and coupled rotations of the thoracic spine, *Clin Biomech* 2(6):311, 1996.
3. Lee D, Vleeming A: Impaired load transfer through the pelvic girdle: a new model of altered neutral zone function. In Vleeming A et al, editors: *Third Interdisciplinary World Congress on Low Back and Pelvic Pain*, ECO, Rotterdam, Netherlands, 1998, ECO.
4. Panjabi MM: The stabilizing system of the spine. I. Function, dysfunction, adaptation, and enhancement, *J Spinal Dis* 5(4):383, 1992.
5. Lee D: Biomechanics of the thorax: a clinical model of in vivo function, *J Manual Manip Ther* 1:13, 1993.

6. Lee D: *Manual therapy for the thorax*, Delta, British Columbia, Canada, 1994, DOPC.
7. Dreyfuss P, Michaelsen M, Pauza D et al: The value of history and physical examination in diagnosing sacroiliac joint pain, *Spine* 21:2594, 1996.
8. Laslett M, Williams W: The reliability of selected pain provocation tests for sacroiliac joint pathology, *Spine* 19(11):1243, 1994.
9. Matyas T, Bach T: The reliability of selected techniques in clinical arthrometrics, *Aust J Physiother* 31:175, 1985.
10. Maher C, Adams R: Reliability of pain and stiffness assessments in clinical manual lumbar spine examination, *Phys Ther* 74:801, 1994.
11. Latimer J, Lee M, Adams R: The effect of training with feedback on physiotherapy students' ability to judge lumbar stiffness, *Manual Ther* 1(5):266, 1996.
12. Vleeming A, Stoeckart R, Volkers ACW, Snijders CJ: Relation between form and function in the sacroiliac joint. I. Clinical anatomical aspects, *Spine* 15(2):130, 1990.
13. Vleeming A, Volkers ACW, Snijders CJ, Stoeckart R: Relation between form and function in the sacroiliac joint. II. Biomechanical aspects, *Spine* 15(2):133, 1990.
14. Snijders CJ, Vleeming A, Stoeckart R: Transfer of lumbosacral load to iliac bones and legs. I. Biomechanics of self-bracing of the sacroiliac joints and its significance for treatment and exercise, *Clin Biomech* 8:285, 1993.
15. Lee D: Rotational instability of the mid-thoracic spine: assessment and management, *Manual Ther* 1(5):234, 1996.
16. Maitland GD: *Vertebral manipulation*, ed 5, London, 1986, Butterworths.
17. Mitchell FL: *The muscle energy manual*, vol 2, *evaluation and treatment of the thoracic spine, lumbar spine, and rib cage*, East Lansing, Mich, 1998, MET Press.
18. Flynn TW: *Thoracic spine and rib cage*, Boston, 1996, Butterworth-Heinemann.
19. Hartman L: *Handbook of osteopathic technique*, ed 3, London, 1977, Chapman & Hall.
20. Richardson CA, Jull GA, Hodges PW et al: *Therapeutic exercise for spinal segmental stabilisation in low back pain: scientific basis and clinical approach*, Edinburgh, 1999, Churchill Livingstone.
21. Lee D: *The pelvic girdle*, ed 2, Edinburgh, 1999, Churchill Livingstone.
22. Vleeming A: Introduction to the Third Interdisciplinary World Congress on Low Back and Pelvic Pain. In Vleeming A et al, editors: Third Interdisciplinary World Congress on Low Back and Pelvic Pain, Rotterdam, Netherlands, 1998, ECO III-IV.
23. Vleeming A, Lee D, Wingerden JP: Joint function: development of an integrated model. Paper presented at the Canadian Orthopaedic Manipulative Therapists Conference, Halifax, November, 1999.

Movement-Impairment Syndromes of the Thoracic and Cervical Spine

CHAPTER

17

Mary Kate McDonnell and
Shirley Sahrmann

Muscle imbalances as they relate to musculoskeletal pain syndromes have been described by Kendall et al,[1] Janda,[2] and Sahrmann.[3] Muscle imbalances often are considered problems of deviation from the normal standards in the length and strength of agonists and antagonists, but impairments in muscle performance are believed to be just one factor that contributes to pain syndromes. Sahrmann and associates have proposed that the primary cause of mechanical pain syndromes is movement patterns that deviate from the normal kinesiological standard.[3] Deviations in movement patterns are believed to result from repeated movements and sustained postures associated with daily fitness or recreational activities. Repeated movements and sustained postures are used therapeutically because they change the anatomical and physiological properties of tissues. A reasonable assumption is that an individual's daily activities also change the properties of the systems involved in movement. Sahrmann[3] has proposed a kinesiopathological model to delineate the systems that produce movement and that are affected by movement. In addition to the muscular and skeletal systems, the nervous system is a major factor in altering movement patterns. The primary changes in muscle induced by repeated movements and sustained postures are alterations in tissue length, strength, and stiffness that affect movement patterns of specific joints and the interaction of multiple joints. The key factor is that the joint develops a high degree of susceptibility to movement in a specific direction. A vicious cycle develops because once a joint motion develops directional susceptibility to movement (joint DSM), the more the joint moves, the more its flexibility increases and the more its kinesiological behavior deviates from the ideal standard. The repeated movements and the slight deviations in movement characteristics lead to microtrauma and eventually to macrotrauma. The result is that the joint movement in the affected direction is associated with pain because of the trauma accompanying the movement.

The first step for the clinician is to identify the type of alterations that can occur in the tissues as the result of repeated movements and sustained postures. The specific alterations of muscle that can occur are increases or decreases in muscle strength, length, and stiffness. Probably the most common understanding of muscle imbalances is the increased strength of an agonist in comparison to its antagonist. One example of this type of imbalance is in quadriceps versus hamstring ratios.[4,5] The imbalance in muscle strength that develops between synergists with offsetting actions is believed to be more common than the imbalance between agonist and antagonist. For example, the medial hamstrings share all the actions of the lateral hamstrings except for medial rotation versus lateral rotation of the hip and the tibia. In the shoulder girdle, the trapezius and the serratus anterior both upwardly rotate the scapula, but the trapezius adducts while the serratus abducts the scapula. Thus an imbalance in the participation of these two muscles will result in the dominant muscle controlling the degree of abduction of the scapula during shoulder flexion. If the scapula does not abduct sufficiently, as indicated by the inferior angle not reaching the midline of the lateral thorax at 180 degrees of shoulder flexion, the consequence will be compensation that contributes to hypermobility in the glenohumeral joint. The obvious intervention is to improve the performance of the less dominant muscle, the serratus anterior, to correct the movement. A similar example can be found in the cervical spine. If the patient has an alignment of cervical lordosis and the rectus capitis posterior and splenius muscles are more dominant than the longus muscle, the neck will extend rather than maintain a constant axis during cervical rotation.

The other alteration in muscle that the therapist must consider is a change in length. Clinicians certainly have long recognized the importance of the development of muscle shortness; however, the increase in muscle length by addition of sarcomeres in series[6] is probably even more important. Probably the most common examples of increases in muscle length are found in the shoulder girdle and the thoracic spine. When patients have depressed shoulders, the upper trapezius has become longer than ideal. In those with a thoracic kyphosis, the thoracic paraspinal muscles are longer than in patients who have an ideal thoracic curve. The result of the addition of sarcomeres in series to a muscle is that its length-tension curve is shifted to the right. Because of this shift in the length-tension curve when the muscle participates in a movement, the segment being moved no longer follows the kinesiological standard for its path of motion. Obviously if the antagonistic muscle is short, another factor that must be addressed by the treatment program is present. The program will require stretching the short muscle as well as shortening the long muscle to restore the kinesiological standard of motion. Therapists should not assume that stretching the short muscle will automatically affect the length of the antagonistic muscle. Corrective exercises must include a program that specifically addresses the long muscle as well as the short muscle. A study in rats in which a muscle was used in a lengthened position for just 30 minutes a day for 7 days was shown to cause an addition of sarcomeres in series and an associated shift in the length-tension curve.[7]

Stiffness is another important property of muscle that has received some attention in the clinical literature[8] but not in relation to pain syndromes. *Stiffness* is defined as the change in tension or unit change in length and has been shown to correlate with muscle volume.[8] Because the musculature of the body can be considered as arrangements of springs in series as well as in parallel, variations in relative stiffness are believed to affect the development of a joint's susceptibility to movement in a specific direction. A clinical example of this concept is found when the rectus femoris or tensor fascia lata muscles are stiffer than the support provided by the abdominal muscles or by the stiffness of the lumbar spine tissues that prevent extension. If a relative stiffness problem is present, stretch of a muscle will cause movement at an adjoining segment. For example, when the patient is lying prone and the knee is passively flexed by the examiner, the stretch of the tensor fascia lata-iliotibial band will cause the pelvis to rotate and tilt anteriorly.

In the ideal situation if the passive tension of the abdominals and/or the lumbar spine is greater than the rectus femoris or the tensor fascia lata, no movement of the pelvis will occur. Some patients who are instructed to actively flex their knee will exhibit no lumbopelvic motion even if it occurred with passive flexion. The lack of pelvic motion can be attributed to automatic contraction of the abdominals to prevent the pelvic motion. In most patients, particularly those with back pain, the pelvic motion occurs with passive and active knee flexion. Many patients with back pain will experience pain associated with the lumbopelvic motion. Manual restriction of the motion usually eliminates the pain.

The performance of multiple tests that demonstrate the association between symptoms and these *compensatory motions*, as they might be termed, has led to the hypothesis that joint DSM is the cause of musculoskeletal pain problems. The condition, in which passive stretch of a muscle causes motion at a joint that should not move, illustrates the concept called *relative stiffness* or *relative flexibility*. This concept states that in a multisegmented system, the body follows the rules of physics and takes the path of least resistance for movement. Thus when several segments are involved in a movement, whether part of the chain of joints involved in a movement or in a joint that should be stabilized, if a segment has become particularly flexible, movement will occur at that segment more easily than at other segments. An example in the thoracic spine of relative stiffness is stiffness of the rectus abdominis muscle in relation to the thoracic paraspinal muscles. The patient with a thoracic kyphosis who has performed many trunk-curls or crunches and who has hypertrophied the rectus abdominis muscle and stretched the thoracic paraspinal muscles exemplifies the thoracic flexor muscle being stiffer than the thoracic extensor muscles. These two muscles can be assessed for their relative stiffness by asking the patient to rock backward while in the quadruped position. When rocking backward, the patient's thoracic spine will flex because the back extensors are more flexible than the rectus abdominis muscle. The latter muscle should stretch as the rib cage tries to elevate during the motion.

The role of motor control in movement patterns is particularly important in cervical and thoracic spine problems. Many individuals have body-language habits that are repeated movements. One example is repeated head nodding or cervical flexion and extension that can contribute to the degeneration of the cervical spine. Individuals with a forward head posture assume this position out of habit and feel very unnatural when they correct their cervical posture. Similarly, individuals with bifocals develop a habit of cervical extension to see through the bottom of their glasses. The movements and the postures are habitual and feel correct. Therefore the patient has to make conscious retraining efforts to avoid the repeated movements and sustained postures that have induced and continue to contribute to the pain. A study by Babyar[9] showed that even after patients with shoulder impingement syndrome no longer had shoulder pain, they still performed excessive elevation of the scapula. Correction of the movement pattern required specific instruction. The most difficult aspect of the treatment program is for the patient to correct long-standing habits.

Biomechanical impairments also contribute to the pain problem by altering the optimal length and strength of musculature as well as by placing excessive stress on bony segments. The force demands on the neck flexors and extensors are altered if the patient has a forward head posture. With the head projecting forward, greater demands on the amount and duration of tension are exerted on the neck extensors and less is placed on the neck flexors than if the head and cervical spine are optimally aligned. If the shoulders are heavy, often the acromial end of the shoulders becomes depressed and the scapula is downwardly rotated. In this alignment, tension placed on the levator scapulae muscle is greater than if the upper trapezius is the correct length and is also supporting the weight of the shoulder girdle. Another biomechanical factor contributing to neck pain is present when body proportions consist of a long trunk and short arms. An individual with this build will have to let the shoulder drop to rest the elbow on an arm rest, whereas the individual with more typical proportions of trunk-to-arm length will not.

The purposes of the examination are to determine the patient's diagnosis and the contributing factors, such as muscle impairments of length, strength, and stiffness; motor control impairments of altered recruitment and habitual movement patterns; and biomechanical impairments. Thus the examination has two main parts. One part consists of tests that assess the relationship among movements, symptoms, and the presence of signs of excessive flexibility. The results of these tests are to establish the diagnosis (i.e., the joint's DSM). As mentioned previously, the other part of the examination is designed to identify the impairments contributing to the joint DSM. These concepts will be illustrated as they apply to mechanical pain problems of the thoracic and cervical spines.

THORACIC SPINE MOVEMENT-IMPAIRMENT SYNDROMES

The prevailing theory in the Movement System (MS) approach to musculoskeletal pain is that the mechanical cause of painful tissues is based on a joint's development of a DSM. This movement, whether an accessory or a physiological movement, is not usually characterized by a large increase in range but just slightly beyond the ideal. In some cases it may just be a posture that is associated with a specific alignment of the joint. The stress or movement in the affected direction is believed to be the cause of pain. Most often, the specific tissues about a joint, such as ligaments, capsule, or joint surfaces causing the pain, are not identified, although differentiation of whether the pain is derived from muscle, nerve, or joint-related structures certainly is desirable. The premise of the MS approach is that because movement or stress occurs too readily at the painful segment, the primary intervention is to prevent the movement, restore alignment of the segment if altered, and if possible, correct factors that contribute to the repeated movement at the painful segment.

At most joints of the body, the movement direction that is most commonly impaired is rotation. Thus most of the syndromes have a component of rotation. Because the degrees of rotation are few in the spine, small increases in range can become problematic. In the spine, lateral flexion is coupled with rotation. Changes in the discs and the ligamentous restraints can contribute to subtle alterations in the degrees of rotation and lateral glide as well as anterior and posterior glide of vertebrae. Thus alterations in the anterior and posterior curves of the spine affect the alignment of the facet joints and the stress placed on the facets joints and ligaments. Because continued stretch can change ligament properties, the optimal control of the joint becomes impaired.

The normal alignment of the thoracic spine varies widely and has been reported to range from 20 to 50 degrees measured as a Cobb angle.[10] Clinical observation suggests that the curve becomes greater in older women than it does in men. Women with osteoporosis usually have a marked increase in their thoracic curve. A curve of less than 20 degrees or greater than 50 degrees is undesirable.

Normally there are only a very few degrees of change in the thoracic spine in either the direction of flexion or extension during forward or back bending. The greatest motion in the thoracic spine is that of rotation. The normal rotation range is 8 degrees at each segment of the upper spine and decreases in the lower three segments to 2 degrees.[11] Thus the motion in one direction in the thoracic spine is about 30 to 35 degrees. During gait, the greatest rotation is between T6 and T7.[12] At this level, the upper and lower vertebral segments are rotating in opposite directions, with the upper half moving in the direction of the arms and the lower segments moving in the direction of the lower extremities. Lateral flexion in the thoracic spine is approximately 6 degrees of motion between each vertebral segment.[12] Lateral flexion is coupled with rotation to the side opposite in the upper and lower thoracic spine. Thus if the lateral flexion is to the right—the concave side—the rotation will be to the left—or the convex side. In scoliosis, the rib hump will develop on the side of the convexity. In the middle thoracic segments, the coupling between lateral flexion and axial rotation is highly variable.

The movement-impairment syndromes are categorized and named according to the movement direction that most consistently produces pain and that is the most susceptible to motion. The movement-impairment syndromes of the thoracic spine in the observed order of frequency are rotation-flexion, rotation, extension, rotation-extension, and flexion. Although thoracic kyphosis is the most common of the spinal alignment impairments, few individuals with this alignment actually complain of pain in the thoracic spine when sitting motionless unless the deformity is very severe. Most often the pain is in the lumbar spine or the thoracolumbar junction when the patient assumes a standing position. These areas become painful because in the upright position, abnormal stresses are placed on these segments as a result of the malalignment. To assume an upright posture, the patient has to lean or shift his spine posteriorly to be able to look forward and to compensate for the thoracic kyphosis. In contrast to the lack of symptoms in the kyphotic spine, symptoms are present when the thoracic spine is straight or in the alignment of extension. The most common cause of pain in the thoracic spine is rotation, which usually occurs at the apex of the thoracic curve.

ROTATION-FLEXION SYNDROME

Symptoms and Associated Diagnoses. Pain in the thoracic spine that may increase when lying down or during activity, such as with reaching. The pain may radiate around the rib cage. In some patients, this pain may be mistaken for chest pain. When all the tests are negative for cardiac dysfunction and signs of rotation are present, this syndrome should be considered. The pain can occur at night when the patient is recumbent and exerts pressure on the spine that results in rotation. Associated diagnoses are scapular muscle strain, rib pain, intercostal nerve radiculopathy, and costochondritis.

Contributing Activities. Contributing activities include throwing, playing tennis or volleyball, canoeing, kayaking, and always working in a position that requires rotation to one side. For example, a nurse may always approach her patients from one side of the bed. The equipment is placed in a position that requires rotation to be able to use it. Another example can be found in therapists who use frequent manual therapy interventions and consistently work from the same side of the patient.

Movement Impairments. In standing or sitting, the rotation range of motion to one side will be greater than to the other side. The rotation range of motion will often be greater than the normal range. The motion will occur at the site of the pain. In the quadruped position, rotation will occur in the thoracic spine when the patient flexes one arm. In the quadruped position, when the patient rocks backward, the thoracic spine may rotate.

Alignment: Structural Variation and Acquired Impairments. Most often the patient has a kyphosis, and because of the rotation the ribs are more prominent on one side than on the other side. In forward bending, asymmetry is evident in the rib area and corresponds to the midthoracic area. In the quadruped position, the thoracic kyphosis is asymmetrical, with one side notably higher than the other. The rib hump will cause the scapula to be in the winged alignment, and the anterior rib cage may be asymmetrical. The patient may also have a scoliosis.

Relative Flexibility and Stiffness Impairments. The thoracic spine is usually the most flexible segment of the spine and is particularly flexible in rotation usually to one side.

Muscle Impairments. The abdominal muscle length is asymmetrical. The external oblique muscle is usually longer or less stiff on the side of the rotation than on the contralateral side. The latissimus dorsi, which attaches from T7-12, may also be short or stiff, which contributes to rotation of the lower thoracic spine in a direction opposite to the upper thoracic spine. Middle and lower trapezius muscles as well as the rhomboid muscles may contribute to rotation, particularly if the patient has participated in unilateral upper extremity activities.

Confirming Tests. Pain with rotation or with unilateral arm movements in the quadruped position is associated with rotation of the thoracic spine. The thoracic spine rotates more to one side than to the other side.

Treatment. The primary objective of intervention is to have the patient stop the rotation motions that are part of daily activities. Often the patient will have pain when first lying down in supine, but if the patient places pillows under the head, shoulders, and upper thorax, the symptoms will not be present. After about 10 minutes some of the pillows will be able to be removed, and the patient will be able to assume a straighter alignment and will not have pain. The quadruped position is useful for exercises because this position markedly reduces the compression on the spine and can enable the patient to decrease the kyphosis. The symmetrical distribution of support in the four-point position also helps the vertebral segments assume the optimal anatomical alignment, thus decreasing the rotation. A useful exercise performed in this position is shoulder flexion while contracting the abdominal muscles to prevent rotation. If the patient experiences some pain in the thoracic spine when attempting to decrease the kyphosis, the patient should allow the spine to flex slightly to alleviate the symptoms. Abdominal exercises that provide control of rotation are also indicated. The patient needs to be carefully instructed in abdominal exercises so that excessive recruitment of the rectus abdominis muscle that would increase the thoracic flexion does not occur. If trapezius, rhomboids, or latissimus dorsi muscles are short, they should be stretched, or if they are stronger on one side, exercises for symmetry should be instituted.

ROTATION SYNDROME

Symptoms and Associated Diagnoses. The patient has a pinching or sharp pain in the thoracic spine region that occurs with subtle movements or when using the arms. He or she may have pain that runs around the rib cage from irritation of the intercostal nerve. Referring diagnoses include thoracic pain, degenerative disc disease, facet syndrome, and costotransverse syndrome.

Contributing Activities. Contributing activities include throwing, playing tennis or volleyball, canoeing, kayaking, or continually working in a position that requires rotation to one side (e.g., working on a computer that is behind a desk, which requires the patient to always rotate to the same side to get to it, or working at a counter with a telephone on the wall behind the counter, which requires the patient to always rotate in the same direction to answer it).

Movement Impairment. Rotation of the thoracic spine causes pain, but there is no obvious spinal malalignment of flexion or extension. A very slight malalignment of lateral flexion may be evident at the level of the pain. There is usually asymmetry in the degrees of rotation to one side versus to the other side.

Alignment: Structural Variations and Acquired Impairments. No obvious structural impairment in the sagittal plane occurs, but there may be a slight malalignment at the vertebral segments that are painful.

Relative Flexibility and Stiffness Impairments. There is rotation of the segment of the thoracic spine that has become the most flexible site for motion.

Muscle Impairments. Hypertrophy or stiffness of the lower thoracic and lumbar paraspinal muscles occurs. Stiffness of the latissimus dorsi, trapezius, rhomboids, and abdominal muscles is asymmetrical.

Confirming Tests. Pain occurs during lateral flexion of the thoracic spine with rotation of thoracic spine or with sitting. In the quadruped position, rotation of the thoracic spine is evident when rocking backward or flexing the shoulder.

Treatment. The patient should be taught to avoid any excessive rotation of the thoracic spine and to avoid any lateral flexion when sitting. Rocking backward should be performed in the quadruped position and shoulder flexion in the same position, and any spinal rotation should be prevented by contracting the abdominal muscles, stretching any stiff muscles of the trunk (e.g., the latissimus dorsi), and improving the control by the abdominal muscles.

EXTENSION SYNDROME

Symptoms and Associated Diagnoses. Pain occurs when the patient is standing erect or trying to maintain a good posture. Midback pain or pain occurs between the shoulder blades. The pain in the interscapular area at rest may be mistaken for a cervical problem.

Contributing Activities. An active effort to stand up very straight contributes to extension syndrome.

Movement Impairments. Pain occurs when the patient is maintaining the thoracic spine in a straight alignment that is relieved by allowing the thoracic spine to flex slightly. This same pattern of pain occurs when patients with a kyphosis attempt to straighten their thoracic spine.

Alignment: Structural Variations and Acquired Impairments. The patient has a straight or flat thoracic spine. The shoulders are usually held back, and the scapulae are adducted. The posture often indicates that the patient is trying too hard to exhibit good posture but has exceeded the normal standards.

Relative Flexibility and Stiffness Impairments. The cervical spine may be too flexible into flexion because the loss of a normal thoracic curve requires the patient to excessively flex the cervical spine to be able to look down.

Muscle Impairments. The thoracic paraspinal muscles may be stiff from prolonged contraction in a shortened position. The rhomboid muscles may also be stiff or short from the faulty attempt to maintain what is believed to be good posture.

Confirming Tests. Pain occurs when the patient is trying to stand straight, and decreased symptoms occur when the patient is relaxing the thoracic spine and allowing it to flex slightly.

Treatment. The patient should be instructed in correct alignment, and the problem of the exaggerated flattening of the thoracic spine should be emphasized.

Extension-Rotation Syndrome

Symptoms and Associated Diagnoses. Pain in the posterior aspect of the midthoracic area occurs with movements of the thorax or sometimes with unilateral arm movements. Pain along the rib cage radiates into the anterolateral aspect of the thorax.

Contributing Activities. Work or recreational activities that involve rotation cause the pain.

Movement Impairments. There is rotation greater to one side than the other. In the quadruped position, there will be rotation in the thoracic spine during shoulder flexion.

Alignment: Structural Variations and Acquired Impairments. The thoracic spine is flat, but there is possible slight malalignment of the thoracic vertebrae in the area of the pain.

Relative Flexibility and Stiffness Impairments. Rotation is the most flexible motion of the thoracic spine.

Muscle Impairments. There are stiff back extensors.

Confirming Tests. There is no pain if rotation is avoided and less pain if the thoracic spine is slightly flexed.

Treatment. Rotational motions of the spine should be avoided, and the restoration of a normal thoracic curve should be encouraged.

Flexion Syndrome

Symptoms and Associated Diagnoses. Few patients have symptoms just from being in the flexed posture. If symptoms are present in an individual with a marked kyphosis, it is primarily from an attempt to correct alignment too rapidly, which may cause the muscles to cramp or cause symptoms associated with vertebral compression. The symptoms may also be from strain of the thoracoscapular muscles that are often abducted because of the kyphosis. Flexion of the lumbar spine contributes to the tendency to rotate excessively. Flexion in the osteoporotic individual also contributes to compression fractures and therefore should be addressed. The flexion syndrome is primarily a postural problem.

Contributing Activities. The flexion syndrome begins during childhood with poor sitting alignment. Young adults with poor sitting postures and with trunk-curl exercises often develop flexion syndrome. Other activities include swimming—particularly butterfly and breast strokes—and cycling on a racing bike. Older adults who do not make an effort to maintain an erect alignment and who have osteoporosis often develop flexion syndrome.

Movement Impairment. There is limited ability to correct the flexion alignment of the thoracic spine.

Alignment: Structural Variations and Acquired Impairments. There is an increased thoracic curve.

Relative Flexibility and Stiffness Impairments. The patient has difficulty reversing the thoracic curve.

Muscle Impairments. In younger adults, shortness of the rectus abdominis is a primary contributing factor. In young men who have done a great deal of weight training the shortness of the back extensors combined with shortness of the rectus abdominis is another contributing factor. Excessive length of the thoracic paraspinal muscles is yet another factor.

Confirming Tests. The patient does not have pain when sitting while allowing the thoracic spine to assume the flexed alignment. The patient experiences pain when standing or attempting to sit up straight.

Treatment. The primary goal is to decrease the thoracic kyphosis. The patient should be supine, lying on the back with the arms overhead, and should be instructed to take a deep breath. Another treatment involves instructing the patient to stand with the lumbar spine against the wall and try to lift his or her chest. The quadruped position allows the thoracic spine to straighten, and rocking backward can be used to emphasize flattening of the thoracic spine. If the patient develops pain or other symptoms, the thoracic spine should be allowed to flex slightly.

DIFFERENTIAL MOVEMENT-IMPAIRMENT DIAGNOSIS

Pain in the interscapular area of the thorax can be from a variety of sources, including medical conditions for which the patient needs to be screened. A variety of texts that incorporate differential diagnoses and appropriate screening methods are available.[13] A common musculoskeletal pain problem that can present as a thoracic spine dysfunction is the scapular abduction syndrome.[3] One form of the scapular abduction syndrome involves strain of the scapular adductor muscles. When patients have this condition, there is some swelling in the paraspinal area on the painful side. With the patient in the supine position, shoulder lateral rotation elicits symptoms in the area between the medial aspect of the scapula and the vertebral spine. In the prone position, there is marked movement of the scapula during shoulder lateral rotation. The shoulder lateral rotators test weak unless the scapula is manually stabilized. The rhomboids and trapezius also test weak. When the patient is in the sitting position, the painful arm should be passively supported so that the shoulder is not pulled forward. This position will help to eliminate or reduce the symptoms. Careful examination will enable the therapist to differentiate thoracic spine mechanical problems from scapular muscle strain.

CERVICAL MOVEMENT-IMPAIRMENT SYNDROMES

In addition to the syndromes that can develop in the thoracic spine, the alignment of the thoracic spine can be an important factor in the pain problems that develop in the cervical spine. As discussed in the introduction of this chapter, musculoskeletal pain syndromes are believed to be caused by deviations from the kinesiological standard in the arthrokinematics and the osteokinematics of joint motion. The result of the deviations is such that joint movement in a specific direction usually causes an increase in symptoms. Just as with the thoracic movement-impairment syndromes, the syndrome is named according to the offending movement direction. The examination is performed to identify the directional specificity of the impairment, the specific movement deviation, and the contributing factors. The standards for normal range of motion are used as the basis for identifying deviations in motion. In general, passive range of motion is greater than active range of motion.[14]

The normal mean range of motion of cervical flexion is 63 degrees for young adults aged 20 to 30 years and 50 degrees for older adults aged 60 to 70 years. The mean range of motion of cervical extension is 79 degrees for young adults but decreases by 32% for older adults aged 70 to 90 years. A variety of studies have shown that cervical range of motion, particularly extension,[15] decreases with age.[14,16,17] Women generally have a greater range of motion than men.[14,16] The normal mean range of motion of cervical lateral flexion is 45 degrees. The normal mean range of motion of rotation about a vertical axis is 70 degrees in one direction in young adults but decreases to 58 to 55 degrees in older adults. A total of 50% of the rotation motion occurs between C1 and C2 because of the rotation of C1 about the odontoid process of C2. The other 50% of the motion occurs at the remaining cervical vertebrae, with each segment contributing approximately 7 degrees of movement.[18,19] In young adults aged 20 to 39 years, the maximal range of intervertebral motion is between C5-6, but in older adults aged 60 to 82 years, this same segment along with C6-7 has the least range of motion.[16,20,] The loss of range of motion at C5-6 and C6-7 is consistent with the greatest amount of disc narrowing also occurring at these levels. The loss of range of motion with aging at the cervical levels that originally had the greatest range is consistent with the belief that over time repetitive motion contributes to degeneration.

Penning[17] suggested that the larger size of the uncinate processes at C2-3, C3-4, and C4-5 reduces some of the shear effects on the discs and ligaments that occurs during the translation motion associated with flexion and extension movements. This is particularly important because a greater amount of translation occurs at the upper cervical segments than at the lower segments. Although less translation motion occurs at C5-6 and C6-7, the smaller uncinate processes of these vertebrae do not provide the same degree of protection from the shear forces that occur during cervical motion.[17]

Adaptive changes in the cervical spine include increased range of motion of axial rotation at C1-2 in the older adult, which may be a compensation for the decreased range of motion at the lower segments.[21] In addition, young competitive swimmers were found to have significant increases in the range of cervical rotation on the side on which they breathe while swimming.[22]

IDEAL ALIGNMENT OF THE UPPER QUARTER REGION

The ideal alignment of the cervical spine consists of an inward curve.[1] Both the lower cervical region (C3-7) and the upper cervical region (Occiput and C1-2) are in a position of extension. The ideal alignment of the thoracic spine is a normal outward curve. The scapulae should be positioned flat on the thorax; in 10 degrees of anterior tilt, rotated 30 degrees anteriorly in the frontal plane, the vertebral borders should be parallel to the spine or in slight upward rotation and positioned approximately 3 inches from the thoracic spine.[23]

The alignment of the thoracic spine can affect the alignment and the movements of the cervical spine. For example, a thoracic kyphosis can increase cervical extension that is one form of the forward head position. When the thoracic spine is kyphotic, the patient adopts the forward head position to maintain the head and eyes in a functional position. A decrease in the normal thoracic curve resulting in a flat thoracic spine can be associated with the spine becoming stiff and losing the range of motion into flexion. When the range of thoracic flexion is limited, the patient often will increase the range of cervical flexion when looking downward. The increased cervical flexion can involve excessive forward translation motion, particularly at the lower cervical segments.

NORMAL (PRECISE) CERVICAL MOVEMENT

Similar to other joints, precise movement in the cervical spine requires optimal arthrokinematics and osteokinematics that are in large part influenced by muscle length, strength, and pattern of participation. All movements of the cervical spine involve coupled motions, which distinguish the motion of the cervical spine from the motion of other vertebral segments. *Coupled motion* is defined as joint movement that always involves motion in two directions.[19] During cervical flexion and extension, the coupled motions are translation and sagittal rotation about a transverse axis. The translation motion is 1 mm between the occiput and the atlas; in the lower cervical spine the total is about 3.5 mm. During flexion, the anterior translation is 1.9 mm, and during extension, the posterior translation is 1.6 mm.[19,24]

Lateral flexion, which has the greatest range—about 10 degrees in one direction at each segment between C2-3, C3-4, and C4-5—is coupled with rotation about a vertical axis. The rotation is toward the same side as the lateral flexion. Thus during lateral flexion to the right, the spinous processes rotate to the left, which is right rotation. This coupling of lateral flexion and rotation is more pronounced than the coupling between the translation motion that occurs during flexion and extension.

Cervical rotation range of motion about a vertical axis is greater between C3-4, C4-5, C5-6—about 11 degrees in one direction and about 9 degrees in the other lower cervical segments. The greatest amount of rotation, about 60%, occurs between the atlas and axis, which equates to about 40 degrees in one direction.[18,19]

Muscle length and participation must be optimal so that the ratio of the coupled motions is appropriate to ensure precise cervical motion. The muscles in the cervical region can be categorized according to their relationship to the instantaneous center of rotation (ICR). Cervical muscles located close to the ICR, the intrinsic muscles, provide more precise control than the extrinsic muscles that are located farther from the ICR. The intrinsic muscles flex or extend the cervical vertebrae with a line of pull of more pure sagittal rotation than translation motion, whereas the extrinsic muscles produce a greater degree of translation motion. The intrinsic muscles that flex (sagittally rotate) the cervical vertebrae include the longus capitis, longus colli, rectus capitis anterior, and rectus capitis lateralis.[25,26] The extrinsic muscles that contribute to forward translational motion of the cervical vertebrae include the sternocleidomastoid and the anterior scaleni.[26] The intrinsic neck extensors located close to the axis of motion include the suboccipitals (rectus capitis posterior major, obliquus capitis inferior, obliquus capitis superior), semispinalis capitis, semispinalis cervicis, splenius capitis, splenius cervicis, longissimus capitis, and longissimus colli.[25] Contraction of the intrinsic neck extensors results in posterior sagittal rotation of the cervical vertebrae.[26] Contraction of the extrinsic neck extensors, the levator scapulae, and the upper trapezius muscles results in posterior translation of the cervical vertebrae.[26] Optimal participation of the intrinsic and extrinsic muscles results in an appropriate ratio of posterior translation and sagittal rotation within the constraints imposed by the shape of the articular surfaces and the extensibility of the ligaments.

During movement of the cervical spine, the ideal muscle strategy would be dominant control by the intrinsic neck muscles so that the movement of the cervical spine is precise. The common clinical observation is dominance of the extrinsic muscles; the effect is excessive translation movement of the cervical spine. Translation motions are associated with shear forces that can injure structures of the neck.

Ideally, the intrinsic suboccipital rotator muscles should control cervical rotation (movement about a vertical axis). The suboccipital muscles that control rotation of the upper cervical region are the rectus capitis anterior, rectus capitis posterior major, obliquus capitis inferior, and the obliquus capitis superior.[25] The intrinsic muscles that control rotation of the lower cervical region are the longus capitis, semispinalis, and splenius.[25] Thus rotation of the head, upper cervical spine, and lower cervical spine require coordination between several sets of muscles. The extrinsic rotator muscles are the sternocleidomastoid, the scaleni, the upper trapezius, and the levator scapulae.[25] If the sternocleidomastoid and the scaleni are the dominant muscles, the motion will be a combination of rotation and potentially excessive side-bending motion. If the levator scapulae and the upper trapezius are the dominant muscles, the motion will be a combination of rotation, side-bending, and extension.

Basic knowledge of the motion at cervical segments, the musculature controlling the motions (with particular emphasis on intrinsic versus extrinsic muscles), and careful attention to observation of alignment and movement patterns are the key components for identifying the cervical movement-impairment syndromes.

CERVICAL MOVEMENT-IMPAIRMENT SYNDROMES

The name of the movement-impairment syndromes is based on the direction of the joint movement that most consistently elicits or intensifies the patient's symptoms. Most often the characteristics of the movement in the offending direction can be observed to deviate from the kinesiological standard. The syndromes in order of observed frequency are cervical extension, rotation-extension, rotation, rotation-flexion, and flexion. At this initial stage of development of the diagnostic categories, no attempt to subcategorize the syndromes according to differences in the behavior of the upper and lower cervical segments has been made. Rather, this information emphasizes the provision of a general format of classification as the potential construct for further development and refinement of the diagnostic categories.

Cervical Extension

Symptoms and Associated Diagnoses. There is pain with cervical extension. The *patient* may have pain in the area of the upper trapezius or the levator scapular muscles. A younger individual with elevated shoulders and a forward posture may awaken with neck pain. The patient probably sleeps with the arm overhead with the head turned away from the arm. This would place the upper trapezius in its shortened position. Associated diagnoses are degenerative disc disease, herniated cervical disc, and facet syndrome.

Contributing Activities. Habitual nodding, forward head posture, and looking through bifocals contribute to cervical extension, as does sleeping with arm overhead, particularly in the prone position.

Movement Impairments. With normal cervical alignment during active extension, excessive posterior translation of one or more of the cervical vertebrae can be observed. This type of motion would be expected if the motion were produced by dominant activity of the levator scapulae. If the patient has degenerative disc disease that causes a marked forward head posture of flexion, the starting position is often excessive anterior translation. The position of flexion and anterior translation interferes with cervical extension. If the patient has degeneration of cervical discs, the structural changes can limit the available extension range of motion. If the forward head posture is the result of increased cervical lordosis, the patient cannot extend because of the lack of available range of motion.

Alignment: Structural Variations and Acquired Impairments. An acquired postural fault of an increased lordosis of both the upper and lower cervical spine is a contributing factor in this syndrome. In the older adult, degeneration of the cervical spine can result in a forward head position with anterior translation of the cervical vertebrae and loss of the normal cervical curve. An older adult with a forward head posture must assume a position of upper cervical extension to look straight ahead. The degree of extension can be exaggerated if the patient also wears bifocal glasses.

A thoracic kyphosis will increase the cervical inward curve and can result in a cervical lordosis. Scapular alignment also affects cervical alignment. Depression or abduction of the scapulae causes the cervicoscapular muscles—the upper trapezius and the levator scapulae—to lengthen. Because the upper trapezius and levator scapulae are primary suspensory muscles of the shoulder girdle, the downward pull from heavy arms exerts compressive force on the cervical facet joints, narrows the intervertebral foramen, and can contribute to traction on the brachial plexus.

Relative Flexibility and Stiffness Impairments. The movement of the lower cervical vertebrae into extension is particularly flexible. The neck extensors are short, and the neck flexors are long, which contributes to cervical lordosis and extension.

Muscle Impairments. There is dominance of the levator scapulae muscle during neck extension, with diminished activity of the intrinsic neck extensors, which contributes to a greater amount of posterior translation motion than if the correct pattern of muscle participation was evident. This common movement impairment can be observed in the following:

1. The quadruped position when the patient performs active neck extension. The attachments of the levator scapulae on the lateral aspect of the cervical vertebrae are particularly prominent before and during the extension. Posterior translation

may be more evident than posterior sagittal rotation during the extension motion (backward movement of the head versus rotation of the head and neck).
2. The quadruped position when the patient performs active neck flexion. The control of the flexion movement is poor. The patient's head and neck do not move smoothly during flexion but demonstrate a "cogwheeling" motion. The movement impairment is attributed to the poor eccentric control of the intrinsic neck extensor muscles.
3. The quadruped position when the patient is rocking back toward the heels. The cervical spine extends as though the head is moving in toward the thorax. The explanation for this observation is that as the patient rocks backward, the scapulae are upwardly rotating, which stretches the levator scapula muscle. If the levator scapula is stiff or short and if the neck flexors, longus colli, and longus capitis are less stiff, the cervical lordosis will increase during the rocking backward movement.
4. The forward head posture. The intrinsic neck flexor muscles are elongated and thus usually test weak. During neck flexion, the activity of the extrinsic neck flexors—the sternocleidomastoid and the scaleni—is dominant, and the lengthened intrinsic neck flexors do not exert optimal counterbalancing control of the motion.

The following tests and observations can be used to assess muscle dominance. In a manual muscle test of the neck flexors,[1] the intrinsic muscles will test weak. When the patient attempts to hold the head and neck in the test position with or without application of resistance, he or she cannot maintain the head in the position of flexion (flattening the inward cervical curve); instead the head moves forward in a translation motion. When this substitution is observed, the extrinsic neck flexors are considered to exert the dominant control. In the upright position, when the patient performs cervical flexion, a greater degree of anterior translation of the cervical spine than sagittal rotation can be observed.

Confirming Tests. The patient has pain in the area of the head and neck. The pain in the levator scapulae area is decreased when the shoulders are passively elevated. The range of cervical flexion is increased with the shoulders passively elevated.

Treatment. The primary objectives of treatment are to limit the degree of cervical extension during daily activities, to improve the control and strength of the intrinsic neck flexor muscles, and to lengthen the cervical extensor muscles. The patient should be taught to avoid excessive extension, particularly posterior translation motion. Patients who wear bifocal glasses are at particular risk because cervical extension is necessary when they try to focus with the lower part of their glasses.

The patient is taught how to maintain correct alignment of the head and neck. The patient can stand or sit with the back and head against the wall; this reference for the correct position can be helpful. If the patient has a thoracic kyphosis, the position will have to be modified. Exercises to strengthen the intrinsic neck extensor muscles, if necessary, and to decrease levator scapulae muscle dominance are also helpful.

The neck extensor muscles can be stretched if required. Patients with elevated shoulders usually have shortness of the upper trapezius and levator scapulae muscles and thus need to perform lower trapezius exercises. If the patient awakens with severe neck pain or has an acute whiplash injury, the use of a cervical collar or even a folded towel around the neck can help to relieve the acute symptoms. If the patient has depressed shoulders, passive elevation of the shoulders by support under the forearm, can help alleviate the symptoms. Exercises to improve the performance of the upper trapezius and serratus anterior are indicated.[3]

Cervical Rotation-Extension

Symptoms and Associated Diagnoses. Pain occurs primarily when the patient rotates the head. The pain is greater or occurs earlier in the range if the head and neck are extended. The pain onset is delayed if the cervical spine is in neutral during rotation. Pain may be present in the neck, the upper trapezius area, or the arm. The associated diagnoses are degenerative disc disease, herniated disc, and facet syndrome.

Contributing Activities. Contributing factors include habitual flexion and extension motion, prolonged time on the telephone holding the receiver between the shoulder and the ear, and repeated overhead shoulder flexion usually involving resistance. Other contributing factors are working in a position that involves a forward head position and heavy weight-training activities that involve overhead lifting.

Movement Impairments. The rotation range of motion is limited; during rotation the motion deviates from the vertical axis, and combination motions such as extension and lateral glide motions are present.

Alignment: Structural Variations and Acquired Impairments. Postural alignment of cervical lordosis or a forward head position is often characteristic of this syndrome. Depressed, downwardly rotated, or forward shoulders are more common than elevated shoulders. Heavy or long arms may be present, or if the patient has a long trunk with short arms, he or she may drop the shoulders to support them on armrests.

Relative Flexibility and Stiffness Impairments. Specific cervical segments are more flexible than other segments, which causes excessive rotation at the flexible segments rather than appropriate distribution of motion from all segments. Often the restriction of these segments results from the tension from the levator scapulae or the upper trapezius muscle. Contraction of the upper trapezius or stretch of the levator scapulae muscles causes cervical rotation, as is evident by palpation of the cervical spinous processes during unilateral shoulder flexion.

Muscle Impairments. Stiff or short neck extensor muscles, dominance of the levator scapulae, and excessive length of the upper trapezius or levator scapulae muscles occur. In individuals with elevated shoulders, the upper trapezius and levator scapulae are short, whereas in individuals with depressed or downwardly rotated shoulders, the upper trapezius is long. In the forward head posture, the neck flexors are long. If the cervical spine rotates during shoulder flexion, the control of the intrinsic neck flexors is insufficient.

Confirming Tests. Passive elevation of the shoulders increases the range of cervical rotation and eliminates the symptoms during rotation. Passive elevation of the shoulders reduces the pain that is present at rest. Unilateral shoulder flexion is associated with rotation of the cervical spinous processes.

Treatment. The primary purpose of the program is to decrease from the shoulder girdle muscles the tension that restricts rotation and contributes to pain. Because the cervical spine is lordotic, correction of the alignment is also necessary. The exercises would be similar to those described previously for the cervical extension syndrome, with the addition of maintaining passive elevation of the shoulders for prolonged periods. The patient should practice cervical rotation with the shoulders passively elevated and should envision rotation about a central axis running through the cervical spine so as to avoid any deviations from the vertical axis. The patient should also try to maintain the normal slight inward curve of the cervical spine during the rotation. As with treatment for all of the syndromes, the patient has to make every effort to perform functional activities while maintaining the optimal alignment when possible and using optimal patterns of movement. Correction of shoulder girdle and thoracic alignment is essential to the treatment program. Emphasis on restoring optimal movement patterns of the shoulder girdle should be made.

Cervical Rotation

Symptoms and Associated Diagnoses. Pain occurs when the head and neck are rotated to one or both sides. The patient may experience clicking and pain during return to neutral from rotation or pain in the lower cervical area with single—arm activities that involve lifting heavy objects. Associated diagnoses are degenerative disc disease, facet syndrome, arthritis, herniated cervical disc, and cervical radiculopathy.

Contributing Activities. Frequent head rotation, frequent golfing, and single-arm activities that involve lifting or carrying heavy objects are contributing factors.

Movement Impairments. Rotation range of motion is limited and painful. During unilateral shoulder flexion, the cervical vertebrae rotate.

Alignment: Structural Variations and Acquired Impairment. The patient usually has elevated or depressed shoulders.

Relative Flexibility and Stiffness Impairments. The cervical spine is more flexible than the levator scapulae, or the upper trapezius muscle is extensible. A lower cervical segment has become more flexible than the other cervical segments.

Muscle Impairments. The levator scapulae and the upper trapezius are either long (depressed shoulders) or short (elevated shoulders). The largest fibers of the upper trapezius muscle arise from the lower half of the ligamentum nuchae, C7, and T1.[27] If depressed shoulders stretch the upper trapezius muscle or the muscle is hypertrophied or stiff, the effect would be restriction of cervical rotation. The extrinsic neck muscles are more dominant than the intrinsic muscles.

Confirming Tests. Passive elevation of the shoulders decreases the pain and improves the range of cervical rotation. Unilateral shoulder flexion rotates the cervical vertebrae. Passive assistance of rotation of the lower cervical vertebrae decreases the pain.

Treatment. The patient should be taught about the effect on the flexible cervical segment of activities that require the use of one arm. Bilateral use of the upper extremities should be encouraged. The patient should make a conscious effort to limit compensatory movement of the upper cervical region. The patient should be instructed in rotating the cervical spine about the correct axis. To move about the correct axis, the patient should visualize a rod running from the top of the head down into the cervical spine and that the head and neck are rotating about this rod. The shoulders should be passively supported in slight elevation, a shrugged position. Correct alignment can be achieved by having the patient sit with the back against the wall and pulling in the abdominal muscles to support a low back position, correcting the thoracic and scapular position (usually by lifting the chest), and then beginning active cervical rotation while maintaining correct alignment of the spine. The therapist can also assist the rotation motion of the segments that are slightly restricted as the patient performs active rotation.

Cervical Rotation-Flexion

Symptoms and Associated Diagnoses. Pain occurs with flexion and with rotation of the cervical spine. Associated diagnoses include degenerative disc disease, herniated disc, and arthritis.

Contributing Activities. Activities that emphasize flattening of the cervical curve and depression of the shoulders, such as ballet, modern dance, and gymnastics. Sleeping with a big pillow or with the head propped up by the armrest of a sofa can also contribute to cervical rotation-flexion impairment syndrome.

Movement Impairment. The lower cervical spine is flat and flexes easily. During unilateral shoulder flexion, one or two segments of the cervical spine concurrently rotate. If the rotation is from lengthening of the levator scapulae muscle, the cervical spinous processes will rotate to the side opposite the shoulder that is flexed. If the contraction of the upper trapezius muscle is the cause of the cervical spine rotation, the spinous processes will rotate to the same side as the shoulder that is flexed.

During cervical axial rotation, the upper cervical vertebrae rotate excessively because of stiffness or restricted range of motion in the lower cervical segments. Similarly, one or two of the lower cervical segments may rotate excessively because of decreased rotation of other lower cervical segments.

Alignment: Structural Variations and Acquired Impairments. There are loss of the normal cervical inward curve and depressed shoulders. Often these patients have a flat thoracic spine. The muscle bulk in the posterior aspect of the neck may be asymmetrical. One scapula may be downwardly rotated.

Relative Flexibility and Stiffness Impairments. The cervical spine flexes more easily than the thoracic spine. The upper trapezius and levator scapulae muscles are less extensible than the flexibility of the cervical spine.

Muscle Impairments. The upper trapezius is lengthened, the neck extensors are lengthened, and the thoracic back extensors may be stiff.

Confirming Tests. Passive elevation of the shoulders increases the cervical rotation range of motion and decreases the pain. The symptoms are decreased when the patient looks down by flexing the thorax rather than the cervical spine. Passively elevating the shoulders and allowing the cervical spine to curve inward decreases the symptoms.

Treatment. The patient's shoulders should be passively elevated. The patient needs to flex the thoracic spine instead of the cervical spine, perform neck extension, and avoid excessive flexion of the cervical spine. The patient can also use a cervical pillow.

Cervical Flexion

Symptoms and Associated Diagnoses. Pain occurs with flexion of the cervical spine. The patient may have pain in the posterior cervical region or upper trapezius or levator scapulae muscles; he or she may also have pain at rest when shoulders are unsupported. Associated diagnoses include degenerative disc disease, herniated disc, arthritis, and cervical radiculopathy.

Contributing Activities. Any activity that emphasizes tucking the chin, flattening the cervical spine, and depressing the shoulders, such as ballet, modern dance, and gymnastics. Attempting to maintain a very straight thoracic spine, standing up very straight, and sleeping with a large pillow or habitually lying with the head propped up are also contributing activities.

Movement Impairments. There is pain with cervical flexion. Because the cervical spine is flat, the range is excessive when flexion is performed. The translation motion during flexion can also be excessive.

Alignment: Structural Variations and Acquired Impairments. There is a decreased cervical inward curve. The thoracic spine is straight. Often the shoulders are depressed.

Relative Flexibility and Stiffness Impairments. The cervical spine flexes more easily than the thoracic spine. The cervical spine is excessively flexible into flexion.

Muscle Impairments. Dominance of intrinsic neck flexors creates a kyphotic cervical curve. There is excessive length of the intrinsic neck extensors. The upper trapezius and levator scapulae muscles are often long.

Confirming Tests. Passively elevating the shoulders and increasing the inward curve of the cervical spine decreases the symptoms. Flexing in the thoracic spine instead of the cervical spine when looking down alleviates the symptoms.

Treatment. The primary objectives of the treatment program are to restore the normal cervical curve and to teach the patient to avoid excessive cervical flexion. The strength and dominance of intrinsic neck extensors increased. Exercises can include prone neck extension in the prone and quadruped positions. As with all cervical spine impairments, the impairments of the scapula must also be corrected. The patient should practice flexing the thoracic spine instead of the cervical spine when looking down and should raise the computer screen and working surface if necessary. A book holder can be used to avoid looking down. The patient can also use a cervical pillow, and can passively support the shoulders so that they are not depressed, and strengthen the intrinsic neck extensors.

SUMMARY

The practice of medicine began to make important strides in improving outcomes when, approximately 150 years ago, patient conditions began to be classified rather than just treated symptomatically. The systematic compilation of signs and symptoms was organized into diagnostic categories that provided the basis for identifying underlying pathophysiology and for deriving appropriate treatment strategies. Many of the painful conditions of the musculoskeletal system originate in repeated movements and sustained postures used in daily activities. These repeated movements and sustained postures change tissues and patterns of movement, which is a reasonable hypothesis consistent with the basis of treatment by physical therapists and the training methods used by athletes and many performing artists. The resulting alteration in movement pattern is believed to cause the pain, and the tissue impairments are believed to be contributing factors. The alteration in movement patterns that deviate from the kinesiological standards for movements of specific joints can be used as the basis of diagnostic categories that direct physical therapy treatment. The movement-impairment syndromes are named for the movement that is believed to cause the pain. The diagnosis directs treatment because the therapist's responsibility is to correct the movement to relieve the symptoms and change the contributing factors that underlie the presence of the movement impairment. The contributing factors are impairments in muscle recruitment and biomechanics. In this classification system, no specific attempt to identify the specific anatomical tissue—except by general category of soft tissue, such as muscle, joint-related tissue, or nerve—is made. The rationale is that the mechanical factors are irritating these tissues and that correction of the movement impairment will allow the affected tissues to heal.

Research to support or refute the rationale for and the specific diagnostic categories described in this chapter is essential. However, the critical importance of developing classification schemes that direct physical therapy treatment warrants dissemination of proposed systems. The proposed system at a minimum offers a method for organizing the results of tests of muscle and movement function. The hypotheses do not involve "leaps of logic" or pseudoscience but are derived from simple anatomical and kinesiological principles. Therapists must begin to think and communicate according to diagnostic categories rather than according to methods of treatment if the profession is to achieve it place as a major provider of health care. The development of theory has provided direction for the advancement of many avenues of science even when the theories have proved incomplete or wrong. Reactions to and investigations of these proposed categories and theories would be welcomed.

References

1. Kendall FP, McCreary EK, Provance PG: *Muscles: testing and function*, Baltimore, 1993, Williams & Wilkins.
2. Janda J: Muscles and motor control in cervicogenic disorders: assessment and management. In Grant R, editor: *Physical therapy of the cervical and thoracic spine*, ed 2, New York, 1994, Churchill Livingstone.
3. Sahrmann SA: *Diagnosis and treatment of movement impairment syndromes*, St Louis, 2000, Mosby.
4. Clanton TO, Coupe KJ: Hamstring strains in athletes: diagnosis and treatment, *J Am Acad Orthop Surg* 6(4):237, 1998.
5. Knapik JJ, Bauman CL, Jones BH et al: Preseason strength and flexibility imbalances associated with athletic injuries in female collegiate athletes, *Am J Sports Med* 19(1):76, 1991.
6. Williams P, Goldspink G: Changes in sarcomere length and physiological properties in immobilized muscle, *J Anat* 127:459, 1978.
7. Lynn R, Morgan DL: Decline running produces more sarcomeres in rat vastus intermedius muscle fibers than does incline running, *J Appl Physiol* 77(3):1439, 1994.
8. Chleboun G, Howell JN, Conatser RR et al: The relationship between elbow flexor volume and angular stiffness at the elbow, *Clin Biomech* 12:383, 1997.
9. Babyar SR: Excessive scapular motion in individuals recovering from painful and stiff shoulders: causes and treatment strategies, *Phys Ther* (76):226, 1996.
10. Bernhardt M, Bridwell KH: Segmental analysis of the sagittal plane alignment of the normal thoracic and lumbar spines and thoracolumbar junction, *Spine* 14(7):717, 1989.

11. Simon SR: *Orthopaedic basic science*, Rosemount, Ill, 1994, American Academy of Orthopaedic Surgeons.
12. Inman VT, Ralston HJ, Todd F: *Human walking*, Baltimore, 1982, Williams & Wilkins.
13. Goodman CC, Snyder TE: *Differential diagnosis in physical therapy*, Philadelphia, 2000, WB Saunders.
14. Chen J, Jasper DC, Solinger AB et al: Meta-analysis of normative cervical motion, *Spine* 24(15):1571, 1999.
15. Kuhlman KA: Cervical range of motion in the elderly, *Arch Phys Med Rehab* 74(10):1071, 1993.
16. Hayashi H, Okada K, Hamada M et al: Etiologic factors of myelopathy: a radiographic evaluation of the aging changes in the cervical spine, *Clin Orthop Rel Res* 214(1):200, 1987.
17. Penning L: Differences in anatomy, motion, development, and aging of the upper and lower cervical disk segments, *Clin Biomech* 3(1):37, 1988.
18. White AA, Panjabi MM: The clinical biomechanics of the occipito-atlanto-axial complex, *Orthop Clin North Am* 9:867, 1978.
19. White AA, Panjabi MM: *Clinical biomechanics of the spine*, ed 2, Philadelphia, 1990, JB Lippincott.
20. Gore DR: Roentgenographic findings of the cervical spine in asymptomatic people, *Spine* 6:521, 1986.
21. Dvorak J, Antinnes JA, Panjabi M et al: Age and gender related normal motion of the cervical spine, *Spine* 17(10 suppl):S393, 1992.
22. Guth EH: A comparison of cervical rotation in age-matched adolescent competitive swimmers and healthy males, *J Orthop Sports Phys Ther* 21(1):21, 1995.
23. Sobush DB: The Lennie test for measuring scapular position in healthy young adult females: a reliability and validity study, *J Orthop Sports Phys Ther* 23(1):39, 1996.
24. Panjabi MM, Summers DJ, Pelker RR: Three-dimensional load displacement curves of the cervical spine, *J Orthop Res* 4:152, 1986.
25. Warwick R, Williams PL: *Gray's anatomy*, ed 35, Philadelphia, 1973, WB Saunders.
26. Porterfield JA, DeRosa C: *Mechanical neck pain: perspectives in functional anatomy*, Philadelphia, 1995, WB Saunders.
27. Johnson G, Bogduk N, Nowitzke A, House D: Anatomy and actions of the trapezius muscle, *Clin Biomech* 9:44, 1994.

Mechanical Diagnosis and Therapy for the Cervical and Thoracic Spine

Stephen May and
Robin A. McKenzie

CHAPTER 18

In 1956 a chance clinical incident stimulated Robin McKenzie to embark on a thorough exploration of symptomatic responses to movements and positions. A patient whose back and leg pain were dramatically reduced after lying in an extended position led him to investigate the behavior of patients' pain when they undertook certain repeated movements or sustained certain postures. He did this in patients with cervical and lumbar, spinal, and peripheral disorders and began to recognize consistent and predictable patterns of symptomatic responses.

These years of experimentation and exploration allowed McKenzie to develop a system of examination and treatment based on mechanical responses to therapeutic loading and to expound a philosophy of self-management that was in marked contrast to the passive therapies that dominated physical therapy practice at the time. Central to the approach were the identification of three mechanical syndromes: the phenomenon of centralization, the use of repeated movements, and the concept of a progression of forces. This progressive system of management encouraged a combination of patient exercises, which could be supplemented with therapist techniques *when necessary*, that was unique at the time because it offered a self-treatment approach to musculoskeletal problems.

Subsequently McKenzie described the approach as it applies to the lumbar, cervical and thoracic spines.[1,2] In these books the method and application of the system is described in detail; this chapter will give a brief overview of the McKenzie system. It will discuss some of the available evidence relevant to the approach, and it will briefly describe the essential components to offer readers a general understanding of this method.

THE EVIDENCE

Since the publication of McKenzie's books, numerous trials that examined various aspects of the system have been conducted. These have included studies examining its reliability, its efficacy, and its use as a tool for diagnosis and prognosis. These studies have made the McKenzie system one of the most researched approaches to diagnosis and treatment within physical therapy.

Many of these trials offer supportive evidence for the approach as a management tool[3-16] and as a prognostic or diagnostic tool.[5,8,13,17-20] However, the methodological quality of some of the efficacy studies is poor, which tends to weaken their findings.[21,22] There is a need for additional trials to clarify the efficacy of the McKenzie approach with rigorous methodology.[23] Nonetheless, a recent review of the evidence[24] and contemporary Danish guidelines[25] recommend the McKenzie exercise program as a useful management approach for back pain. Unfortunately, most of the available evidence relates to the lumbar spine, whereas research concerning the cervical spine is far less abundant.

NONSPECIFIC SPINAL PAIN

As has been demonstrated in the lumbar spine, morphological changes can be present in the cervical spine in asymptomatic people; thus imaging studies by themselves are an insufficient basis on which to make a diagnosis. For instance, disc degeneration that is visible on radiography and that results in narrowing of the joint space and development of bony sclerosis and anterior and posterior osteophytes is very common in the population over age 40 years without symptoms.[26,27] Asymptomatic herniated discs, even those causing spinal cord impingement, have been identified in the thoracic and cervical spine with the use of computed tomography and magnetic resonance imaging.[28,29] For any such technology to be used in diagnosis, it clearly must be combined with a thorough clinical examination.

Despite the advent of advanced imaging techniques, the majority of spinal disorders cannot be given a specific diagnosis.[30] Diagnoses may be based on symptoms, radiological findings, or a physiopathological hypothesis and thus frequently lack consistency and uniformity. For this reason the Quebec Task Force on Spinal Disorders recommended a classification system based substantially on symptom location.[30] More recent guidelines for back pain also suggest broad-based diagnostic categories, including the following: serious spinal pathology, nerve root problems, and simple backache.[31,32]

McKenzie identified three nonspecific mechanical syndromes that describe symptom response in relation to loading strategies (i.e., posture or movement). By classifying patients according to one of these subgroups based on the mechanics of their condition rather than a pathological hypothesis, it is possible to determine the direction and force of mechanical therapy required.

THREE MECHANICAL SYNDROMES IN NONSPECIFIC NECK PAIN

POSTURAL SYNDROME

Because the symptoms of postural syndrome are intermittent and easily abolished, few patients come to the clinic with pain of postural origin. However, many patients have postural components that need to be addressed in the overall management of their problems.

Symptoms of postural origin will be felt locally around the spine but may radiate and may be felt concurrently in the cervical, thoracic, and lumbar regions. The individual is able to move fully and freely. Sustained loading in static postures, most commonly when sitting or working in other positions with prolonged neck flexion, brings on the pain. It is abolished once the patient moves from this position, and he or she remains symptom free when moving. Examination will generally reveal nothing abnormal, with full movements and no pain. Typically these individuals are young and sedentary and undertake little exercise—for example, school children may be brought to the clinic by concerned parents.

McKenzie[1,2] suggested that a conceptual model allowing an understanding of pain behavior of this nature is to be found in soft tissues exposed to sustained loading. After prolonged mechanical deformation and creep-loading, mechanical nociception will occur if collagen is excessively strained.[33] At a microscopic level it is supposed that pain is generated by the compression of nerve endings as they are squeezed between deformed collagen fibers.[33] Pain results from excessive mechanical strain, but once this is released, pain abates immediately; thus no lasting tissue damage that would provoke an inflammatory response has occurred. Any of the periarticular soft tissues could be involved. Pain of similar origin can be evoked by bending a finger fully backward and holding it there for several minutes.

Some studies have found no relationship between extreme cervical resting postures or the cervicothoracic kyphosis and the occurrence of neck pain.[34,35] However, Griegel-Morris et al[36] found that subjects with more marked kyphosis and rounded shoulders had increased incidence of interscapular pain, and those with a protruded head posture had increased incidence of cervical, interscapular, and headache pain. Cervical headache sufferers have been shown to exhibit a more protruded or forward head posture than nonheadache populations.[37] None of these studies looked at the direct relationship between posture and pain and thus failed to explore the symptomatic response to certain mechanical loading strategies. In studies that have examined posture and pain simultaneously, cervical flexed postures have been shown to directly affect symptom production and magnification when studied simultaneously.[16,38,39] Harms-Ringdahl[38] showed that healthy volunteers who maintained flexion of the lower cervical and thoracic spine perceived pain within two to 15 minutes. This then increased with time, eventually forcing them to discontinue the posture, which caused the symptoms to cease. Pain was generally localized around the neck and upper scapulae but radiated into the arms in a few individuals.

Dysfunction Syndrome

There are characteristic histories in patients with dysfunction syndrome. They may have been involved in a motor vehicle accident (MVA) or surgery, had a previous history of neck pain (with or without referral into the arm) that has improved but not resolved, or be older and display the symmetrical loss of movement commonly found in those with cervical spondylosis. Pain is always intermittent and always provoked by the same end-range movements or positions. This consistency of response to mechanical loading is the key characteristic of this syndrome. Pain will appear at the point of limitation of movement. Once the limited painful movement is released, the pain will abate but can be reliably provoked each time it is repeated. Symptoms are thus produced only at end range, never during the movement. The intensity and localization of the pain is similarly consistent over time.

McKenzie[1,2] proposed a conceptual model explaining that this symptomatic response to loading strategies could be found in the behavior of soft tissues subjected to years of poor postural habits or to the repair process. The aging process may lead to a gradual reduction in mobility and adaptive shortening of soft tissues that are not exercised from time to time through the full range of movement. Alternatively, imperfect healing leading to structural impairment can occur after external trauma or an intervertebral joint derangement, which leaves an area of inextensible scarred tissue. This restricts mobility and provokes pain when normal mechanical strain is applied to this abnormal tissue.

The pain in dysfunction syndrome thus arises from mechanical deformation of structurally impaired tissue. The inability to determine which tissue is at fault need not be of concern to the clinician. Any of the soft tissues of or about the cervical joints, similar to other tissues in the body, respond to injury by repair, which may result in the formation of contractures and adhesions.[40-42] Trauma, however, is not essential for the formation of abnormal tissue, which also may arise because of intervertebral joint derangement or the contracture that occurs with degenerative changes.[43] McCarthy et al[43] describe one of six types of pain in osteoarthritis as follows, "Pain at end range of movement: this is a sensation of discomfort and stiffness, accompanied by pain as the joint comes to the end of its limited range of movement; it may be related to contraction of the capsule limiting movement." In many individuals, this curtailed range of movement and stiffness, which accompanies the degenerative process, is not associated with pain, but in some it is.

Derangement Syndrome

The third subgroup comprises by far the most common cause of pain in those who seek treatment for neck and thoracic pain as well as back pain. For instance, in a series of 319 patients, 2.2% were classified as having postural syndrome, 18.5% as having dysfunction syndrome, and 79.3% as having derangement syndrome.[44] A history of past episodes of similar neck pain is common, although in between times the patient has full and free range of movement, unlike patients with dysfunction syndrome. The problem may commonly arise insidiously and may radiate into the arm—or in more severe cases, it may refer pain and paraesthesia into the distal part of the limb. Over time, symptoms may resolve spontaneously, or they may gradually worsen.

Symptoms may be constant or intermittent, but they generally show a marked sensitivity to different mechanical loading. If the pain is constant, the patient may be incapable of finding any pain-free position. Symptoms may be produced, aggravated, abolished, or eased in different positions or at different times of day. The pain may change location, from central to lateral, from right to left, from spinal to peripheral, and vice versa. Some movements or just one may be painfully blocked. At times movements may be painful to perform, whereas at other times the same movements provoke no pain—again, unlike patients with dysfunction syndrome. A key characteristic of the derangement syndrome is this variability of presentation, which can seem baffling to patients. The intensity, location, and frequency of symptoms as well as the disturbance of movement will often alter over time, with different activities, and in the course of a single day.

On physical examination, repeated movements or sustained positions can increase or decrease, produce or abolish, or centralize or peripheralize the patient's symptoms. Pain is felt during the movement, at end-range, or both, and the physical obstruction to movement will increase or decrease in tandem with the symptoms. Rapid and lasting changes in symptoms and range of movement commonly will occur, and in more chronic conditions this may require a longer time period. These lasting alterations in symptomatic and mechanical presentations are characteristic of derangement. Severe constant symptoms referred into the forearm and accompanied by neurological signs and symptoms are more likely to prove resistant to mechanical therapy.

As suggested by this description, the ways in which derangements can present are very varied. There may be central intermittent neck pain with a loss of cervical extension, scapular and arm ache with restriction of extension and ipsilateral movements; intermittent pain and paraesthesia in the whole of the arm; or severe constant brachialgia. These possible presentations describe worsening scenarios and a pathological continuum in which initially there is articular derangement only but in which nerve root involvement later occurs as well.

A Conceptual Model

A possible conceptual model to explain this symptomatic and mechanical behavior may be found in the cervical intervertebral disc. Discogenic pain may be the cause of neck and radiating pain into the upper limb. If deformation of the disc then causes irritation of the nerve root, radicular signs and symptoms into the hand may result.

Cervical discs are innervated structures—at least in the outer part of the annulus fibrosus—and thus are a possible source of pain.[45,46] Direct stimulation or injection of cervical discs at surgery or with discography has reproduced patients' pain in the head, throat, neck, shoulder, scapular, anterior chest wall, and arm.[47,48] Scapular pain is commonly reported, either unilaterally or bilaterally.[49-51] It is described as a diffuse severe aching sensation that does not extend below the elbow and is distinct from the sharp lancinating pain that accompanies brachialgia.[47] Severe and familiar pain commonly can be provoked by cervical discography in patients with chronic neck and radiating pain.[48,52] Discography is a technique that has been used for many decades to make decisions about surgical interventions; its ability to provoke patients' symptoms is key in this role.[49-51,53-55] Although cervical discogenic pain is a clinical fact, with symptomatic discs commonly able to generate neck, scapular, and arm pain, the nature of its pathology is less clear.

Morphological patterns of inner and outer annular disruption, leakage of contrast material, and disc bulging have been observed in asymptomatic volunteers and painless discs.[48,52] It would seem that the pathological process in the cervical spine is different from that in the lumbar spine.[52,56] The cervical disc is not simply a smaller version of the lumbar disc; essential differences in the biomechanics, morphology, degeneration, and pathology exist.[57-61] Notable distinctions between the two regions include the early obliteration of the nucleus pulposus as a distinct entity, the paucity of the posterior annulus, and the development of the uncovertebral 'joints' and clefts in the posterior annulus, which can dissect the disc from side to side. Notwithstanding the findings of these cadaveric studies, clinical work reveals that the disc is still capable of displacement, protrusion, and extrusion.

Studies using magnetic resonance imaging or computed tomographic scans have demonstrated the regression of disc herniations that can accompany the resolution of cervical radiculopathy with conservative treatment.[62-64] In 60 patients with radicular (n = 52) and medullary signs (n = 8), operative findings were herniated discs in 77%.[65] Bulging, incompetent discs in the presence of a narrow spinal canal can apparently produce radicular or long tract signs, which are resolved or markedly improved after surgery.[66] Cervical disc herniations at surgery have been classified as nuclear and annular and subligamentous or epiligamentous.[67] The literature gives other examples of disc protrusions or sequestrations that cause radicular and myelopathic signs and symptoms in patients undergoing cervical discectomy.[68-71]

The nature of cervical disc herniations has not received much study. The herniated mass has been shown to be predominantly cartilaginous end-plate in one group of patients.[72] To determine the pathogenesis of herniations, these authors also studied degenerative changes in cadavers. Horizontal clefts were present in 97% of discs examined, most commonly in the posterior two thirds of the disc; vertical clefts were found in 49%. In a third of discs from individuals who were over 35 years of age, a portion of the end-plate was detaching or already avulsed. They concluded that cervical disc herniations are commonly due to avulsed fragments of cartilaginous end-plate material being displaced down vertical and horizontal fissures.

These studies show that, despite marked differences between the cervical and lumbar intervertebral discs, they are still capable of causing radiating discogenic pain and referred neurogenic pain. Cervical provocation discography has revealed symptomatic discs in 50% to 60% of populations studied; sizeable proportions also had symptomatic zygapophyseal joints diagnosed by joint blocks.[73,74] However, the typical pain patterns of zygapophyseal joints tend to be located adjacent to the spine with a limited spread of pain,[75,76] whereas cervical discs have commonly been shown to radiate pain into the arm.[47,48] The studies by Cloward[47] also showed that the site of stimulation of the disc reflected the localization of perceived pain. If the disc was stimulated centrally, pain was felt centrally; if stimulation was only a centimeter to left or right, pain was perceived laterally. In other words, a cervical derangement starting centrally will cause central pain, whereas one placed laterally will cause lateral pain that may spread down the arm.

It is clear that discs are commonly involved in cervical pain, although the exact mechanism of pain production is not fully elucidated. McKenzie's conceptual model suggests that more intense stimulation of the intervertebral joint and nerve root complex can cause pain to peripheralize down the arm and that it can be centralized if this process can be reversed, centralization of the pain can be achieved. It is a theoretical model to explain a common clinical observation. It has not been scientifically validated, and better explanations for this phenomenon may arise in the future. Regardless of the ultimate worth of this conceptual model, the clinical usefulness of other aspects involved in the McKenzie approach will not be diminished.

ESSENTIAL COMPONENTS TO MECHANICAL DIAGNOSIS AND THERAPY

In this section, key aspects of the approach will be described, and the relevant evidence will be presented. Topics discussed will be the following:

- The centralization phenomenon
- Therapeutic loading strategies in the cervical spine
- Self-treatment
- Progression of forces
- Symptomatic responses
- Recurrent nature of neck pain
- Patient education
- Repair and remodeling: soft tissue response to injury

CENTRALIZATION PHENOMENON

McKenzie[1,2] used the term *centralization* to describe the phenomenon whereby the performance of certain repeated movements or sustained positions causes radiating symptoms from the spine to move proximally up the limb and toward the midline of the spine. Conversely, other movements—commonly in the opposite direction—may cause pain to radiate distally, away from midline or into the limb; this was termed *peripheralization.* These changes in location only occur in the derangement syndrome. Centralization describes an improving situation, whereas peripheralization describes a worsening one.

These symptom responses can be used to direct management. Movements or positions that cause centralization should be used therapeutically. Those positions or movements that cause peripheralization should be temporarily avoided. Sometimes pain can be reduced and abolished within a few hours; on other occasions, days or weeks may be necessary. Sometimes, there is a concurrent and short-term increase in proximal pain as the distal pain disappears.

Analysis of the centralization response to repeated movement shows that it often predicts a good response to therapy in both acute and chronic patients.[13,17,19,20] Thus it allows the identification of patients with reversible mechanical disorders who will respond well to mechanical therapy and the identification of the direction of force for treating the disorder. Very often, movements or positions in one direction reduce or centralize symptoms, whereas movements or positions in the opposite direction worsen them; this predilection for a particular movement has been termed *directional preference*.[14] Centralization has been noted in between 50% and 90% of chronic and acute back pain patients.[12,13,15,17-19,77]

Most studies to date have been conducted on lumbar patients; however, one study[20] included both acute neck and back patients. This study classified the subjects as a centralization group if there was an immediate change in pain location during the physical examination, as a partial reduction group if centralization occurred over the episode of care, and a noncentralization group if there was no change in pain location or if peripheralization occurred. In the cervical patient group, 25% were classified as centralizers, 46% as partial centralizers, and 25% as noncentralizers (the total did not equal 100%). Although the reduction of symptoms occurred more slowly in the partial centralization group—and not always in direct response to loading strategies—this group and the centralization group had greater improvements in pain intensity and function than the noncentralization group did ($p < 0.001$). There was no statistically significant difference in these improvements between the two groups. Thus, as in the lumbar spine, centralization in the cervical spine is a predictor of a good prognosis.

In an unpublished study Donelson et al[78] examined the effect of repeated movements in the sagittal plane on neck and referred pain. Some 45% of subjects experienced a decrease in pain intensity and/or centralization testing movements in one direction and a worsening of symptoms when testing in the other. Of the patients demonstrating this directional preference, 67% preferred extension and retraction, whereas 33% preferred flexion and protrusion. Of the remaining patients, 14% showed a preference for extension but not retraction, and 12% were worse with flexion and protrusion but not better with extension and retraction. This suggests that the identification of directional preference is as relevant to the treatment of neck pain as it is to back pain.

Therapeutic Loading Strategies in the Cervical Spine

Another key concept in the McKenzie approach is the use of repeated movements. These form an essential part of the initial physical examination and subsequently play a vital role in management strategies. By analyzing symptomatic responses in the form of centralization, peripheralization, or alteration in pain intensity, physical therapists can safely apply the appropriate direction of movement as a home treatment plan. These symptomatic responses are rarely revealed by one movement but usually only become apparent *after* a series of repeated movements. In fact, a single movement very often appears to aggravate the pain, whereas the pain is reduced after repetition. This paradoxical pain behavior is apparent only if repeated movements are used. Sometimes, sustained loading rather than repeated movements may be needed. Although treatment generally starts in a loaded position, if symptoms are more acute or severe, an unloaded starting position is sometimes necessary.

Movements in the sagittal plane are generally explored first because the largest proportion of patients have a directional preference for extension or retraction.[78] If on testing these movements increase the pain, cause peripheralization, or fail to alter symptoms, then movements in the frontal plane are explored.

Movements used in the sagittal plane reflect the paradoxical coupling pattern of movement in the cervical spine.[79] Retraction produces lower cervical extension and upper cervical flexion, whereas protrusion produces lower cervical flexion and upper cervical extension. Maximal extension is produced in the lower cervical spine by extension but by protrusion at Occ-C2; maximal flexion is produced in the lower cervical spine by flexion but by retraction at Occ-C2. These movement patterns have clinical relevance (e.g., in the use of retraction before restoration of lower cervical extension or in the treatment of headaches associated with a protruded head posture).[37]

Self-Treatment Philosophy

Another key element in the McKenzie approach is the use of patient-generated forces as the treatment of first choice. If the patient is able to resolve the problem using a regular exercise program and advice on altering postural loading, he or she can become independent of therapists. Static and dynamic patient-generated forces, when properly implemented, can be successfully applied to many patients.

This approach has numerous advantages.[80] At best, therapists can provide mobilization or manipulation once every 24 hours; the patient applying self-management loading strategies can regularly, throughout the day, apply self-mobilization techniques and constantly monitor postural stresses. Furthermore by first repeatedly testing the effect of movement in certain directions, the safety of that loading strategy can be assured. Should the need arise for mobilization or manipulation in the same directional plane, these can be confidently used without fear of harm.

Use of passive therapies, which include therapist-generated mobilization and manipulation, engender patient dependency. Contemporary guidelines about spinal care stress the importance of patient responsibility for management.[31,32] This responsibility can be encouraged if the patient is offered an approach that is based on self-management techniques. Therapist-directed treatment approaches have the obvious implication that the patient is incapable of affecting his or her own cure and that this depends entirely on the attentions of the therapist. This may make good business sense, but in the light of the recurrent, episodic, and prolonged histories that many patients suffer with musculoskeletal problems, it does not appear to be in the patient's best interest.

In back-pain patients, psychosocial issues have been highlighted as predictors of chronic symptoms. Factors such as fear-avoidance behavior, passive coping strategies, anxiety about pain, low self-efficacy, and external health locus of control have been found to be associated with or predictive of disability and chronic symptoms.[81-84] Although similar studies relative to cervical spine problems have not been conducted, it is likely that a biopsychosocial model of pain is relevant to both areas. Passive treatment strategies are more likely to exacerbate these issues, whereas an active treatment approach in which the patient is the key participant is more likely to help confront them.

Progression of Forces

Many patients respond to self-treatment procedures and do not require any other input. However, some patients may require increased force to get the desired result.

This increased force may come in the form of many repetitions of home exercises, or it could include therapist-generated techniques. McKenzie[1,2,80] thus proposed a *progression of forces* in which higher levels of force are introduced only when improvements do not occur. Thus therapist procedures are rarely used as a first choice of treatment. Failure to gain lasting centralization or reduction of pain with self-treatment exercises leads to the use of mobilization and, if necessary, manipulation for the desired end. This reluctance to use therapist techniques allows the patient to attain personal responsibility and management for his or her problem, the advantages of which have already been discussed.

Symptomatic Responses

Spinal problems commonly show mechanical sensitivity to different positions and movements—that is, they are *activity-related.*[30] In the McKenzie system, treatment is guided by the response of symptoms to the loading strategies. In the derangement syndrome, certain postures or movements worsen or peripheralize the pain; those activities are, as far as is reasonably possible, temporarily avoided. Movements and activities that involve the opposite direction often centralize or reduce the symptoms; these are used in the home exercise program.

In the dysfunction syndrome, the patient's pain is provoked by certain movements. Each time the patient repeats the movement, his or her pain is produced; in treatment, this movement is used to remodel the painful limitation of movement. Management strategies are thus based on the patient's symptomatic responses. This is a more reliable guide than any conceptual model.

Numerous studies have shown that assessment based on pain responses is generally much more consistent between examiners than assessment based on palpation or visual observation. Judgments about the presence or absence of centralization and peripheralization have been shown to be reliable between clinicians, with kappa values of 0.5 to 0.79.[85,86] Symptomatic response to single-test movements have been shown to have a fair-to-good level of reliability (kappa values, 0.31 to 0.76[87,88]) and repeated test movements a good level of reliability (kappa value, 0.74[89,90]). The relative consistency with which different clinicians judge symptom behavior stands in marked contrast to judgments based on palpation or observation. Studies that have examined therapists' ability to palpate the same lumbar segment, the amount of passive accessory motion available, the presence of fixations, or the presence of a lateral shift by observation have found a low level of reliability between clinicians (kappa values, 0.19 to 0.28).[89,91-95] (The level of reliability derived from kappa values previously given is based on Altman's interpretations of these values.[96])

Thus the use of symptom responses to guide treatment direction is based on an examination process that has been shown to have a level of reliability between therapists that is considerably better than decisions based on palpation or observation.

The value of being guided by symptomatic responses will be reinforced by the patient's mechanical presentation. Just as the sudden onset of pain is accompanied by gross losses of movement, so is the improvement of symptoms concurrent with the range of movement returning to normal. In this way the symptomatic and mechanical presentations should worsen and improve in tandem and provide two methods by which to assess the efficacy of treatment.

Recurrent Nature of Neck Pain

Neck pain is extremely common in the general population, with prevalence rates very similar to that of back pain. Lifetime prevalence has been estimated at 67%, point prevalence at 22%, and 6-month prevalence at 40% to 55%.[97,98] Long histories of neck problems are common,[99] and patients with neck pain frequently have repeated episodes. A past history of neck pain is one of the highest risk factors for a future episode.[98] No evidence suggesting that rates of prevalence or incidence are affected at all by any intervention could be found. Given that spinal problems so often have a recurrent, episodic, and prolonged history, the most logical approach would seem to be providing patients with self-applied management strategies. If the patient is provided with appropriate management strategies, his or her responsibility for dealing with the problem becomes feasible, and self-treatment allows the patient to develop independence and long-term benefit. This is certainly a more rational expenditure of health resources than is offering short-term symptomatic relief for which the patient is dependent on the therapist.

Patient Education

To facilitate self-treatment, patients must be provided with appropriate information. It is the therapist's responsibility to ensure that patients gain enough understanding to be able to manage their problems independently. Education thus is a key aspect of the McKenzie approach; indeed, this should be seen as an essential element of any therapeutic encounter.

The value of simple advice and a home exercise program has been compared to normal outpatient physical therapy in a group of patients with acute neck sprain after traffic accidents.[6,7] Patients in the advice group were assessed once by a physical therapist and told about posture correction, pain relief, and regular neck exercises involving retraction and lateral movements; patients in the physical therapy group were given up to 18 appointments during which they received modalities, traction, active and passive mobilization and instruction about posture and home exercises. Both these groups had significant improvements in pain and mobility at 1 and 2 months, whereas a rest and collar group did not.[7] However, when these patients were reevaluated 2 years later, there were significant differences in the persistence of symptoms between the advice group and the two other groups.[6] Whereas 44% and 46% of the physical therapy and rest groups, respectively, had chronic neck pain, only 23% in the advice group had recurrent pain. In this instance more was clearly less; numerous sessions of physical therapy were less effective than one advice session in which patients were encouraged to take responsibility for management of their problems. This trial has major cost-effectiveness implications.

Tissue Repair and Remodeling

The effects of immobilization on connective tissues and joint structures have been widely documented.[100,101] Commonly noted changes as a result of stress deprivation include increased random deposition of collagen fibrils and crosslinks, thinning of and pannus formation over cartilage, loss of tensile strength, formation of adhesions and contractures in and between soft tissues, degradation of the ligament-bone interface, and generalized osteoporosis of bone. In summary, the effect of stress deprivation is to weaken and atrophy ligament, tendon, muscle, and bone; to degrade surfaces and tissue interfaces; and to cause disorganized tissue to bond randomly together.

Conversely, early motion after injury and exercise in general have been shown to strengthen connective tissue and muscle and accelerate return to normal function.[102,103] It is said that the phenomenon by which bone alters its shape and density according to the mechanical stresses placed on it, known as *Wolff's law*, should in fact be applied to all musculoskeletal tissue.[101,102] It highlights the truism that these tissues and structures will reflect the functional stresses put on them. Progressively increased loads will strengthen tissues and enhance function; stress deprivation will cause atrophy and impair function.

The role of rest in musculoskeletal medicine has been reevaluated in recent years. Once a mainstay of orthopedic management of many conditions, its possible role in the development of chronic spinal disability and iatrogenic illness has been exposed.[104,105] Physical therapy is also emerging from a recent past during which there was considerable dependence on a similar philosophy of rest and the use of passive modalities. Given that the most commonly used of these modalities, ultrasound, cannot be justified by the evidence, therapists will hopefully also be relinquishing this approach. Several systematic reviews of ultrasound[106,107] and more recent randomized placebo controlled trials involving acute ankle sprains and shoulder disorders[108,109] show that this treatment is of no benefit by itself or as an adjunct to exercise in treating pain or affecting return to function. Continuing to use this modality in the light of this evidence is difficult to justify. Furthermore, it does not appear rational given the understanding of musculoskeletal tissues outlined earlier, which need a program of progressive mechanical loading to maximize function after a brief period of rest during the very acute stage.

The McKenzie approach to musculoskeletal medicine reflects this concept, which is vital in understanding the management of musculoskeletal conditions. During the acute stage, therapeutic forces must not disrupt healing or cause further tissue damage, but as this subsides, mechanical loading is required to enhance the repair and remodeling processes. Once a problem becomes chronic, normalization of function will be achieved only through the use of progressive therapeutic forces. The McKenzie system offers a logical and structured way in which this can be achieved that is accessible to both therapist and patient.

MECHANICAL DIAGNOSIS AND THERAPY

A good history and physical examination are essential in making the appropriate classification. This process is described in full elsewhere.[1,2] Once patients have been classified into one of the three nonspecific mechanical syndromes—postural, dysfunction, or derangement—then an appropriate management strategy can be proposed. This is based on the patient's symptomatic responses to mechanical loading strategies. The indications for and directions in which to apply therapeutic exercises will be exposed during the physical examination.

POSTURAL SYNDROME

The only treatment required for patients with pain entirely of postural origin is regular avoidance of the offending posture. A thorough explanation must be provided. It must be demonstrated to the patient that sustained end-range loading, usually in sitting, produces his or her symptoms and that a change of posture can abolish the pain, which will not return as long as the offending position is avoided. Freedom from pain is achieved by avoiding end-range stress on normal tissues. Exercises, passive mobilization, manipulation, or electrotherapy are not appropriate.

Only the patient is able to affect a change in his or her symptoms in the postural syndrome. The essential components of management are thus education as to the cause of the problem and the adoption of corrective postures. Patients with postural pains only will be rarely encountered in the clinic, but postural stresses may exacerbate symptoms in other syndromes.

Dysfunction Syndrome

The pain from dysfunction syndrome arises when abnormal tissues are stressed at a premature end range. The abnormality may have arisen because of previous trauma (e.g., car crash) or a previous derangement, or it may have arisen spontaneously as a result of the degenerative process. A certain movement or movements consistently provoke the pain. The problem has persisted, often for many months or more, and the patient, commonly uncertain about the right course of action, has avoided the painful movement. This may only serve to worsen the condition as immobility results in further tissue shortening.

Rather than avoid loading or stressing the scarred, contracted, or shortened tissue, it is necessary to remodel it by applying regular and frequent stressing movements. To be effective, therapeutic motion must be to the end of the available range and must actually provoke the patient's symptoms. Unless the pain is produced, the exercises will not be of value. Once the movement is released, the pain will abate, and no lasting aggravation of symptoms should occur, although it may feel uncomfortable for 5 to 10 minutes. This symptomatic response to loading strategies is highly characteristic of the dysfunction syndrome: pain is produced at end-range movement but does not last. The appropriate exercises need to be repeated every couple of hours. There will be no rapid change in symptoms or range of movement, but gradually over a few weeks to a few months, range will improve and pain will decrease.

A thorough explanation must be given to the patient to justify this exercise protocol to him or her. A change can only be effected by the performance of the appropriate movements on a regular basis every day. Without commitment, change is unlikely. It can be explained that tissues are contracted or scarred and need remodeling, that this process should provoke pain, but that no lasting pain or peripheralization of pain should occur. The healing process is complete, and the pain being caused is not a sign of further tissue damage. A time frame should be provided to avoid unrealistic expectations. The value of other interventions is limited; only the patient, by applying the appropriate therapeutic exercise with enough force and frequency, can cause remodeling to occur and make a change.

Derangement Syndrome

The therapeutic exercise in derangement syndrome must have the opposite effect on symptoms from that experienced by patients with dysfunction syndrome and must decrease or centralize symptoms that are present. As discussed earlier, this may occur rapidly during the application of the appropriate loading strategy, or it may occur over days of repeated therapeutic exercise.[20] The first stage is to reduce the derangement; this is accomplished by regularly applying movements that reduce, abolish, or centralize the patient's symptoms. For this purpose end-range—usually sagittal plane movements—are first used. If there is no change in symptoms after 24 hours, force progressions may be used. These techniques include increasing the number and frequency of repeated movements over a test period as well as therapist techniques. Frontal plane movements and techniques are applied if there is no change or if the symptoms are worsened or peripheralized.

Once the appropriate direction and nature of loading strategy has been identified, this is repeated regularly every 2 to 3 hours, as long as it continues to have the same effect. Positions that cause the symptoms to return should be temporarily avoided. Reduction of derangement is maintained by postural correction and avoidance of aggravating movements. Once the reduction of the derangement is maintained, all movements and positions should be tested to ensure that function is full and that the patient is confident to move freely. Advice concerning avoidance of further episodes and similar appropriate action should another episode occur should be given.

Two studies that support the clinical relevance of the derangement model in the cervical spine have already been mentioned.[20,78] These show that use of repeated movements can reduce or centralize the pain and that the latter is associated with a good prognosis. These studies also show that centralization and directional preference are relevant to the cervical spine and that extension movements are the most common directional preference shown.

A recent study has also shown the role that loading strategies can have in compression of cervical nerve roots.[16] After being in a posture of sustained neck flexion, patients experienced significant increases in cervical radicular symptoms ($p < 0.01$), whereas after 20 neck retractions, there was a significant reduction in radicular pain ($p < 0.001$). Flexion also significantly reduced the H-reflex, whereas retraction significantly increased it. This is a measure of compression of the nerve root, with suppression of the H reflex reflecting more compression, more interference with the nerve, and more pain. There were no such changes in an asymptomatic comparison group. This study confirms the relevance of directional preference in constructing management strategies; flexion postures here are seen to aggravate symptoms, whereas early range lower cervical extension reduces them.

Nonresponders

Some patients may not be easily classified into one of the three mechanical syndromes. In patients who have chronic symptoms, mechanical responses can be obscured by psychological or social factors.[30] Such patients may not benefit from specific exercise therapy but rather may require a generalized exercise and strengthening program.[110,111] Back pain with a more severe, specific pathology that failed to improve with conservative therapy could be predicted by the response to mechanical therapy.[5] Patients with neck pain caused by herniated cervical intervertebral discs have been shown to do well with a general aggressive nonsurgical management approach.[112] Duration or severity of symptoms should never be used to exclude patients from a trial of mechanical diagnosis and therapy; however, these studies make clear the value of a generalized exercise approach for patients with neck pain if specific exercises are not beneficial.

In cervical disc disease, in addition to reports of soft disc herniations, hard disc lesions are often reported.[113-118] This refers to degenerative changes in the motion segment that lead to the growth of osteophytes, which may then cause compression of nerve roots or the spinal cord. These are forms of irreversible central and lateral stenosis, as are found in the lumbar spine. The value of conservative treatment for these specific pathologies of the cervical spine is unknown but probably is rather limited.

CONCLUSION

This chapter has sought to give a brief description of the McKenzie approach to the management of neck pain; however, for a fuller description readers are referred elsewhere.[1,2] Essential elements in the system are a classification scheme for musculoskeletal pain that is sensitive to mechanical loading strategies and that attempts to expose this mechanical responsiveness through thorough history taking and repeated movements. This evaluation is based on symptomatic responses, such as centralization or the reduction of pain, as well as on mechanical responses, such as changes in function or range of movement. This allows therapists to offer their patients another essential element of the system, a rational and logical basis for home management.

In these days of evidence-based practice, it is vital that physical therapy establishes the reliability of examination techniques and the efficacy of treatment interventions. This chapter has sought also to present some of the available evidence concerning various aspects of the McKenzie approach. As a management system for musculoskeletal care, mechanical diagnosis and therapy have been exposed to a reasonable degree of research. Certain elements of the approach, such as the reliability of recognizing symptomatic responses and the use of centralization as a prognostic indicator, are reasonably well supported in the literature. The active, patient-centered management strategy, which is at the heart of the McKenzie approach, is validated by efficacy trials, the natural history of spinal problems, the response of musculoskeletal tissues to injury, and the biopsychosocial model of pain; however, further randomized controlled trials of good quality need to be conducted to confirm that this is indeed so.

Training in the McKenzie approach is essential to use the method properly. Detail beyond the scope of this chapter can be gained by course attendance and further reading.[1,2] However, a prerequisite for a detailed understanding is a grasp of the concepts presented in this chapter, which are the foundation for the approach.

References

1. McKenzie RA: *The lumbar spine: mechanical diagnosis and therapy*, Waikanae, New Zealand, 1981, Spinal Publications.
2. McKenzie RA: *The cervical and thoracic spine: mechanical diagnosis and therapy*, Waikanae, New Zealand, 1990, Spinal Publications.
3. Ponte DJ, Jensen GJ, Kent BE: A preliminary report on the use of the McKenzie protocol versus Williams protocol in the treatment of low back pain, *J Orthop Sports Phys Ther* 6:130, 1984.
4. Nwuga G, Nwuga V: Relative therapeutic efficacy of the Williams and McKenzie protocols in back pain management, *Physiother Pract* 4:99, 1985.
5. Kopp JR, Alexander AH, Turocy RH et al: The use of lumbar extension in the evaluation and treatment of patients with acute herniated nucleus pulposus, *Clin Orthop Rel Res* 202:211, 1986.
6. McKinney LA: Early mobilisation and outcome in acute sprains of the neck, *Br Med J* 299:1006, 1989.
7. McKinney LA, Dornan JO, Ryan M: The role of physiotherapy in the management of acute neck sprains following road-traffic accidents, *Arch Emergency Med* 6:27, 1989.
8. Alexander AH, Jones AM, Rosenbaum DH: Nonoperative management of herniated nucleus pulposus: patient selection by the extension sign: long-term follow-up, *Orthop Trans* 15:674, 1991.
9. Stankovic R, Johnell O: Conservative treatment of acute low-back pain: a prospective randomised trial—McKenzie method of treatment versus patient education in "mini back school," *Spine* 15:120, 1990.
10. Stankovic R, Johnell O: Conservative treatment of acute low-back pain: a 5-year follow-up study of two methods of treatment, *Spine* 20:469, 1995.
11. Cherkin DC, Deyo RA, Battie M et al: A comparison of physical therapy, chiropractic manipulation, and provision of an educational booklet for the treatment of patients with low back pain, *New Eng J Med* 339:1021, 1998.

12. Delitto A, Cibulka MT, Erhard RE et al: Evidence for use of an extension-mobilization category in acute low back syndrome: a prescriptive validation pilot study, *Phys Ther* 73:216, 1993.
13. Donelson R, Silva G, Murphy K: Centralization phenomenon: its usefulness in evaluating and treating referred pain, *Spine* 15:211, 1990.
14. Donelson R, Grant W, Kamps C, Medcalf R: Pain response to sagittal end-range spinal motion: a prospective, randomised, multicentered trial, *Spine* 16:S206, 1991.
15. Williams MM, Hawley JA, McKenzie RA, van Wijmen PM: A comparison of the effects of two sitting postures on back and referred pain, *Spine* 16:1185, 1991.
16. Abdulwahab SS, Sabbahi M: Neck retractions, cervical root decompression, and radicular pain, *J Orthop Sports Phys Ther* 30:4, 2000.
17. Long AL: The centralization phenomenon: its usefulness as a predictor of outcome in conservative treatment of chronic low back pain, *Spine* 20:2513, 1995.
18. Donelson R, Aprill C, Medcalf R, Grant W: A prospective study of centralization of lumbar and referred pain: a predictor of symptomatic discs and anular competence, *Spine* 22:1115, 1997.
19. Sufka A, Hauger B, Trenary M et al: Centralization of low back pain and perceived functional outcome, J Orthop Sports Phys Ther 27:205, 1998.
20. Werneke M, Hart DL, Cook D: A descriptive study of the centralization phenomenon: a prospective analysis, *Spine* 24:676, 1999.
21. Belanger AY, Despres MC, Goulet H, Trottier F: The McKenzie approach: how many clinical trials support its effectiveness? WCPT 11th International Congress Conference Proceedings, London, July 28-August 2, 1991.
22. Rebbeck T: The efficacy of the McKenzie regimen: a meta-analysis of clinical trials. Proceedings of 10th Biennial Conference of Manipulative Physiotherapists Association of Australia, Melbourne, Australia, Nov 26-29, 1997.
23. Faas A: Exercises: which ones are worth trying, for which patients, and when? *Spine* 21:2874, 1996.
24. Maher C, Latimer J, Refshauge K: Prescription of activity for low back pain: what works? *Aust J Physio* 45:121, 1999.
25. Danish Institute for Health Technology Assessment: Low-back pain: frequency, management and prevention from an HTA perspective, Danish Health Technology Assessment 1(1), Copenhagen, 1999.
26. Friedenberg ZB, Miller WT: Degenerative disc disease of the cervical spine: a comparative study of asymptomatic and symptomatic patients, *JBJS* 45A:1171, 1963.
27. Gore DR, Sepic SB, Gardner GM: Roentgenographic findings of the cervical spine in asymptomatic people, *Spine* 11:521, 1986.
28. Awwad EE, Martin DS, Smith KR, Baker BK: Asymptomatic versus symptomatic herniated thoracic discs: their frequency and characteristics as detected by computed tomography after myelography, *Neurosurgery* 28:180, 1991.
29. Teresi LM, Lufkin RB, Reicher MA et al: Asymptomatic degenerative disk disease and spondylosis of the cervical spine: MR imaging, *Radiology* 164:83, 1987.
30. Spitzer WO, LeBlanc FE, Dupuis M et al: Scientific approach to the assessment and management of activity-related spinal disorders: a monograph for clinicians—report of the Quebec Task Force on Spinal Disorders, *Spine* 12:S1, 1987.
31. Bigos S, Bowyer O, Braen G et al: *Acute low back problems in adults*, clinical practice guideline No. 14, AHCPR Publ No 95-0642, Rockville, Md, 1994, Agency for Health Care Policy and Research, Public Health Service.
32. Clinical Standards Advisory Group: *Back pain*, London, 1994, HMSO.
33. Bogduk N: The anatomy and physiology of nociception. In Crosbie J, McConnell J, editors: *Key issues in musculoskeletal physiotherapy*, Oxford, England, 1993, Butterworth-Heinemann.
34. Grimmer K: The relationship between cervical resting posture and neck pain, *Physiotherapy* 82:45, 1996.

35. Refshauge K, Bolst L, Goodsell M: The relationship between cervicothoracic posture and the presence of pain, *J Manual Manip Ther* 3:21, 1995.
36. Griegel-Morris P, Larson K, Mueller-Klaus K, Oatis CA: Incidence of common postural abnormalities in the cervical, shoulder, and thoracic regions and their association with pain in two age groups of healthy subjects, *Phys Ther* 72:425, 1992.
37. Watson DH: Cervical headache: an investigation of natural head posture and upper cervical flexor muscle performance. In Boyling JD, Palastanga N, editors: *Grieve's modern manual therapy*, ed 2, Edinburgh, 1994, Churchill Livingstone.
38. Harms-Ringdahl K: On assessment of shoulder exercise and load-elicited pain in the cervical spine: biomechanical analysis of load-EMG methodological studies of pain provoked by extreme position, *Scand J Rehab Med* S14:1, 1986.
39. Gooch L, Lee HB, Twomey LT: In vivo creep of the cervical spine. Proceedings of the 7th Biennial Conference of the Manipulative Physiotherapists Association of Australia, Blue Mountains, New South Wales, November 27-30, 1991.
40. Evans P: The healing process at cellular level: a review, *Physiotherapy* 66:256, 1980.
41. Hardy MA: The biology of scar formation, *Phys Ther* 69:1014, 1989.
42. Hunter G: Specific soft tissue mobilization in the treatment of soft tissue lesions. *Physiotherapy* 80:15, 1994.
43. McCarthy C, Cushnaghan J, Dieppe P: Osteoarthritis. In Wall PD, Melzack R, editors: *Textbook of pain*, ed 3, Edinburgh, 1994, Churchill Livingstone.
44. Robinson M: *The McKenzie method of spinal pain management.* In Boyling JD, Palastanga N, editors: Grieve's modern manual therapy, ed 2, Edinburgh, 1994, Churchill Livingstone.
45. Bogduk N, Windsor M, Inglis A: The innervation of the cervical intervertebral discs, *Spine* 13:2, 1988.
46. Mendel T, Wink CS, Zimny ML: Neural elements in human cervical intervertebral discs, *Spine* 17:132, 1992.
47. Cloward RB: Cervical discography: a contribution to the etiology and mechanism of neck, shoulder and arm pain, *Ann Surg* 150:1052, 1959.
48. Schellhas KP, Smith MD, Gundry CR, Pollei SR: Cervical discogenic pain: prospective correlation of MRI and discography in asymptomatic subjects and pain sufferers, *Spine* 21:300, 1996.
49. Cloward RB: Cervical discography: technique, indications, and use in diagnosis of ruptured cervical discs, *Am J Roentgenol* 79:563, 1958.
50. Roth DA: Cervical analgesic discography: a new test for the definitive diagnosis of the painful-disk syndrome, *JAMA* 235:1713, 1976.
51. Whitecloud TS, Seago RA: Cervical discogenic syndrome: results of operative intervention in patients with positive discography, *Spine* 12:313, 1987.
52. Parfenchuck TA, Janssen ME: A correlation of cervical MRI and discography/CT discograms, *Spine* 19:2819, 1994.
53. Kikuchi S, Macnab I, Moreau P: Localization of the level of symptomatic cervical disc degeneration, *JBJS* 63B:272, 1981.
54. Smith GW: The normal cervical discogram with clinical observations, *Am J Roentgenol* 81:1006, 1959.
55. Stuck RM: Cervical discography, *Am J Roentgenol* 86:975, 1961.
56. Bogduk N: Point of view, *Spine* 19:2824, 1994.
57. Taylor JR, Twomey LT: Functional and applied anatomy of the cervical spine. In Grant R, editor: *Physical therapy of the cervical and thoracic spine*, ed 2, New York, 1994, Churchill Livingstone.
58. Mercer SR, Jull GA: Morphology of the cervical intervertebral disc: implications for McKenzie's model of the disc derangement syndrome, *Manual Ther* 2:76, 1996.
59. Mercer S, Bogduk N: The ligaments and anulus fibrosus of human adult cervical intervertebral discs, *Spine* 24:619, 1999.
60. Bland JH, Boushey DR: Anatomy and physiology of the cervical spine, *Semin Arthritis Rheum* 20:1, 1990.

61. Hirsch C, Schajowicz F, Galante J: Structural changes in the cervical spine: a study on autopsy specimens in different age groups, *Acta Orth Scand* S109:1, 1967.
62. Bush K, Chaudhuri R, Hillier S, Penny J: The pathomorphologic changes that accompany the resolution of cervical radiculopathy, *Spine* 22:183, 1997.
63. Maigne JY, Deligne L: Computed tomographic follow-up study of 21 cases of nonoperatively treated cervical intervertebral soft disc herniation, *Spine* 19:189, 1994.
64. Mochida K, Komori H, Okawa A et al: Regression of cervical disc herniation observed on magnetic resonance imaging, *Spine* 23:990, 1998.
65. Perneczky G, Bock FW, Neuhold A, Stiskal M: Diagnosis of cervical disc disease: MRI versus cervical myelography, *Acta Neurochir* 116:44, 1992.
66. Vassilouthis J, Kalovithouris A, Papandreou A, Tegos S: The symptomatic incompetent cervical intervertebral disc, *Neurosurgery* 25:232, 1989.
67. Isu T, Iwasaki Y, Miyasaka K et al: A reappraisal of the diagnosis in cervical disc disease: the posterior longitudinal ligament perforated or not, *Neuroradiology* 28:215, 1986.
68. Manabe S, Tateishi A: Epidural migration of extruded cervical disc and its surgical treatment, *Spine* 11:873, 1986.
69. O'Laoire SA, Thomas DGT: Spinal cord compression due to prolapse of cervical intervertebral disc (herniation of nucleus pulposus), *J Neurosurg* 59:847, 1983.
70. Nakajima M, Hirayama K: Midcervical central cord syndrome: numb and clumsy hands due to midline cervical disc protrusion at the C3-4 intervertebral level, *J Neurol Neurosurg Psych* 58:607, 1995.
71. Young S, O'Laoire S: Cervical disc prolapse in the elderly: an easily overlooked, reversible cause of spinal cord compression, *Br J Neurosurg* 1:93, 1987.
72. Kokubun S, Sakurai M, Tanaka Y: Cartilaginous endplate in cervical disc herniation, *Spine* 21:190, 1996.
73. Aprill C, Bogduk N: The prevalence of cervical zygapophyseal joint pain: a first approximation, *Spine* 17:744, 1992.
74. Bogduk N, Aprill C: On the nature of neck pain, discography, and cervical zygapophysial joint blocks, *Pain* 54:213, 1993.
75. Dwyer A, Aprill C, Bogduk N: Cervical zygapophyseal joint pain patterns. I. A study in normal volunteers, *Spine* 15:453, 1990.
76. Aprill C, Dwyer A, Bogduk N: Cervical zygapophyseal joint pain patterns. II. A clinical examination, *Spine* 15:458, 1990.
77. Karas R, McIntosh G, Hall H et al: The relationship between nonorganic signs and centralization of symptoms in the prediction of return to work for patients with low back pain, *Phys Ther* 77:354, 1997.
78. Donelson R, Grant W, Kamps C, Richman P: *Cervical and referred pain response to repeated end-range testing: a prospective, randomized trial*, New York, 1997, North American Spine Society.
79. Ordway NR, Seymour RJ, Donelson RG et al: Cervical flexion, extension, protrusion, and retraction: a radiographic segmental analysis, *Spine* 24:240, 1999.
80. McKenzie RA: A perspective on manipulative therapy, *Physiotherapy* 75:440, 1989.
81. Burton AK, Tillotson KM, Main CJ, Hollis S: Psychosocial predictors of outcome in acute and subchronic low back trouble, *Spine* 20:722, 1995.
82. Jensen MP, Turner JA, Romano JM, Karoly P: Coping with chronic pain: a critical review of the literature, *Pain* 47:249, 1991.
83. Klenerman L, Slade PD, Stanley IM et al: The prediction of chronicity in patients with an acute attack of low back pain in a general practice setting, *Spine* 20:478, 1995.
84. Philips HC, Grant L, Berkowitz J: The prevention of chronic pain and disability: a preliminary investigation, *Behav Res Ther* 29:443, 1991.
85. Kilby J, Stigant M, Roberts A: The reliability of back pain assessment by physiotherapists, using a 'McKenzie algorithm,' *Physiotherapy* 76:579, 1990.
86. Fritz JM, Delitto A, Vignovic M, Busse RG: Interrater reliability of judgments of the centralization phenomenon and status change during movement testing in patients with low back pain, *Arch Phys Med Rehabil* 81:57, 2000.

87. McCombe PF, Fairbank JCT, Cockersole BC, Pynsent PB: Reproducibility of physical signs in low-back pain, *Spine* 14:908, 1989.
88. Strender LE, Sjoblom A, Sundell K et al: Interexaminer reliability in physical examination of patients with low back pain, *Spine* 22:814, 1997.
89. Donahue MS, Riddle DL, Sullivan MS: Intertester reliability of a modified version of McKenzie's lateral shift assessment obtained on patients with low back pain, *Phys Ther* 76:706, 1996.
90. Spratt KF, Lehmann TR, Weinstein JN, Sayre HA: A new approach to the low-back physical examination: behavioral assessment of mechanical signs, *Spine* 15:96, 1990.
91. McKenzie AM, Taylor NF: Can physiotherapists locate lumbar spinal levels by palpation? *Physiotherapy* 83:235, 1997.
92. Billis EV, Foster NE, Wright CC: Inter-tester and intra-tester reliability of three groups of physiotherapists in locating spinal levels by palpation, *Physiotherapy* 85:375, 1999.
93. Binkley J, Stratford PW, Gill C: Interrater reliability of lumbar accessory motion mobility testing, *Phys Ther* 75:786, 1995.
94. Mootz AD, Keating JC, Kontz HP et al: Intra- and interobserver reliability of passive motion palpation of the lumbar spine, *J Manip Physiol Ther* 12:440, 1989.
95. Gonnella C, Paris SV, Kutner M: Reliability in evaluating passive intervertebral motion, *Phys Ther* 62:436, 1982.
96. Altman DG: *Practical statistics for medical research*, London, 1991, Chapman & Hall.
97. Cote P, Cassidy JD, Carroll L: The Saskatchewan health and back pain survey: the prevalence of neck pain and related disability in Saskatchewan adults, *Spine* 23:1689, 1998.
98. Leclerc A, Niedhammer I, Landre MF et al: One-year predictive factors for various aspects of neck disorders, *Spine* 24:1455, 1999.
99. Gore DR, Sepic SB, Gardner GM, Murray MP: Neck pain: a long-term follow-up of 205 patients, *Spine* 12:1, 1987.
100. Akeson WH, Amiel D, Abel MF et al: Effects of immobilization on joints, *Clin Orthop Rel Res* 219:28, 1987.
101. Bland JH: Mechanisms of adaptation in the joint. In Crosbie J, McConnell J, editors: *Key issues in musculoskeletal physiotherapy*, Oxford, England, 1993, Butterworth-Heinemann.
102. Akeson WH, Amiel D, Woo SLY et al: Concepts of soft tissue homeostasis and healing. In Mayer T, Mooney V, Gatchel R, editors: *Contemporary conservative care for painful spinal disorders*, Philadelphia, 1991, Lea & Febiger.
103. Frank C, Akeson WH, Woo SLY et al: Physiology and therapeutic value of passive joint motion, *Clin Orthop Rel Res* 185:113, 1984.
104. Allan DB, Waddell G: An historical perspective on low back pain and disability, *Acta Orth Scand* 60:S234, 1989.
105. Waddell G, Feder G, Lewis M: Systematic reviews of bed rest and advice to stay active for acute low back pain, *Br J General Pract* 47:647, 1997.
106. Gam AN, Johannsen F: Ultrasound therapy in musculoskeletal disorders: a meta-analysis, *Pain* 63:85, 1995.
107. van der Windt DAWM, van der Heijden GJMG, van den Berg SGM et al: Ultrasound therapy for musculoskeletal disorders: a systematic review, *Pain* 81:257, 1999.
108. Nyanzi CS, Langridge J, Heyworth JRC, Mani R: Randomised controlled study of ultrasound therapy in the management of acute lateral ligament sprains of the ankle joint, *Clin Rehab* 13:16, 1999.
109. van der Heijden GJMG, Leffers P, Wolters PJMC et al: No effect of bipolar interferential electrotherapy and pulsed ultrasound for soft tissue shoulder disorders: a randomised controlled trial, *Ann Rheum Dis* 58:530, 1999.
110. Jordan A, Bendix T, Nielsen H et al: Intensive training, physiotherapy, or manipulation for patients with chronic neck pain, *Spine* 23:311, 1998.
111. Randlov A, Ostergaard M, Manniche C et al: Intensive dynamic training for females with chronic neck/shoulder pain: a randomized controlled trial, *Clin Rehab* 12:200, 1998.
112. Saal JS, Saal JA, Yurth EF: Nonoperative management of herniated cervical intervertebral disc with radiculopathy, *Spine* 21:1877, 1996.

113. Lunsford LD, Bissonette DJ, Jannetta PJ et al: Anterior surgery for cervical disc disease. I. Treatment of lateral cervical disc herniation in 253 cases, *J Neurosurg* 53:1, 1980.
114. Lunsford LD, Bissonette DJ, Zorub DS: Anterior surgery for cervical disc disease. II. Treatment of cervical spondylotic myelopathy in 32 cases, *J Neurosurg* 53:12, 1980.
115. Epstein JA, Epstein BS, Lavine LS et al: Cervical myeloradiculopathy caused by arthrotic hypertrophy of the posterior facets and laminae, *J Neurosurg* 49:387, 1978.
116. Gore DR, Sepic SB: Anterior cervical fusion for degenerated or protruded discs: a review of 146 patients, *Spine* 9:667, 1984.
117. Mosdal C: Cervical osteochondrosis and disc herniation: eighteen years use of interbody fusion by Cloward's technique in 755 cases, *Acta Neurochir* 70:207, 1984.
118. Odom GL, Finney W, Woodhall B: Cervical disc lesions, *JAMA* 166:23, 1958.

CHAPTER

19 Neck and Upper Extremity Pain in the Workplace

Barbara McPhee and
David R. Worth

Musculoskeletal complaints are ubiquitous; almost everyone experiences symptoms of these conditions at some time in their lives, with the likelihood of occurrence increasing with age. The population at large perceives these conditions as a normal part of life, and this has led to a tendency to consider them as inevitable rather than potentially preventable.

Musculoskeletal disorders arising in the workplace are proving to be a particularly perplexing problem because they are poorly understood and research into their nature, causes, and prevention is difficult and inadequate. Although designed to do otherwise, workers' compensation and health care systems, interacting with personal and social factors, may encourage some workers to continue to receive disability payments and discourage an early return to work after injury. As a result, it is increasingly recognized in many industrialized countries that musculoskeletal disorders are costing industry and the community dearly, both in human and financial terms.

In industrialized countries, low back pain is estimated to account for more than 50% of the total cost of work-related musculoskeletal disorders, amounting to many billions of dollars annually, and may represent more than 50% of total injury costs.[1] In the mid-1980s occupational back pain was estimated to represent over 20% of all reported cases of work-related disability in the United States, accounting for 32% of compensation payments at a sum amounting to over $11.1 billion, and the costs have continued to rise.[2]

These figures take no account of the personal and social disruption that back pain creates for those it affects, as well as for their immediate family and friends; nor do they account for the frustration and feelings of futility engendered in health care and social welfare professionals who try unsuccessfully to rehabilitate the worker for a return to work. It appears that in many industrialized countries, the traditional medical approach to the management of work-related back pain has failed in a significant percentage of cases. Unfortunately, less attention and money have been directed at preventing work-related back pain than seems justified by the cost of these disorders once they occur.

Increasing reports of pain, discomfort, and dysfunction of the neck and upper extremities associated with repetitive work in fixed or awkward postures indicate that these conditions are no less a problem than back pain in terms of diagnosis and management, although there is now anecdotal evidence that prevention programs for them can be very cost effective.[2] In the United States, the reporting of "disorders associated with repeated trauma" has more than tripled since 1984. Although this category includes chronic noise-induced hearing loss as well as disorders of the neck and upper extremities, it does not include back pain.[2] The same document points out that there were 147,000 new cases of these disorders reported in 1989, which accounted for 52% of all recordable occupational illnesses reported to the Occupational Safety and Health Administration (OSHA) in that year. In 1981 and 1984 noise-induced hearing loss and neck and upper extremity disorders accounted for 18% and 28%, respectively, of occupational illnesses. It has been suggested that their real incidence rate may be 130% higher than the reported rate.

In Norway in the mid-1980s, it was estimated that approximately 60% of sick leave was attributable to musculoskeletal disorders of all kinds.[3,4] These conditions also were responsible for a significant number of early retirements and work pensions. In 1983 statistics from the Swedish Occupational Injury Information System revealed that more than 50% of reported cases of occupational diseases were related to ergonomic factors in the workplace, such as physically heavy work, manual materials handling, repetitive work, and unsuitable work postures.[5] Employees exposed to these factors had up to 26 days more sick leave than other workers. Researchers have noted that repetitive jobs with unsuitable work postures have replaced more varied tasks, and that the prevalence of symptoms in the neck and shoulders seems to be increasing.[5]

HISTORY

EARLY RESEARCH

Ramazzini,[6] in 1713, described disorders in craftsmen, tradesmen, scribes, and notaries that resembled musculoskeletal complaints of today. Apart from Ramazzini's observations, comparatively little was published on work-related musculoskeletal disorders before the 1970s. One notable exception to this was the literature generated by the perplexing problem of craft palsies or occupational cramp.[7] In 1959 Hunter[8] listed 49 different occupational groups in which the hands could be affected by such cramps. The causes of these conditions are not well understood, and although they seem less prevalent now, they undoubtedly still exist.

From the 1920s to the 1960s, papers were published describing the clinical aspects of work-related musculoskeletal disorders of the upper limb and shoulder girdle, with authors speculating on their causes.[9-15] The work factors listed as the probable causes of the conditions described were speed and intensity of muscle effort, persistent strain, overuse of muscles, unaccustomed work often occurring after a change of job or equipment or on returning from a vacation, and trauma. One researcher suggested that the conditions appeared to increase in frequency during periods of economic stress, such as during the Great Depression. The medical conditions were described with care, but their prevention in the workplace seemed to have been secondary to their identification and treatment. By the middle of the twentieth century, musculotendinous injuries, notably tenosynovitis and peritendinitis, were recognized as being induced by certain types of work in workers' compensation legislation in most industrialized countries.

Gradually, attempts were made to identify the disorders more precisely, and suggestions were made for their prevention, particularly in relation to the growing and costly problem of low back pain. In 1970 van Wely[16] reported that a team of health and safety professionals demonstrated that they could predict, with reasonable accuracy, which tasks and work postures would lead to symptoms in operators and what parts of the worker's body would be affected. Van Wely also described how these disorders might have been prevented, emphasizing two approaches: the ergonomic design of tools, furniture, and equipment and the thorough training of workers in correct postures and work techniques. These observations and recommendations were a turning point in the study and prevention of work-related musculoskeletal disorders.

In 1976 Herberts and Kadefors[17] in Sweden demonstrated fatigue electromyographically in the shoulder muscles of welders, thereby supporting the belief that fatigue was an important factor in the etiology of the shoulder pain commonly experienced by older welders. An earlier electromyographic (EMG) study[18] showed that excessive loads were being placed on the shoulder and arm muscles of workers using pneumatic hammers and bolt guns. It was tempting to assume that such loads, over a period of time, could lead to early degenerative changes in the musculoskeletal structures involved.

In Japan the study of a wide range of work-related disorders of the neck and upper extremity, known in that country as *occupational cervicobrachial disorders (OCDs)*, began in the late 1960s in groups as diverse as cash-register operators, industrial workers, film rollers, crèche attendants, nurses, keyboard operators, telephone operators, and clerks writing with ballpoint pens.[19-26] Japanese research has formed the basis of many of the descriptive studies of work-related disorders in other countries. Maeda[27] was the first to develop a system of collecting subjective data on symptoms of OCD using body charts. Maeda, Horiguchi, and Hosokawa[28] also extensively researched various factors associated with the signs and symptoms of OCD. Much of their approach and progress in identifying factors associated with the development of OCD was made possible by the early work of the Japan Association of Industrial Health. It defined *OCD* and outlined causative factors, clinical features, and stages of such disorders and the health services required to control them.

Awareness of work-related musculoskeletal disorders in Australia came with the work of Perrott.[29] Using a biomechanical model of injury and its prevention, he described how unnecessary movement, shear strain, torsion, and muscle imbalance could be minimized.

Peres,[30] also in Australia, described injuries resulting from chronic fatigue resulting from intense effort, monotony, and the lack of variety of work. He emphasized the detrimental effects of a static muscle load resulting from poor posture and recommended a preventive strategy based on the redesign of work practices, early reporting of symptoms, redeployment, and task alternation. Peres recognized that most cases of injury from process work occurred in women and suggested that this was the result of their weaker musculature and the greater number of women engaged in process work. However, he pointed out that men were not immune to such injury and described overuse conditions in male canecutters, metal workers, milkers, and carpenters.

Much of the pioneering work in Australia on the association between work postures, repetitive manual work, and symptoms of neck, arm, trunk, and leg discomfort was done by Ferguson.[7,31-35] Asked to investigate an outbreak of unspecified upper limb injuries in 77 women working in an electronics factory, Ferguson analyzed injury records, examined the subjects, and undertook task analysis. He found that the injuries fell into two broad groups: well-defined clinical syndromes, such as supraspinatus tendonitis and tennis elbow and ill-defined symptom complexes. The latter group comprised the majority of cases seen, yet this was the first time such injuries had been reported in the literature in Australia.

Interestingly, Ferguson described the conditions in his subjects and postulated the causes for them in much the same way as had the Japanese researchers, although there was no contact between the two groups at that time. Ferguson broadened the view that these injuries were cases of tenosynovitis and peritendinitis crepitans to include a wide variety of musculotendinous injuries in the arm, which he called *repetition injuries.* Later the term *strain* was added by another chronicler of these disorders in Australia,[36] and the term *repetition strain injury (RSI)* replaced tenosynovitis as the umbrella term used for a range of neck and upper limb disorders believed to be associated with work.

In further work Ferguson examined personality, social, and work organization factors and associated medical conditions in relation to the etiology of the disorders he was investigating, as well as the intervention and prevention procedures for them.[33-35] In a study of telephone operators,[34] it was concluded that the frequent complaints of discomfort, aching, and other symptoms were caused by static loads on joints and muscles resulting from the fixed forward bending postures determined by the nature and design of the visual, auditory, and manipulative tasks of these peoples' work.

Ferguson drew attention to the long recovery periods in many cases of RSI, postulating a number of reasons for this, but reached no firm conclusions. However, he felt that malingering was unlikely in these cases, because most workers exhibited a desire to return to work for financial reasons. He took a broad view of the prevention of RSI, suggesting that social and work organization as well as biomechanical factors were important. He stressed the need for the adequate investigation of injuries and for epidemiological studies and pointed out that musculoskeletal injuries were very costly whether or not they were responsible for lost time.

RECENT RESEARCH

For the past 20 years the increasing number of complaints of disorders of the neck and upper extremities being reported by workers in an increasing range of industries around the world has prompted a more systematic approach to research. It is now well accepted that repetitive work with the hands or the feet can lead to these complaints. The use of high forces and the need for fixed postures compound the effects on the workers.

Two groups of disorders have emerged: the more clearly defined and diagnosable conditions, most particularly of the elbow, lower arm, and hand, which are commonly associated with heavy, repetitive work with the hands, and the less well defined shoulder and neck disorders seen in workers who undertake light repetitive work in fixed postures, such as computer operators, as well as those who do heavy work.

Repetitive manual activities required continuous stabilizing around the shoulder girdle by muscles such as the trapezius. In cases in which this load is increased by the need to use force or to sit fixed in one position for long periods, the load and rate of fatigue are increased manyfold. With an increased variety of movements within a job, the effects of muscle fatigue can be substantially diminished; the less variety, the greater the risks of fatigue, discomfort, pain, and injury.

The jobs listed in the following section are manually repetitive for a large percentage of the working day and are likely to load the musculature of the upper limbs, upper trunk, and neck to a degree that requires frequent rest breaks to enable recovery and prevent premature fatigue. In some jobs the taking of rest breaks can occur routinely within the work cycle; in others such breaks may have to be imposed through a reorganization of work. Such breaks are necessary to offset fatigue. When they do not occur (often coinciding with increased workloads and an increasing pace of work that require an increased frequency and length of breaks), workers will begin to experience symptoms of fatigue that may eventually lead to injury in the more susceptible.

WORK FACTORS

Substantial evidence now indicates that various risk factors, present in different forms and different combinations in many jobs, do lead to higher than expected frequencies of neck and upper extremity disorders. The untrained observer can deduce that jobs involving heavier work such as press operations, sewing machining, packaging, meat and poultry processing, and assembling are strenuous and potentially harmful even for the capable and skilled individual.

The difficulties of so-called light work involving continuous, high-speed, repetitive hand and finger movements, often in fixed and awkward postures, are not as obvious as those of heavier jobs. However, in contrast to the case for much of the repetitive and physically demanding work in industry, there has been an exponential increase in the numbers of these "light" jobs and in the percentage of workers undertaking them. This in itself should be ample justification for paying more attention to the potential health hazards of such work. The causes of occupational musculoskeletal conditions arising from "light," white collar jobs are complex, and there may be a need to reclassify these conditions. They also appear to be less amenable to simple preventive strategies than the better-known, more traditionally identified conditions described in the orthopedic literature.

Among white collar workers, and particularly office workers performing keyboard-based tasks, it is likely that the increased prevalence of musculoskeletal disorders is the result of the following factors:

1. The rapid introduction of computer technology without due regard for how human operators will work within such systems
2. The concomitant, increasingly repetitive, and fixed nature of tasks that were formerly more varied in terms of postures and movements
3. Increasing awareness by workers of occupational health and safety issues, without the concomitant changes in attitude required by planners and managers to meet increasingly better standards of working conditions and services to workers

In Australia an unprecedented number of disorders of the upper limb and neck were reported in the office workforce in the mid-1980s.[37,38] Whereas there had been an endemic level of shoulder, arm, and hand disorders in the manufacturing, food processing, and garment-making industries before this time, there arose a growing number of white collar workers reporting symptoms from what had previously been considered light, relatively undemanding work. These complaints reached epidemic proportions in 1985 to 1986 and brought much attention to the previously unrecognized problems of the shoulder and neck region. Although there was much speculation about the causes of these problems and debate about the nature of the resulting disorders, researchers in many parts of the world are only now reaching plausible hypotheses and explanations for the occurrence of these phenomena. An excellent review of research literature on shoulder and neck complaints, as well as guidelines for practitioners in managing these complaints, are recommended reading.[39,40]

Associations between work and an increased prevalence of neck and upper extremity disorders have been found in engineering assembly and process workers[18,31,41-53]; meat and poultry workers[54-61]; food packing[62]; sewing machinists and garment workers[63-66]; cashiers, accounting machine operators, and key punchers[67-72]; video data terminal (VDT) and data entry operators[73-86]; mail workers[87-88]; and musicians.[89] Most researchers now agree that physical loading of the musculoskeletal system, sometimes in conjunction with psychological stress, precipitates the initial symptoms of such disorders, which may resolve spontaneously, come and go intermittently without further development, or gradually or rapidly progress to the point at which the individual cannot continue to work under the same conditions. The progression of such disorders is likely to relate to the extent of physical loading they impose, both acutely and cumulatively; to the psychological factors such as personal or work stresses; and to the adequacy with which their causes and symptoms are addressed, both within and outside the workplace.

Individual Factors

Individuals exposed to hazards in occupational situations react differently to them. This also can be said of individuals' reactions to stressful and/or repetitive movements and prolonged fixed postures. An operation that is difficult and even damaging for one person may not constitute a risk for another. The higher the levels of physical stress, the greater will be the number who succumb to injury. Susceptibility to strain appears to be a continuum, with the highly susceptible at one end and the highly resilient at the other. If so, there is an argument for screening out susceptible individuals before permitting them to work at jobs known to cause symptoms; but this is not easy, nor is it usually acceptable. There must be some understanding of why some people are resilient and others are not.

Although there appears to be no strong recent evidence that personal (individual) factors might influence this resilience, writers of some of the earlier papers on work-related musculoskeletal injury did speculate that anatomical, physiological, and psychological factors were associated with the development of disorders of the neck and upper limbs. For instance, it was suggested that the anatomy of the wrist in some people might have a bearing on the way in which stresses are transmitted within and through it.[14] Physiologically, deficiencies in the peripheral circulation were considered by some investigators as being the direct cause of fatigue and subsequent strain,[90] whereas others considered muscle strength to be responsible for these effects.[19] Psychological factors such as personality, anxiety, and mood also have been implicated in the reduced capacity to withstand stress.[30,80,91]

However, much more evidence is needed in the area of personal factors before they can be used to determine which individuals may be at greater risk of developing musculoskeletal disorders as the result of their work. On the other hand, scientific evidence increasingly points to links between certain types of work and workplaces and to differences in individual methods of work[50,85] and the incidence of disorders of the neck and upper extremities. It seems that any individual has an increased risk of strain when new demands are made on the individual; the individual habitually works beyond his or her capacity; or personal, social, or environmental factors reduce the individual's tolerance to physical stress.

The relationship between physical workload and its effects on functional capacity and the development and severity of symptoms appears to be modified by temporal factors, such as the length of the working day, periods worked without breaks, and the percentage of the working day spent doing repetitive activities in fixed postures. In addition, personality, mood, the perception of load, work pressures, job satisfaction, and other personal factors may alter the individual's response to early signs of fatigue and discomfort. The following factors need to be considered in preventing these disorders[85]:

1. External load factors (task and workplace design and work organization) required by a task, including number of movements, static muscle work, force, work postures determined by equipment and furniture, and time worked without a break
2. Factors that influence load but that may vary between individuals, including work postures adopted, static muscle work used, unnecessary force used, number and duration of pauses taken, and speed and accuracy of movements
3. Factors that alter the individual's response to a particular load (workplace, individual, and social factors), including age; sex; physical capabilities; environmental factors such as vibration, cold, noise, and other contaminants; previous repetitive work and job experience; and psychosocial variables

CLASSIFICATION OF DISORDERS AND THEIR SIGNS AND SYMPTOMS

Three main groups of musculoskeletal or soft tissue disorders give rise to neck and upper extremity pain in workers. These are traumatic, degenerative, and abusive use disorders (Table 19-1).

Traumatic Disorders

Traumatic disorders, although not as common as degenerative or abusive use syndromes, constitute a group of disorders that, under Australian Workers' Compensation law,[92] may be regarded as work-induced injuries. These disorders are characterized by their causal relationship to a discrete traumatic incident. Such an incident may be unrelated to a work process and may occur at or on the way to or from the workplace. Typical examples are cervical spine injuries in "journey accidents" and soft-tissue injuries or fractures resulting from falls or other accidents during the work period.

It may be argued that these musculoskeletal injuries were not caused by the work process, but they are generally considered to be work related. They may result in a

Table 19-1 Classification of Disorders Associated with the Neck and Upper Extremity Pain in Workers

Traumatic	Degenerative	Abusive Use
Acute soft tissue injury	Intervertebral disc disease	Postural overload syndrome
Fracture	Cervical spondylosis	
Dislocation	Arthrosis	Overuse syndrome
Subluxation	Seronegative spondyloarthropathy	Environmental condition syndromes
Laceration		
Traumatic arthritis	Rheumatoid arthritis	
Traumatic bursitis	Inflammatory joint disease	
Reflex sympathetic dystrophy	Soft tissue disease	
Burns	Bony necrosis	

temporary or permanent, total or partial, painful disability for the worker. This may cause economic and other loss and hardship to both the worker and employer. Often, it is difficult for the traumatically injured worker to remain at work or to return to work after a substantial absence.

Box 19-1 provides an expanded list of commonly encountered traumatic disorders leading to neck and upper extremity pain in the workplace. It is not within the scope of this chapter to describe these traumatic disorders in detail. This has been adequately done in many orthopedic texts.[93-97] However, it is important to point out that acute soft tissue injuries of the cervical spine often have a devastating effect on the worker when he or she returns to work, despite an absence from work during which the final symptoms of such injuries may have resolved.

Once a return-to-work program has commenced, it is essential that care be taken to protect the worker's cervical spine from work-induced postural strain and trauma. This requires that management personnel, supervisors, line foremen, fellow workers, and health care professionals recognize that the worker has a physical disability. The worker who returns after having a serious injury and who has not for some time experienced the rigors of work is likely to suffer well-recognized symptoms. Adding work and production pressures to this person's daily activities puts the injured soft tissue at risk, and increased static and dynamic loading on ligaments and muscles may aggravate symptoms of the injury.

Degenerative Musculoskeletal Disorders

The group of disorders known as *degenerative musculoskeletal disorders* is typified by clinical, radiological, or EMG evidence of degenerative changes in the joints or soft tissues of the musculoskeletal system. Notwithstanding their not being work-induced disorders, they are often preexisting conditions, the symptoms of which may be precipitated or aggravated by incidents at work, and may predict the onset of a work-related injury. These conditions may lead to neck and upper extremity pain in workers.

The significant difference between the degenerative and the traumatic groups of musculoskeletal disorders is in the time and nature of their onset. The onset of a traumatic disorder is usually sudden and related to a specific incident, whereas the onset of a degenerative disorder is usually insidious and not incident related. Again, it is not within the scope of this chapter to discuss the management of these disorders. Degenerative disorders commonly related to neck and upper extremity pain in the workplace include the following:

Cervical spinal intervertebral disc lesions
Cervical spondylosis and related disorders
Cervical spinal zygapophyseal joint arthrosis
Thoracic outlet syndrome
Diseases of the joints (e.g., rheumatoid arthritis, ankylosing spondylitis)
Frozen shoulder
Tennis elbow, golfer's elbow, medial or lateral humeral epicondylitis
Olecranon bursitis
Olecranon-trochlear arthritis
Aseptic necrosis of the lunate bone
Arthrosis of the trapezio—first metacarpal joint
Compression syndromes (e.g., carpal tunnel syndrome)
Tenosynovitis (e.g., rheumatoid or de Quervain's stenosing tenosynovitis)
Trigger finger

Box 19-1

Commonly Seen Traumatic Disorders Leading to Neck and Upper Extremity Pain in the Workplace

Acute cervical spine soft tissue injuries

Fracture in the cervical and cervicothoracic spine

Cervical radiculopathy

Axillary nerve compression

Suprascapular nerve entrapment

Fracture and fracture dislocation in the upper limb and shoulder girdle

Glenohumeral instability

Shoulder bursitis

Acute tear of the rotator cuff mechanism of the shoulder joint

Shoulder impingement syndrome

Distal biceps or long head of biceps rupture

Triceps tendon rupture

Fracture at the elbow

Traumatic arthritis of the elbow

Traumatic bursitis at the elbow

Traumatic ulnar nerve neuritis at the elbow

Ulnar nerve entrapment at the elbow or wrist

Traumatic arthritis at the wrist

Ligamentous strain or rupture at the wrist

Ruptured or lacerated tendons of the wrist or hand

Trapeziometacarpal joint instability

Scapholunate dissociation

Scaphoid fracture

Pisiform fracture

Hook of hamate fracture

Distal radioulnar joint subluxation

Extensor carpi ulnaris subluxation

Injuries or degeneration of the triangular fibrocartilage complex

Tears at the lunotriquetral joint

Midcarpal instability

Volar plate injuries in the hand

Ligamentous and capsular injuries of the fingers

Sesamoiditis at the metacarpophalangeal joint of the thumb

Fingertip injuries

Reflex sympathetic dystrophy after trauma

Amputations and stump pain

Dupuytren's contracture
Ganglion
Osteoarthritis of the scaphotrapeziotrapezoid joints
Scapholunate advanced collapse
Kienböck's disease
Pisotriquetral arthritis
Radiocapitellar arthritis

Abusive Use Disorders

This group of disorders is noted for their lack of specific diagnosis. They present with widespread symptoms that include pain, paresthesias, loss of coordination and hand function, weakness of grip, intermittent swelling, and occasionally, apparent vascular disturbance. However, there are some specific conditions that may arise from abusive use of the upper limb, head, and neck, and they include the following:
Flexor or extensor carpi ulnaris tendonitis
Radial or posterior interosseous nerve entrapment
Triceps tendonitis
Ulnar neuritis
Pronator syndrome: anterior interosseous and pronator teres syndrome
Biceps tendonitis
Adverse neural tension
Vibration syndrome
Cold exposure syndrome

There are three major subgroups of abusive use disorders: (1) postural overload syndromes, (2) overuse syndrome, and (3) environmental condition syndromes. Environmental condition syndromes include vibration and cold exposure.

Postural Overload Syndromes. Postural overload syndromes arise from tasks done in postures that mechanically disadvantage the muscular system. Muscles involved in these syndromes may be grouped into three categories as follows:

1. Muscles primarily performing the tasks (prime movers)
2. Muscles synergistically contracting to facilitate the prime movers (synergists)
3. Muscles statically contracting to maintain body balance to permit the prime movers and synergists to act in the performance of the task (stabilizers)

The following example serves to demonstrate situations in which muscles in all three categories may act at a mechanical disadvantage. A keyboard operator who has not been taught correct keyboard techniques and posture is likely to approach the keys with the wrist kept at approximately 30 to 45 degrees of extension. In this position, lift-off occurs in the following sequence: (1) The extensor carpi ulnaris, extensor carpi radialis longus, and brevis muscles contract statically to maintain the wrist posture while the extensor digitorum communis extends the metacarpophalangeal joints; (2) at the same time, the flexor digitorum sublimis and profundus flex the proximal and distal interphalangeal joints; and (3) the fingers then strike the keys as a result of contraction of the interossei and lumbricals, which flex the metacarpophalangeal joints when the extensor digitorum communis relaxes. This is referred to as *handhammer function.*

The problem occurs when the prime mover for lift-off, the extensor digitorum communis, fails to relax sufficiently, or contract eccentrically, to permit efficient key striking. This is caused by the maintained posture of wrist extension producing inner-range static contraction of the extensor digitorum communis, which then acts as a synergist to the wrist extensors, thus failing to fully relax during key striking. The result is inner-range dynamic and static overload of the extensor digitorum communis as a prime mover for lift-off (dynamic) and a synergist to wrist extension (static).

Such long-term, inner-range postural overload leads to adaptive shortening of the extensor digitorum communis. If this keyboard operator also has a chronic head forward posture with an increased cervical and thoracic spinal curvature, spinal stability will be maintained by excessive static contraction of the long extensor muscles of the spine (stabilizers). These muscles contract in their outer range for long periods, resulting in symptomatic overload. Therefore the keyboard operator is likely to exhibit the following symptoms and signs:

Middorsal aching
Suprascapular pain
Aching of the upper cervical spine
Suboccipital pain
Headache
Pain radiating into the upper arm
Lateral epicondylar ache and pain
Posterior forearm pain
Hand pain
Loss of power grip strength
"Pins and needles" sensation in the suprascapular region and forearm
Loss of coordination and hand precision skills

The strategies for preventing these problems include maintenance of the normal curvatures of the thoracic and cervical spine and proper adjustment of the operator's chair and sitting posture. Detailed instruction in safe keyboard operation involves adjusting the keyboard and chair height relationships to permit lift-off and keystroke to occur within approximately 5 degrees of wrist flexion. The work environment must include office furniture that is adjustable and permits optimal posture.

Overuse Syndrome. As with postural overload syndromes, overuse syndrome also is clearly demarcated from traumatic and degenerative disorders because it is not yet known to present with any identifiable pathology reported in clinical or research medicine. It is listed under abusive use disorders in this discussion because its symptoms appear to correlate well with the performance of specific tasks.

Overuse syndrome has been defined as "established pain and tenderness in muscle and joint ligaments of the upper extremity, produced by hand-use-intensive activity for long periods and use which is clearly excessive for the individuals affected."[98] Overuse syndrome is not caused by repetitive use alone. It is associated with abusive use whereby the intensity of the work performed by a muscle, multiplied by the duration of this work, exceeds the capacity of the muscle. The intensity of the work, which is the product of the force of the load and the distance through which the load is lifted, is affected by the velocity of muscle contraction. The intensity of muscle work also is affected by the quality of the muscle contraction. In ballistic movements, agonist and antagonist muscle groups coordinate to accelerate or decelerate a particular segment of the upper extremity.

Although it is not the purpose of this chapter to discuss in detail the physiology of work, it is important to emphasize that the "ability of muscle fibers to maintain a high tension, and the individual's subjective feeling of fatigue, are highly dependent on the blood flow through the muscle."[99] Workers who must perform highly coordinated, high-velocity, intense muscular work over long periods are at risk of exceeding the preoxygenation capacity of the muscle group being used and therefore the capacity to persist in managing workloads. Muscles may then become painful.

Symptoms. The symptoms of overuse syndrome are local pain in muscles, ligaments, and joints; weakness of the affected limb; "pins and needles" or heaviness; and loss of responsiveness (e.g., the tendency to strike wrong keys). This may be a description of loss of coordination and proprioception.

Signs. The signs of overuse syndrome are tenderness in the muscles and particular structures, swelling over the affected muscle group, weakness of precision and power grip, and loss of coordination, particularly proprioception. Both postural overload and overuse syndromes are related to the nature of a work method and the physical and organizational environment in which the work is done. Therefore consideration of the interaction of biomechanical, physiological, and psychological effects are necessary to determine the efficiency with which work is performed.

Environmental Condition Syndromes. Exposure to vibration is a common problem when using power tools. If used for sufficiently long periods or at high levels, such tools may cause discomfort, reduced work efficiency, and musculoskeletal complaints. There is controversy about the methods used to reduce exposure to vibration, but some standards for such exposure, albeit inadequate, are available.

The physiological effects of vibration from a handheld tool may include tissue strain or compression, the severity of which depends on how the vibration is transmitted to the tissue and whether resonance or attenuation occurs.[100] The severity of the effects of hand-transmitted vibration as a component of work is influenced by the magnitude of the vibration (frequency × amplitude), the duration of exposure per working day, rest spells and breaks, the posture of the hands and arms (i.e., wrist, elbow, and shoulder joint angles), the direction of vibration through the arms, and any predisposing health factors.

Exposure of the hand and fingers to cold profoundly affects their strength, dexterity, and sensitivity. The grip forces required to hold hand tools are significantly higher at reduced hand temperatures. Occupations such as poultry processing or boning result in frequent contact with cold objects by the gloved hand.[97] Cooling factors include the ambient temperature (0° to 5° C), cold gloves and clothing, and direct contact with cold objects (0° to 2° C) that significantly reduces the skin temperature of the hands (0° to 5° C). The frequency and duration of cold exposure are key factors in an analysis directed toward preventing its effects on the hand.

SUMMARY

To clearly understand the etiology and consequently the management of work-related pain, a thorough understanding of the diagnostic criteria for accurately categorizing such pain is essential. For example, tenosynovitis may follow a crushing injury to the hand, may be associated with rheumatoid arthritis, or may be a consequence of postural overload syndrome. The management of primary tenosynovitis is simple and well documented and should not present a long-term problem. However, the prevention of aggravation and recurrence of this condition depends on its cause and the control of aggravating factors.

The categorization of discrete diagnoses of work-related injury into a collective group such as RSI,[101] OCD, or cumulative trauma disorder (CTD) can be misleading, and clearly is technically incorrect. It also has discouraged the correct and accurate diagnosis of these disorders and has made a complex set of signs and symptoms appear to be deceptively simple. The classification offered in this chapter (Table 19-1) is an attempt to solve a diagnostic dilemma, to broaden our overview, and to allow us to deal with these painful disorders a little more scientifically and effectively.

PREVENTION

Despite the problems in diagnosing work-related musculoskeletal disorders, their varying classification, and difficulties treating many of the work-related disorders of the neck and upper extremity, it is important to remember that many of these conditions are preventable. The complex interaction of work, personal, and social factors that may give rise to complaints related to the neck and upper extremities in workers means that ergonomics is an essential component of any program for preventing these problems.

Ergonomics considers the design of work and its organization, as well as the design of the workplace in relation to the capabilities and limitations of the worker. A range of freely available publications now deal specifically with the prevention of these disorders,[102-110] all of which outline different strategies for accomplishing this, including the extensive application of principles of ergonomics. Where unavoidable problems arise, appropriate case management should aim at minimizing the severity of a condition and returning the patient to work, with necessary modifications, as soon as possible.

The prevention of work-related musculoskeletal disorders can be considered under the three main headings of primary, secondary, and tertiary prevention, as follows:

Primary prevention. Aiming at eliminating or minimizing risks to health or well-being

Secondary prevention. Alleviating the symptoms of ill health or injury, minimizing residual disability, and eliminating or at least minimizing factors that may cause recurrence

Tertiary prevention. Rehabilitating patients with disabilities to the fullest possible function and modifying the workplace to accommodate any residual disability

The effective implementation and evaluation of measures for preventing musculoskeletal disorders in the workplace may require a multidisciplinary approach involving ergonomics, occupational health, epidemiology, engineering, administration, and management. A prevention program will require cooperation, organization, and commitment, most particularly from senior management. It may be expensive in the short term because of the need to purchase new equipment or rearrange the work and the workplace, and it may temporarily reduce production. Often there is a reluctance on the part of management to accept short-term costs and organizational upheaval for the long-term benefit of a prevention program. Nevertheless, such an approach may be necessary for the successful long-term control of work-related musculoskeletal disorders and their associated costs.

Ergonomic Analyses in the Workplace

To avoid mismatches between workers and their jobs, there must be some understanding of the demands of a particular kind of work and the capacity of each worker to meet those demands. Measurement of workload and its effects on individuals and groups is for physical therapists one of the more challenging aspects of the management of neck and upper extremity disorders. Measurement can be accomplished in the following areas: workplace measurement and assessment, including task analysis; workload measurement (individuals or groups); and symptom recording.

Workplace Measurement and Assessment, Including Task Analysis. Workplace measurement and assessment techniques measure or assess the adequacy of the workplace and ability of the required tasks to accommodate workers' physical and mental capabilities and limitations. Many well-known methods are described and discussed in a number of textbooks on ergonomics. Several are particularly useful for physical therapists.[109,111,112] A wide range of techniques is available, but each may need tailoring to local requirements and conditions. Some training in ergonomics for physical therapists is essential if they are to develop measurement methods that are valid, reliable, and usable.

Measurement of Workload. Again, many of the techniques for measuring workload are described in detail in the textbooks previously cited. They attempt in different ways to record and analyze loads on the body during work. Two better-known methods are *Posture Targeting* and *Ovako Working Postures Analyzing System* (OWAS).[111] Another method developed especially for the assessment of loads on the upper limbs is called *Rapid Upper Limb Assessment (RULA)*. This method is easy to use and is described in detail, along with worksheets and score cards, in McAtamney and Corlett's publication.[109]

Symptom Recording. Body charts are a practical method for collecting information about symptoms of neck and upper extremity disorders in the workplace. Although specific conditions of the neck and upper extremities have been identified as being associated with particular types of work, growing numbers of workers, especially those engaged in so-called light, highly repetitive work, such as VDT operators, are complaining of ill-defined symptom complexes, the causes of which are not yet fully determined. These conditions are seldom adequately defined or described; however, many may be manifestations of local muscle fatigue and overload of related structures. Others appear to result from postural overloading, particularly of the neck, and may involve referred symptoms. In the absence of specific diagnoses, the delineation of these conditions can be aided by the use of body charts that a worker or clinician may complete.

Body charts have enabled researchers and those concerned with control of musculoskeletal disorders in the workplace to gain a clearer picture of symptom patterns and their prevalence without having to categorize them as medical conditions. Furthermore, it has enabled a systematic approach to the prevention of such disorders by identifying occupational groups with a high prevalence of symptoms in the neck and upper extremities and by pinpointing elements of these groups' jobs that may be associated with symptom development.[85,113]

Functional Capacity Assessments

Mismatches often occur between the demands of a job and the worker's capacity to undertake the work safely. Therefore medical practitioners and physical therapists must understand in some detail the demands of various tasks (workload measurement or assessment) and the capabilities of individual workers to perform these tasks (assessment of functional capacity) and must appreciate that these capabilities are likely to change over time.

In cases in which particular work puts unreasonable demands on workers, it is vital that advice be given on how risks of injury can be reduced through better workplace layout or design, more adequate training, or more efficient work organization. Consideration will have to be given to modification of work to accommodate individuals with reduced physical capacity. As a last resort, it may be necessary to advise people who are physically unsuited for certain work against undertaking that work and suggest that they seek less demanding jobs.

Specific Task Training and Education in Ergonomics

Most jobs can be done in a variety of ways, and one way will usually be less stressful and fatiguing than others. It is important that the most efficient methods be identified for each job and that these methods be taught only to new employees and those learning a new job or using new equipment. Even with training, however, employees may slip into inefficient practices, and these should be monitored and corrected by on-the-job supervision.

For the development of correct work techniques and postures, together with training and on-the-job supervision, supervisors should be consulted to help define these factors. Wherever possible, training should be organized and run by a training officer or someone else skilled in teaching others. Education is an especially important aspect of ergonomics. If money, time, and expertise are used to produce an ergonomically sound workplace, then employees should understand why it has been so designed and how it can best be used.

Task Variation and Job Rotation

Task variation, or multiskilling, is highly desirable and can be achieved through job enlargement, which requires careful job and task design to enable a number of different types of activities to be incorporated into a single job description, or (less effectively) through job rotation. Job rotation is a ready way of spreading the load of particularly stressful jobs among a large group of employees, but it does have drawbacks. It works only in settings in which jobs are sufficiently different to provide physical and mental variety. Moreover, many employees do not like rotating for a number of reasons, even when it is in their best interests to do so. Furthermore, job rotation can mask the real causes of the problems created by a particular kind of work and may only prolong the period before such problems arise. Job rotation also means that employees have to learn more skills and therefore require more training and supervision. Consequently, rotation should be seen only as a temporary solution while engineering, work design, and organizational problems are being resolved. Job enlargement (enrichment) is a much more acceptable alternative for providing task variation but requires careful planning and longer training periods.

Work Rates

Human performance varies among individuals and over time. Work rates should therefore be realistic to accommodate the physical and psychological capacities of the slowest workers. This is particularly important in machine-paced work.

Minimizing Aggravating Factors

Organizational difficulties of various kinds can arise in any enterprise. Mechanical and technical breakdowns and inefficiencies can have a disruptive effect on employees and usually involve periods of extra workload to make up for lost production or output. As an example, instances of poor quality control may require reworking of a product or product component, thereby expending time that results in no additional productivity. Therefore machine and equipment adjustment and maintenance are most important to the smooth and efficient operation of any system. Other organizational factors, such as the need for overtime, shift work, and peak loading, as well as bonus payments and other incentive schemes, often require higher outputs than the employees of an organization can safely manage and should be avoided through the use of careful planning.

Pause Exercises

Pause exercises (pause gymnastics), originally a Scandinavian concept,[114] are gaining acceptance increasingly in other countries.[115] They are rhythmic, free or set movements performed during the working day to help alleviate the effects of fixed work postures and repetitive movements. They usually include a series of full-range movements, sometimes done to music, designed to meet the needs of particular working groups. Set movements should vary from time to time to avoid boredom and should be performed moderately slowly and carefully to ensure maximal benefit.

Because the nature of work varies a great deal from time to time and among different groups of people, pause exercise movements should be designed to take these factors into account. Performance of the exercises should be supervised initially and at regular intervals by a professional trained in anatomy and exercise physiology, such as a physical therapist. Such a person can ensure that movements are performed correctly and can identify individual difficulties so that they can be investigated and treated early. Pause exercises programs aim to do the following:

- Encourage changes of posture from those adopted for the majority of the work day
- Strengthen and stretch muscles that might be weak or tight
- Stimulate circulation and help reduce feelings of fatigue at the end of the working day

A comprehensive review of the safety and effectiveness of a range of exercise programs for VDT and office workers is recommended reading.[116]

Work Pauses

The importance of pauses during physical activity is widely acknowledged. Although there is little information about the actual benefits of work pauses, there is sufficient evidence to suggest that they are an essential part of certain tasks if unnecessary fatigue is to be avoided.[117,118] They can be self-regulated or fixed and supervised, but to be effective, their duration and frequency must be appropriate to the levels of activity and fatigue experienced by the persons using them. For example, more frequent, longer breaks may be required toward the end of a day or a week, and the system must be flexible to accommodate different circumstances. Individually regulated breaks are the most desirable, but workers often have to be encouraged to pause from work even when they are tired. They must be positively discouraged from accumulating breaks.

Pause exercises and regulated work pauses are only temporary solutions for alleviating the effects of fixed, repetitive, or demanding work. In the long term, work should be designed to allow variation in tasks and movements and to allow regular pauses throughout the day.

Evaluation of Prevention Programs

As mentioned previously, a number of publications produced by government agencies,[102-108] universities,[109] and journals[110] address the prevention, control, and management of neck and upper limb disorders. All deal with the identification of potentially harmful workloads, methods for measuring these workloads and assessing their impact, and control or prevention procedures suitable for different types of work. Nearly all of these publications recommend monitoring of the effectiveness of such prevention programs, although the criteria for monitoring are not discussed. Methods by which a formal evaluation of quite extensive programs might be undertaken have not been addressed at all in any of the publications, and this seems to be a glaring oversight. When so many resources and so much time can be devoted to controlling these disorders, it would seem important to build some sort of evaluation into a prevention program, if only to help sell it to increasingly cost-conscious managers.

Some attempts have been made to evaluate the outcome of programs for preventing neck and upper extremity disorders, the most notable of which was undertaken in Norway and included a cost-benefit analysis.[119] In 1975 an intervention study was initiated in a Norwegian electronics factory in response to an unusually high rate of sick leave in the preceding 2 years and increasing complaints of musculoskeletal disorders of the upper limb, neck, shoulder, and back.[120] This study attempted to discover the reasons for the increasing rates of complaints and to evaluate the impact of ergonomic changes undertaken at the factory from 1975 onward.

It proved more difficult to argue that the ergonomic changes led directly to a reduction in musculoskeletal disorders than to show that the former work situations at the factory contributed to the occurrence of the disorders. Nevertheless, there was evidence that the changes had a positive influence on health and were associated with decreasing complaints of symptoms. However, a more recent study of assembly workers in Sweden demonstrated the effectiveness of instruction in correct work techniques to new workers in reducing the number of days lost because of arm-neck-shoulder complaints.[51] This highlights an important area that has had little attention in the literature, namely, the beneficial effects of training and education of workers, supervisors, and managers in what they can do for themselves to control musculoskeletal disorders arising from work practices.

A group of investigators in the United States attempted with some degree of success to establish an intervention program in a manufacturing industry.[121] Although the statistical analyses were never reported, complaints of disorders appeared to decrease, whereas the productivity in some jobs increased significantly. The changes implemented by the program included organizational rearrangements, such as the introduction of job rotation in selected areas and the provision of gloves to some workers, and engineering controls, such as the introduction of rotatable jigs and suspended tool retractors and the redesign of components. Many of the researchers' recommendations were rejected as being not feasible, but some of the easier, less costly changes were made. In addition to this, some workers modified or redesigned tools that helped decrease injuries and increase productivity. Generally, the changes that proved most successful were those in which the front-line supervisor participated and acted on recommendations.

More recently, an American company reported in a commercial newsletter on a program that is applying the *OSHA Guidelines for Meatpacking Plants*[108] to a baking company. However, although it seems that the response to the program has been positive, no evaluation has been undertaken at this stage. A common feature of intervention programs such as this is occupational health professionals' interest and participation in them. In the program described, these professionals provided statistical and epidemiological surveillance of injuries and complaints, and thereby provided the mechanism by which the success of the program could be measured, however imprecisely.

The difficulties of measuring the effects of changes in ergonomics or of any preventive health care program in the workplace are not insurmountable, but it is impossible to eliminate the influence of other factors that may alter the way in which people work or perceive their work. In the case of musculoskeletal disorders, part of the problem is related to the "Hawthorne effect" (a change in performance of subjects merely because they are part of a study), part is related to the ubiquitous and ill-defined nature of the conditions being studied, and part is related to the numerous sources of bias and confounding variables that arise in the workplace. Nevertheless, as increasing numbers of work-related musculoskeletal disorders are reported, there is an urgent need to convincingly demonstrate that certain preventive measures are effective against these disorders.

REHABILITATION

The general concept of medical rehabilitation is of well-established, institutionalized care given by large, multidisciplinary centers that is usually associated with mainstream health care systems. Worker rehabilitation may be included in the services offered by these centers, but only when an injury or illness has become chronic. Specialist on-site worker rehabilitation centers that provide occupational health services and are funded by employers or centers that are funded privately or by the government and are located in nearby areas are now common in many countries. These centers cater to the particular needs of workers to enable them to return to work as early as possible and with a minimum of disability. This involves not only an understanding of occupationally related medical conditions and their treatment but also a consideration of workplace factors that may have led to a worker's condition and that may have to be modified before a return to work is possible. Such an approach requires liaison with managers and supervisors and a knowledge of the individual client's work and work process. Consequently, it is desirable for professionals working in occupational health services or worker rehabilitation centers to be trained in occupational health and safety.

In general terms, it may be estimated that a workforce of 300 or more full-time employees in a manufacturing company would justify the employment of a part-time physical therapist, visiting doctor, and full-time occupational health nurse, although this would vary according to the nature of the industry and its occupational health and safety programs. Worker rehabilitation can be considered as having two stages: therapeutic intervention and vocational rehabilitation.

THERAPEUTIC INTERVENTION

The treatment of many of the conditions listed in Box 19-1 has been detailed in textbooks of physical therapy and medicine and are not described here. Injuries at the worksite largely affect the musculoskeletal system and soft tissue and require attention as soon as possible after they occur. It is preferable that primary care for such injuries occurs at the workplace and in accordance with the statutory regulations of relevant legislation, such as occupational health and safety and workers' compensation acts.

An occupational health nurse is the most appropriate person to undertake immediate primary care; where this is not possible, it may be necessary to refer the worker to an appropriate health service. Workers in most countries are not compelled to attend the employer's chosen health service but instead may attend one of their own choice. This may be a general practitioner or family physician, hospital, community health center, or alternative practitioner such as a chiropractor or acupuncturist. Whatever the choice, it is preferable that the practitioner have some training and experience in occupational health and safety. Physical therapy, occupational therapy, and medical review may follow immediate primary care.

Vocational Rehabilitation

The objective of vocational rehabilitation is the return of the injured worker to as full and productive a life as possible from an occupational point of view. The realization of this objective is a multifaceted process including attention to a number of areas, including the following:

- Therapeutic rehabilitation and activities of daily living
- Workplace and job analysis
- Coordination of all medical, legal, and medicolegal activities
- Administrative and production demands
- Psychological factors
- Matters of workers compensation
- Rehabilitation counseling
- Vocational assessment
- Work trial assessment
- Vocational counseling
- Job placement
- Redeployment placement
- Funded work trials
- Interaction with other employment and rehabilitation agencies
- Constant monitoring and documentation of progress
- Manipulation of criteria used to determine progress
- Reporting and other factors

The injured worker should be referred to a vocational rehabilitation consultant as soon as the worker's medical advisers believe, on medical grounds, that the worker can perform some duties within his or her physical and emotional capacity. This occurs before the worker is fit to return to normal duties. The usual timing of such a referral is within 21 days of a medical assessment in which it is determined that a return to full recovery will be protracted and that it is in the worker's best interests to return to some productive work in the interim period. This may be referred to as "early referral to a rehabilitation consultant."

On referral, the rehabilitation consultant visits the worker to assess his or her current physical and emotional status and ability to perform activities of daily living. The consultant confirms this assessment by contacting all health personnel concerned with the worker. It is important at this stage to establish the worker's current employment profile—the summation of the worker's functional capabilities. This is best achieved by using a functional-capacity assessment, which should be undertaken by physical or occupational therapists experienced in such assessments.

The tools and technology used to accomplish functional-capacity assessment vary tremendously; however, it is essential that some universal criteria be applied. These include high validity and reliability; standardized equipment and protocols; ability to assess the level of worker participation; ability to assess workday endurance; ability to assess static, dynamic, and mobility tolerances; weighted activities; and specific upper limb function in terms of frequency, duration, and intensity. This assessment is followed by a job analysis done at the workplace to determine whether the worker can return to the duties previously performed. If the usual duties are no longer appropriate for the worker, alternative duties have to be found. These may be of a transitional nature, thereby allowing the worker to undertake certain duties for short periods only.

It is the rehabilitation consultant's responsibility to recommend suitable modifications in the workplace to the worker's employer and to ensure that these modifications are made to avoid exacerbation of the worker's preexisting condition or the creation of a new injury. These changes include those of an ergonomic nature, with particular attention given to the biomechanical aspects of work methods and to those of an administrative nature, including work flow and incentive schemes. By making these recommendations, the rehabilitation consultant can actively help prevent injury within the workplace.

The worker's successful return to work will depend on the consultant's successful manipulation of the major criteria: the frequency, duration, and intensity of work-related operations. Space here does not allow a detailed consideration of these criteria, but it should be noted that they can be manipulated in a variety of ways. The method of performing duties is modified in accordance with the categories set out previously. In this way, using the example cited earlier in the chapter, a keyboard operator would be instructed in correct task performance to avoid particular forms of pathomechanical operation.

For example, postures would be corrected to avoid postural overload syndromes, techniques would be modified to avoid overuse syndromes, and so on. The worker would return to work after the medical advisor had issued an appropriate certificate permitting such duties as would be set out in a rehabilitation plan prepared by the rehabilitation consultant. The rehabilitation consultant would be present at the workplace when the worker returned to work to supervise the induction. The program would be recorded and given to the worker, the medical advisers, the employer, the worker's legal representatives, and any other personnel necessary for the smooth management of the program.

The program would be modified according to the criteria previously outlined, at times coinciding with the medical review of the worker. In this way the person responsible for certifying the worker's fitness to perform certain duties would be informed prospectively of the changes to be made in the rehabilitation program as progress was achieved. Ideally, this should also permit the worker to progress through a program of transitional alternative duties to normal duties, although in some cases the progression may be to permanent alteration of duties.

This process takes place under the watchful eye of the rehabilitation consultant, who monitors progress and documents changes in the program. It is necessary for the consultant to regularly review the worksite situation.

Success in the occupational placement of injured workers is directly related to the time of their referral. Early referral should be considered mandatory because when a worker's final recovery will be protracted and yet the worker still can perform some physical duties, the earlier the referral, the better the outcome of both treatment and placement.

The interaction between those who provide vocational rehabilitation and those who provide therapeutic rehabilitation is not only essential but also the most efficient and effective way of ensuring a comprehensive return-to-work program for an injured worker.

References

1. Nachemson AL: Models of prevention: early care programmes. In Abstracts of the second International Conference on Musculoskeletal Injuries in the Work Place, Copenhagen, May 27-29, 1986.
2. Occupational Safety and Health Administration (OSHA), US Department of Labor: Proposed rules, *Fed Regis* 57:149, 1992.
3. Westgaard RH, Aarås A: *Static muscle load and illness among workers doing electro-mechanical assembly work:* a report, Oslo, 1980, Institute of Work Physiology.

4. Westgaard RH, Aarås A: Postural muscle strain as a causal factor in the development of musculo-skeletal illnesses, *Appl Ergonom* 15:162, 1984.
5. Kilbom Å: Occupational disorders of the musculoskeletal system, *Newsletter of the National Board of Occupational Safety and Health*, Stockholm, 82(4) and 83(1), 1983.
6. Ramazzini B: *DeMorbis artificum (diseases of workers)*, 1713, Chicago, 1940, University of Chicago Press (Translated by WC Wright).
7. Ferguson D: An Australian study of telegraphists' cramp, *Br J Ind Med* 28:280, 1971.
8. Hunter D: *Health in industry*, London, 1959, Penguin.
9. Blood W: Tenosynovitis in industrial workers, *Br Med J (Clin Res)* 2:468, 1942.
10. Flowerdew RE, Bode OB: Tenosynovitis in untrained farm workers, *Br Med J (Clin Res)* 2:637, 1942.
11. Howard NJ: Peritendinitis crepitans: a muscle-effort syndrome, *J Bone Joint Surg* 19:447, 1937.
12. Reed JV, Harcourt AK: Tenosynovitis: an industrial disability, *Am J Surg* 62:392, 1943.
13. Smiley JA: The hazards of rope making, *Br J Ind Med* 8:265, 1951.
14. Thompson AR, Plewes LW, Shaw EG: Peritendinitis crepitans and simple tenosynovitis: a clinical study of 544 cases in industry, *Br J Ind Med* 8:150, 1951.
15. Conn HR: Tenosynovitis, *Ohio State Med J* 27:713, 1931.
16. Van Wely P: Design and disease, *Appl Ergonom* 1:262, 1970.
17. Herberts P, Kadefors R: A study of painful shoulders in welders, *Acta Orthop Scand* 47:381, 1976.
18. Carlsöö S, Mayr J: A study of the load on joints and muscles in work with a pneumatic hammer and a bolt gun, *Scand J Work Environ Health* 11:32, 1974.
19. Komoike Y, Horiguchi S: Fatigue assessment on key punch operators, typists and others, *Ergonomics* 4:101, 1971.
20. Onishi N, Nomura H, Sakai K: Fatigue and strength of upper limb muscles of flight reservation system operators, *J Hum Ergol (Tokyo)* 2:133, 1973.
21. Nishiyama K, Nakaseko M, Hosokawa M: Cash register operators' work and its hygienical problems in supermarket, *Sangyo Igaku* 15:229, 1973.
22. Ohara H, Aoyama H, Itani T: Health hazard among cash register operators and the effects of improved working conditions, *J Hum Ergol (Tokyo)* 5:31, 1976.
23. Onishi N, Nomura H, Sakai K et al: Shoulder muscle tenderness and physical features of female industrial workers, *J Hum Ergol (Tokyo)* 6:87, 1976.
24. Onishi N, Sakai K, Itani T et al: Muscle load and fatigue of film rolling workers, *J Hum Ergol (Tokyo)* 6:179, 1976.
25. Ono Y, Masuda K, Iwata M et al: Fatigue and health problems of workers in a home for mentally and physically handicapped persons. Proceedings of the Eighth International Ergonomics Association Congress, Tokyo, 1982.
26. Nakaseko M, Tokunaga R, Hosokawa M: History of occupational cervicobrachial disorder in Japan, *J Hum Ergol (Tokyo)* 11:7, 1982.
27. Maeda K: Concept and criteria of occupational cervicobrachial disorder in Japan. Proceedings of seminar on ergonomics and repetitive tasks, Nordic Council of Ministers, Helsinki, Oct 19-23, 1981.
28. Maeda K, Horiguchi S, Hosokawa H: History of the studies on occupational cervicobrachial disorder in Japan and remaining problems, *J Hum Ergol (Tokyo)* 11:17, 1982.
29. Perrott JW: Anatomical factors in occupational trauma, *Med J Aust* 1:73, 1961.
30. Peres NJC: Process work without strain, *Australian Factory*, July 1, 1961.
31. Ferguson D: Repetition injuries in process workers, *Med J Aust* 2:408, 1971.
32. Ferguson D, Duncan J: A study of the effect of equipment design on posture. Scientific proceedings of the Australian and New Zealand Society of Occupational Medicine, Melbourne, Oct 1972.
33. Duncan J, Ferguson D: Keyboard operating posture and symptoms in operating, *Ergonomics* 17:651, 1972.
34. Ferguson D: Posture, aching, and body build in telephonists, *J Hum Ergol (Tokyo)* 5:183, 1976.

35. Ferguson D, Duncan J: A trial of physiotherapy for symptoms in keyboard operating, *Aust J Physiother* 22:61, 1976.
36. *Repetition strain injury in the Australian public service: task force report*, No 16, Canberra, Australia, 1985, Australian Government Publishing Service.
37. Worksafe Australia: *Repetition strain injury (RSI): a report and model code of practice*, Canberra, Australia, 1986, Australian Government Publishing Service.
38. Stone W: Occupational repetition strain injuries, *Aust Fam Phys* 13:9, 1984.
39. Winkel J, Westgaard R: Occupational and individual risk factors for shoulder-neck complaints. I. Guidelines for the practitioner, *Int J Indust Ergonom* 10:79, 1992.
40. Winkel J, Westgaard R: Occupational and individual risk factors for shoulder-neck complaints. II. The scientific basis (literature review) for the guide, *Int J Indust Ergonom* 10:85, 1992.
41. Kuorinka I, Koskinen P: Occupational rheumatic diseases and upper limb strain in manual jobs in a light mechanical industry, *Scand J Work Environ Health Suppl* 5(3):39, 1979.
42. Herberts P, Kadefors R, Andersson G et al: Shoulder pain in industry: an epidemiological study on welders, *Acta Orthop Scand* 52:299, 1981.
43. Kvarnstrom S: Occurrence of musculoskeletal disorders in a manufacturing industry with special attention to occupational shoulder disorders, *Scand J Rehabil Med* 8(suppl):1, 1983.
44. Kvarnstrom S: Diseases of the musculo-skeletal system in an engineering company, *Scand J Rehabil Med* 8(suppl):61, 1983.
45. Kvarnstrom S: Occupational cervicobrachial disorders in an engineering company, *Scand J Rehabil Med* 8(suppl):77, 1983.
46. Kvarnstrom S: Occupational cervicobrachial disorder: a case-control study, *Scand J Rehabil Med* 8(suppl):101, 1983.
47. Silverstein BA, Fine LJ, Armstrong TJ: Hand-wrist cumulative trauma disorders in industry, *Br J Ind Med* 43:779, 1986.
48. Silverstein BA, Fine LJ, Armstrong TJ: Occupational factors and carpal tunnel syndrome, *Am J Ind Med* 11:343, 1987.
49. Christensen H: Muscle activity and fatigue in the shoulder muscles of assembly plant employees, *Scand J Work Environ Health* 12:587, 1986.
50. Kilbom Å, Persson J, Jonsson BG: Disorders of the cervicobrachial region among female workers in the electronics industry, *Int J Indust Ergonom* 1:37, 1986.
51. Jonsson BG, Persson J, Kilbom K: Disorders of the cervicobrachial region among female workers in the electronics industry, *Int J Indust Ergonom* 3:1, 1988.
52. Parenmark G, Engvall B, Malmkvist A-K: Ergonomic on-the-job training of assembly workers: arm-neck-shoulder complaints drastically reduced amongst beginners, *Appl Ergonom* 19:143, 1988.
53. Ohisson K, Attewell R, Skerfving S: Self-reported symptoms in the neck and upper limbs of female assembly workers, *Scand J Work Environ Health* 15:75, 1989.
54. Armstrong TJ, Foulke J, Joseph B et al: Investigation of cumulative trauma disorders in a poultry processing plant, *Am Ind Hyg Assoc J* 43:103, 1982.
55. Viikari-Juntura E: Neck and upper limb disorders among slaughterhouse workers, *Scand J Work Environ Health* 9:283, 1983.
56. Falck B, Arnio P: Left-sided carpal tunnel syndrome in butchers, *Scand J Work Environ Health* 9:291, 1983.
57. Roto P, Kivi P: Prevalence of epicondylitis and tenosynovitis among meatcutters, *Scand J Work Environ Health* 10:203, 1984.
58. Streib EW, Sun SF: Distal ulnar neuropathy in meat packers, *J Occup Med* 26:842, 1984.
59. Finkel ML: The effects of repeated mechanical trauma in the meat industry, *Am J Ind Med* 8:375, 1985.
60. Magnusson M, Ortengren R, Andersson G et al: An ergonomic study of work methods and physical disorders among professional butchers, *Appl Ergonom* 18:43, 1987.
61. Magnusson M, Ortengren R: Investigation of optimal table height and surface angle in meatcutting, *Appl Ergonom* 18:146, 1987.

62. Luopajärvi T, Kuorinka I, Virolainen M et al: Prevalence of tenosynovitis and other injuries of the upper extremities in repetitive work, *Scand J Work Environ Health* 5(suppl)3:48, 1979.
63. Punnett L, Robbins JM, Wegman DH et al: Soft tissue disorders in the upper limbs of female garment workers, *Scand J Work Environ Health* 11:417, 1985.
64. Brisson C, Vinet A, Vezina M et al: Effect of duration of employment in piecework on severe disability among female garment workers, *Scand J Work Environ Health* 15:329, 1989.
65. Sokas RK, Spiegelman D, Wegman DH: Self-reported musculoskeletal complaints among garment workers, *Am J Ind Med* 15:197, 1989.
66. Westgaard RH, Janus T: Individual and work-related factors associated with symptoms of musculoskeletal complaints. II. Different risk factors among sewing machine operators, *Br J Ind Med* 49:154, 1992.
67. Maeda K, Hünting W, Grandjean E: Localised fatigue in accounting machine operators, *J Occup Med* 22:810, 1980.
68. Hünting W, Grandjean E, Maeda K: Constrained postures in accounting machine operators, *Appl Ergonom* 11:145, 1980.
69. Hünting W, Laubli T, Grandjean E: Postural and visual loads at BDT workplaces. I. Constrained postures, *Ergonomics* 24:917, 1981.
70. Nishiyama K, Nakaseko M, Hosokawa M: Cash register operators' work and its hygienical problems in supermarket, *Sangyo lgaku* 15:229, 1973.
71. Ohara H, Aoyama H, Itani T: Health hazard among cash register operators and the effects of improved working conditions, *J Hum Ergol (Tokyo)* 5:31, 1976.
72. Margolis W, Kraus, J: The prevalence of carpal tunnel syndrome symptoms in female supermarket checkers, *J Occup Med* 12:953, 1987.
73. Smith M, Cohen B, Stammedohn L: An investigation of health complaints and job stress in video display operations, *Hum Factors* 23:387, 1981.
74. Grandjean E, Hünting W, Nishiyama K: Preferred VDT workstation setting, body posture, and physical impairments, *J Hum Ergol* 11:45, 1982.
75. Grandjean E, Hünting W, Piderman M: VDT workstation design: preferred settings and their effects, *Hum Factors* 25:161, 1983.
76. Grandjean E: Postures and the design of VDT workstations, *Behav Informat Technol* 3:301, 1984.
77. Kukkonen R, Luopäjarvi T, Riihimaki V: Prevention of fatigue among data entry operators. In Kvalseth TO, editor: *Ergonomics of workstation design*, London, 1983, Butterworth-Heinemann.
78. Ong CN: VDT workplace design and physical fatigue: a case study in Singapore. In Grandjean E, editor: *Ergonomics and health in modern offices*, Oxford, England, 1984, Taylor & Francis.
79. Sauter SL: Predictors of strain in VDT-users and traditional office workers. In Grandjean E, editor: *Ergonomics and health in modern offices*, London, 1984, Taylor & Francis.
80. Björkstén M: Musculoskeletal disorders among medical secretaries. Abstracts of the XXI International Occupational Health Congress, Dublin, September 9-14, 1984.
81. Hagberg M, Sundelin G: Discomfort and load on the upper trapezius muscle when operating a word processor, *Ergonomics* 29:1637, 1986.
82. Rossignol A, Morse E, Summers V et al: Video display terminal use and reported health symptoms among Massachusetts clerical workers, *J Occup Med* 29:112, 1987.
83. Jeyaratnam J, Ong CN, Kee WC et al: Musculoskeletal symptoms among VDU operators. In Smith MJ, Salvendy G, editors: *Work with computers: organizational, management, stress and health aspects*, Amsterdam, 1989, Elsevier Science Publishers.
84. Linton SJ, Kamwendo K: Risk factors in the psychosocial work environment for neck and shoulder pain in secretaries, *J Occup Med* 31:609, 1989.
85. McPhee BJ: Musculoskeletal complaints in workers engaged in repetitive work in fixed postures. In Bullock M, editor: *Ergonomics: the physiotherapist in the workplace*, Edinburgh, 1990, Churchill Livingstone.

86. Kamwendo K, Linton SJ, Mortiz U: Neck and shoulder disorders in medical secretaries, *Scand J Rehabil Med* 23:57, 1991.
87. Wells JA, Zipp JF, Schuette PT et al: Musculoskeletal disorders among letter carriers, *J Occup Med* 25:814, 1983.
88. Jørgensen K, Fallentin N, Sidenius B: The strain on the shoulder and neck muscles during letter sorting, *Int J Indust Ergonom* 3:243, 1989.
89. Fry HJH: Overuse syndrome of the upper limb in musicians, *Med J Aust* 144A:182, 1985.
90. Welch R: The measurement of physiological predisposition to tenosynovitis, *Ergonomics* 16:665, 1973.
91. Welch R: The causes of tenosynovitis in industry, *Ind Med* 41:16, 1972.
92. Workers' Compensation Act of South Australia, Section 9, 1971.
93. Cyriax J: *Textbook of orthopaedic medicine*, ed 7, vol 1, London, 1978, Baillière Tindall.
94. Grieve, GP: *Common vertebral joint problems*, Edinburgh, 1981, Churchill Livingstone.
95. Watson-Jones R: *Fractures and joint injuries*, Edinburgh, 1962, Churchill Livingstone.
96. Holh M: Soft tissue neck injuries. In The Cervical Spine Research Society Editorial Sub-Committee, editors: *The cervical spine*, Philadelphia, 1983, JB Lippincott.
97. Millender LH, Louis DS, Simmons BP, editors: *Occupational disorders of the upper extremity*, New York, 1992, Churchill Livingstone.
98. Fry HJH: Overuse syndrome of the upper limb in musicians, *Med J Aust* 144(4):182, 1985.
99. Astrand PO, Rohdahl K: *Textbook of work physiology: physiological bases of exercise*, ed 2, New York, 1977, McGraw-Hill.
100. Kjelberg A, Wickstrom B: Whole-body vibration; exposure time and acute effects—a review, *Ergonomics* 28(3):535, 1985.
101. Browne CD, Nolan BM, Faithfull DK: Occupational repetition strain injuries: guidelines for diagnosis and management, *Med J Aust* 3:329, 1984.
102. Worksafe Australia: *National code of practice for the prevention and management of occupational overuse syndrome*, Canberra, Australia, 1990 (first published 1986), Australian Government Publishing Service.
103. Worksafe Australia: *Guidance note for the prevention occupational overuse syndrome in keyboard employment*, Canberra, Australia, 1989, Australian Government Publishing Service.
104. Worksafe Australia: *Guidance note for the prevention occupational overuse syndrome in the manufacturing industry*, Canberra, Australia, 1992, Australian Government Publishing Service.
105. New Zealand Department of Labour: *Occupational overuse syndrome: guidelines for prevention*, Wellington, New Zealand, 1991, OS&H, Department of Labour.
106. New Zealand Department of Labour: *Occupational overuse syndrome treatment and rehabilitation: a practitioner's guide*, Wellington, New Zealand, 1992, OS&H, Department of Labour.
107. Health and Safety Executive (UK): *Work related upper limb disorders—a guide to prevention*, London, 1990, Her Majesty's Stationery Office.
108. US Department of Labor (Occupational Safety and Health Administration): *Ergonomics program management guidelines for meatpacking plants*, Washington, DC, 1991 US Printing Office (reprinted).
109. McAtamney L, Corlett EN: *Reducing the risks of work related upper limb disorders: a guide and methods*, University of Nottingham, UK, 1992, Institute for Occupational Ergonomics.
110. Luopajärvi T: Ergonomic analysis of workplace and postural load. In Bullock M, editor: *Ergonomics: the physiotherapist in the workplace*, Edinburgh, 1990, Churchill Livingstone.
111. Wilson JR, Corlett EN: *Evaluation of human work*, London, 1990, Taylor & Francis.
112. Kuorinka I, Jonsson B, Kilbom Å et al: Standardised Nordic questionnaires for the analysis of musculoskeletal symptoms, Appl Ergonom 18:233, 1987.
113. McPhee B: *Report to the National Health and Medical Research Council on a travelling fellowship*, Sydney, 1980, Commonwealth Institute of Health.
114. Gore A, Tasker D: *Pause gymnastics*, Sydney, 1986, CCH.
115. Lee K, Swanson N, Sauter S et al: A review of physical exercises recommended for VDT operators, *Appl Ergonom* 23:387, 1992.

116. Rohmert W: Problems of determining rest allowances. I. *Appl Ergonom* 4:91, 1973.
117. Rohmert W: Problems of determining rest allowances. II. *Appl Ergonom* 4:158, 1973.
118. Spilling S, Eitrheim J, Aarås A: Cost benefit analysis of work environments: investment at STK's telephone plant at Kongsvinger. In Corlett EN, Wilson J, Manenica I, editors: *The ergonomics of working postures*, London, 1986, Taylor & Francis.
119. Westgaard RH, Aarås A: The effect of improved workplace design on the development of work-related musculoskeletal illnesses, *Appl Ergonom* 16:91, 1985.
120. McGlothlin JD, Armstrong TJ, Fine LJ et al: Can job changes initiated by a joint labor-management task force reduce the prevalence and incidence of cumulative trauma disorders of the upper extremity? Proceedings of the 1984 International Conference on Occupational Ergonomics, Toronto, 1984.
121. King B: Strategies to combat carpal tunnel syndrome, *Ed Welch on Workers' Compensation* (bimonthly newsletter), East Lansing, Mich, 1992.

Efficacy of Manual Therapy in the Treatment of Neck Pain

CHAPTER 20

Bart W. Koes and
Jan Lucas Hoving

NECK PAIN

Neck pain occurs frequently in Western societies. The reported point prevalence varies from 9.5% to 35%, although the most common point prevalence is approximately 10% to 15%. If the 12-month period prevalence is considered, however, figures of up to 40% have been reported.[1] The reported prevalence is usually somewhat higher for women compared with men. Neck pain is a prominent reason for visiting a health care provider (e.g., a primary care physician, physical therapist, or manual therapist). A recent study has shown that once nonspecific neck pain becomes chronic, two of five patients will consult their general medical practitioner, with a third of these patients being referred to an allied health practitioner.[2] Apart from the personal suffering for the patients at issue, the cost to society as a result of neck pain is enormous.

The majority of the costs occur because of sick leave and disability and the related loss of productive capacity. Borghouts et al[3] estimated the total costs for neck pain in 1996 in the Netherlands to be $686 million (calculated in U.S. dollars). Of these costs, 50% were derived from disability pensions, with direct medical costs accounting for 23%. Of the direct medical costs, 84% were attributable to allied health (mostly physical therapy). The total number of days lost because of neck pain has been estimated at 1.4 million.[3]

Neck pain is typically characterized by self-reported pain experienced in the cervical region. The pain may or may not be accompanied by limited range of motion in the cervical spine. Often, disorders of the cervical spine include neck pain with or without radiation to the upper limb and headache. The complaints also may lead to limitation in daily functioning, including work activities. The pain may arise from several structures in the cervical region, including the joints and the soft tissues. In most cases, however, it is not possible to identify the pain-generating tissue. Although there are several potential underlying pathologies that may give rise to neck pain (e.g., systemic rheumatic diseases, infections, malignancies, and fractures), in most cases no clear cause of the pain can be found. The condition is therefore often labeled as *nonspecific neck pain*. In the literature one may find many different descriptions of nonspecific neck pain such as *cervical osteoarthritis, occupational cervicobrachial disorder, tension neck syndrome, thoracic outlet syndrome, cervical spondylosis,* and *mechanical neck pain.* The reality is that valid and reproducible diagnostic criteria for these classifications are usually lacking.[4,5]

Although the history in some cases suggests a causal basis for the neck pain, in most cases the basis for the neck pain is unclear. It is likely that patients with nonspecific neck pain comprise several subgroups with different causes and different prognostic profiles; however, to date no clear, valid, and reproducible classification system has been developed. A classification system that may be useful is one consisting of 11 categories based on a regional description of the pain, the pattern of radiation, the duration of the complaints, paraclinical findings, and the response to treatment. This system was developed by the Quebec Task Force on Spinal Related Disorders and published in 1987.[6] Although the system has not yet been well validated, at present it seems an acceptable approach.

Little is known about the clinical course of acute neck pain. For patients with more than a 6-month history, neck pain improvement rates of up to 50% have been reported, with a mean reduction of pain and analgesic use of about 30% (in a 6-month follow-up period). A less favorable prognosis has been associated with high pain levels and a previous history of neck pain.[7]

MANUAL THERAPY

One of the many therapeutic interventions available for the management of neck pain is manual therapy. Worldwide, manual therapies are applied quite often. Different forms and techniques exist.[8] A common feature of all of these different techniques is the use of the hands during the therapy. Gross et al[9] described manual therapy as "all procedures in which the hands are used to mobilize, adjust, manipulate, apply traction, massage, stimulate, or otherwise influence the spine and paraspinal tissues."

This chapter is limited to a consideration of two forms of manual therapy: spinal manipulation and spinal mobilization. *Spinal manipulation* has been defined as "a passive maneuver in which specifically directed manual forces are applied to vertebral articulations of the body."[9] Two forms of spinal manipulation are described: (1) long-lever manipulations, which consist of a high-velocity thrust exerted on a point of the body some distance away from the area where it is expected to have its beneficial effect, and (2) short-lever manipulations, which consist of a high-velocity thrust directed specifically at an isolated joint.[9,10] Spinal mobilization, on the other hand, may be described as a nonthrust form of manipulation directed at joint dysfunction.[9,10]

The osteopath and chiropractic professionals have traditionally applied spinal manipulation and mobilization. Today, various professions, including medical doctors, physical therapists, manual therapists, and massage therapists, as well as chiropractors and osteopaths, use and apply spinal manipulation and mobilization in daily practice.

RATIONALE

The rationale for the use of spinal manipulation and mobilization is not fully understood. The intervention in the treatment of neck pain is aimed at the reduction of pain and the improvement of mobility and function for the patient. Gross et al[9] described the following potential working mechanisms for understanding the beneficial effects of spinal manipulation and mobilization:

1. Mechanical alteration of tissues. This hypothesis is that as a consequence of the restoration of joint mobility, the detrimental effects of immobilization of joints will be minimized. It is acknowledged, however, that the means by which spinal motion is restored are not fully understood and will need further exploration.
2. Neurophysiological effects. This hypothesis proposes that mechanoreceptors are stimulated as a consequence of the spinal manipulation, thereby having an effect through the large diameter fibers in modulating pain. In addition, several other neuromuscular mechanisms have been suggested. Again, the actual mechanism of pain relief is poorly understood.
3. Psychological influences. The implication of this hypothesis is that the laying on of hands has strong psychological effects for a patient.[11] This may occur directly or indirectly via the neuromuscular system (through muscle tension reduction).[9]

For all three postulated working mechanisms, only a little empirical evidence has been collected. Further studies are needed. A more extended description of the potential working mechanisms for the efficacy of manual therapy is presented in Chapter 12.

EFFICACY OF SPINAL MANIPULATION AND MOBILIZATION

Irrespective of the biological or theoretical rationale, it is both possible and necessary to determine the efficacy of spinal manipulation and mobilization. Stimulated by a series of publications by the Evidence-Based Medicine Working Group of McMaster University,[12] there is now a worldwide interest in evidence-based practice, with the emphasis very much on health care intervention based on scientific evidence derived from sound clinical studies. Evidence-based medicine or practice is not confined to the medical profession; increasingly it is being used in physical therapy and manual therapy. Consequently, there is an increasing interest in the determination of the efficacy, including the side effects and costs of common interventions in the field of physical therapy. This section of the chapter focuses on the determination of efficacy of spinal manipulation and mobilization with neck pain.

Randomized Clinical Trials of Spinal Manipulation and Mobilization for Neck Pain

To address the question of whether spinal manipulation and mobilization are effective in the management of patients with neck pain, this discussion is restricted to the assessment of evidence from randomized clinical trials. Since the 1950s the randomized clinical trial has been widely recognized as the "gold standard" for intervention studies into the efficacy of new or existing treatments. The characteristics of this trial design are the use of one or more control groups and the use of a randomization procedure to divide the participating patients among the study groups. In addition, much effort is placed on the adequate blinding of patients, the treating physicians or therapists, and the outcome assessment. Other research designs, such as that using a patient series without a control group or studies designed as a controlled clinical trial with no

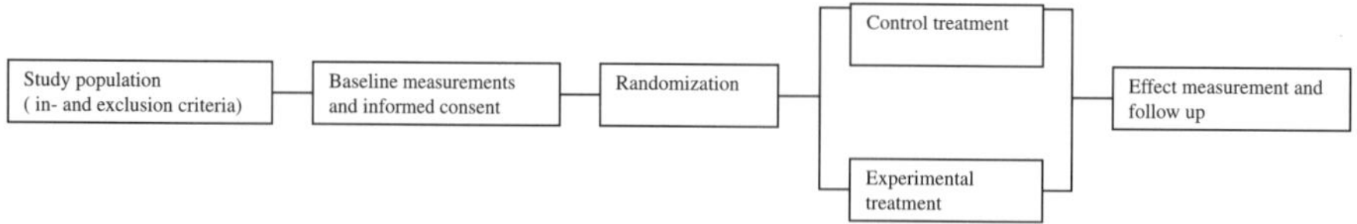

Figure 20-1
Design of a randomized controlled trial.

randomization are much more susceptible to various forms of bias (e.g., selection bias, information bias, and confounding). The basic scheme of a randomized clinical trial is shown in Figure 20-1.

Identification, Scoring, and Determination of Outcome

Relevant randomized control trials (RCTs) were identified via literature searches in existing databases such as MEDLINE and Embase and by screening the reference lists of (review) articles that were identified. To be considered in this chapter, publications had to meet the following criteria:

1. The study was a relevant RCT.
2. One of the study groups received spinal manipulation or mobilization with or without cointerventions.
3. The study population consisted of patients with nonspecific neck pain.
4. The article was published in English, Dutch, or German.

All trials were subsequently scored according to the criteria listed in Table 20-1. The criteria are based on generally accepted principles of intervention research.[13,14] To each criterion a weight was attached. The maximum score was set at 100 points for each study, with higher scores indicating higher methodological quality. Two reviewers, independently of each other, assessed the methodological quality of the studies.

A study was determined to be positive if the authors concluded (in their abstract or conclusions) that manipulation was more effective than the reference treatment. In some cases the authors reported favorable outcomes for manipulation in only a subgroup of the study population. In a negative study the authors reported no differences between the study treatments or even better results in favor of the reference treatment. *Short-term outcome* refers to effect measurements made during or just after the intervention period. *Long-term outcome* refers to outcome measurements made at least 3 months after randomization.

Results

A total of 10 randomized clinical trials were identified for inclusion in this chapter. Table 20-2 shows the trials and their method scores. Three trials[15-17] included patients with acute neck pain. Seven trials included patients with subacute and chronic neck pain.[18-30]

No single trial scored 60 or more points, and only three studies had a methodological score greater than 50 points, indicating poor quality generally. Table 20-2 demonstrates that the most prevalent methodological shortcomings were the improper description of subjects dropping out of the trial *(D)*, the small size of the population *(F)*, the lack of a placebo group *(J)*, the insufficient blinding of patients *(L)*, and the absence of the blinded effect measurements *(N)*.

Table 20-1 Criteria List for the Methodological Assessment of Randomized Clinical Trials of Manipulation for Neck Pain*

Criteria	Weight
Study Population (30)	
A: Homogeneity	2
B: Comparability of relevant baseline characteristics	5
C: Randomization procedure adequate	4
D: Dropouts described for each study group separately	3
E: <20% loss to follow-up	2
<10% loss to follow-up	2
F: >50 subjects in the smallest group	6
>100 subjects in the smallest group	6
Interventions (30)	
G: Interventions included in protocol and described	10
H: Pragmatic study	5
I: Cointerventions avoided	5
J: Placebo controlled	5
K: Mentioning good qualification of manipulative therapist	5
Effect (30)	
L: Patients blinded	5
M: Outcome measures relevant	10
N: Blinded outcome assessments	10
O: Follow-up period adequate	5
Data Presentation and Analysis (10)	
P: Intention-to-treat analysis	5
Q: Frequencies of most important outcomes presented for each treatment group	5

*For details, see the appendix at the end of the chapter.

Table 20-3 presents the main characteristics of the trials. Manipulation and mobilization were given alone or in combination with other therapeutic modalities. The reference treatments were mainly analgesics, neck collars, and other physiotherapeutic interventions.

Acute Neck Pain

All three trials evaluating the efficacy of manipulation and mobilization in patients with acute neck pain and whiplash had method scores of less than 50 points. Nordemar and Thörner[15] reported a "remarkably quick symptom reduction" in some patients treated with manual therapy, but no significant differences were found with use of a collar alone. McKinney[16] and Mealy et al,[17] on the other hand, reported positive effects of mobilization in combination with other conservative interventions (exercises, heat, ice, and analgesics in the case of Mealy et al and heat, cold, short-wave diathermy, hydrotherapy, traction, education, and analgesics in the case of McKinney) compared with the control treatments (rest, collar, and analgesics in the case of Mealy et al and rest, education, analgesics, and collar, in the case of McKinney).

Table 20-2 Randomized Trials on the Efficacy of Manipulation and Mobilization for Acute and Chronic Neck Pain in Order of Methods Score

	Scores for Methods Criteria																	
	A	B	C	D	E	F	G	H	I	J	K	L	M	N	O	P	Q	Total Score
Author	2	5	4	3	4	12	10	5	5	5	5	5	10	10	5	5	5	100
Acute Neck Pain																		
Nordemar[15]	1	3	—	3	4	—	5	5	5	—	—	—	4	—	3	5	5	43
McKinney[16]	1	2	1	3	—	—	5	5	—	5	—	—	4	4	3	—	5	38
Mealy[17]	1	2	4	—	2	—	—	5	—	—	—	—	4	—	3	—	5	26
Subacute and Chronic Neck Pain																		
Koes[18-21]	1	3	2	3	2	—	10	5	5	—	—	5	4	4	5	—	5	54
Jordan[22]	2	4	2	3	2	—	10	—	5	—	5	—	8	2	5	—	5	53
Cassidy[23,24]	1	5	2	3	4	—	10	—	—	—	5	—	4	4	3	5	5	51
Sloop[25]	1	1	2	3	4	—	—	—	—	—	5	5	8	8	—	5	—	42
Brodin[27-29]	-	1	4	—	2	—	5	5	5	—	5	—	4	—	3	—	5	39
Vernon[30]	—	1	2	—	4	—	5	—	—	—	5	3	2	2	3	5	5	37
Howe[26]	—	3	2	—	—	—	5	5	—	—	—	—	4	2	3	—	5	29

Table 20-3 Characteristics of RCTs Evaluating Manipulation and Mobilization for Patient with Neck Pain

Author	Disorder	Index Treatment	Reference Treatment	Results
Acute Neck Pain				
Nordemar[15]	Nonradiating acute cervical pain	(I) Mobilization, analgesics, advisement to rest, collar and manual traction for 30 minutes three times a week for 2 weeks (n = 10).	(R1) Analgesics, collar, advised to rest and TNS for 15 minutes three times a week for 2 weeks (n = 10). (R2) Analgesics, collar, and advisement to rest for 2 weeks (n = 10).	Mean (SD) on pain VAS after 1 and 6 weeks (I) 18 (25), 0 (R1) 17 (19), 0; (R2) 35 (45), 0. No significant differences. A total of 3-month follow-up yielded similar results to those at 6 weeks (according to author).
McKinney[16]	Acute whiplash injury	(I) Mobilization: combination of heat or cold applications, short-wave diathermy, hydrotherapy, traction and active and passive repetitive movements according to McKenzie and Maitland and postural exercises for three 40 minute sessions per week for 6 weeks (n = 71). Patients in all three groups received a cervical collar and standard analgesics.	(R1) Rest and analgesics: rest period 10-14 days and general advice regarding mobilization (n = 33). (R2) Advice: instructions regarding analgesics use, heat and cold applications, relaxation, collar use, exercises. One treatment session of 30 minutes (n = 66).	Median pain score on a VAS at baseline and after 1 and 2 months: (I) 5.3, 3.3, 1.9, (R1) 5.6, 5.0, 3.0, (R2) 5.3, 3.4, 1.8. Both (I) and (R2) significantly better than (R1) at 1 and 2 months.
Mealy[17]	Acute neck pain (whiplash)	(I) Maitland mobilization and analgesic and physical therapy modalities and exercises (n = 31).	(R) Analgesics and collar, advice on rest and exercises (n = 30).	Mean pain on VAS after 4 and 8 weeks: (I) 2.85, 1.69; (R) 5.08, 3.49. Group I significantly better.

TNS, Transcutaneous nerve stimulation; *SD*, standard deviation; *VAS*, visual analog scale; *NRS*, numerical rating scale; *CI*, cumulative incidence.

Continued

Table 20-3 Characteristics of RCTs Evaluating Manipulation and Mobilization for Patient with Neck Pain—cont'd

Author	Disorder	Index Treatment	Reference Treatment	Results
Chronic Neck Pain				
Koes[18-21]	Chronic nonspecific neck complaints	(I) Manual therapy: manipulation and mobilization maximum 3 months (n = 13).	(R1) Physiotherapy: exercises, massage, modalities, max 3 months (n = 21). (R2) Continued treatment by general practitioner, maximum 3 months (n = 16). (R3) Detuned short-wave diathermy (10 minutes) and detuned ultrasound, (10 minutes) twice a week for 6 weeks (n = 14).	Mean score on severity of main complaint (10 point NRS; blinded outcome assessor) at baseline and after 3, 6 and 12 weeks: (I) 7.15, 4.50, 3.23, 2.09, (R1) 7.29, 4.85, 3.45, 3.30, (R2) 7.19, 5.77, 4.85, 3.31, (R3) 7.21, 5.18, 3.75, 1.90. Mean (SD) score on physical functioning (10 point NRS; blinded outcome assessor) at baseline and after 3, 6 and 12 weeks: (I) 6.11, 3.34, 2.22, 1.20, (R1) 5.61, 3.86, 2.95, 2.52, (R2) 5.29, 4.20, 2.84, 2.86, (R3) 5.71, 3.68, 2.12, 1.26. No significant differences.
Jordan[22]	Chronic nonspecific neck pain	(I) Manipulation by chiropractor: high-velocity and low-amplitude spinal manipulation of the apophyseal joints of the cervical spine, manual traction, instruction, education, 15-20 minutes twice per week for 6 weeks (n = 40).	(R1) Intensive training: stretching, isometric strengthening, instruction, education, ergonomic advice, 60-75 minutes twice per week for 6 weeks (n = 40). (R2) Physiotherapy: individual treatment plan, active and passive, hot packs, massage, ultrasound, manual traction, exercise, ergonomic advice, education, 30 minutes twice per week for 6 weeks (n = 39).	Median (90% CI) pain level at baseline, and after 6 weeks (posttreatment), 4 and 12 months: (I) 13 (10-15), 6 (4-7), 6 (5-8), 6 (6-8), (R1) 12 (10-15), 6 (3-9), 4 (3-10), 6 (4-9), (R2) 12 (10-15), 6 (3-8), 4 (3-10), 8 (6-11). Median (90% CI) disability level at baseline, and after 6 weeks, 4 and 12 months: (I) 8 (7-10), 4 (4-5), 6 (4-7), 5 (3-6), (R1) 8 (7-10), 5 (4-7), 5 (3-7), 5 (4-7), (R2) 9 (8-11), 4 (3-6), 5 (3-8), 6 (4-7). Median (90% CI) patient's perceived effect post-treatment and after 4 and 12 months: (I) 2 (1-5), 3 (1-5), 3 (1-4), (R1) 2 (1-4), 3 (1-4), 3 (1-4), (R2) 2 (1-4), 3 (1-4), 3 (1-4). Median (90% CI) doctor's global assessment post-treatment (I) 2 (1-4), (R1) 2 (1-4), (R2) 2 (1-4). No significant differences.

Cassidy[23,24]	Unilateral mechanical neck pain	(I) Manipulation: a single low-amplitude and high-velocity thrust manipulation to the cervical spine (n = 52).	(R) Mobilization: mobilization technique to the cervical spine using isometric contractions, followed by stretching (n = 48).	Mean pain severity (SD) VAS pretreatment to posttreatment (I) 37.7 (25.9), 20.4 (21.2); (R) 31.0 (19.9), 20.5 (21.0). Percentage of patients with improvement in neck pain was 85% (I) and 69% (R). No statistical differences found. Manipulation was reported to be more effective than mobilization, however.
Sloop[25]	Chronic cervical spondylosis or chronic nonspecific neck pain	(I) Manipulation after amnesic dose of 20 mg of diazepam intravenously by rheumatologist experienced in manipulation techniques, one session (n = 21).	(R) Placebo: amnesic dose of 20 mg diazepam intravenously (n = 18).	Number of patients (%) improved after 3 weeks: (I) 12 (57%), (R) 18 (28%); not significant. Mean (SD) improvement in pain intensity (VAS) after 3 weeks: (I) 5 (32), (R) 18 (31); not significant. No differences in range of motion and activities of daily living.
Brodin[27-29]	Chronic neck pain with or without radiating pain to the upper extremity	(I) Specific manual mobilization (described by Stoddard), massage, electrical stimulation, manual traction, heat for nine times over 3 weeks of treatment. In addition, education ("cervical school") for 3 hours (n = 23).	(R1) Analgesics, massage, electrical stimulation, manual traction, heat, education ("cervical school") for 3 hours, and mock manual therapy (n = 17). (R2) Analgesics (n = 23).	Percentage of patients pain free after 1 week of treatment: (I) 48%, (R1) 12%, and (R2) 22%. Significant differences in favor of mobilization compared to the other two interventions.
Vernon[30]	Chronic mechanical neck pain	I) Manipulation: a single rotational high-velocity and low-amplitude thrust (n = 5).	(R) Mobilization: rotational mobilizations into the elastic barrier, 1 session (n = 4).	Percentage of change from pretreatment to posttreatment pressure pain threshold in four standardized neck tender points: from 44%-56% improvement for (I) up to 0.8% improvement for (R). Statistically significant differences were reported in favor of group I.
Howe[26]	Neck pain resulting from lesion cervical spine	(I) Manipulation (high-velocity, low-amplitude) and/or injection plus azapropazone for one to three treatments for 1 week (n = 26).	(R) Azapropazone (n = 26).	Percentage of patients with immediate pain improvement: (I) 68%, (R) 6% posttreatment. No significant differences after 1 and 3 weeks.

TNS, Transcutaneous nerve stimulation; *SD*, standard deviation; *VAS*, visual analog scale; *NRS*, numerical rating scale; *CI*, cumulative incidence.

Chronic Neck Pain

Only three of the seven trials evaluating manipulation and mobilization in patients with chronic neck pain scored more than 50 points.[18-24] Koes et al[18-21] compared manipulation and mobilization (provided by specifically trained physical therapists) to nonmanipulative physical therapy, usual care by a general practitioner, and a "placebo." The manipulative and nonmanipulative physical therapy showed better short-term results of overall improvement and physical functioning than the other two groups, but this difference was not statistically significant. The second study[22] compared manipulation with physical therapy and intensive training. All three groups improved substantially over time. There were, however, no statistically significant differences between the three groups. Cassidy et al[23,24] compared manipulation with mobilization but found no significant differences between these treatment approaches in the management of chronic neck pain.

The four RCTs with method scores below 50 produced mixed findings. Sloop et al[25] compared a single manipulation (provided by a rheumatologist experienced in spinal manipulation) after an amnesic dose of diazepam with a "placebo" in which only diazepam was given. These authors reported no significant differences between the groups. Brodin,[27-29] Howe and Newcombe,[26] and Vernon et al,[30] on the other hand, all reported positive results after manipulation.

Manipulation Versus Mobilization

Only two RCTs directly compared the efficacy of manipulation with mobilization.[23,24,30] Cassidy et al[23,24] compared rotational manipulation with mobilization (muscle energy) in patients with unilateral neck pain (mostly chronic: >6 months). The manipulation group reported more pain improvement (85% versus 69%), and the improvement in cervical range of motion (ROM) also was greater in the manipulation group. However, the differences were not statistically significant. Vernon et al[30] compared rotational manipulation with mobilization (oscillation) in patients with chronic neck pain (2 weeks' to 8 years' duration). The manipulation group improved with respect to rise in pain pressure threshold immediately after treatment (40% to 55%). There was no change in the mobilization group. The difference was statistically significant. Based on these two studies (one positive, one negative), it is not possible to draw firm conclusions regarding the relative efficacy of manipulation compared with mobilization. Further studies in this area are definitely needed.

SIDE EFFECTS OF SPINAL MANIPULATION AND MOBILIZATION

Besides the positive effects of therapeutic intervention, it is important to consider the potential side effects when assessing the value of that intervention. Manipulation of the cervical spine, especially the high-velocity thrust techniques, has been associated with potential (severe) side effects in a number of case reports in the literature. Some authors have addressed this issue in a number of systematic reviews of the literature to get more precise estimates of the potential risk involved when applying cervical spinal manipulation.[31,32] Estimates are reported for severe neurovascular compromise ranging from 1 in 50,000 to 1 in 5 million manipulations.[33] Because these data are usually not based on systematic (prospective) registration of the number of side effects after manipulation (the numerator) and on the actual number of manipulations applied (the denominator), the estimated risks may be far from accurate. Di Fabio[31] found a total of 177 case reports of injuries associated with cervical manipulation in the literature in the period 1925 to 1997. The type of complications range from arterial dissection (pseudoaneurysm, arterial spasm, rupture; approximately 19% of cases) to Wallenberg's syndrome (approximately 13% of the cases) and spinal cord injury (9%). Death occurred in 18% of cases. In 46% of the case reports the type of manipulation applied was not described. Where the direction of the manipulation was given, those most often described were rotational thrusts (23%). Dabbs and Lauretti[34] suggested that the risk of complication is 100 to 400 times greater from using nonsteroidal antiinflammatory medications than from receiving cervical manipulation.

DISCUSSION

The value of a literature review relates directly to the success in obtaining the results of all studies (RCTs) that have been conducted. There are, for example, indications that small clinical trials with positive results are more likely to be published.[35] Although the authors have put considerable effort into obtaining all the available published RCTs incorporating manipulation and mobilization in the treatment of neck pain, it remains possible that we have missed some RCTs, the results of which might differ from the ones included in this chapter. In this area of research, no agency registers the trials that are being or will be carried out. Consequently, at present there is no way of detecting trials that may not have been published because of negative results.

We identified only 10 RCTs evaluating manipulation and mobilization for patients with neck pain. Most of these had major methodological flaws. The most common flaws are presented in Table 20-1. Clearly, more attention needs to be given to the description of dropouts, the size of the study population, the use of placebo groups, and blinded effect measurements in RCTs conducted in the future. There have been a number of reviews published on the efficacy of manipulation and mobilization for neck pain.[10,31,36,37] The conclusion of these authors varied depending on the focus of the review article. Some stated that because of the limited number of RCTs of acceptable quality, there is only limited evidence available to support the efficacy of manipulation and mobilization,[35,36] although promising results are reported in some studies. Others[10] conclude that manipulation and mobilization probably provide at least short-term benefit for some patients with neck pain. Di Fabio[31] concluded that the literature does not demonstrate that the benefits of manipulation of the cervical spine outweigh the risks.

Some authors statistically pooled the results of (subsets) of the RCTs.[10,35,36] We chose not to statistically pool the results of the available trials because it was deemed inappropriate to combine data from studies with widely varying methodological quality. The reason for not pooling the results of the subgroup of trials with a relatively high methodological score with those with a low score is that we do not think that the patient characteristics and treatments used in these trials show sufficient similarity to permit statistical pooling of their data.

The trials reported in this review considered manual therapies in general. The frequency of the application of manipulation and mobilization showed large differences, however. Although most of the trials consisted of a series of manipulative interventions over time, three trials investigated the effect of a single manipulative thrust.[25,26,30] At present we do not have a clear insight into dose-response relationships. However, if a long-term effect is desired, one could question whether a single manipulation would be a sufficient dose, especially if the patient has chronic neck pain.

Five studies, including the ones with relatively higher methodology scores, reported no treatment being superior. The absence of positive findings might in part, however, be the result of relatively small study populations, thus making it difficult to detect existing treatment differences between manipulations and reference treatments. However, the results of the trials presented indicated that neither manipulation nor mobilization was consistently better than other therapeutic approaches. Possibly, manipulation, mobilization, or a combination of the two is effective only in certain subgroups of patients with neck pain. If this is indeed so, it remains unclear which subgroups will benefit because there are positive and negative studies for patients with both acute and chronic pain. Clearly, research is urgently needed, and such research must take into account the methodological flaws in previous RCTs.

References

1. Ariens GAM, Borghouts JAJ, Koes BW: Neck pain. In Crombie IK, editor: *Epidemiology of pain,* Seattle, 1999, IASP Press.
2. Borghouts JAJ et al: The management of chronic pain in general practice: a retrospective study, *Scan J Prim Health Care* 17:215, 1999.
3. Borghouts JAJ et al: Cost-of-illness of neck pain in the Netherlands in 1996, *Pain* 80:629, 1999.
4. Buchbinder R et al: Classification systems of soft tissue disorders of the neck and upper limb: do they satisfy methodological guidelines? *S J Clin Epidemiol* 49(2):141, 1996.
5. Buchbinder R, Goel V, Bombardier C: Lack of concordance between the ICD-9 classification of soft tissue disorders of the neck and upper limb and chart review diagnosis: one steel mill's experience, *Am J Ind Med* 29:171, 1996.
6. Spitzer WO, Leblanc FE, Dupuis M, editors: Scientific approach to the assessment and management of activity-related spinal disorders, *Spine* 7(suppl):1, 1987.
7. Borghouts AJ, Koes BW, Bouter LM: The clinical course and prognostic factors of non-specific neck pain: a systematic review, *Pain* 77:1, 1998.
8. Farrell JP, Jensen GM: Manual therapy: a critical assessment of role in the profession of physical therapy, *Phys Ther* 72(12):843, 1992.
9. Gross AR, Aker PD, Quartly C: Manual therapy in the treatment of neck pain, *Rheum Dis Clin N Am* 22:579, 1996.
10. Hurwitz EL et al: Manipulation and mobilization of the cervical spine: a systematic review of the literature, *Spine* 21:1746, 1996.
11. Coulehan JL: Adjustment, the hands, and healing, *Cult Med Psychiatry* 9(4):353, 1985.
12. The Evidence-Based Medicine Working Group: Evidence-based medicine: a new approach to teaching the practice of medicine, *JAMA* 268:2420, 1992.
13. Feinstein AR: *Clinical epidemiology: the architecture of clinical research,* Philadelphia, 1985, WB Saunders.
14. Meinert CL: *Clinical trials: design, conduct and analysis,* New York, 1986, Oxford University Press.
15. Nordemar R, Thörner C: Treatment of acute cervical pain: a comparative group study, *Pain* 10:93, 1980.
16. McKinney LA: Early mobilisation and outcome in acute sprains of the neck, *Br Med J* 299:1006, 1989.
17. Mealy K, Brennan H, Fenelon GC: Early mobilization of acute whiplash injuries, *Br Med J* 292:656, 1986.
18. Koes BW et al: The effectiveness of manual therapy, physiotherapy, and continued treatment by the general practitioner for chronic nonspecific back and neck complaints: design of a randomized clinical trial, *J Manip Physiol Ther* 14:498, 1991.
19. Koes BW et al: The effectiveness of manual therapy, physiotherapy, and treatment by the general practitioner for nonspecific back and neck complaints, *Spine* 17:28, 1992.

20. Koes BW et al: A blinded randomized clinical trial of manual therapy and physiotherapy for chronic back and neck complaints: physical outcome measures, *J Manip Physiol Ther* 1:16, 1992.
21. Koes BW et al: A randomized clinical trial of manual therapy and physiotherapy for persistent back and neck complaints: subgroup analysis and relationship between outcome measures, *J Manip Physiol Ther* 16:211, 1993.
22. Jordan A et al: Intensive training, physiotherapy, or manipulation for patients with chronic neck pain: a prospective, single-blinded, randomized clinical trial, *Spine* 23:311, 1998.
23. Cassidy JD et al: The effect of manipulation on pain and range of motion in the cervical spine: a pilot study, *J Manip Physiol Ther* 15:495, 1992.
24. Cassidy JD, Lopes AA, Yong-Hing K: The immediate effect of manipulation versus mobilization on pain and range of motion in the cervical spine: a randomized controlled trial, *J Manip Physiol Ther* 15:570, 1992.
25. Sloop PR et al: Manipulation for chronic neck pain: a double-blind controlled study, *Spine* 7:532, 1982.
26. Howe DH, Newcombe R: Manipulation of the cervical spine, *J R Coll Gen Pract* 33:574, 1983.
27. Brodin H: Cervical pain and mobilization, *Med Phys* 6:67, 1983.
28. Brodin H: Cervical pain and mobilization, *Int J Rehab Res* 7:190, 1984.
29. Brodin H: Cervical pain and mobilization, *Manual Med* 2:18, 1985.
30. Vernon HT et al: Pressure pain threshold evaluation of the effect of spinal manipulation in the treatment of chronic neck pain: a pilot study, *J Manipulative Physiol Ther* 13:13, 1990.
31. Di Fabio RP: Manipulation of the cervical spine: risks and benefits, *Phys Ther* 79(1):50, 1999.
32. Assendelft WJJ, Bouter LM, Knipschild PG: Complications of spinal manipulation: a comprehensive review of the literature, *J Fam Pract* 42(5):475, 1996.
33. Rivett DA, Milburn P: A prospective study of complications of cervical spine manipulation, *J Manip Physiol Ther* 4:166, 1996.
34. Dabbs V, Lauretti WJ: A risk assessment of cervical manipulation vs NSAIDs for the treatment of neck pain, *J Manip Physiol Ther* 18:530, 1995.
35. Dickersin K, Scherer R, Lefebre C: Identifying relevant studies for systematic reviews, *Br Med J* 309:1286, 1994.
36. Aker PD et al: Conservative management of mechanical neck pain: systematic overview and meta-analysis, *Br Med J* 313:1291, 1996.
37. Gross AR et al: Conservative management of mechanical neck disorders: a systematic overview and meta-analysis, *Online J Curr Clin Trials* 5: Doc. 200 + 201, 1996.

Appendix

OPERATIONALIZATION OF THE CRITERIA FROM TABLE 20-1

Each criterion must be applied independently of the other criteria.

A Description of inclusion and exclusion criteria (1 point). Restriction to a homogeneous study population (1 point).

B Comparability for duration of complaints, value of outcome measures, age, recurrence status, and radiating complaints (1 point each).

C Randomization procedure described (2 points). Randomization procedure that excludes bias (e.g., sealed envelopes) (2 points).

D Information from which group and with reason for withdrawal.

E Loss to follow-up: all randomized patients minus the number of patients at main moment of effect measurement for the main outcome measure, divided by all randomized patients multiplied by 100.

F Smallest group immediately after randomization.

G Manipulative treatment explicitly described (5 points).
All reference treatments explicitly described (5 points).

H Comparison with an existing treatment modality.

I Other physical therapy modalities or medical interventions are avoided in the design of the study (except analgesics, advice on posture, or use at home of heat, rest, or a routine exercise scheme).

J Comparison with a placebo therapy.

K Mentioning of qualified education and/or experience of the manipulative therapist(s).

L Placebo controlled: attempt for blinding (3 points), blinding evaluated and fully successful (2 points).
Pragmatic study: patients fully naive (3 points), or time restriction (no manipulative treatment for at least 1 year) (2 points), naiveness evaluated and fully successful (2 points).

M Use (measured and reported) of pain, global measure of improvement, functional status (activities of daily living), spinal mobility, medical consumption (2 points each).

N Each blinded measurement mentioned under point M earns 2 points.

O Moment of measurement during or just after treatment (3 points).
Moment of measurement 6 months or longer after treatment (2 points).

P When loss to follow-up is less than 10%: All randomized patients for most important outcome measures, and on the most important moments of effect measurement minus missing values, irrespective of noncompliance and cointerventions.

Q When loss to follow-up is greater than 10%: Intention-to-treat as well as an alternative analysis that accounts for missing values. For most important outcome measures, and on the most important moments of effect measurement.

CHAPTER 21

Reflections on Clinical Expertise and Evidence-Based Practice

Ruth Grant

Taking time to stand back and reflect is always important, particularly at the beginning of a new century. The intent of this chapter is to capture some reflections on the changing nature of work, the exponential increase in access to information, and the way that knowledge is valued, managed, and used. It also reflects on the centrality of lifelong learning for health and growth not only of an individual, but also of a profession, and reflects on the synergy, or lack thereof, between clinical practice and the evidence base for it.

CHANGES IN THE NATURE OF WORK

Technological change and other changes stemming from the globalization of economies around the world are now having a profound effect on the nature of work in its broadest sense: the way it is organized and the skills it requires.[1] These changes are now so rapid that many students graduating from universities today can be expected to have up to five distinctly different careers in their working lifetimes. They may also anticipate that their working life span may be shorter, with a greater portion of their life spent in active retirement. They are keen to learn, acquire new knowledge, and particularly age successfully.

Further change is predicted by Ellyard[2] (a futurist and strategic analyst) in his book, *Ideas for a New Millennium*, published in 1998. Ellyard states, "If one looks at the rates of globalisation and technological change . . . it seems reasonable to deduce that in the next 25 years, up to 70 per cent of all job categories are likely to change, half of the existing job categories will disappear, the other half will consist of new jobs that do not yet exist. Other jobs will keep their present names but the nature of the work will change."[2]

For example, numerous changes have occurred in the banking industry because of technological change; this is particularly true about the job of a bank teller. In the banking industry the cost of a transaction at an automated teller machine or over the Internet is one-twentieth that of an over-the-counter transaction at the bank. Using this example, we can begin to see why Ellyard[2] was prepared to predict the future of work in the way that he did.

Where would we place the physical therapy profession in Ellyard's prediction? As physical therapists, we would no doubt place our profession in Ellyard's last category: our titles may remain the same but the nature of our work will change. However, 25 years from now, will our profession have been very successful in establishing a sound and comprehensive clinical research base for diagnosis, assessment, and treatment to ensure a continuing professional relevance and vital contribution to patient care? Or will the changes not be of our making and serve to constrain the profession? To what extent, a quarter of a century from now, will clinicians have access to, and have adopted, the outcomes of sound research so that evidence-based practice will be the norm? To what extent will the decision making by physical therapists in the management of their patients continue to be based predominantly on clinical experience and biomedical or pathophysiological explanations? The challenge is that the evidence base remains to be established for much of the practice of medicine as well as of physical therapy. Sackett et al,[3] writing in 2000, stated that "conventional wisdom" had it "that only about 20% of [medical] clinical care was based in solid scientific evidence." Estimates of the extent to which physical therapists are currently practicing evidence-based diagnosis, assessment, and treatment are unknown.

CHANGES IN ACCESS TO AND AMOUNT OF INFORMATION

The exponential growth in access to information is already a feature (and will continue to be a feature) of life in the twenty-first century. The implications of this fact are staggering. Although it took 34 years for 50 million people worldwide to have access to the radio and 15 years for the same number of people to have access to television, it has taken only *4 years* for 50 million people worldwide to become users of the Internet. Traffic on the Internet is estimated to double every 100 days; seven people become Internet users every second. It was predicted that 1 billion people would be using the Internet in 2001.[4] In an analysis of how users used the Internet, it was found that 88% used it to get information, 83% to communicate (i.e., e-mail), 80% to do research, and 75% to "surf the Net."[4] Not surprisingly, many of the people surveyed used the Internet for more than one of these purposes.

Biomedical and health information via the worldwide web is one example of the knowledge explosion. Patients will increasingly expect their health care provider of whatever persuasion to have up-to-date knowledge of their condition, the efficacy and risks associated with different treatment approaches, and perhaps even the evidence base for the choice of treatment recommended or given—information the patients themselves can access from the web. The exponential growth in access to information globally has the potential to change a profession.

A *profession* or *professional group* may be defined as a group having knowledge that is not available to others; a professional knowledge base sets that profession apart from others. As health information becomes increasingly accessible to patients, a lot of knowledge will no longer be unique to a profession; in fact, much of this information (e.g., disease processes, interventions and associated risks, medications, and therapies in both conventional and alternative medicine) is already available on the Internet. As a result, our patients may be better informed than ever before. When a patient is *well* informed, the partnership between the therapist and patient can be enormously powerful and the patient's own sphere of influence as a healthy lifestyle advocate very profound. Knowing simple key facts about nutrition and exercise, for example, can significantly affect a patient's health and morbidity. Thus access to the "information superhighway" and the resultant increase in patient knowledge can challenge the definition of *profession* in interesting ways and may change the concept of professional responsibility.

One of the truly great challenges that physical therapists face (along with other health professionals) in the twenty-first century is keeping up-to-date with clinically important new information relevant for the way they diagnose and treat patients, not least because of the sheer volume of clinical and relevant biomedical literature. For example, in 1955, there were just two randomized controlled trials of physical therapy.[5,6] In April 2001, there were 2400 listed on the Physiotherapy Evidence Database (PEDro)[7] of the Centre for Evidence-Based Physiotherapy at the University of Sydney. (Web addresses for all databases referred to in this chapter are given at the end of the chapter.)

The volume of clinical literature in medicine was so big in 1995 that Davidoff et al[8] estimated that general physicians who wanted to keep abreast of the journals relevant to their practice would have to examine 19 articles a day, 365 days a year. However, from polls of medical grand rounds' audiences at a number of medical schools in the United Kingdom, Sackett et al[9] found that 75% of medical interns had not read anything about the problems presented by their patients in the previous week and were being taught by senior consultants, up to 40% of whom also had not read anything in the previous week. Even self-reports of medical clinicians' average weekly reading times showed (perhaps not surprisingly) that there was simply no way that medical practitioners could keep abreast of their fields of medicine using traditional approaches, such as perusing journals. This situation, we could predict, is by no means unique to medicine.

The constant but unfilled need for clinically important new information leads to a progressive decline in clinical competence. (Again, the medical profession has been the most intensively researched in this respect.) This progressive decline has been shown in medicine in the knowledge about the care of hypertension, for example. Evans et al[10] and Ramsey et al[11] demonstrated a statistically and clinically significant negative correlation between medical practitioners' knowledge of up-to-date care of hypertension and the years that had elapsed since graduation from medical school. Significantly, Sackett et al[9] showed that the decision to start antihypertensive agents in these patients was better predicted by the number of years since graduation from medical school than by the severity of the target organ damage in the patient.

CHANGES IN WAYS OF ACCESSING INFORMATION

Globalization and technological change have resulted in an exponential increase in access to information concomitant with a knowledge explosion. Health professionals, including medical practitioners and physical therapists, struggle to keep abreast of the published literature relevant to their practice. Health information is now more accessible via the Internet than ever before, and it is available to all who have an interest in it: health professionals, patients, and members of the general public. For the clinician, keeping up-to-date now clearly requires electronic information-searching skills (or access to others with these skills) and critical appraisal skills, particularly for the evaluation of published clinical research trials found through searches; this is in addition to the time needed to keep up-to-date.

Interestingly, Ellyard[2] proposes a new professional: the "knowledge navigator." Technology, Ellyard argues, is making the old demarcation between teacher and librarian more and more blurred. The knowledge navigator emerges from an integration of the traditional role of teacher and librarian. Knowledge navigators, Ellyard[2] states, "could assist learners [clinicians] to seek and find knowledge by gaining access to a wide variety of knowledge resources and to enrich and affirm that knowledge and learning where appropriate. There is also another future role . . . as a mentor who is responsible for assisting and inspiring personal development." Even though they have yet to emerge as a distinct professional group, knowledge navigators already exist. It is vital that physical therapists use them and the services they offer.

Much is being done (and much of this is closely aligned with evidence-based practice) to assist the clinician to quickly and efficiently locate the best evidence to inform practice. The PEDro database is an excellent example of the work of knowledge navigators, although the physical therapists responsible for developing, maintaining, and extending PEDro in the Centre for Evidence-Based Practice at the University of Sydney would probably not yet be familiar with the term. PEDro provides physical therapists (and others) with the most comprehensive database of physical therapy clinical trials, including randomized controlled trials and systematic reviews. Importantly, this site provides for the user, publications that have been critically appraised and given a quality rating. The database includes over 1700 randomized controlled trials, approximately 250 systematic reviews, and over 200 other papers. The knowledge navigators who created PEDro have also identified core journals of evidence-based physical therapy practice and ranked them by trial quality.[12]

CHANGES IN PRACTICE: EVIDENCE-BASED PRACTICE

Thompson-O'Brien and Moreland[19] define *evidence-based practice* as the process of using the results of sound research (as determined by critical appraisal) to guide clinical care within the context of the individual client and local environment. Sackett[3] (the "father" of evidence-based medicine) defines it as "the integration of best research evidence with clinical expertise and patient values."

For many physical therapists (and indeed medical practitioners) evidence-based practice has tended to become synonymous with clinical practice treatment choices determined by evidence from randomized controlled trials and from systematic reviews in such a way and to such an extent, that the clinician's clinical experience and the patient's individual needs and values take second place. Support can be found for this view in that although there has been a large increase in the number of randomized controlled trials, there is still not enough evidence to comprehensively guide practice or to answer many clinical questions. Furthermore, the evidence available is often not of sufficient quality to guide clinical decision making. Indeed, it may be argued that randomized controlled trials generally measure outcomes deemed important by the researcher and are less likely to include outcome measures that patients deem important.[13-18]

This is why it is important to remember Sackett's definition of evidence-based medicine ("the integration of best research evidence with clinical expertise and patient values"). By *best research evidence,* Sackett et al[3] mean clinically relevant research, especially from patient-centered clinical research into, for example, the accuracy and precision of diagnostic tests or the efficacy of particular treatment approaches. This is only one of the key components of Sackett's definition. Clinical expertise and patient values are also key components. *Clinical expertise* is "the ability to use our clinical skills and past experience to rapidly identify each patient's unique health state and diagnosis, their individual risks and benefits of potential interventions and their personal values and expectations," and *patient values* are "the unique preferences, concerns and expectations each patient brings to a clinical encounter, and which must be integrated into clinical decisions if these are to best serve the patient." These authors then go on to emphasize, "When these three elements are integrated, clinicians and patients form a diagnostic and therapeutic alliance which optimises clinical outcomes and quality of life." Thus an adherence to the outcomes of randomized controlled trials of physical therapy *alone* in patient management would not in itself be evidence-based practice. Attention to clinical expertise and patient values is critical as well.

Many clinicians fear that use of an evidence-based practice approach equates with a downgrading of clinical expertise and attention to patient needs and values; the definition by Sackett et al[3] should allay such fears. It remains very important however, that physical therapists know how to access best evidence where this is available and to incorporate it in their care of patients whenever possible. Where such an evidence base does not exist, the physical therapist needs to ensure that clinical decision making is based on a systematic, critically evaluative examination, treatment, and assessment approach and is based on up-to-date biomedical knowledge and pathophysiological considerations. The practicing clinician also needs to be able to ask key questions of critical clinical relevance so that knowledge navigators can explore them and particularly so that researchers within the profession can address them.

CHALLENGES FOR ESTABLISHING EVIDENCE-BASED PRACTICE

Sackett et al[3] have identified four "realizations" that explain the rapid spread of evidence-based medicine and that have been attested to by practicing clinicians. (These realizations are just as relevant for manual therapists or physical therapist clinicians as they are for medical practitioners.) They are as follows:

- A daily need for valid information about diagnosis, prognosis, treatment, and preventative measures
- The inadequacy of traditional sources for this information because they "are out of date (textbooks), frequently wrong (experts), ineffective (electronically delivered continuing professional education) or too over whelming in volume, or too variable in their validity for practical clinical use (medical journals)"[3]
- The disparity between diagnostic skills and clinical judgment, which increases with experience, and up-to-date knowledge and clinical performance, which appear to decline with experience
- The inability to set aside more than 30 minutes per week for relevant reading and study and a virtual inability to be able to find and assimilate the latest evidence when with patients

These realizations or challenges, it could be argued, are almost too overwhelming for busy clinicians in full-time practice if they are to be able to identify the current evidence base (or lack thereof) for what they do and to be better informed. The following actions are strongly recommended to help professionals develop and use an evidence-based practice approach:

1. Use scarce reading time wisely. For example, identify a clinical problem commonly seen in practice (rather than a rare one) and specifically devote reading time to become familiar with the evidence base for its treatment. Using scarce reading time to browse through professional journals for evidence one hopes to recall when it is needed later is not the best use of this time.
2. Have or rapidly develop information-search skills and Internet-access skills. If clinicians are to use scarce reading time effectively, they must develop basic search skills, computer literacy, and Internet-access skills. Mature clinicians without these

skills can arrange for a "knowledge navigator" to assist them. (Examples are a faculty member at the physical therapy school, a librarian at the university library, a clinician with advanced search skills and with similar interests in the area of physical therapy practice.)

Many physical therapists are familiar with MEDLINE (the largest biomedical database), and many begin their searches there. MEDLINE is available on the Internet and is free. It may be accessed through the search engine PubMed, which has a user-friendly search interface; simply typing in *physical therapy*, *neck pain*, and *clinical trial* in the search window, for example, allows a thorough search of these topics. However, many physical therapy journals are not available on MEDLINE but are indexed in another biomedical database, Cumulative Index to Nursing and Allied Health Literature (CINAHL). CINAHL also requires access through the search engine Ovid, which unlike PubMed, requires user fees. Most biomedical libraries provide access to Ovid because it opens the door to a number of databases (CINAHL and EMBASE/Excerpta Medica amongst them) and to a number of secondary information sources or distilled information sources (see point 4).

3. Develop skills to critically appraise clinical research. Many recent physical therapist graduates have critical appraisal skills. Many mature physical therapists, experienced clinicians though they may be, may not. This provides an opportunity for a group of similarly placed clinicians to organize customized continuing professional education to achieve such skills. There are useful published articles (e.g., Greenhalgh[20] and Guyatt et al[21]), and the excellent book by Sackett et al[3] is also invaluable. The second edition has a CD that contains clinical examples, critical appraisals, and background papers from 14 other health disciplines, including physical therapy. These examples can be substituted for the medical practice examples and critical appraisals in the book as one learns about integrating evidence-based practice in one's own clinical setting. There are also Internet sites that help with the critical appraisal of studies, including the Centre for Evidence-Based Physiotherapy (which maintains the Physiotherapy Evidence Database, PEDro). PEDro also has a tutorial to educate users about study validity.

   The importance of educating clinicians to be critical consumers of published clinical research is illustrated by the following example. An intensive evidence-based practice, week-long workshop is a core component of the studies for physical therapists undertaking the advanced specialization Master of Physiotherapy degree at the University of South Australia (in manipulative physiotherapy, sports physiotherapy, or orthopedics and manual therapy, for example). Successful completion of the assessments integral to the workshop results inter alia, in these graduate students becoming accredited PEDro critical appraisers (and early knowledge navigators, to use Ellyard's term). Given that the majority of the physical therapists undertaking these Masters programs are international students, the benefits are extending well beyond Australian shores.

4. Be familiar with distilled literature sources or secondary sources of information in which research studies have already been critically appraised. The important things to know are what these sources are and how to access them. A recently published special issue of *Physiotherapy Theory and Practice* on evidence-based practice[22] is strongly recommended because it introduces the physical therapist to these distilled literature sources. Particularly recommended in this regard are the papers by Walker-Dilks[23] and O'Brien.[24]

   Walker-Dilks[23] states, "Distilled literature sources are becoming popular because they are fast and easy to search, the content has been reviewed for quality and the information is presented in a more usable format." Amongst these sources is the Cochrane Database of Systematic Reviews. Abstracts of these reviews (which summarize and report evidence from clinical trials) are freely available at the Cochrane Website. In addition, there is the Controlled Clinical Trials Register, which is also under the Cochrane banner. Importantly, these include trials reported in journals not indexed in MEDLINE. The Cochrane Library is the electronic source of secondary information produced by the Cochrane Collaboration, an international organization that prepares, maintains, and disseminates systematic reviews of controlled trials. One important "field" of the Cochrane Collaboration is "Rehabilitation and Related Therapies."

Secondary sources of information also include abstract journals. Only high-quality studies that meet defined criteria are included, and these are presented in a structured abstract form. Evidence-Based Medicine is one of these. It is a joint publication by the American College of Physicians and the BMJ Publishing Group; another is the ACP journal produced by the American College of Physicians. Both of these abstract journals are available in CD form in Best Evidence, which is updated annually. It is important to realize that a number of these distilled literature sources need to be accessed using a front-end search engine that requires user fees. Ovid is such a search engine that provides, through its "Evidence-Based Medicine Reviews," access to not only Best Evidence but also the Cochrane Database of Systematic Reviews. User fees may be prohibitive for clinicians, but many libraries provide this access.

Walker-Dilks[23] states that some journals are now including structured abstracts within their individual issues; these are often accompanied by a commentary from an experienced clinician or expert in the field. Three examples are the Critically Appraised Papers (CAPs) section of each issue of the *Australian Journal of Physiotherapy*, the Evidence-Based Orthopedics section of the *Journal of Bone and Joint Surgery* (American volume), and the Patient-Oriented Evidence that Matters (POEMs) component of the *Journal of Family Practice.*

The Internet also provides excellent secondary sources of information such as the Physiotherapy Evidence Database (PEDro). Finally, it is important not to forget that the second edition of *Evidence-Based Medicine* by Sackett et al[3] also has its own website. This website will update the book's contents and resource lists as new evidence or strategies come to light. It also provides links to other evidence-based websites and resources.

CONCLUSION

Many challenges remain. First, when physical therapists do not have comprehensive evidence from randomized controlled trials of physical therapy interventions or well-designed qualitative studies for guidance, they should ensure that they are using validated outcome measures in determining the effects of treatment. They need to be careful wherever possible to ensure that the assessment and treatment approaches used are based on good clinical research. When this is not possible, they need to ensure that they are systematic in clinical decision making and that the treatments provided for patients are based on sound biomedical and pathophysiological knowledge. Second, physical therapists engaged in clinical research must ensure that they get the evidence from sound research to the clinician and into clinical practice. Third, they need to be cognizant of the fact that, overwhelming though the logic may be, there is no clear evidence as yet, that evidence-based practice improves quality of care. Physical therapy as a profession will prosper in the twenty-first century if physical therapists pay due heed and ensure that their practice "integrates the best research evidence with clinical expertise and patient values."[3]

References

1. Rifkin J: *The end of work*, New York, 1995, GP Putman's Sons.
2. Ellyard P: *Ideas for the new millennium*, Melbourne, 1998, Melbourne University Press.
3. Sackett DL, Straus SE, Richardson WS et al: *Evidence-based medicine*, ed 2, Edinburgh, 2000, Churchill Livingstone.
4. Dolence MG: Emerging strategies for 21st century higher education: condition report, Global Learning Systems, Clarememont, Calif, 2001, Michael G Dollenz and Associates.
5. Coyer AB, Curwen IH: Low back pain treated by manipulation: a controlled series, *Br Med J* 1:705, 1955.
6. Harris R, Millard JB: Paraffin-wax baths in the treatment of rheumatoid arthritis, *Ann Rheum Dis* 14:278, 1955.
7. Sherrington C, Moseley A, Herbert R et al: Guest editorial, *Physiother Theory Pract* 17:125, 2001.
8. Davidoff F, Haynes B, Sackett D et al: Evidence based medicine: a new journal to help doctors identify the information they need, *Br Med J* 310:1085, 1995.
9. Sackett DL, Richardson WS, Rosenberg W et al: *Evidence-based medicine*, ed 1, Edinburgh, 1998, Churchill Livingstone.
10. Evans CE, Haynes RB, Birkett NJ et al: Does a mailed continuing education program improve clinician performance? Results of a randomised trial in antihypertensive care, *JAMA* 255:501, 1986.
11. Ramsey PG, Carline JD, Inui TS et al: Changes over time in the knowledge base of practicing internists, *JAMA* 266:1103, 1991.
12. Maher C, Moseley A, Sherrington C et al: Core journals of evidence-based physiotherapy practice, *Physiother Theory Pract* 17:143, 2001.
13. Di Fabio R: Myth of evidence-based practice, *J Orthop Sports Phys Ther* 29:632, 1999.
14. Feinstein AR, Horwitz RI: Problems in the "evidence" of "evidence-based medicine," *JAMA* 103:529, 1997.
15. Greenhalgh T: Narrative based medicine: narrative based medicine in an evidence based world, *Br Med J* 318:323, 1999.
16. Herbert RD, Sherrington C, Maher C et al: Evidence-based practice: imperfect but necessary, *Physiother Theory Pract* 17:201, 2001.
17. Ritchie JE: Using qualitative research to enhance the evidence-based practice of health care providers, *Aust J Physiother* 45:251, 1999.
18. Ritchie JE: Case series research: a case for qualitative method in assembling evidence, *Physiother Theory Pract* 17:127, 2001.
19. Thompson-O'Brien MA, Moreland J: Evidence-based information circle, Physio Can 50:171, 1998.
20. Greenhalgh T: How to read a paper: assessing the methodological quality of published papers, *Br Med J* 315:305, 1997.
21. Guyatt GH, Sackett DL, Cook DJ: User's guide to the medical literature. II. How to use an article about therapy or prevention: are the results of the study valid? *JAMA* 270:2598, 1993.
22. *Physiotherapy Theory and Practice*, 17(3), 2001.
23. Walker-Dilks C: Searching the physiotherapy evidence-based literature, *Physiother Theory Pract* 17:137, 2001.
24. O'Brien MA: Keeping up-to-date: continuing education, practice and improvement strategies, and evidence-based physiotherapy practice, *Physiother Theory Pract* 17:187, 2001.

Websites

American College of Physicians: http://www.acponline.org/journals/acpjc/jcmenu.htm
Best Evidence CD (updated annually): http://www.acponline.org/catalog/electronic/best_evidence.htm
BMJ Publishing Group and the American College of Physicians: http://ebm.bmjjournals.com
Cochrane Database of Systematic Reviews: http://www.update-software.com/cochrane/cochrane-frame.html (This is within the Cochrane Library, which also includes the Controlled Clinical Trials Register.)
MEDLINE through PubMed: http://www4.ncbi.nlm.nih.gov/PubMed/
Ovid (which requires a user fee): Ovid: http://www.ovid.com/ (The site includes a Cumulative Index to Nursing and Allied Health Literature [CINAHL] and EMBASE/Excerpta Medica.)
PEDro: http://www.cchs.usyd.edu.au/pedro/
Sackett et al: *Evidence-based medicine*, ed 2: http://hiru.mcmaster.ca/ebm.htm

Index

A

Abdominal wall, palpation of, 132
Abusive use disorder, musculoskeletal disorders associated with, 383–385
Active physiological mobility test, motion in thorax examined with, 320–321
Activity, role of upper limb neurodynamic test in, 210
Adolescent, complex regional pain syndromes in, 316–317
Adrenal gland, brain stress response and, 303
Adrenocorticotropin hormone, brain stress response and, 303*f*
Aging
  cervical disc affected by, 19
  thoracic injury and, 21–22
Alar ligament test, 131
Allodynia, mechanical, complex regional pain syndromes treatment and, 315
Amputation, phantom pain and, 205
Amygdala, sympathetic nervous system function and, 296
Analgesia
  brain stress response and, 303–304
  manipulation-induced, 218, 221–224
    animal model for, 232
    future research for, 232–233
    neurophysiological basis of, 233
    nonopioid, 221
    opioid, 221
    sympathetic nervous system and, 295, 304
  mobilization-induced, 230–232
  mobilization techniques and, 304–305
  nonopioid, 220, 230–232
    periaqueductal gray matter and, 304
  opioid, 220, 230–232
    periaqueductal gray matter and, 304
  patient-controlled, 202
  periaqueductal gray matter and, 219–220, 304
  somatotopic organization of, 223–224

Page numbers followed by *b* indicate boxes; *f*, figures; *t*, tables.

Analgesia—cont'd
  stimulation-produced, 220
  sympathetic nervous system and, 304–305
  tolerance for, 230, 231
Analgesic drugs, use of, patient examination and, 111
Analgesic tolerance, 231
  definition of, 230
Anesthesia, cervicogenic headache treated with, 252
Ankylosing spondylitis, thoracic pain and, 79
Annulus fibrosus
  innervation of, 63
  whiplash injury and, 41
Anteroposterior oscillatory pressure, intervertebral movement examined with, 135
Anticoagulant drugs, use of, patient examination and, 111
Anxiety, work-related musculoskeletal disorders and, 379
AP. *see* Anteroposterior oscillatory pressure
APA. *see* Australian Physiotherapy Association
Arm
  disorders of, risk factors for, 378
  innervation of, 126
  pain in
    keyboarding associated with, 384
    repetitive work associated with, 376
  referred pain in, 278
  upper, pain in, 70
Arterial dissection, 144–145
  cervical spine manipulation as cause of, 409
Arterial spasm, cervical spine manipulation as cause of, 409
Arteriovenous fistula, causes of, 14
Artery
  carotid
    determination of integrity of, 111
    dissection of, 152
    innervation of, 63–64
  injury to, cervical spine manipulation as cause of, 409

Artery—cont'd
of neck, 63
subclavian, thoracic outlet syndrome and, 131
vertebral, 14
assessment of change in blood flow in, 152
blood flow in, 153
cervical manipulation and injury to, 147–148
cervical spine movement and, 138
change in flow velocity in, 144
dissection of, 144–145
location of, 9
mechanism of injury to, 149–151
occlusion of, 154
peak flow velocity of, 154
symptoms of dissection of, 151
uncovertebral osteophytes and, 20
volume flow rate of, 155
vertebrobasilar
determination of integrity of, 111
risk factors for dissection of, 151
Arthralgia, zygapophyseal joint, 278
Arthritis
neck and upper extremity pain associated with, 380*t*
olecranon-trochlear, neck and upper extremity pain associated with, 381
Arthrokinematic analysis, thoracic motion evaluated with, 323
Arthrokinematics, definition of, 46*t*
Arthrosis, neck and upper extremity pain associated with, 380*t*
Articular system, dysfunction of
cervicogenic headache associated with, 243–244
cervicogenic headache management and, 257
Aspirin, use of, patient examination and, 111
Atlantoaxial joint, 11–12
articulation of, 159
cervical flexion movement and, 12
cervical spine anatomy and, 8–9
innervation of, 62, 63*f*
kinematics of, 27–29
palpation of, 168–169
range of motion of, 28*t*
Atlantooccipital joint, 10–11
cervical flexion movement and, 12
cervical spine anatomy and, 8–9
dislocation of, 10
innervation of, 62, 63*f*
kinematics of, 26–27
palpation of, 134
range of motion of, 27
Atlas
axial rotation of, 28
palpation of, 134
physical examination of, 159
Atlas-axis complex
extension and right rotation of, 165*f*
flexion and left rotation of, 165
flexion and right rotation of, 164*f*
headache symptoms and palpation of, 172
palpation of, 165–167
testing extension and right rotation of, 163
testing of, 161–163
Australian Physiotherapy Association
clinical guidelines for cervical manipulation from, 143–147
premanipulative testing protocol from, 138–143
Autonomic function, interaction of, with motor function, 227–229
Axial rotation
cervical vertebra range of motion and, 31
description of, 32
range of, 29
thoracic, 46
Axis of rotation
cervical, 36–38
instantaneous, 36–38

B

B cell, innervation of, immune response and, 306
Back pain
derangement syndrome as cause of, 358
psychosocial issues and, 362
repeated movements and, 361
workplace injury and, 374
Biomechanical factors, diagnosis of patient and, 99
Blood flow, cerebral, vertebral artery and, 149
Blood pressure, analgesia and, 225
Body, upper, hypermobility of, 196–197
Body alignment, chronic disorders and, 183
Body chart
tracking of symptoms and, 107–108
workload measurement with, 387
Bone, effect of immobilization on, 364
Bone scan, patient medical examination and, 112
Bony anomaly, palpation examination of, 134–135

Bony necrosis, neck and upper extremity pain associated with, 380*t*
Brain
immune system interaction with, 306*f*
pain control and, 303
Brain stress response, description of, 302–304
Brain-stress response, 305
Brainstem
descending pain inhibitory system from, 224
ischemia of, cervical manipulation as cause of, 150, 151
sympathetic nervous system function and, 296
Brown-Sequard's syndrome, 110
Burn, neck and upper extremity pain associated with, 380*t*
Bursitis, neck and upper extremity pain associated with, 380*t*, 381
Butterfly vertebra, formation of, 8

C

Cadence, cervical spine movement and, 36
CAN. *see* Central autonomic network
Cancer, history of, patient examination and, 111
Capsaicin, hyperalgesia effect of, 232
Capsular fibrosis, joint compression caused by, 328
Carotid system, cerebral blood flow and, 149
Carotid tubercle, cervical spine anatomy and, 12
Carpal tunnel syndrome
cervical spine osteoarthritis and, 299
management of, 209
upper limb neurodynamics test and, 204
Cartilage plate, spinal development and, 6
Causalgia, diagnostic criteria for, 309*t*
Central autonomic network, sympathetic nervous system function and, 296
Central nervous system. *see also* Nervous system
bed of, 128
cervicothoracic region examination and, 127
muscles and regulation of, 184–187
pain originating from, 97
upper limb neurodynamics test and, 205
Centralization, repeated movements and, 360–361
Centre for Evidence-Based Physiotherapy, 418
Cerebellum, sensory homunculus and, 204
Cerebrovascular accident, cervical manipulation and, 147
Cervical disc. *see* Disc, cervical
Cervical motion segment, diagram of, 37*f*
Cervical osteoarthritis, 399
Cervical spine
alignment of, 345
anatomy of, 3–25
anterior view of, 16*f*
biomechanics of, 26–44
cadence of motion of, 36
cervicogenic headache and examination of, 300
clinical guidelines for manipulation of, 143–147
combined movements of
active examination and, 124*f*
in examination and treatment, 159–181
development of, 4–6
disorders of
diagnosis of, 274
neck pain and, 399
examination of, 105–137
by combined movements, 160–161
examination of routine movements in, 120
extension of, example of active movement for, 121*f*
extension syndrome in, 347–348
flexion movement of, 12, 18
flexion syndrome in, 351–352
high
combined movements of, 159–172
palpation of, 163–170
hypomobility of, 284
incidence of injury to, 4
injury to
anatomy of, 20–22
mechanisms of, 20–21
innervation of, 20, 22, 61–72
kinesthesia of, neck pain and, 250
longitudinal ligament in, 63
lordosis in, extension syndrome and, 347
lower, 12–20
examination of, 179–181
extension in, 36
flexion in, 36
kinematics of, 29–42
treatment of, 180–181
manipulation of
assessment during, 146
clinical guidelines for, 143–147
clinical trials of, 401–408
complications of, 148–149

Cervical spine—cont'd
manipulation of—cont'd
contraindications for, 140
efficacy of, 401–408
informed consent for, 146–147
rotary, injury associated with, 150
screening test prior to, 152–155
side effects of, 408–409
vascular complications associated with, 150
vertebral artery injury associated with, 147–148
manual therapy techniques applied to, 217–238
measures of motion of, population characteristics and, 244*t*
mechanical diagnosis and therapy for, 355–373
middle
movements of, 172–179
palpation of, 174
treatment of, 175–178
mobilization of
analgesic effects of, 222
clinical trials of, 401–408
efficacy of, 401–408
hyperalgesia and, 221
side effects of, 408–409
sympathetic nervous system affected by, 226
motion segments in, 14–15
movement-impairment syndromes of, 335–354, 344–345, 346–352
movement of, muscle involvement in, 346
muscle flexibility and, 191
muscle spasm and treatment of, 182
osteoarthritis in, carpal tunnel syndrome and, 299
pain in
case study of, 284–289
zygapophyseal joint arthralgia as cause of, 278
pain patterns of, 61–72
passive movement techniques for, 274
premanipulative testing of, 138–158
range of motion of, 14–15, 30*t*, 32*t*, 34–35, 345
disc fissuring and, 17
relative stiffness of, 337
rotation-extension syndrome in, 349–350
rotation-flexion syndrome in, 351
rotation of, during physical examination, 119
rotation syndrome in, 350–351
screening questions about, 110
Cervical spine—cont'd
screening tests for, 152–155
stability of, muscle control for, 247
syndromes associated with, management of, 273–294
therapeutic loading strategies in, 361–362
upper, anatomy of, 8–12
whiplash injury and, 40, 41*f*
Cervical spondylosis, 400
neck and upper extremity pain associated with, 380*t*, 381
Cervical syndrome, 278–292
case study of, 279–281
history of, 275
isolation of, 273–274
management of, 273–294
Cervical vertebra, rotation of, zygapophyseal joint and, 34
Cervico-encephalic syndrome, 23
Cervicogenic disorders, muscle and motor control in, 182–199
Chest
mobility of, in child, 48
pain in, sources of, 78
referred pain patterns in, 78*f*
Chest wall
cervical spine referred pain and, 65
referred pain and, 77
Child
complex regional pain syndromes in, 316–317
mobility of chest in, 48
muscle imbalance in, 188
Chordoma
formation of, 8
notochord cells and, 7
Cigarette smoking, vertebrobasilar artery dissection and, 151
CINAHL. *see* Cumulative Index to Nursing and Allied Health Literature
Cineradiograph, high-speed, range of motion study with, 34–35
Circle of Willis, vertebral artery and, 150
Clinical expertise, definition of, 416
Clinical Guidelines for Premanipulative Procedures for the Cervical Spine, 143–147
Clinical reasoning
characteristics of, 94, 105
definition of, 85, 101
physical examination and, 106
in physical therapy, 85–104
process of, in physical therapy, 86

Clinical trials
design of, 402
neck pain treatment and, 401–408
physiotherapy, database of, 416
of spinal manipulation and mobilization, 401–408
CNS. *see* Central nervous system
Cobb angle, 338
Cochrane Database of Systematic Reviews, 419
Cognition, physical therapist skills and, 91
Cold exposure syndrome, abusive use disorders and, 383
Cold pack, cervicogenic headache treated with, 252
Collaborative reasoning, definition of, 90
Compensatory reflex response, 184
Complex regional pain syndrome, 308–316
Complex regional pain syndromes
in adolescents, 316–317
in children, 316–317
clinical diagnosis of, 310–312
diagnostic criteria for, 309*t*
management of, 312–314
pathophysiology of, 309–310
physical therapy for management of, 312–316
types of, 308
Compression
cervical spine examination and, 125
movement with, in cervical spine examination, 126
Compression syndrome, neck and upper extremity pain associated with, 381
Computed tomography
atlas rotation studied with, 28–29
cervical vertebra range of motion measured with, 31
patient medical examination and, 112
Connective tissue, laxity of, hypermobility associated with, 196
Consent
express, before cervical manipulation, 147
implied, before cervical manipulation, 147
Controlled Clinical Trials Register, 419
Corticosteroid drugs, cervicogenic headache treated with, 253
Corticotropin-releasing hormone, brain stress response and, 303*f*
Costochondral joint, unstable, 326
Costotransverse joint
anterolateroinferior glide of, 325*f*
arthrokinematic glide at, 331
midthorax rotation and, 54
Costotransverse joint—cont'd
pain from, 77
palpation of, 134
rheumatoid arthritis and, 80
stability of, tests for, 326
thoracic
fixated, 331–332
mobility tests for examination of, 323
Costovertebral joint
effect of aging on, 48
thoracic range of motion and, 47
Coupled motion, definition of, 46*t*, 345
Craniocervical flexion test, cervicogenic headache diagnosis with, 248, 249*f*
Craniovertebral hypermobility, tests for, 131–132
Craniovertebral instability, symptoms of, 111
CRPS. *see* Complex regional pain syndrome
Crush, neural syndromes associated with, 299
CT. *see* Computed tomography
Cubital tunnel syndrome, 211
cervical spine osteoarthritis and, 299
Cumulative Index to Nursing and Allied Health Literature, search skills for use of, 418
Cytokine
description of, 305
role of, 306

D

Data, collection of, hypothesis development and, 88–89
De Kleyn's test, 153
Death, cervical spine manipulation as cause of, 409
Defense reaction, description of, 302–304
Defense reflex, neck and shoulder muscles affected by, 185
Degenerative joint disease
cervicogenic headache associated with, 239
joint pain associated with, 80
Degenerative spondylosis, effects of, 19
Dens
atlantoaxial joint complex and, 12
axis vertebra formation and, 11
Dens/atlas osseous stability test, 131
Derangement syndrome
description of, 358–359
therapy for, 363, 366
Dermatome, definition of, 66
Diagnosis
of cervicogenic headache, 238–252
in physical therapy, 89–90

Diagnostic reasoning, definition of, 89
Diencephalon, sympathetic nervous system function and, 296
Differentiation, principles of, active examination and, 119
Diplopia, vertebrobasilar insufficiency associated with, 144
Directional preference, movement patterns and, 361
Disability
  definition of, 95
  hypothesis categories and, 105
  patient subjective examination and, 106
Disc
  C6, symptoms of disorder of, 108
  C7
    symptoms of disorder of, 108
    symptoms typical of lesion of, 107*t*
  cervical
    bulging of, 19
    fissuring of, 17–18
    herniated, 359–360
    innervation of, 62–63, 64*f*, 359
    lumbar disc compared to, 359
    neck and upper extremity pain associated with lesions of, 381
    nucleus pulposus formation and, 15
    referred pain and, 66
    regional characteristics of, 16
  cervical intervertebral, structure of, 32
  degeneration of, nonspecific spinal pain and, 356
  fissuring of, 19
  intervertebral
    herniation of, 79
    innervation of, 22, 62–63
    right rotation thoracic fixation and, 332
    spinal development and, 6
    spine range of motion and, 15
  lumbar
    axial load of, 16
    cervical disc compared to, 15, 359
  thoracic
    innervation of, 76*f*
    pain from, 77
Disc disease, neck and upper extremity pain associated with, 380*t*
Dislocation, neck and upper extremity pain associated with, 380*t*
Distraction
  cervical spine examination and, 125
  movement with, in cervical spine examination, 126
Dizziness
  cervical manipulation as cause of, 143
  limitation on physical examination caused by, 114
  vertebrobasilar insufficiency associated with, 138, 139, 140, 144
Doppler ultrasound, premanipulative screening with, 152, 153
Dowager's hump, 284
Drop attacks, vertebrobasilar insufficiency associated with, 144
Drugs, use of, patient examination and, 111
Dupuytren's contracture, neck and upper extremity pain associated with, 382
Dura matter
  cervical, cervicogenic headache and, 250–251
  thoracic, pain from, 77
Dynamic stability, thoracic mobility and, 326
Dysarthria, vertebrobasilar insufficiency associated with, 144
Dysfunction
  definition of, 95
  hypothesis categories and, 105
  patient subjective examination and, 106
  psychological, 98
  sources of, 98–99
  hypothesis categories and, 106
Dysfunction syndrome
  description of, 357–358
  mechanical deformation of tissue and, 358
  therapy for, 363, 366
Dysphagia, vertebrobasilar insufficiency associated with, 144

E

Earache, screening questions about, 110
Elbow
  extension of, hypermobility and, 197
  flexion of, 195
Embolus, cervical manipulation as cause of, 151
Embryo, human, spinal development and, 5*f*
Emotion, limbic system and regulation of, 185
Environment, diagnosis of patient and, 99
Environment condition syndrome, 385
  neck and upper extremity pain associated with, 380*t*
Ergonomics
  cervicogenic headache management and, 257

Ergonomics—cont'd
complex regional pain syndromes management and, 315
education in, 388
history of, 376
measurement of effects of, 390–391
workplace, 386–387
Ethical reasoning, definition of, 90
Evidence-based practice
establishment of, 417–418
physiotherapy and, 416–419
Examination
palpation, 134–135
passive, 133–136
physical (*see* Physical examination)
subjective
assessment of vertebrobasilar insufficiency during, 144
clinical guidelines for cervical manipulation and, 144–145
components of, 117
Excerpta Medica, search skills for use of, 418
Exercise
instruction for, 90
pause, worker injury prevented by, 389
therapeutic
derangement syndrome treated with, 366–367
dysfunction syndrome treated with, 366
Extensibility, testing of muscle tightness and, 191–193
Extension
active examination of, 119
atlantooccipital joint kinematics during, 26–27
cervical
coupled motions in, 345
screening questions about, 109
of cervical vertebra, 34, 36
functional spinal unit and, 49
low cervical, 124*f*
of lower cervical spine, 36
of lower thorax, 58–59
of midthoracic spine, 120
of midthorax, 50–52
between occiput and atlas, 159
passive physiological movement and, 133
range of motion of cervical spine and, 30*t*
restricted, cervicogenic headache diagnosis and, 244
right rotation combined with
high cervical spine testing by, 161
testing with, 160–162
Extension—cont'd
rotation and, vertebral artery affected by, 153
sustained, vertebral artery affected by, 153
thoracic, 46
example of, 122*f*
upper limb neurodynamic test and, 207
Extension-rotation syndrome, 342
Extension syndrome, 341–342
cervical, 347–348

F

Facet, cervical vertebral, angles of, 13–14
Fainting, vertebrobasilar insufficiency associated with, 144
FASTRAK System, 45
Fatigue, work-related musculoskeletal disorders and, 376
Female, whiplash syndrome and chronic pain in, 20
Fibrosis, capsular, joint compression caused by, 328
Finger, repetitive movement and injury to, 378
Flexibility
movement for, complex regional pain syndromes management with, 314–315
testing of muscle tightness and, 191–193
Flexion
active examination of, 119
atlantooccipital joint kinematics during, 26–27
cervical
coupled motions in, 345
example of, 121*f*
screening questions about, 109
upper limb tension test and, 129
cervical contralateral, upper limb tension test and, 129
of cervical vertebra, 34, 36
craniocervical, testing control of, 265–266
elbow, testing of, 195
functional spinal unit and, 49
head, muscle weakness and, 194
ipsilateral, upper limb tension test and, 129
lateral (*see* Lateral flexion)
in lower cervical spine, 36
of lower thorax, 58–59
of midthoracic spine, 120
of midthorax, 47–49
of mobile thorax, 48
between occiput and atlas, 159

Flexion—cont'd
passive physiological movement and, 133
range of motion of cervical spine and, 30*t*
restricted, cervicogenic headache diagnosis and, 244
right rotation combined with
high cervical spine testing by, 160
testing with, 160–161
shoulder, scapula abduction and, 336
thoracic, 46
bilateral restriction of, 329–330
example of, 122*f*
unilateral restriction of, 330–331
trunk, screening questions about, 110
Flexion syndrome, 342–343
cervical, 351–352
Focal dystonia, receptive field and, 204
Force, progression of, patient self-treatment and, 362–363
Forearm, pain in, 70
keyboarding associated with, 384
Formen magnum, location of, 9
Fracture
burst, 21
end-plate, 21
neck and upper extremity pain associated with, 380*t*
Frontal lobe, descending pain inhibitory system from, 224
FSU. *see* Functional spinal unit
Functional capacity, assessment of, in workplace, 387–388
Functional capacity assessment, worker vocational rehabilitation and, 392
Functional fingerprint, definition of, 301
Functional limitation, definition of, 95
Functional spinal unit, 49, 51–52

G

Ganglion, neck and upper extremity pain associated with, 382
Glenohumeral joint
abduction at, 195
dysfunction of, cervicogenic headache and, 250
hypermobility in, 336
muscle imbalance and, 188
Golfer's elbow, neck and upper extremity pain associated with, 381
Graphesthesia, complex regional pain syndromes diagnosis with, 311
Growth plate, spinal development and, 6
Guyon's tunnel syndrome, cervical spine osteoarthritis and, 299

H

Hand
dysesthesia in, 110
pain in, 70
keyboarding associated with, 384
repetitive movement and injury to, 378
Handhammer function, 383
Head
axial rotation of, 27
cervical spine referred pain and, 65
flexion-extension of, 28
flexion of, muscle weakness and, 194
forward posture of, 286*f*, 288
cervical headache associated with, 357
cervicogenic headache associated with, 243
cervicogenic headache diagnosis and, 243
movement pattern affected by, 337
neck pain associated with, 357
muscles of, 184
disorders of, 187
pain in, cervical extension syndrome and, 348
position of, patient examination and, 117
posture of, muscle imbalance evaluation and, 190
referred pain to, 239
rotation of, hypermobility and, 197
stability of, muscle control for, 247
symmetry of, patient examination and, 118
Headache
cervical, 22
abnormal instantaneous axis of rotation and, 38
forward head posture and, 357
treatment of, 170–171
cervical extension and, 124
cervical origin, 159, 239
cervicogenic
articular system dysfunction and, 243–244
causes of, 239
cervical musculoskeletal dysfunction and, 241–251
definition of, 239
diagnostic criteria for, 239
differential diagnosis of, 238–252
forward head posture associated with, 243
incidence of, 239
management of, 239–270
management program for, 257
migraine without aura differentiated from, 240

Headache—cont'd
  cervicogenic—cont'd
    muscle dysfunction associated with, 247–249
    musculoskeletal characteristics of, 252
    physical therapy for treatment of, 254*t*–256*t*
    symptoms of, 239
    thoracic spine involvement in, 300
    treatment of, 252–258
  differential diagnosis of, 238–252
    manual examination in, 244–245
  keyboarding associated with, 384
  migraine
    cervicogenic headache differentiated from, 240
    differential diagnosis of, 238–252
    incidence of, 239
    vertebrobasilar artery dissection and, 151
  migraine without aura
    classification criteria of, 240*t*
    differential diagnosis of, 238–252
  physical dysfunction and classification of, 242*t*
  school, causes of, 188
  screening questions about, 110
  tension
    classification criteria of, 240*t*
    differential diagnosis of, 238–252
    incidence of, 239
    muscle tone and, 183
  unilateral, intervertebral source for, 135
  unilateral symptoms of, 171
  vertebral artery dissection associated with, 145, 151
Heart rate, analgesia and, 225
Heat pack, cervicogenic headache treated with, 252
Hematoma, cervical manipulation as cause of, 151
Hemivertebra, development of, 8
Hemorrhage, cervical manipulation as cause of, 151
High-arm cross, hypermobility assessment with, 197
Hormone replacement therapy, patient examination and, 112
Horner's syndrome, 152, 300
Hydrotherapy
  complex regional pain syndromes management with, 314
  complex regional pain syndromes treated with, 317
Hypermobility
  assessment of, 196
  constitutional, 196–197
  craniovertebral
    physical examination and, 110
    tests for, 131–132
  muscular, 196–197
  passive examination and, 133
Hypertension, vertebrobasilar artery dissection and, 151
Hypertonus, neck muscles and, 184
Hypoalgesia, definition of, 228
Hypomobility, passive examination and, 133
Hyporeactive immobility, 220
Hypothalamic-pituitary-adrenocortical axis, brain stress response and, 303*f*
Hypothalamic system, defense reflex and, 185
Hypothalamus
  brain stress response and, 303
  sympathetic nervous system function and, 296
Hypothesis
  about prognosis, 100
  development of, perception and, 87–88
  of muscle imbalance, 130
Hypothesis categories
  clinical knowledge and, 94–101
  definition of, 94
Hypothetico-deductive process, 88

I

IAR. *see* Instantaneous axis of rotation
ICR. *see* Instantaneous center of rotation
IHS. *see* International Headache Society
Illness
  sympathetic nervous system and, 305–307
  systemic, cytokines and, 306
Illness script, knowledge base and, 93
Immune system
  brain interaction with, 306*f*
  inhibition of, 306
  sympathetic nervous system and, 301, 305–307
  sympathetic nervous system integration with, 297
Impairment, definition of, 95
Implied consent, before cervical manipulation, 147
Inflammation
  neurogenic, sympathetic nervous system and, 307
  palpation for examination of, 134
Inflammatory joint disease, neck and upper extremity pain associated with, 380*t*

Information
  access to, 415–416
    physical therapy and, 414–415
  growth of, physical therapy and, 414–415
Informed consent, patient
  before cervical manipulation, 146–147
  cervical manipulation and, 140, 141
Injury
  cervical spine, 20–22
  early motion after, 364
  facet, in thoracic articular column, 22
  history of, cervical syndromes associated with, 274
  repetition, work-related, 377
  work-related
    evaluation of programs for prevention of, 389–390
    prevention of, 386–391
  worker, functional capacity assessment and, 387
Instance script, knowledge base and, 93
Instantaneous axis of rotation, 36–38
  abnormal, 38–39
    neck pain associated with, 39
  biological basis of, 39–40
  compression forces and, 40
  location of, 39
  whiplash injury and, 40
Instantaneous center of rotation, 345–346
Insular cortex, sympathetic nervous system function and, 296
Interactive reasoning, definition of, 90
International Association for the Study of Pain
  complex regional pain syndromes algorithm by, 313
  criteria for regional pain syndromes by, 308, 309
  headache classification from, 242*t*
International Headache Society
  classification criteria for migraine without aura from, 240
  diagnostic criteria from, 238
  physical dysfunction in headache classification from, 242*t*
Internet
  growth of, 414
  health information available on, 415
  search skills for use of, 417–418
Interpretation, hypothesis development and, 87–88
Intervertebral joint
  direction of movement and, 277
  movement of, 172, 277
  palpation of, 134
Intervertebral joint—cont'd
  regular movement of, 173
  test movements of, pain response to, 274
Intervertebral space, opening one side of, 277
Interview, patient, 106
  routine screening questions for, 109–110
Irritability, limitation on physical examination caused by, 113
Ischemia, brainstem, cervical manipulation as cause of, 150, 151

J

Jefferson's fracture, 11
Job rotation, worker injury prevented by, 388
Job satisfaction, work-related musculoskeletal disorders and, 379
Joint
  atlantoaxial (*see* Atlantoaxial joint)
  atlantooccipital (*see* Atlantooccipital joint)
  cervical
    cervicogenic headache and dysfunction of, 244
    function of, 3
  compression of, causes of, 328–329
  degenerative changes in, 381
  directional susceptibility to movement in, 334
  diseases of, neck and upper extremity pain associated with, 381
  dysfunction of, cervicogenic headache associated with, 243–244
  effect of immobilization on, 364
  facet, hemarthrosis in, 21
  hypomobility of, restoration of movement in, 276
  impaired rotation of, 338
  interbody, cervical spine and, 14
  intervertebral (*see* Intervertebral joint)
  irritable, mobility regained in, 276
  Luschka, 16–17
  mobilization of, pain modulated by, 233
  occipitoatlantal (*see* Occipitoatlantal joint)
  painful, muscle spasm and, 182
  palpation of, 134
  peripheral, examination of, 132
  relationship of, with muscles, 182
  relative stiffness of, 337
  segmental, dysfunction of, 244
  uncovertebral, 16–17
  zygapophyseal (*see* Zygapophyseal joint)
Joint block, cervicogenic headache diagnosis and, 242

Journal
abstract, information in, 419
professional, information in, 419

K

Keyboarding
disorders associated with, 383–384
musculoskeletal disorders associated with, 378
Kienbock's disease, neck and upper extremity pain associated with, 382
Kinematics
atlantoaxial, 27–29
atlantooccipital, 26–27
definition of, 26
of lower cervical spine, 29–42
Kinesthesia, cervical, cervicogenic headache and, 250
Kinetics, definition of, 26
Knowledge
base of, 92–94
clinical, 93
organization of, 94–101
definition of, 92
organization of, 92–94
physical therapist level of, 91
tacit, 92
Kyphosis
cervicothoracic, 357
neck pain and, 357
thoracic, 339
thoracic osteoporotic, 20
thoracic spine, 345
Kyphotic deformity, 284
wry neck and, 289–290

L

Laceration, neck and upper extremity pain associated with, 380*t*
Lateral epicondylalgia, manipulation-induced analgesia and, 221
Lateral flexion
active examination of, 119
cervical, coupled motions in, 345
in flexion position, 176
low cervical, 124*f*
of middle cervical spine, 172
of midthoracic spine, 120
in neutral position, 176
of occiput, 160
passive physiological movement and, 133
right
in flexion position, 178*f*
in neutral position, 177*f*
Lateral flexion—cont'd
thoracic, 123*f*, 339
upper limb neurodynamic test and, 207
Lateral glide technique
autonomic function affected by, 225
sympathetic nervous system response to, 222*t*
Leg, pain in, repetitive work associated with, 376
Ligament
atlantoaxial joint complex and, 12
in atlantoaxial region, 62
axis vertebra and, 11
cervical, innervation of, 61
effect of immobilization on, 364
laxity of, hypermobility associated with, 196
longitudinal
innervation of, 22
thoracic extension and, 51
nuchal, 9
thoracic, pain from, 77
transverse, atlantoaxial joint and, 11
Light-headedness, vertebrobasilar insufficiency associated with, 144
Limb, upper
cervical spine referred pain and, 65
pain in, 70
Limbic system, role of, in motor control, 185
Locus ceruleus, brain stress response and, 303
Lordosis, lumbar, patient examination and, 117
Low-load craniocervical flexion test, cervicogenic headache diagnosis with, 248
Lower cervical syndrome, 23
Lumbar lordosis, patient examination and, 117
Lymphoid tissue, innervation of, immune response and, 306

M

Magnetic resonance imaging, patient medical examination and, 112
Manipulation
mobilization compared to, 276
spinal
clinical trials of, 401–408
definition of, 400
efficacy of, 401–408
mobilization compared to, 408
neck pain managed with, 400–408
side effects of, 408–409
as treatment technique, 276

Manipulative Physiotherapists Association of Australia, 141–143
Manipulative therapy, cervicogenic headache treated with, 252, 253
Manipulative thrust technique, complications associated with, 150
Manual therapy. *see also* Physical therapy
  analgesia induced by, 218
    future research on, 232–233
  autonomic function affected by, 224–226
  cervical spine and, 217–238
  clinical reasoning in, 85–104
  definition of, 320
  elevation of pressure pain threshold associated with, 222–223
  mechanical alteration of tissue in, 401
  midthorax treatment with, 328–333
  models of, 217–218
  motor function affected by, 227
  neck pain treated with, 399–412
  neurophysiological effects of, 401
  pain-inhibitory effect of, 229
  psychological influences of, 401
  sympathetic nervous system affected by, 225–226
  for thorax, 320–334
  upper limb-neurodynamic test and, 201–202
Maximum possible effect, evaluation of analgesia and, 231
McKenzie system, 355–368
Mechanical neck pain, 400
Median nerve
  mechanosensitivity of, 203
  upper limb neurodynamic test and, 200
Medical expertise, development of, 93
Medical history, patient examination and, 112–113
Mediolateral translation stability test, thoracic mobility and, 327
MEDLINE, search skills for use of, 418
Medulla oblongata, sympathetic nervous system function and, 296
Membrana tectoria, 11
Memory, knowledge base and, 92
Meningomyelocele, description of, 7
Meniscoid inclusion, 18
Menopause, patient examination and, 111
Mesoderm, spinal development and, 4
Mesodermal column
  development of, 4
  formation of, 7
  growth of, 7
Metacarpophalangeal joint, postural overload syndrome and, 383
Metacognition, physical therapist skills and, 91
MIA. *see* Analgesia, manipulation-induced
Microfracture, trabecular, 21
Midbrain
  descending pain inhibitory system from, 224
  periaqueductal gray region of, 219
  sympathetic nervous system function and, 296
Midthorax, 47–58
  biomechanics of, trunk rotation and, 57
  definition of, 46
  flexion in, 47–49
  lateral bending of, 54
  manual therapy for, 328–333
  rotation of, example of, 56*f*
  rotational instability of, 327
Migraine. *see* Headache, migraine
Mind-disease influence, 305
Mobility, active physiological, of thorax, 321
Mobilization
  active, role of upper limb neurodynamic test in, 209–211
  manipulation compared to, 276
  passive, 277
    complex regional pain syndromes management and, 315–316
    neurodynamic tests and, 208–209
  spinal
    clinical trials of, 401–408
    definition of, 400
    efficacy of, 401–408
    manipulation compared to, 408
    side effects of, 408–409
  as treatment technique, 276
Monocyte, innervation of, immune response and, 306
Motion
  cervical, range of, 345
  coupled, definition of, 345
  range of (*see* Range of motion)
Motor control, in cervicogenic disorders, 182–199
Motor cortex, sensory homunculus and, 204
Motor function
  effect of manual therapy on, 227
  interaction of, with autonomic function, 227–229
Motor test, complex regional pain syndromes diagnosis with, 311

Movement
abnormal, physical examination and, 116
active
neurodynamics test and, 207
role of upper limb neurodynamic test in, 210
active physiological, during physical examination, 119–122
amplitude of, 277
cervical
description of, 345–346
measures of, 244*t*
muscle involvement in, 346
cervical extension syndrome and impairment of, 347
cervical flexion syndrome and impairment of, 352
cervical rotation-extension syndrome and impairment of, 349
cervical rotation-flexion syndrome and impairment of, 351
cervical rotation syndrome and impairment of, 350
combined
active examination and, 123–125
in cervical spine examination and treatment, 159–181
examination by, 160–163
lower cervical spine examined by, 179–180
middle cervical spine examined by, 173
middle cervical spine treated with, 175–178
patient response to, 179
differentiation of, 118
direction of, position of joint and, 276–277
directional preference of, 361
extension-rotation syndrome and impairment of, 342
extension syndrome and impairment of, 341–342
flexion syndrome and impairment of, 343
impairment syndromes of spine and, 335–354
irregular, of middle cervical spine, 174
isometric, complex regional pain syndromes management with, 314–315
of middle cervical spine, 172–179
examination of, 173
motor control role in, 337
muscle imbalance and, 187–188
neck, cervicogenic headache and, 243

Movement—cont'd
pacing of, role of upper limb neurodynamic test in, 210
pain response to, 274–275
passive
for cervical syndromes, 274–278
neurodynamics test and, 207
as treatment technique, 276
patterns of, evaluation of, 193–196
pause exercise, 389
physical examination and, 117
prehension pattern in, 186
range of
cervicogenic headache diagnosis and, 244
pain response to, 274–275
regular, description of, 173–174
repeated
McKenzie exercise program and, 361–362
muscle affected by, 334
neck pain and, 361, 367
repetition of, in cervical examination, 125
repetitive
hand and finger injury associated with, 378
individual reaction to, 379
rotation-flexion syndrome and impairment of, 339
rotation syndrome and impairment of, 341
slider, role of upper limb neurodynamic test in, 210–211
speed of, cervical examination and, 125
sustaining of, in cervical examination, 124
symptoms assessed in relation to, 275–276
technique of, 277–278
tensioner, role of upper limb neurodynamic test in, 210–211
upper body, muscle imbalance and, 189–196
Movement-impairment syndrome
cervical, 344–345, 346–352
compensatory motion and, 337
differential diagnosis of, 343–344
muscle imbalance associated with, 334
thoracic spine, 338–343
MPAA. *see* Manipulative Physiotherapists Association of Australia
MPE. *see* Maximum possible effect
Muscle
axioscapular, dysfunction of, 250
axis vertebra and, 11

Muscle—cont'd
biceps, innervation of, 127
central nervous system regulation and, 184–187
cervical
innervation of, 61
performance of, 130
cervical extension syndrome and impairment of, 347–348
cervical flexion syndrome and impairment of, 352
cervical flexor
motor control of, 267–270
spine support and control by, 248
testing and retraining of, 265–270
cervical range of motion and, 346
cervical rotation-extension syndrome and impairment of, 349
cervical rotation-flexion syndrome and impairment of, 351
cervical rotation syndrome and impairment of, 350
cervicogenic disorders and, 182–199
contraction of, headache differential diagnosis and, 246–247
deltoid, innervation of, 127
digastric, tightness in, 187
dorsal neck, spine support and control by, 248
dysfunction of, cervicogenic headache management and, 257
effect of immobilization on, 364
extension-rotation syndrome and impairment of, 342
extension syndrome and impairment of, 342
extensor, spine support and control by, 248
extensor pollicis longus, innervation of, 127
finger flexor, innervation of, 127
flexion syndrome and impairment of, 343
flexor, weakness in, 188
flexor and extensor, action of, 27
hamstring, imbalance of quadriceps to, 334
hypermobility of, 196–197
hypertonic
joint compressed by, 330
joint compression caused by, 328
imbalance of, 187–188
cervicothoracic disorders and, 130
evaluation of, 189–196
hypothesis of, 130
implications for treatment of, 197–198
in lower body, 188

Muscle—cont'd
imbalance of—cont'd
movement-impairment syndromes and, 335–336
movement-impairment syndromes associated with, 335
impaired function of, treatment of, 198
inferior oblique, 12
interscapular, evaluation of, 189
intrinsic, innervation of, 127
laxity of, hypermobility associated with, 196
length of
coupled motions and, 345
headache differential diagnosis and, 246
movement-impairment syndromes and, 336
levator scapula
evaluation of tightness of, 192*f*
extensibility of, 191
levator scapulae, tightness in, 187
longus capitus, spine support and control by, 248
longus colli, spine support and control by, 248
lumbrical, innervation of, 127
masseter, tightness in, 187
multisegmental, spine control by, 247
mylohyoid, weakness in, 188
neck, 183–183
cervicogenic headache management and, 258
hypertonus of, 184
relaxation of, 184
neck flexor
spine support and control by, 248
testing and retraining of, 2650270
pain production and, 183–187
pectoralis, tightness in, 187
pectoralis major
evaluation of, 190
evaluation of tightness of, 192*f*, 193*f*
extensibility of, 191
performance of
cervical spine examination and, 130
physical examination and, 117
physical examination and evaluation of, 115
postural overload syndrome and, 383
quadriceps, imbalance of hamstring to, 334
relationship of, with joints, 182
rhomboid
evaluation of, 189
weakness in, 188

Muscle—cont'd
rotation-flexion syndrome and impairment of, 339–340
rotation syndrome and impairment of, 341
scalene, 13
tightness in, 187
scapular elevator, innervation of, 127
serratus anterior
evaluation of, 190
imbalance of trapezius to, 336
scapular position affected by, 250
weakness in, 188
winging of scapula and, 195
shoulder, 183–184
innervation of, 127
shoulder girdle, 184
cervicogenic headache management and, 258
spasm in, pain associated with, 192
sternocleidomastoid
testing of, 191
tightness in, 187
stiffness of, movement-impairment syndromes and, 336
suprahyoid, weakness in, 188
temporalis, tightness in, 187
tenderness in, headache diagnosis and, 245–246
thoracic
pain from, 77
performance of, 130
thoracic pain from, 80
tightness in, movement affected by, 187
tightness of
hypermobility and, 196
testing of, 191–193
trapezius
evaluation of, 189
evaluation of tightness of, 192*f*
extensibility of, 191
imbalance of serratus anterior to, 336
repetitive manual work and injury to, 377
scapular position affected by, 250
tightness in, 187
weakness in, 188
triceps, innervation of, 127
trigger point in, headache differential diagnosis and, 245–246
weakness of, movement patterns affected by, 193–196
Muscle spasm, neck, 184
Muscle stretching, cervicogenic headache treated with, 252
Muscle tightness, headache differential diagnosis and, 246
Muscle tone, pain production and, 182–183
Musculoskeletal system
cervicogenic headache and characteristics of, 252
disorders of
abusive use as cause of, 383–385
classification of, 380–385
degenerative, 381–382
history of research of, 375–378
physical loading and, 379
prevention of, 386–391
risk factors for, 378
worker education for prevention of, 390
in workplace, 374–398
dysfunction of
cervicogenic headache and, 241–251
muscle imbalance and, 197
physical loading of, disorders associated with, 379
physiology of, 26
treatment of pain in, 202
Myelopathy, spinal cord compromise and, 110
Myotome
definition of, 66
mesodermal column formation and, 7

N

Naloxone
manual therapy analgesia and, 230–231
opioid analgesia and, 220
opioid analgesia blocked by, 230
Narrative reasoning, definition of, 90
Nausea
cervical manipulation as cause of, 143
vertebrobasilar insufficiency associated with, 144
Neck
arteries of, 63
disorders of, risk factors for, 378
dysfunction of, repetitive work associated with, 374
flexion of, compression and, 125
limbic system effect on, 185
manual therapy for, 217
movement restriction of, cervicogenic headache and, 243
muscle imbalance and, 188
muscles in, 183–184
disorders of, 187
somatic pain and, 61
pain in (*see* Neck pain)
position of, patient examination and, 117

Neck—cont'd
range of motion of, 29, 34–35
relaxation of, 184
stability of, muscle control for, 247
Neck pain, 61, 399–400
abnormal instantaneous axis of rotation and, 39
acute, clinical trials for, 403–408
cervical extension syndrome and, 348
cervicogenic headache and, 249
cervicothoracic kyphosis and, 357
chronic, clinical trials for assessment of therapy for, 408
classification system for, 400
clinical trials for assessment of efficacy of therapy for, 404*t*, 405*t*–407*t*
clinical trials of therapy for, 401–408
conceptual model for, 359–360
costs associated with, 399
criteria for assessment of clinical trials of manipulation for, 403*t*
derangement syndrome as cause of, 358
disorders associated with, 380*t*, 382
dysfunction syndrome and, 357–358
forward head posture and, 357
manual therapy for treatment of, efficacy of, 399–412
mechanical, 400
mechanical strain as cause of, 357
mechanical syndromes in, 356–360
non-specific, 399
prevalence of, 399
recurrent nature of, 363–364
repeated movement for reduction of, 367
repeated movements and, 361
repetitive work associated with, 374, 376
role of muscles in, 183
unilateral, 275
vertebral artery dissection associated with, 145, 151
in workplace, 374–398
Neck sprain syndrome, 23
Nerve
cervical
distribution of pain from, 69
roots of, 20
cervical sinuvertebral, 63*f*
dorsal rami, somatic pain and, 61
entrapment of, abusive use disorders and, 383
function of, impairment of, 126
mobility of, examination of, 128
palpation of, 129–130
complex regional pain syndromes diagnosis with, 312
Nerve—cont'd
physical compromise of, cervicogenic headache and, 250–251
sinuvertebral, 22
thoracic dorsal rami, 73–74
thoracic sinuvertebral, 75–77
ulnar, impingement of, 299*f*
ventral rami
ligaments innervated by, 61
location of, 62*f*
Nerve bed, description of, 128
Nerve block, cervicogenic headache diagnosis and, 242
Nerve conduction, tests of, 127
Nerve root
C6, compression of, 108
cervical radicular pain and involvement of, 291
Nervous system
autonomic, function of, 224
central (*see* Central nervous system)
conduction in, physical examination and, 117
dysfunction of, cervicogenic headache management and, 257
examination of, 126–130
peripheral
cervicothoracic region examination and, 127
nerve bed of, 128
physical examination and evaluation of, 115
sympathetic
analgesia and, 304–305
efferent, 307–316
illness and, 302–307
immune response and, 305–307
inflammation and, 307
inhibition of, 220
manual therapy and, 225–226
new concepts of, 296
organization of, 302*f*
pain and, 295–296
pain perception and, 228
peripheral, 296–302
spinal, 296–302
tissue repair and, 307
upper limb neurodynamic test and, 203–205
Neural conduction, impairment of, 126–127
Neural tissue, distortion of, 299
Neural tube
spinal development and, 4, 5*f*
vertebral column growth and, 7

Neurodynamic procedure, cervical spine examination and, 124
Neurodynamic test
complex regional pain syndromes diagnosis by, 312
median nerve affected by, 207–208
passive mobilization and, 208–209
upper limb, 200–214
Neurodynamics
tissue health explained by, 208
upper limb test and, 200–214
Neuroendocrine system
chronic pain and, 98
sympathetic nervous system integration with, 297
Neuroimmune system, chronic pain and, 98
Neuromeningeal tissue, test movements of, pain response to, 274
Neuron
postganglionic, 300
preganglionic, 300
sympathetic nervous system function and, 298
Nociceptor
brain stress response and, 303–304
mechanical, 223
peripheral, manipulation-induced analgesia and, 218
thermal, 223
Nonsteroidal antiinflammatory drugs
cervicogenic headache treated with, 252, 253
complications associated with use of, 148
patient examination and, 112
Noradrenaline, mechanical nociception and, 223
Noradrenergic system, analgesia and, 304
Notochord
development of, 4
spinal development and, 5*f*
vertebral column growth and, 7
Notochordal cell, nucleus pulposus formation and, 15
NSAID. *see* Nonsteroidal antiinflammatory drugs
NTS. *see* Nucleus tractus solitarii
Nucleus pulposus, development of, 15–16
Nucleus tractus solitarii, sympathetic nervous system function and, 296
Numbness
occipital, source of symptoms and, 110
radiculopathy indicated by, 68
Nystagmus, vertebrobasilar insufficiency associated with, 139

O

Occipitoatlantal complex
examination of, by combined movements, 160–161
headache symptoms and palpation of, 172
palpation of, 165
testing extension and right rotation of, 162*f*
testing flexion and right rotation of, 161*f*
Occipitoatlantal joint
articulation of, 159
movement of, 160
Occiput
lateral flexion of, 160
physical examination of, 159
Occupational cervicobrachial disorder, 376, 399
Occupational health nurse, in workplace, 391
OCD. *see* Occupational cervicobrachial disorder
Odontoid process, axis vertebra formation and, 11
Oral contraceptive, vertebrobasilar artery dissection and, 151
Ossification, spinal development and, 6
Osteoarthritis
cervical, 399
neck and upper extremity pain associated with, 382
pain associated with, 358
Osteokinematic analysis, motion in thorax and, 320
Osteokinematics, definition of, 46*t*
Ovako working postures analyzing system, workload measurement with, 387
Overpressure, use of, in active examination, 120
Overuse syndrome, 384–385
neck and upper extremity pain associated with, 380*t*
OWAS. *see* Ovako working postures analyzing system

P

PA. *see* Posteroanterior oscillatory pressure
PAG. *see* Periaqueductal gray matter
Pain
arm
cervical rotation for diagnosis of, 124
repetitive work associated with, 376
autonomic function and, 228–229
categories of mechanisms of, 95–97
central, 97

Pain—cont'd
centralization of, 360–361
cervical
case study of, 275, 284–289
muscle spasm and, 182
referred, 65
zygapophyseal joint arthralgia as cause of, 278
cervical radicular, 290–292
of cervical spine, 61–72
cervicogenic, posteroanterior glide technique for, 229
chronic, 98
management of, 202
whiplash injury associated with, 21
compressing movement and, 275
control of, brain areas associated with, 303
discogenic, 284–289, 360
conceptual model for, 359–360
distribution of, cervical nerve and, 69
end-of-range of movement and, 275
inhibitory systems for, 219–220
instantaneous axis of rotation and, 39
interaction of, with autonomic function and motor function, 227–229
interscapular, 21
irritability of, symptoms assessed in relation to, 276
leg, repetitive work associated with, 376
manipulation-induced analgesia and control of, 218
mechanical stimulus and, 108
mechanisms of, 95–98
medial scapular, 289
muscle as pathogenic factor in, 183–187
muscle tone and, 182
musculoskeletal
biomechanical impairments associated with, 337
joint directional susceptibility to movement and, 337
movement system approach to, 338
sympathetic nervous system and, 295
treatment of, 202
neck
biomechanical impairments associated with, 337
cervical extension syndrome and, 348
incidence of, 183
manual therapy for, 217
mechanical strain as cause of, 357
mechanical syndromes in, 356–360
unilateral, 275
vertebral artery dissection associated with, 145

Pain—cont'd
neck—cont'd
vertebral artery dissection indicated by, 151
night, diagnosis and, 109
nociceptive, 97, 98
nonspecific spinal, description of, 356
patterns of, in chest, 78*f*
peripheral neurogenic, 97
peripheralization of, 360–361
phantom-limb, 204–205
pressure, elevation of threshold of, 222
radicular, 68–71
cervical, 69
lumbar, 69
referral patterns of, 22–23
referred, 64–65
to head, 239
herniated disc and, 360
patterns of, 66–67, 77–78
provocation of, 277
test movement for diagnosis of, 275
scapular, 359
cervical rotation for diagnosis of, 124
segmental inhibitory mechanisms for, 218
severity of, symptoms assessed in relation to, 276
somatic, cervical spine and, 61–64
somatic motor, 97–98
somatic referred, 64–65
definition of, 65
radiculopathy and, 68
stretching movement and, 275
suboccipital, keyboarding associated with, 384
suprascapular
keyboarding associated with, 384
treatment of, 175
sympathetic nervous system and, 295–296, 307–316
thoracic
derangement syndrome as cause of, 358
muscle spasm and, 182
pathology of, 79–80
in thoracic region, sources of, 77
threshold for, elevation of, 222
through range of movement, 275, 278
trunk, repetitive work associated with, 376
understanding of behavior of, 357
upper extremity
disorders associated with, 380*t*, 382
in workplace, 374–398
visceral referred, definition of, 65

PAIVM. *see* Passive accessory intervertebral movement
Pallor, vertebrobasilar insufficiency associated with, 145
Palpation
abnormal, physical examination and, 116
cervical examination and, 134–135
complex regional pain syndromes diagnosis by, 312
of lower cervical spine, 179–181
of middle cervical spine, 174
of rib, 179–180
testing with, 163–170
unilateral headache symptoms and, 171
Parabrachial nucleus, sympathetic nervous system function and, 296
Paraesthesia, occipital, source of symptoms and, 110
Paravertebral ganglia
somatic tissues innervation and, 300
sympathetic nervous system function and, 298
Passive accessory intervertebral movement, 135–136
Passive accessory mobility test, examination of thoracic motion with, 323–328
Passive physiological intervertebral movement, 133
Passive physiological mobility test, examination of thoracic motion with, 322
Pathobiological mechanism, hypothesis categories and, 105
Patient
communication with, by physical therapist, 89
general health of, 111
information sources available to, 414
informed consent from, 140
interaction of, with therapist, 86
medical evaluation of, 112
medical history of, 112–113
personal profile of, 106
physical examination of, 105
prognosis for, 100–101
self-treatment by, 362
subjective examination of, 106–112
therapist observation of, 87
Patient education
about neck pain, 364
musculoskeletal pain treatment and, 202
physical therapy intervention and, 90
promotion of, 91
Pattern-recognition, process of, hypothesis development and, 88
PEDro. *see* Physiotherapy Evidence Database
Pelvis
motion in, 337
posture affected by, 186
rotation of, 336–337
Perception, hypothesis development and, 87–88
Periaqueductal gray matter
brain stress response and, 303–304
columnar structure of, 219
dorsal system, 304
mediation of analgesia in, 304
pain modulation and, 233
sympathetic nervous system function and, 296
ventral system, 304
Peripheralization, repeated movements and, 360–361
Peritendinitis, work-related, 375, 377
Personality, work-related musculoskeletal disorders and, 379
Phantom-limb pain, 204–205
Physical examination
active, 118–126
assessment during, 136
assessment of vertebrobasilar insufficiency during, 144
cervical headache and, 170–171
cervicogenic headache diagnosis by, 244–245
components of, 117–118
data collection during, 89
description of, 115–118
full, 114–115
interpretation of results of, 146
limitations on, 113
planning for, 113–115
precautions about, 110–112
premanipulative procedures for cervical spine and, 145–146
premanipulative testing protocol and, 139
signs of potential involvement in, 116–117
subjective, 106–112
Physical therapist
collaboration with patient by, 91
communication with patient by, 89
interaction of, with patient, 86
Physical therapy. *see also* Manual therapy
cervicogenic headache treated with, 252, 254*t*–256*t*
changing nature of, 413–421
for child with complex regional pain syndromes, 316

Physical therapy—cont'd
  chronic neck pain treated with, 408
  clinical reasoning in, 85–104
  clinics in, 295–320
  collaborative reasoning in, 87*f*
  complex regional pain syndromes managed with, 312–316
  contraindications to, 100, 110–112
  diagnosis in, 89–90
  evidence-based practice in, 416–419
  future of, 413–421
  intervention in, 90–91
  lack of benefit of, 365
  reassessment in, 90–91
  scan inquiries in, 88
  search strategies in, 88
Physiotherapy Evidence Database, 415, 416, 419
Pituitary gland, brain stress response and, 303
Plasma extravasation, inflammation and, 307
PNF. *see* Proprioceptive neuromuscular facilitation
Pons, sympathetic nervous system function and, 296
Posterior gliding, forward head posture and, 286*f*
Posteroanterior glide technique
  autonomic function affected by, 225
  cervicogenic pain treated with, 229
  example of, 280*f*
  motor function affected by, 227
  sympathetic nervous system response to, 222*t*
Posteroanterior oscillatory pressure
  example of, 287*f*
  spinous process examined with, 135
Posteroanterior pressure, in right rotation and flexion, 176
Postfacilitation inhibition, muscle imbalance and, 197
Postisometric relaxation, muscle imbalance and, 197
Postural overload syndrome, 383–384
  neck and upper extremity pain associated with, 380*t*
Postural reflex, 185
Postural syndrome
  neck pain associated with, 356–357
  therapy for, 365–366
Posture
  abnormal, cervicogenic headache diagnosis and, 242
  body, muscle dysfunction and, 198
Posture—cont'd
  central nervous system regulation of, 184
  cervical, patient examination and, 117
  flexion syndrome and, 343
  forward head, 285*f*, 288
    cervical headache associated with, 357
    cervicogenic headache diagnosis and, 243
    movement pattern affected by, 337
    neck pain associated with, 357
  head, muscle imbalance evaluation and, 190
  physical examination and, 117
  reflexes and, 185
  sitting, patient examination and, 118
  sources of symptoms and, 109
  symptoms assessed in relation to, 276
  thoracic, patient examination and, 117
Posture targeting, workload measurement with, 387
PPIVM. *see* Passive physiological intervertebral movement
Ppt
  see Pressure pain threshold
Pragmatic reasoning, definition of, 90
Predictive reasoning, definition of, 90
Prefrontal cortex, sympathetic nervous system function and, 296
Premanipulative Testing Protocol, 138–143
  description of, 139
  evaluation of, 140–143
Pressure pain threshold, 223–224
  headache differential diagnosis and, 245–246
  maximum possible effect and, 231
Primitive vertebral column, spinal development and, 4
Procedural reasoning, definition of, 89
Profession, definition of, 414
Prognosis, hypothesis categories and, 106
Pronator syndrome, abusive use disorders and, 383
Proprioception, loss of, radiculopathy indicated by, 68
Proprioceptive neuromuscular facilitation, 184
Proteoglycan, cervical disc and, 16
Protocol for Premanipulative Testing of the Cervical Spine, 138–143
Proximal crossed syndrome, 188
Pseudoaneurysm, cervical spine manipulation as cause of, 409
Psychological factors, work-related musculoskeletal disorders and, 379

Psychosocial factors, diagnosis of patient and, 99
Psychosocial features, patient subjective examination and, 106
PubMed, search skills for use of, 418
Pulse, peripheral, examination of, 131
Push up, muscle weakness evaluation and, 194

Q

Quebec Task Force on Spinal Related Disorders, 400

R

Radial nerve neural tissue provocation test, 225
Radiculopathy, description of, 68–69
Radiofrequency therapy, cervicogenic headache treated with, 252
Radiography
  biplanar
    atlas rotation studied with, 28
    cervical vertebra range of motion measured with, 31
  patient medical examination and, 112
Randomized control trial
  criteria for assessment of, 403*t*
  neck pain therapy assessed with, 404*t*, 405*t*–407*t*
  neck pain therapy assessment and, 402
Range of motion
  abnormal, 38
  of atlantoaxial joint, 28*t*
  of atlantooccipital joint, 27
  cervical, 345
  cervical movement-impairment syndromes and, 344
  of cervical spine, 30*t*, 32*t*
  intersegmental, 35
  of neck, 29, 34–35
  thoracic, 47
Range of movement
  altered, passive examination and, 133
  cervical spine anatomy and, 14–15
  cervicogenic headache diagnosis and, 244
Rapid upper limb assessment, workload measurement with, 387
RCT. *see* Randomized control trial
Reasoning
  clinical (*see* Clinical reasoning)
  collaborative, in physical therapy, 87*f*
  types of, 89–90
Receptive field, concept of, 204
Rectus capitis posterior minor, location of, 9
Reflex response, compensatory, 184
Reflex sympathetic dystrophy
  diagnostic criteria for, 309*t*
  neck and upper extremity pain associated with, 380*t*
Reflexes, testing of, 127
Rehabilitation
  vocational, 392–393
  worker, 391–393
Relaxation, postisometric, 184
Repetition strain injury, work-related, 377
Respiratory rate, analgesia and, 225
RF. *see* Receptive field
Rheumatoid arthritis
  neck and upper extremity pain associated with, 380*t*
  thoracic pain and, 80
Rib
  midthoracic rotation and, 57
  palpation of, 179–180
  posterior rotation of, 50
  right rotation thoracic fixation and, 332
  segmental mobility of thorax and, 323–324
  thoracic rotation and, 50–51
  thoracic vertebra motion and, 321
Righting reflex, 185
Rotation
  active examination of, 119
  cervical
    muscle control of, 346
    during physical examination, 119
    physical examination and, 145
  contralateral, in midthorax, 55
  costovertebral joint and, 48
  extension and, vertebral artery affected by, 153
  flexion combined with, high cervical spine testing by, 160
  instantaneous center of, 345–346
  ipsilateral, in midthorax, 55
  low cervical, 124*f*
  of lower thorax, 59
  of middle cervical spine, 172
  midthoracic, 55–58, 120, 123*f*
  passive physiological movement and, 133
  pelvis, 336–337
  range of motion and, cervical movement-impairment syndromes and, 344
  restricted, cervicogenic headache diagnosis and, 244
  right
    in flexion position, 176, 177*f*
    in neutral position, 175–176

Rotation—cont'd
sustained, vertebral artery affected by, 153
thoracic, 46, 324
during physical examination, 119
range of, 338
unilateral restriction of, 331
of thoracic vertebra, 321
upper limb neurodynamic test and, 207
Rotation-extension syndrome, cervical, 349–350
Rotation-flexion syndrome, 339–340
cervical, 351
Rotation syndrome, 340–341
cervical, 350–351
Rotoscoliosis, segmental, 330
RSI. *see* Repetition strain injury
RULA. *see* Rapid upper limb assessment

S

Scan inquiry, definition of, 88
Scapholunate advanced collapse, neck and upper extremity pain associated with, 382
Scapula
abduction of, 336
dysfunction of, cervicogenic headache and, 250
innervation of, 22
position of, patient examination and, 117
rotation of, 195
winging, 190
causes of, 195
Scapular abduction syndrome, 343
Scheuermann's disease, 21
Sclerotome, definition of, 66
Scoliosis
dysfunction of pelvis and, 186
thoracic spine rotation and, 339
Screening test, cervical manipulation and, 152–155
SD. *see* Standard deviation
Seatbelt injury, right rotation thoracic fixation and, 332
Segmental costal stability test, thoracic mobility and, 326–327
Segmental spinal stability test, thoracic mobility and, 326
Self-care, musculoskeletal pain treatment and, 202
Self-mobilization, McKenzie exercise program and, 362
Self-motivation, musculoskeletal pain treatment and, 202
Self-treatment
McKenzie exercise program and, 362
progression of force in, 362–363
Sensation, impairment of, complex regional pain syndromes diagnosis and, 311
Sensorimotor stimulation, description of, 198
Sensory homunculus, description of, 203
Sensory test, complex regional pain syndromes diagnosis with, 311
Seronegative spondyloarthropathy, neck and upper extremity pain associated with, 380*t*
Serotonin, thermal nociception and, 223
Sharp-Purser test, 131
Shoulder
abduction of, 195
elevated, muscle tightness indicated by, 190*f*
innervation of, 127
limbic system effect on, 185
muscles in, 183–184
scapula abduction in, 336
Shoulder crossed syndrome, 188
Shoulder girdle
cervical spine referred pain and, 65
elevation of, 195
muscles in, 184
pain in, 70
position of, patient examination and, 118
repetitive manual work and injury to, 377
work-related musculoskeletal disorders of, 375
Sick leave, worker, musculoskeletal disorders and, 375
Skin
conductance of
analgesia and, 225
manipulation-induced analgesia and, 226
temperature of
analgesia and, 225
manipulation-induced analgesia and, 226
Slider movement, description of, 210–211
Slump test, 127, 128–129
complex regional pain syndromes diagnosis with, 312
Smoking. *see* Cigarette smoking
SNS. *see* Nervous system, sympathetic
Soft tissue
degenerative changes in, 381
effect of immobilization on, 364

Soft tissue—cont'd
neck and upper extremity pain associated with, 380*t*
palpation of, 134
texture of, physical examination and, 117
Soft tissue disease, neck and upper extremity pain associated with, 380*t*
Somatosensory cortex, receptive fields of, 204
Somatosensory homunculus, description of, 203
Somite
mesodermal column formation and, 7
spinal development and, 4, 5*f*
Spina bifida, description of, 7
Spinal cord
compromise of, signs of, 110
degenerative disc and, 20
determination of integrity of, 111
growth of, 7
injury to, cervical spine manipulation as cause of, 409
reflex pathways in, 301
Spine
cervical (*see* Cervical spine)
development of, 4–6
cartilaginous stage of, 6
mesodermal stage of, 4–5
osseous stage of, 6
function of, 3
growth of, 6
lumbar, examination of, by combined movements, 160–161
manipulation of
for neck pain, 400–408
side effects of, 408–409
midcervical, thoracic movement and, 52
midthoracic, examination of routine movements in, 120
mobilization of
for neck pain, 400–408
side effects of, 408–409
normal movement of, physical examination and, 114–115
segmentation of, 7–8
stability of, muscle control for, 247
thoracic (*see* Thoracic spine)
thoracolumbar, 3
vertebral abnormalities in, 7–8
Spinous process, palpation of, 134
Spleen, innervation of, immune response and, 306
Spondylosis
cervical spine as site of, 284
degenerative, effects of, 19
Stability test, thoracic mobility examined with, 324–326
Staged craniocervical flexion test, motor function affected by, 227
Standard deviation
cervical spine range of motion measurement and, 30
range of axial rotation measurement and, 29
range of motion studies and, 27
Standing, analysis of muscles in, 189–190
Stereognosis, complex regional pain syndromes diagnosis with, 311
Sternocostal joint, unstable, 326
Sternum, right rotation thoracic fixation and, 332
Steroid drugs, use of, patient examination and, 111
Stiffness
muscle, definition of, 336
testing of muscle tightness and, 191–193
Straight leg raise test, complex regional pain syndromes diagnosis with, 312
Stress
behavioral response to, 305
limbic system and, 185
pain associated with, 97
reproduction of patient symptoms by, 116–117
work-related musculoskeletal disorders and, 379
Stroke, cervical manipulation and, 147, 151
Structural differentiation, concept of, 207
Subluxation, neck and upper extremity pain associated with, 380*t*
Substance P, inflammation and, 307
Supraspinous fossa, referred pain in, 278
Sweating, vertebrobasilar insufficiency associated with, 145
Sympathetic ganglia, sympathetic nervous system function and, 298
Sympathetic outflow, description of, 298
Sympathetic slump test, complex regional pain syndromes diagnosis with, 312
Sympathoexcitation, definition of, 228
Symptoms
behavior of, 99, 108–112
character of, 107–108
depth of, 107–108
hypotheses about, 99
mechanical stimulus of, 108–109
pattern of, 109
provocation of, limitation on physical examination caused by, 113

Symptoms—cont'd
reproduction of, during physical examination, 117
severity of, 107–108
site of, 107–108
source of, structural stability and, 110–111
sources of, 98–99
hypothesis categories and, 106
of vertebrobasilar insufficiency, 139
assessment of, 144
Systolic/diastolic ratio, vertebral artery blood flow and, 153

T

T cell, innervation of, immune response and, 306
Task analysis, prevention of injuries in workplace and, 386–387
Tautness, testing of muscle tightness and, 191–193
Teaching, reasoning and, 90
Tectorial membrane test, 131
Telencephalon, sympathetic nervous system function and, 296
Temperature test, complex regional pain syndromes diagnosis with, 311
Tendon, effect of immobilization on, 364
Tendonitis, abusive use disorders and, 383
Tennis elbow, neck and upper extremity pain associated with, 381
Tenosynovitis
neck and upper extremity pain associated with, 381
work-related, 375, 377
Tension neck syndrome, 399–400
Tensioner movement, description of, 210–211
Thalamus, sensory homunculus and, 204
Thoracic osteoporotic kyphosis, 20
Thoracic outlet syndrome, 131, 400
neck and upper extremity pain associated with, 381
Thoracic spine
alignment of, 338, 345
biomechanics of, 45
cervicogenic headache and examination of, 300
examination of, 46, 105–137
examination of routine movements in, 120
extension of, example of active movement for, 122*f*
extension-rotation syndrome in, 342
extension syndrome in, 341–342
Thoratic spine—cont'd
flexion of, example of active movement for, 122*f*
flexion syndrome in, 342–343
injury to, 21–22
innervation of, 73–81
kyphotic, 345
lateral flexion in, 339
low, examination of, 122
mechanical diagnosis and therapy for, 355–373
movement-impairment syndromes of, 335–354, 338–343
muscle flexibility and, 191
muscle spasm and treatment of, 182
pain patterns in, 73–81
relative stiffness of, 337
rotation-flexion syndrome in, 339–340
rotation of
during physical examination, 119
range of, 338
rotation syndrome in, 340–341
screening questions about, 110
upper, examination of routine movements in, 120
Thoracolumbar outflow, description of, 298
Thorax
bilateral restriction of flexion of, 329–330
biomechanics of, 45–60
examination of segmental motion in, 320–328
lower, 58–59
biomechanics of, 58–59
definition of, 46
rotation of, 59
manual therapy for, 320–334
mobile, 322
extension of, 50
flexion and, 48
flexion in, 49*f*
osteokinematic analysis of, 320
range of motion of, 47
rotation fixation of, 332
rotation of, 324
segmental mobility of, 323
stability tests for, 324–326
stiff, 49, 321
extension of, 51
unilateral restriction of flexion of, 330–331
unilateral restriction of rotation of, 331
Thrombosis, cervical manipulation as cause of, 151

Thrust technique
fixated costotransverse joint treated with, 331
side effects of, 408
thoracic fixation treated with, 332
Thumb, hyperextension of, hypermobility and, 197
Thymus, innervation of, immune response and, 306
Tinnitus, vertebrobasilar insufficiency associated with, 144
Tissue. *see also* Soft tissue
contracted, stretching of, 277
effect of immobilization on, 364
examination of, complex regional pain syndromes diagnosis with, 311
manual therapy for mechanical alteration of, 401
neural, distortion of, 299
Tonic neck reflex, 185
Torticollis, description of, 289
Traction
cervical, 292
cervical spine pain treated with, 286
cervicogenic headache treated with, 252
longitudinal, applied to thorax, 329
nerve root pain in cervical spine treated with, 291
Transcutaneous electrical nerve stimulation
cervicogenic headache treated with, 252
complex regional pain syndromes management with, 314
Transverse ligament test, 131
Trauma
cervical, vertebrobasilar insufficiency associated with, 145
cervicogenic headache associated with, 239
complex regional pain syndromes associated with, 308
in child, 316
fixated costotransverse joint caused by, 331
musculoskeletal disorders associated with, 375
Trigeminocervical nucleus, headache and, 239
Trigger finger, neck and upper extremity pain associated with, 381
Trigger point
headache differential diagnosis and, 245–246
muscle imbalance and, 187
pain production and, 183
testing of muscle tightness and, 191
Trigger point therapy, cervicogenic headache treated with, 252
Trunk
biomechanics of lower thorax and, 59
motion of, thoracic flexion and, 53
pain in, repetitive work associated with, 376
rotation of, midthorax biomechanics and, 57

U

ULNT. *see* Upper limb neurodynamic test
Ultrasound
lack of benefit of, 365
premanipulative screening with, 152, 153
ULTT. *see* Upper limb tension test
Uncinate process
function of, 32–34
growth of, 16
thoracic flexion and, 52
Uncovertebral joint of Luschka, 16–17
Uncovertebral osteophytes
elderly patient and, 19
vertebral arteries affected by, 20
Uncovertebral region, computed tomography scan of, 33*f*
Upper crossed syndrome, 185, 186*f*
Upper extremity
disorders of, risk factors for, 378
pain in
disorders associated with, 380*t*, 382
workplace and, 374–398
repetitive work associated with, 374
work-related musculoskeletal disorders of, 375
Upper limb neural tissue provocation test, 225
Upper limb neurodynamic test, 200–214
aim of, 200
assessment in manual therapy with, 206–208
clinical relevance of, 206–207
complex regional pain syndromes diagnosis with, 312
future of, 211
in patient-management strategies, 208–211
Upper limb tension test, 129–130, 200

V

VA. *see* Artery, vertebral
Vascular system
integrity of, 130
physical examination and, 117
testing of, 131

VBI. *see* Vertebrobasilar insufficiency
Ventrolateral medulla, sympathetic nervous system function and, 296
Vertebra
  arthritic, oblique view of, 19
  axis, 11
  butterfly (*see* Butterfly vertebra)
  centers of ossification in, 6
  cervical
    axial rotation of, 34
    description of, 12
    diagram of, 13*f*
    extension of, 34
    facets of, 12–13
    flexion of, 34
    function of, 3
    movement of, 18
    range of motion of, 30–31, 34–35
  injury to, aging and, 21–22
  position of, palpation examination of, 134–135
  thoracic
    extension of, 50–52, 58–59
    flexion of, 48, 58–59
    innervation of, 76*f*
    mediolateral translation between, 327
    pain from, 77
    right rotation fixation and, 332
    rotation of, 47, 57*f*, 321
    side-flexion of, 52, 53
Vertebra prominens, 12
Vertebral column
  abnormalities in, 7–8
  growth of, 6
Vertebrobasilar artery dissection, risk factors for, 151–152
Vertebrobasilar insufficiency
  dizziness associated with, 138, 139, 140
  inducement of, cervical manipulation and, 142
  limitation on physical examination caused by, 114
  source of symptoms and, 110
  testing for, 130, 131
Vibration syndrome, abusive use disorders and, 383
Viscera
  physical examination and, 117
  thoracic, examination of, 132
Vision, blurred, vertebrobasilar insufficiency associated with, 144
Vocational retraining, complex regional pain syndromes management and, 315
Vomiting, vertebrobasilar insufficiency associated with, 144

W

Walking, patient examination and, 118
Wallenberg test, 153
Wallenberg's syndrome, 151
Whiplash injury
  cervical spine affected by, 41*f*
  cervical spine injury caused by, 20
  cervicogenic headache and, 249
  chronic pain associated with, 21
  clinical trials for, 403–408
  mechanism of, 40
Wolff's law, 364
Work, repetitive, injury associated with, 377, 378–379
Worker
  education of, injury prevention and, 390
  rehabilitation of, 391–393
  sick leave for, 375
  therapeutic intervention for, 391–392
  vocational rehabilitation of, 392–393
Workers' compensation, musculoskeletal disorders in workplace and, 374
Workload, measurement of, worker injury and, 387
Workplace
  changes in nature of, 413–414
  evaluation of programs for injury prevention in, 389–390
  neck and upper extremity pain in, 374–398
  occupational health nurse in, 391
  prevention of injuries in, 386–391
World Wide Web. *see* Internet
Wrist
  postural overload syndrome and, 383
  repetitive movement and injury to, 379
Wry neck, 188
  case study of, 282–283
  differentiation between types of, 290
  discogenic, 289–290

Z

Zygapophyseal joint, 17–19
  acute locking of, 282–283
  arthralgia of, 278
  arthropathy of, case study of, 275
  axial rotation of, 32
  cervical vertebra rotation and, 34
  computed tomography scan of, 33*f*
  disorder of, case study of, 279–281
  hypomobility of, 276
  innervation of, 22, 61, 75
  locked, wry neck compared to, 289
  midthoracic rotation and, 58
  midthorax extension and, 50
  midthorax rotation and, 54

Zygapophyseal joint—cont'd
movements of, 172
pain from, 77
pain in, manipulation-induced analgesia and, 221
pain patterns of, 360
posteroanterior gliding of, 280*f*, 281*f*
recurrent locking of, 283
referred pain and, 66, 68
referred pain patterns of, 79*f*
Zygapophyseal joint—cont'd
stiff thorax and, 49
thoracic
glide of, 329
mobility tests for examination of, 323
mobilization of, 331*f*
thoracic side-flexion and, 52
thoracic vertebral movement and, 48
whiplash injury and, 41, 42

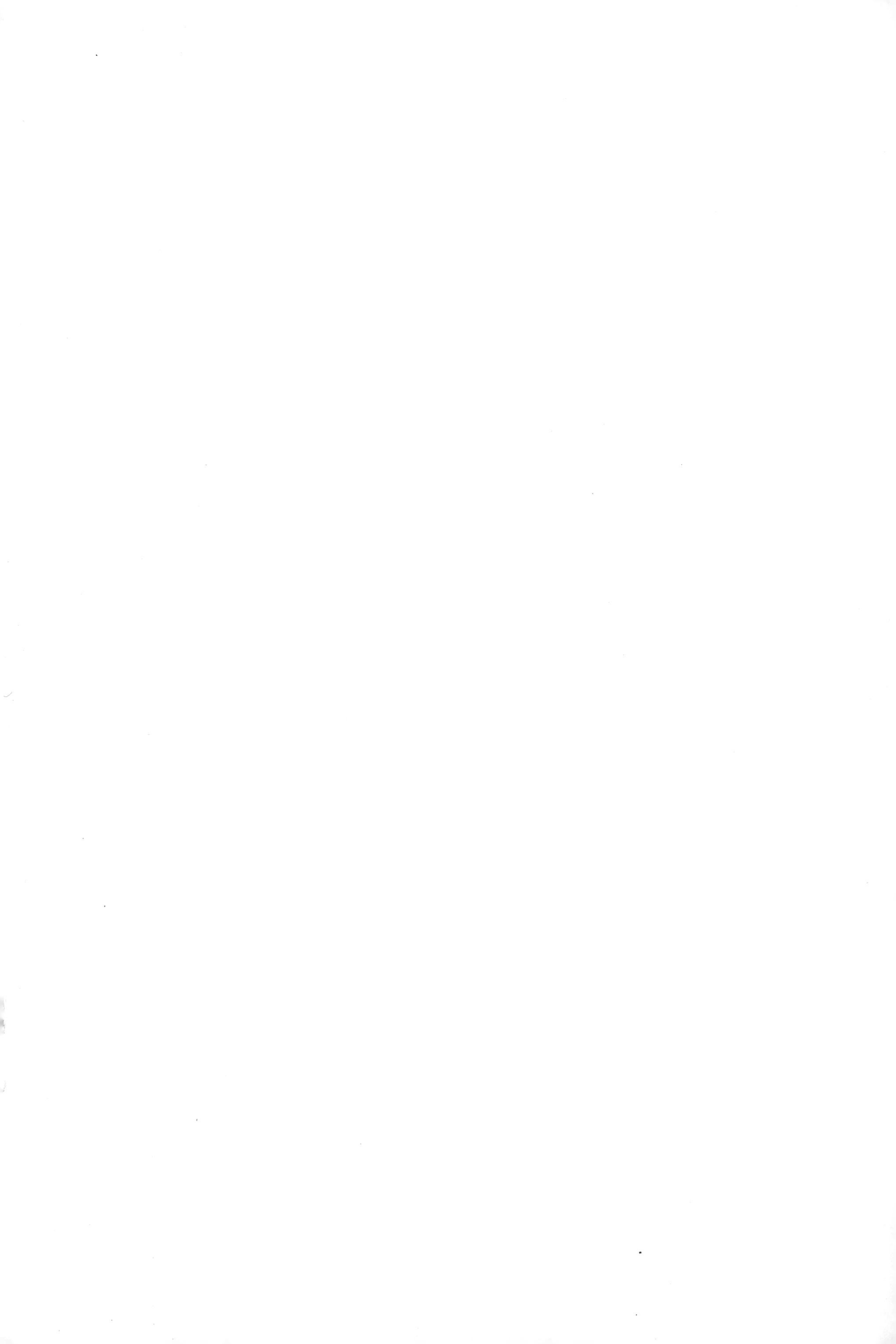